Textbook of Clinical Psychiatry
An Interpersonal Approach

Textbook of Clinical Psychiatry

An Interpersonal Approach

Second Edition

A. H. CHAPMAN, M.D.
Visiting Lecturer, The Greater Kansas City Mental Health Foundation; Formerly, Associate Clinical Professor of Psychiatry, University of Kansas School of Medicine; Attending Psychiatrist, St. Mary's Hospital, Menorah Medical Center, and Research Hospital and Medical Center, Kansas City, Missouri

With Contributions by

JOHN M. DAVIS, M.D.
Professor of Psychiatry, University of Chicago School of Medicine; Director of Research, Illinois State Psychiatric Institute, Chicago, Illinois

and

ELZA M. ALMEIDA, R.N., M.S.
Consultant in Psychiatric Nursing to the Division of Patient Care Services, Menorah Medical Center, Kansas City, Missouri

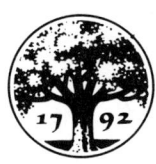

J. B. Lippincott Company
Philadelphia Toronto

SECOND EDITION
Copyright © 1976, by J. B. Lippincott Company

Copyright © 1967, by J. B. Lippincott Company

This book is protected by copyright and, with the exception of brief excerpts for review, no part of it may be reproduced in any form by print, photoprint, microfilm or any other means without written permission from the publisher.

Small portions of the text of this publication have been adapted from *The Physician's Guide to Managing Emotional Problems,* by the same author, published and copyrighted by the J. B. Lippincott Company in 1969, and from *Management of Emotional Problems of Children and Adolescents,* Second Edition, by the same author, published and copyrighted by the J. B. Lippincott Company in 1974.

ISBN 0-397-52072-7

Library of Congress Catalog Card No. 75-29428

Printed in the United States of America

5 4 3 2 1

Library of Congress Cataloging in Publication Data

Chapman, Arthur Harry,
   Textbook of clinical psychiatry.

   Includes bibliographies and index.
   1. Psychiatry. I. Davis, John M. II. Almeida, Elza M., joint author. [DNLM: 1. Mental disorders. WM100 C466t]
RC454.C45   1975   616.8'9   75-29428
ISBN 0-397-52072-7

To the memory of my father, Harry Chapman,
and
my first teacher in psychiatry, Eugen Kahn,
late Sterling Professor of Psychiatry, Yale University

Preface

This book seeks to provide medical students and physicians with a comprehensive textbook of psychiatry written from the interpersonal point of view. It aims to cover the entire range of psychiatric disorders in clear, simple language. It aspires to be a guidebook for the student, a ready reference for the practicing physician and a source of information for the professional worker in associated medical fields.

Psychiatric developments that have occurred since the publication of the first edition have been added, and many parts of the book have been rewritten to reflect changing viewpoints and new information in psychiatric practice and theory. For his contribution of new material on experimental and biochemical aspects of treatment with medications (Chapter 22), I would like to thank John M. Davis, M.D., Professor of Psychiatry at the University of Chicago School of Medicine, and Director of Research at the Illinois State Psychiatric Institute in Chicago, Illinois. I would also like to thank Elza M. Almeida, R.N., M.S., Consultant in Psychiatric Nursing to the Division of Patient Care Services at the Menorah Medical Center in Kansas City, Missouri, for her collaboration in the revision of sections on behavior therapy, psychiatric records, mental retardation, and psychotherapeutic environments in Chapters 3, 5, 7, 20, 21, and 25.

The interpersonal approach to psychiatry views most psychiatric illness as the result of the patient's interpersonal problems with significant people in his environment. The stressful interpersonal relationships may have taken place mainly in the patient's past life, or they may to a large extent be current difficulties with people. Most psychiatric illnesses are caused by various combinations of both past and current interpersonal traumas. Even those psychiatric disturbances caused by organic brain disease, such as cerebral arteriosclerosis, are colored by the patient's pre-existing personality structure and interpersonal life. The full presentation of the interpersonal approach, as it interprets the causes and treatment of the entire range of psychiatric illness, is the task of this book.

The material of this book is drawn from two main sources. First, it relies upon my total experience in studying and treating psychiatrically ill persons and in teaching psychiatry to medical students and young physicians. Second, it incorporates the reviewed material on slightly over 2500 patients seen during the years of a busy consultative and therapeutic clinical practice. In this way I have attempted to infuse a sound basis of personal clinical experience. Dr. Davis's extensive research in the biochemical and psychopharmacologic aspects of psychiatric illnesses, as well as his clinical work, gives particular value to his contributions, and Ms. Almeida's clinical experience enables her to deal effectively with the therapeutic organization of psychiatric hospital services and with various other subjects.

This book is directed to the medical student who is seeking a clear textbook of psychiatry, to the practicing physician who wants to have a prompt aid at hand and to the worker in associated medical fields who wants information on emotional illnesses. If it fills some of these needs, it will justify the time required to read it and the effort taken to write it.

A. H. CHAPMAN

Contents

Part One: The Interpersonal Basis of Psychiatry 1

  1 The Interpersonal Approach to Psychiatry 3
     The Interpersonal Approach to Personality Development 4

  2 The Historical Evolution of Modern Psychiatry 25
     Concepts of Mental Illness From Ancient Times to the Renaissance 25
     The Beginnings of Modern Psychiatry 26
     Psychiatric Development in the Nineteenth Century 27
     Psychiatric Development in the Twentieth Century 29

  3 Various Concepts of Emotional Functioning 40
     General Terms and Concepts 40
     Affects and Their Disturbances 45
     Disturbances of Thought Processes 48
     Other Disturbances of Thought Processes 49
     Disturbances of Perception 51
     Disturbances of Memory 54
     Disturbances of Consciousness 56
     Concepts of Body Constitution and Personality Structure 57
     Various Concepts of Personality Functioning 58
     Freudian-Psychoanalytic Concepts 58
     Behavior Theory and Behavior Therapy 70
     Various Other Concepts Concerning Emotional Functioning 72

Part Two: Psychiatric Evaluation of the Patient 77

  4 The Psychiatric Examination 79
     Interview Examination of the Patient 80
     Obtaining Information from the Patient's Family 93
     Examination of the Uncommunicative Patient 94

  5 Further Examination Procedures 97
     Psychological Testing 97
     Special Interview Technics 101
     Physical Evaluation 103
     Formulation of the Psychiatric Diagnosis 104
     Special Problems in Handling Psychiatric Diagnoses and Records 107

Part Three: The Interpersonally Caused Disorders 109

Section One: The Neuroses 110

    6 Anxiety Neurosis 112
        Clinical Characteristics of Anxiety Neuroses 112
        Interpersonal Causes of Anxiety Neuroses 114
        The Clinical Course of Anxiety Neuroses 119
        Treatment of Anxiety Neuroses 120
        The Role of Anxiety in Other Kinds of Neuroses 122

    7 Phobic Neurosis 124
        Clinical Characteristics of Phobic Neuroses 124
        Interpersonal Causes of Phobias 126
        Clinical Course of Phobic Neuroses 129
        Treatment of Phobic Neuroses 130

    8 Obsessive and Compulsive Neuroses 135
        Clinical Characteristics of Obsessive and Compulsive Neuroses 135
        Interpersonal Causes of Obsessive and Compulsive Neuroses 139
        Clinical Course of Obsessive and Compulsive Neuroses 144
        Treatment of Obsessive and Compulsive Neuroses 145

    9 Hysterical Neuroses: Conversion and Dissociative Types 148
        Clinical Characteristics of Conversion Hysteria 148
        Clinical Characteristics of Dissociative Hysteria 152
        Interpersonal Causes of Conversion and Dissociative Hysteria 154
        Clinical Course of Conversion and Dissociative Hysteria 157
        Treatment of Conversion and Dissociative Hysteria 158
        Clinical Problems Related to Conversion Hysteria 164

   10 Other Neurotic Syndromes 168
        Depressive Neurosis 168
        Neurasthenic Neurosis 175
        Depersonalization Neurosis 175
        Hypochondriacal Neurosis 176

Section Two: Psychosomatic Illness 181

   11 The Common Psychosomatic Illnesses 183
        The Multiple Levels of Disorder in Psychosomatic Illness 183
        Various Psychosomatic Illnesses 185
        The Comprehensive Management of Psychosomatic Illness 203

Section Three: Personality Disorders 209

   12 The Various Personality Disorders 211
        The Common Personality Disorders 213
        Other Personality Disorders 224
        Personality Disorders Associated with Sexual Disturbances 227

   13 Personality Disorders Contributing to Alcoholism and Drug Abuse 237
        Personality Disorders Associated with Alcoholism 237
        Personality Disorders Associated with Narcotic Addiction 246
        Personality Disorders Associated with Other Forms of Drug Abuse 252

Section Four: Psychotic Disorders 259

    14 Schizophrenia 261
           Clinical Characteristics of Schizophrenia 261
           Clinical Course of Schizophrenia 265
           Interpersonal Causes of Schizophrenia 271
           Treatment of Schizophrenia 275

    15 Severe Depressions 280
           Clinical Characteristics of Severe Depressions 281
           Interpersonal Causes of Severe Depressions 284
           Treatment of Severe Depressions 287
           Suicide: A Clinical and Public Health Problem 290

    16 Manic Psychoses 294
           Clinical Characteristics of Manic Disorders 294
           Interpersonal Causes of Manic Disorders 297
           Treatment of Manic Disorders 298

    17 Other Psychotic Disorders 303
           Paranoia and Involutional Paranoid State 303
           Psychoses of Association 308
           Postpartum and Postoperative Psychoses 309

Part Four: Psychiatric Disturbances Caused by Organic Brain Disorders 313

    18 The Common Organic Brain Disorders 315
           The Basic Symptoms in Organic Brain Disorders 315
           Organic Brain Disorders Caused by Cerebral Arteriosclerosis and
              Senile Brain Degeneration 318
           Organic Brain Disorders Caused by Head Trauma 323
           Organic Brain Disorders Caused by Brain Damage in the Prenatal,
              the Natal and the Postnatal Periods 331
           Organic Brain Disorders Associated with Chronic Alcoholism 337

    19 Other Types of Organic Brain Disorders 343
           Organic Brain Disorders Caused by Intoxication by Drugs and Chemicals . 343
           Organic Brain Disorders Caused by Circulatory Disturbances 349
           Organic Brain Disorders Caused by Intracranial Neoplasms 350
           Organic Brain Disorders Caused by Metabolic Disturbances 351
           Organic Brain Disorders Caused by Intracranial Infections 352
           Organic Brain Disorders Caused by Syphilis of the Central Nervous System 354
           Organic Brain Disorders Caused by Degenerative Central Nervous System
              Diseases 356
           Organic Brain Syndromes Caused by Convulsive Disorders 358
           Organic Brain Disorders Caused by Severe General Infections 359
           Some Basic Principles for the Management of Organic Brain Disorders ... 360

Part Five: Mental Retardation 363

    20 Mental Retardation and the Management of Mentally Retarded Patients ... 365
           Clinical Features of Mental Retardation 365
           Special Mental Retardation Syndromes 371
           The Management of Mentally Retarded Patients 376

Part Six: Treatment Methods in Psychiatry ... 383

21 Psychotherapy and Psychotherapeutic Environments ... 385
The Basic Processes in Psychotherapy ... 385
The Major Types of Psychotherapy ... 390
Special Modifications of Psychotherapy ... 399
Psychotherapeutic Environments ... 405

22 Experimental and Biochemical Aspects of Treatment with Medications ... 410
Antipsychotic Drugs ... 410
Antidepressant Drugs ... 425
Minor Tranquilizers (Antianxiety Medications) and Sedative-Hypnotics ... 432
Lithium and Miscellaneous Other Medications ... 437

23 Physical Methods of Treatment ... 441
Electroshock Therapy ... 441
Insulin Coma Therapy ... 445
Psychosurgery ... 446
Other Physical Methods of Treatment ... 447

24 Special Technics in Child and Adolescent Psychiatry ... 449
The Child Guidance Clinic Approach to the Emotional Problems of Children and Adolescents ... 449
Special Technics of Treatment in Child and Adolescent Psychiatry ... 452
Other Treatment Services for Children and Adolescents ... 456

Part Seven: Other Aspects of Psychiatry ... 459

25 Special Problems of Interpersonal Adjustment ... 461
Special Problems of Adjustment in Children ... 461
Special Problems of Situational Adjustment in Adulthood ... 471
Special Problems of Sexual Adjustment ... 481

26 Legal Aspects of Psychiatry ... 491
The Person and His Responsibility for Criminal Acts ... 493
The Person and Psychiatric Hospitalization Procedures ... 495
The Person and His Capacity for Making Wills, Contracts and Other Important Decisions ... 501
The Person and Privileged Communications to Psychiatrists and Other Mental Health Professional Workers ... 503
The Legal Responsibilities and Liabilities of Psychiatrists and Other Mental Health Professional Workers ... 505

Index ... 507

Textbook of Clinical Psychiatry
An Interpersonal Approach

Part One

The Interpersonal Basis of Psychiatry

In the first chapter of this section we shall outline the interpersonal approach to psychiatry. We shall discuss the interpersonal development of personality structure, and we shall trace some of the ways in which unhealthy interpersonal relationships can lead to psychiatric problems. In the second chapter we shall outline the historical evolution of modern psychiatry. The third chapter covers some further concepts and terms used in psychiatry in discussing patients and explaining their difficulties.

1

The Interpersonal Approach to Psychiatry

Psychiatry deals with unhealthy interpersonal relationships and unhealthy disturbances in emotions and ideas. This definition of psychiatry is broad, but a definition of modern psychiatry must be wide enough to include such diverse fields as marital difficulties, child rearing problems, neuroses and psychoses. Psychiatry embraces the study of the causes, nature and courses of these interpersonal and emotional disturbances, and the methods of treating and preventing them.

Most psychiatric difficulties are the result of interpersonal problems of the patient with crucial persons in his environment. The traumatic interpersonal relationships may have occurred mainly in his past life, or to a large extent they may be current stresses with people. Usually, a psychiatric disturbance is the result of the combination of both past and current unhealthy interpersonal relationships. The respective importance of past and present stresses varies much from patient to patient. The most important relationships in producing emotional disturbances are the intimate relationships of the patient's life. These include his relationships with his parents, siblings, marital partner, children, close friends and others with whom he has intimate, prolonged relationships. Stressful situations with colleagues or superiors at work, or unhealthy relationships in broader social and cultural groups may also be important.

The interpersonal experiences of childhood have much importance, for the experiences of the childhood years are making their impressions on an unmarked slate. The experiences of later years affect the individual through the previously laid down personality structure. However, the experiences of adolescence and early adult life also play a significant part in determining emotional health or illness, and the soundness or unhealthiness of interpersonal situations throughout the individual's later life continues to play an appreciable role. Any psychiatric illness is the result of many life experiences, though some experiences play a much larger role than others. Any emotional illness may be likened to a tree with many roots. Some roots are large, others are small, some are deep and some are superficial, but they all contribute to the tree.

In any psychiatric disturbance the roles of different life experiences vary immensely. Some persons have experienced such extensive emotional stress in childhood that even minor stresses in adult life may precipitate psychiatric illness. Other persons emerge from the formative years of life with a relatively healthy personality structure and become emotionally disturbed only if subjected to prolonged, severe interpersonal stress in adult life. There is a broad middle ground of persons whose personalities have certain features that lead to psychiatric illness only if they are exposed to particular kinds and severities of trauma. For instance, a passive, dependent woman may adjust well if she marries a dominant but kind and considerate man. The same person may have much psychiatric illness if she marries a dominating but brutal and exploiting man. The interpersonal approach to psychiatry emphasizes that the patient must be viewed in the setting of all his life experiences—past and present—to understand a psychiatric illness and plan its treatment.

The interpersonal approach recognizes that the individual does not understand the meaning of many of his experiences and may have much difficulty in coming to grips with them on a conscious level of awareness. In many psychiatric disturbances much of the work of treatment is aimed at helping the person to understand fully his life experiences and emotions, and to resolve them in the context of the patient-therapist relationship. The interpersonal approach views both conscious and unconscious thoughts and feelings as playing important roles in emotional health or illness. The interchange between conscious and unconscious thoughts and feelings is viewed as somewhat fluid. We shall discuss this subject at somewhat greater length later in this chapter in the section titled *The Various Levels of Awareness.*

Even those psychiatric illnesses mainly caused by organic brain disease, such as cerebral arteriosclerosis, are best studied as occurring against the background of the patient's pre-existing personality structure and interpersonal life. The problems of the various forms of mental retardation can be understood best by a comprehensive view of their effects on the individual's capacity for interpersonal living and his emotional and intellectual adjustments with people. A person's life has emotional and intellectual significance mainly in the context of the long chain of interpersonal relationships in which he has lived.

THE INTERPERSONAL APPROACH TO PERSONALITY DEVELOPMENT

The interpersonal approach to psychiatry becomes clearer as one traces the various stages of personality development. Therefore, in the following sections of this chapter we shall trace some aspects of the interpersonal development of the individual from birth to adulthood, and we shall discuss the impact of his interpersonal life on his developing personality structure and his emotional functioning. Our main purpose in tracing this development is to explain the interpersonal approach to psychiatry; many other aspects of personality development and functioning are covered in later chapters.

Personality consists of the long-term, characteristic ways in which an individual interacts with the people around him, and the ways he feels and thinks about himself and others.

We can evaluate an individual's personality only in the context of an interpersonal relationship with him. Only by observing his actions and interacting with him do his ways of feeling, thinking and relating to people become evident to us. In order to understand him we must set up an interpersonal relationship between him and ourselves. Treatment of any emotional problems he has can occur only in the setting of an interpersonal relationship in which we are not only observers, but also active participants. If we see a person sitting on the other side of a bus we can have no concept of his personality. We can begin to understand him only if we begin to interact with him, both verbally and nonverbally.

This is a central point in the interpersonal approach to psychiatry. *All psychiatric observations, theories and treatment technics must be developed out of interpersonal activity between patients and participant-observer therapists.* The things that go on between people—those things which we can see, hear and feel—constitute the only valid data wtih which psychiatric concepts and treatments can be built.

Much of the current disarray in psychiatry arises from the fact that many psychiatric schools of thought are built on elaborate, highly speculative theories about what goes on *in some vague thing called the mind of the patient.* Such mental things cannot be seen, heard, felt or observed in any objective way. The doctrines of these diverse psychiatric schools of thought are, therefore, set up in such ways that they can neither be proved nor disproved; they must forever remain matters of faith. Their principles may be likened to the axiom, "All events are controlled by Divine Providence"; much human experience can be marshalled both to substantiate and refute this statement, but since it cannot be proved or disproved it must always remain in the realm of speculation and faith. The interpersonal approach to psychiatry, however, with its emphasis on directly observable interactions between people, puts us on much firmer ground, both in understanding patients and in devising ways to treat them.

We shall now outline the development of personality in the context of the individual's significant interpersonal relationships.

The First Year of Life

The first interpersonal world of a child is the family into which he is born, and the two most important people in shaping that interpersonal environment are his mother and father. Hence, the qualities and kinds of interpersonal relationships that the parents give the child during his developing years have great significance in molding his personality structure.

Even during the first few months of his life the child is sensitive to the feelings and attitudes of the people who are caring for him. In an inarticulate way, the child perceives whether he is cared for in a tender, loving manner or in a cold and irritable manner. The child cannot put his feelings and experiences into words, of course, for the capacity to make his feelings and ideas articulate develops only much later. However, he acutely senses the attitudes of the people around him by their physical handling of him, by the tones of voice in which they speak to him, and by the tenderness, or the absence of it, that characterizes each thing that is done for him.

The child reacts in various ways to these early interpersonal contacts. The child who is treated with tenderness and love responds with relaxed comfort in the mother-child relationship and in his contacts with the other people who care for him. On the other hand, the fearful, insecure mother often betrays her anxiousness during her care of the child, and he may in turn be tense and fretful. The rejecting, hostile mother who treats her child in a cold, irritable manner may induce feelings of apathetic withdrawal or fitful rage.

Most psychiatrists feel that the experiences of the first year of life may play a role in determining the nature of later emotional functioning. The child who finds love and tenderness in his early life is likely to feel warmly toward people, and is well started in the development of a comfortable capacity for close interpersonal relationships. On the other hand, coldness and hostility in the care of an infant may sow the first seeds of painful withdrawal from interpersonal relationships. Moreover, the interpersonal experiences of early life often continue into later years. For example, the hostility or coldness of some parents, often arising out of their own personality problems, does not stop abruptly at the end of the first year. Such unhealthy interpersonal relationships frequently continue, though perhaps in modified form, through the child's developing years.

I recall a 16-year-old boy in whom marked emotional deprivation in early life played a significant role in later psychiatric illness. During the first 12 months of his life he was cared for in an orphanage in which he was not given tender, affectionate care. The basic necessities of cleanliness and nutrition were given to him in a cold, mechanical manner, but other than these perfunctory attentions he was left to himself. At the end of one year of such emotional deprivation he was an apathetic, withdrawn baby who could not sit up or stand. He whined passively in his crib in fearful withdrawal from people. At the age of 12 months he was adopted from the orphanage by a childless couple who gave him much attention and affection. Over a several-year period he emerged from his withdrawn, fearful state and became a pleasant boy with good intelligence. However, he remained somewhat shy, and an underlying tenseness persisted in many areas of his interpersonal life. When he was 16 he accepted a summer job working for a relative of his parents in a nearby town. Away from the emotional security of his parental home, he became very anxious, but he persisted in his work. He became progressively more frightened and, after proceeding through a short period of marked panic, he developed a paranoid schizophrenic illness with florid auditory hallucinations and delusions. Under hospital treatment, he recovered. The severe emotional damage this boy suffered during the first year of life undoubtedly played a significant role in forming the emotional problems that under later stresses led to his schizophrenic illness.

However, if the emotional stresses of the first year of life are mild or moderate and of short duration, their unhealthy effects often may be erased by later periods of healthier interpersonal life. Of course, a child should receive the most secure, affectionate environment his parents can offer during his early life, but the failings of upset parents over brief periods of time can be corrected by more secure relationships soon afterward.

During the first year of life the mother, or the person who plays her role, is the most important person in the child's interpersonal world. The activities of feeding, bathing, rocking and tenderly caring for the child fall to her, and the vast bulk of the child's interpersonal life in the first few months of his life is with his mother. Hence, the mother's basic personality, her attitudes toward the child, and the emotional comfort or stressfulness of her life at this time are important.

During the first year, the father and other members of the family play secondary roles. The influence of the father is felt to a large extent through his relationship with the mother. The father who gives the mother a secure, affectionate marital relationship helps the mother to give relaxed, loving care to the child. On the other hand, the father who by his emotional problems or marital instability causes emotional turmoil in the mother may prevent her from giving the child the full measure of comfortable, affectionate care he needs. In a similar manner, other children in the family and other relatives may influence the child's emotional security by the roles they play in the interpersonal lives of the parents. During the latter part of the first year of the child's life the father and other members of the family begin to have more interpersonal activities with the child, and their warmth and love, or the lack of it, begin to play an increasing role in the child's emotional life and developing personality structure.

During the latter part of the first year of life the child begins to develop his first rudimentary concepts of himself. He has inarticulate sensations about whether he is a worthwhile, a valueless, or a strangely unfit person. To these early vague concepts a person has of himself Harry Stack Sullivan, one of the main developers of the interpersonal approach to psychiatry, gave the terms the "good-me", the "bad-me," and the "not-me." Sullivan's terminology has not been widely accepted, but his ideas have had a profound effect on the evolution of 20th century psychiatry. The infant's dim impressions about "good-me," "bad-me" and "not-me," or the confused combinations of them he develops, are strengthened or modified throughout childhood and early adolescence. They play central roles in determining whether in later life he feels that he is a capable person with good interpersonal capacities, a defective person who in various ways cannot relate comfortably to people, or an eerily estranged individual who cannot form relationships at all (or only in gravely distorted ways). Hence, their effect on emotional health or sickness is marked.

The Second and Third Years

During the second and third years of life the child begins to extend his world of interpersonal relationships. He learns to walk, and his increased mobility enables him to enter into many kinds of new relationships with both children and adults. He begins to acquire the training a broader social life requires; he becomes toilet trained and he learns to eat at a common table with others. Most important of all, he begins to learn to talk, and this ability opens broad avenues in his relationships with others and in his capacity to make his feelings and thoughts clearer both to others and to himself.

The development of speech has far-reaching consequnces. For, in addition to expressing what a person feels and does, *speech also molds his feelings and actions*. This basic fact is overlooked in many schools of psychiatric thought. For example, to a child reared in an affectionate, outgoing family, the word "love" means close, tender feelings toward others and harmonious activities with them. To a child reared in a cold, sternly rigid family, the word "love" means duty, mechanical performance of obligations to near persons, and closeness bred of social custom rather than warm emotions. To a child reared in a hostile or chaotic family, "love" may have grossly distorted connotations, or no clear meaning at all. Moreover, the meanings which the developing child attaches to such words as "mother," "father," "friend," and others are usually carried into his adolescence and adult life, and they affect both what he expects of "mothers" and "fathers" and how he acts when he becomes one himself. Until feelings and thoughts are crystallized in words, a person cannot handle them well, but the ways in which he forms his feelings and thoughts into words affect his subsequent concepts of himself, other persons, and the things that occur between people.

The child's interpersonal activities with his parents and his siblings, and with other children and adults, expand rapidly during his second and third years. In this period, as in all his previous and subsequent childhood, he continues to need the warm, secure affection of his parents to give him the basis for emotional comfort in many new types of relationships both inside and outside the family. The child who has received secure affection and a feeling of being a loved and esteemed person approaches the world with reasonable self-confidence and reaches out for sound relationships with people in healthy ways. The rejected, frightened or insecure child who has been reared in a hostile, anxious or unstable parental atmosphere views interpersonal relationships with unhealthy feelings of emotional withdrawal, fearfulness or angry rebellion.

During the first year of his life, the parents do many things for the child. They make virtually no demands, and do not require that he perform any specific tasks. In the second and third years the parents begin to make various demands and expect him to conform to certain rules of family life. They expect him to become toilet trained, to learn to feed himself, to avoid excessive breakage and damage of household goods, to get along reasonably well with his brothers and sisters, and to learn many other requirements of social living. The child who has been reared with reasonable love and affection, coupled with firm limitations by the parents on his undesirable acts, begins to respond to his parents' expectations and demands. On the other hand, the child who has received much harshness and coldness, or who has received erratic and ineffective limitations on undesirable behavior, may be resistant and rebellious. Children require much love and reasonable, firm limitations as they gradually develop into interpersonally comfortable, well adjusted persons.

During the first year, love and tender care were the child's most important needs. During the second and third years the parents must begin to put limitations on any untoward behavior. They should apply such limitations with reasonable firmness and consistency. The world is full of realistic limitations that a person must obey to live a successful social life. If he fails to obey these restrictions and limitations in later life, he will have serious difficulties in his social adjustments.

Harry Stack Sullivan gave special attention to the role of parents in imposing limitations and discipline on a child during the long process of transforming him from a skillful animal into a well adjusted human being. Sullivan pointed out the dangers of inadequate or erratic limitations on children. However, he emphasized that discipline, though it may cause pain or inconvenience to the child, should never produce anxiety in him. For example, a parent may, for legitimate reasons, spank a child (pain) or deprive him of television time (inconvenience), but he should never tell the child that he is a bad or inadequate person, since these things lower his self-esteem and mobilize anxiety.

The capacity of adults to follow the complex restrictions of social living comfortably is much influenced by how well their parents were able in a reasonable way to impose on them the many limitations of childhood. When the limitations of childhood have been inadequate, or when they have been imposed with coldness and brutality, the child's capacity to follow the limitations of adult life may be impaired. The limitations on the behavior of children are imposed to a large extent by the authority and correction of their parents; the limitations of adulthood are mainly self-imposed. A child does not hit his little sister because he fears the reprimand or punishment of his parents; a well adjusted adult does not hit other people because he has internal standards and principles that limit such behavior. Successful interpersonal living requires that the developing child gradually learns to take upon himself the task of imposing the limitations that his parents enforced in his earlier years.

The successful imposition of limitations on a child should be done against the background of the parents' basic love for the child. Limitations without love are often harsh and insensitive. They may lead to a sullen withdrawal of the child from his relationship with his parents, and this sullen negativism may be carried into many other relationships in later life. Limitations without love may lead in other children to rebellion and defiance, which may erupt as gross delinquency in adolescence or later. On the other hand, when the child has few limitations placed on his behavior and is unrealistically allowed to do whatever he pleases, he may emerge from childhood with a defective sense of the necessary limitations of adult life. I recall a patient who in childhood had few restrictions put on her behavior. Her unaffectionate father ignored her, and her passive, indecisive, anxious mother could not restrain the child in any way. As an adult, this patient was a demanding woman who had great difficulty imposing even the most common self-disciplines on herself. She could not tolerate the slightest resistance of her husband to her demands and wishes, and she could not endure even minor disobedience from her children. Marked marital and child-rearing problems caused her eventually to seek psychiatric help. Inadequate limitations during the formative years, especially when coupled with inadequate love, may be as unfortunate in their results as excessive limitations.

Many studies of child development have led to the conclusion that the formation of ethical and moral standards is based to a large extent on the reasonable limitations that parents impose on their children during the early years. At that time their parents place limitations and restrictions on their behavior and enforce them by reasonable discipline, and even punishment, when needed. From adolescence onward, the individual, if he is to live successfully in society, must place these restrictions and limitations on himself. In a sense, he must internalize the limitations and discipline of his parents into his own personality structure and impose them on himself.

Consensual Validation

How does a person correct unhealthy attitudes, personality problems and old interpersonal traumas, and develop sound ways of emotional living? One of the basic means by which this occurs is the process which Harry Stack Sullivan called *consensual validation* (literally, the gradual *validation* of concepts and interpersonal patterns by multiple kinds of *sensory* experiences).

In consensual validation a person *evaluates aspects of himself and his relationships with others in numerous interpersonal situations and from many points of view.* A person thus corrects personality warps that have arisen in previous interpersonal relationships by re-evaluating both them and his current ones in fresh ways; he also alters his conceptions of himself in the process. These changes may be put into words or they may not; that is, the individual may or may not be articulately aware that he is actively correcting personality warps and emotional problems in healthier day-to-day life situations. In the following example the person is not clearly aware that he is healing old personality difficulties in sounder current life circumstances.

During the first five years of life a child may have suffered much emotional rejection and depreciation by a hostile mother, and as a result he feels that he is a worthless, inferior person who is incapable of forming sound relationships with people and unworthy of them. However, from the age of five onward a series of new experiences begins and he starts to view himself in the context of multiple new interpersonal situations; that is, consensual validation begins. His father, who until that time had traveled much in his work and had seen little of the boy, begins to spend more time with him, and when the subject of Mother comes up, Father says, "Well, you've just got to put up with that. She's critical of everybody and everything." In school the boy has new interpersonal relationships with teachers and classmates who treat him as a worthwhile person. He also spends more time playing in neighborhood homes and yards where he is considered a valued person. Thus, throughout the rest of childhood and during his adolescence he is able to appraise both his own personality and his relationships with others in many new situations, and by the process of consensual validation he develops a healthier concept of himself and better capacities to relate to people. These improvements, moreover, open the way to ever-increasing numbers of comfortable relationships with people, which in turn give wider scope for the spontaneous operation of consensual validation.

However, the capacity of consensual validation to heal personality problems is affected by many variables. If a father shares and reinforces a mother's unhealthy attitude toward a child, if his siblings adopt similar behavior toward him, and if his opportunities for corrective contacts in wider social circles outside the family are limited, then there is little possibility for consensual validation to help. Also, the degree of personality warp is important; small ones are more easily corrected than large ones. Another factor is the age at which consensual validation begins to operate to a significant extent; if it begins in childhood or early adolescence, it has a much greater impact than if it begins in middle adolescence or afterwards. However, *consensual validation can have significant healthy effects at any time during life, including all of adulthood and, in some circumstances, in old age.*

Consensual validation (*validating* concepts and interpersonal relationships through the medium of many kinds of *sensory* experiences) also plays a major role in the day-to-day resolution of many common difficulties of living. When a person can openly discuss problems in his marriage and with his children, misunderstandings on his job, and conflicts in his social life, he often obtains broader views, and his distortions may be corrected. Although language plays a large part in this process, much that is useful is seen and felt and never put into words. Consensual validation helps by both verbal and nonverbal means and on both conscious and unconscious levels.

As we shall point out in our discussions of psychotherapy, consensual validation forms an important aspect of the work of psychiatrists and other mental health professional workers (as well as, in some cases, family physicians and other nonpsychiatric physicians) in dealing with neuroses, personality disorders, psychosomatic illnesses, situational adjustment problems and other emotional difficulties. Wider perspectives and fresh insight help patients to comprehend themselves and their life situations in healthier ways.

The concept of consensual validation implies that since emotional problems arise in sick interpersonal relationships, they can be resolved by healthy ones. These healthy relationships include both the spontaneous ones that occur in varied social experience and the professional ones that occur in psychotherapy and counseling.

Ages Three Through Seven

From the age of three onward into later childhood, the interpersonal world of the child expands rapidly. He begins to form new relationships with other relatives, the neighborhood children, children in nursery school and grade school, and people in other social groups into which he is gradually introduced. An important aspect of these expanding interpersonal circles is learning to share people with other people. The child's first interpersonal circle includes only his mother and himself. Then he learns that he cannot have all his mother's time and attention exclusively. He has to share her with his father, who appears on the child's interpersonal horizon. Sometimes a child resents sharing his mother with the father and may have competitive feelings for the mother's attention. In a reasonably well-adjusted family such feelings resolve themselves in time, and the child forms affectionate relationships with both his parents.

A child may have some difficulty sharing his parents with his brothers and sisters. Competitive rivalry for the parents' attention may arise between the various children in a family. However, when each child has a feeling of affectionate security in the love of his parents, coupled with the parents' capacity for imposing limitations and giving reasonable freedom to each child, such jealousies and rivalries resolve themselves. The process of sharing people with other people goes on throughout life. For example, the child must learn to share the attention of the teacher with the other children in the classroom. The child must learn that he cannot dominate the schoolroom situation, but must share its activities and privileges with other children. Thus, in ever widening interpersonal circles, the process of sharing people with other people goes on throughout life.

Individual brief incidents in the child's

life do not have a serious effect on his personality. The persistent day-to-day, year-to-year emotional environment of the child forms the child's character structure, not brief isolated incidents. The parent who says that his child was well adjusted until he had a frightening experience at the age of 6, and that the child has been shy and fearful ever since, is merely finding a scapegoat on which to blame the defective interpersonal environment in which the child was reared.

Thus, the child's personality structure gradually develops in the matrix of the interpersonal relationships of his life. Out of the cumulative results of his daily interactions with the important people in his environment arise his personality strengths or weaknesses, his emotional security or anxiousness, and his warm capacity for interpersonal relationships or his interpersonal limitations. When the child's interpersonal environment is hostile, insecure or unstable, a child slowly evolves his fears, his doubts about his worth and ability, his depressiveness or his psychosomatic distresses. The seriousness of any developing personality problems depends largely on the severity and persistence of the damaging interpersonal relationships and the ways in which later interpersonal relationships accentuate or diminish these difficulties.

I recalled a 23-year-old patient who throughout her childhood and adolescence had been subjected to daily hostile haranguing and depreciation by her mother. The mother favored the patient's two older brothers, and the painful stresses of this patient's relationship with her mother were made more devastating by the open favoritism shown the brothers. Her father was an austere lawyer who treated the patient with mechanical coldness and in general reinforced the mother's attitudes. The patient grew up with the feeling that she was unloved and unlovable, and that her depreciation by her parents was justified by her lack of talent or attractiveness. She retreated into painful shyness and in time her social awkwardness seemed to prove the validity of her mother's scorn, and her social isolation blocked her from other interpersonal relationships that might have had healthy influences on her. Much unconscious resentment toward her parents smoldered behind a frightened façade of passive withdrawal, and whenever her resentments threatened to break into open expression she struggled with feelings of profound guilt and terror. She retreated into studious intellectuality as a way of shunning people, and in scholastic achievement she sought a way of finally winning the approval of her family. At 23, when she was facing final examinations in graduate school, she became terrified of possible failure, which would seem the final confirmation of her feelings of utter worthlessness. She went through a depressive illness in which she attempted suicide twice. Under prolonged treatment she recovered, and in time she developed a more realistic evaluation of herself. In psychiatric interview treatment, she gradually understood how her problems arose out of the unhealthy interpersonal relationships that had dominated her emotional life, and she resolved her emotional turmoil.

Anxiety and Security

Harry Stack Sullivan emphasized the role of *anxiety*, and its opposite, *security*, in personality development and emotional functioning. *Anxiety* is a feeling of apprehension, alarm and desolation which may range in degree from mild discomfort to panic, and *security* is a feeling of comfortable, secure well-being.

Anxiety arises when the basic needs of the individual for affection, esteem, physical safety and many other things are not met. Anxiety may occur in an infant with a cold, hostile mother, or in a child with a rejecting father, or in an adolescent who is struggling to channel his burgeoning sexuality and independent strivings into socially acceptable channels. Similarly, it may occur in an adult whose needs for tender closeness are not being met in a bad marriage, or in an elderly person who perceives in himself the first dreaded signs of senile forgetfulness, or in people undergoing myriad other kinds of experiences. Anxiety is so painful that an individual tries, often in ways he does not clearly understand, to dispel it by one or many kinds of emotional and interpersonal reactions. Thus, the child of cold, rejecting parents may become passive and ingratiating to seek the tenderness that never comes and to avoid the hostility that is always imminent, or he may retreat into a solitary life of daydreams and lonely activities, or he may thrash back in wild rebellion that punishes his parents and defeats his own best interests. In sick, distorted ways he is seeking *security* (relief from anxiety) by trying to make a bad parent-child relationship better, or by fleeing from it into an inner world, or by smashing it altogether by chaotic counter-hostility.

If this child's ingrained interpersonal way of trying to avoid anxiety becomes passive deference to people, or shy withdrawal, or diffuse hostility that alienates people and keeps them always distant from him, he has a high risk of carrying this pattern of interacting with people into late adolescence and adulthood. He carries it into his marital relationship, his child-rearing activities, his vocational activities, and many other kinds of interpersonal relationships.

In addition, severe anxiety has a special characteristic: by crippling a person in his relationships with people, it hampers his abilities to work out his problems with them. For example, a person in a panic cannot comfortably discuss and solve a marital problem, or a vocational difficulty, or a social misunderstanding. Similarly, lesser states of anxiety limit an individual's problem-solving capacities in lesser, but important, ways.

However, during his developing years, or even in adult life, a person may develop healthy ways of dispelling anxiety and relating to people. A mother who was cold and rejecting for many months to her child during his infancy because of a marital crisis of her own, may overcome her problems and later give her child secure affection. The fretful, tense infant responds by gradually becoming a more comfortable, *secure* child. If unhealthy, anxiety-producing relationships do not last too long and are corrected by later secure relationships, the pent-up anxiety in the developing person can be resolved.

When anxiety is not resolved, and, in addition to the accumulated tenseness inside a person, is daily increased by the sick relationships in which he is living, it may in time produce many kinds of emotional and physical symptoms. It does this through unhealthy emotional reactions (of which the individual is usually unaware), which Harry Stack Sullivan called *security operations*. Through these security operations the individual is attempting in sick ways to rid himself of anxiety and to achieve at least fleeting security. Thus, security operations may give anxiety limited release in phobias, obsessions, hysterical disorders, psychosomatic illnesses, schizoid personality disturbances and many other kinds of difficulties (which we shall discuss at length throughout much of the rest of this book). In extreme cases security operations break down altogether and the individual develops a psychosis—schizophrenia, or mania, or depression. Sullivan's term *security operation* is somewhat akin to the Freudian-psychoanalytic term *defense mechanism*, which is dealt with at length in Chapter 3.

In an artificial, oversimplified way we may think of anxiety and security as being on opposite ends of a seesaw. When one end is high the other is low. One of the main goals of interpersonal life is to achieve and maintain reasonable amounts of security while keeping anxiety at low levels.

Self-Image Formation

An important facet of an individual's developing personality structure is the self-image he gradually develops of himself. Each person has within himself a concept about what kind of person he feels himself to be. He carries within himself a mental picture of the kind of person he thinks he is. This is known as the self-image. No one's self-image is entirely accurate; sometimes the individual has many mistaken ideas and feelings about himself. However, the emotionally healthy person has a reasonable concept of what he is like.

The self-image includes ideas about capabilities, talents and capacities to get along with people. The individual has certain ideas about his physical appearance and whether he considers himself to be handsome or ugly. In the self-image are bound up many things affecting his self-confidence, self-esteem and happiness. In many instances the individual is not consciously aware of various aspects of his self-image concept.

A person may have unhealthy distortions in his self-image. A man who is talented and capable may secretly fear that he has little ability. He may feel that he manages to scrape by only by working hard. Individuals may view themselves as unlovable, inadequate, inferior, unable to hold the affection of people, and other things, as the result of mistaken self-images. Distortions in a person's self-image often contribute to the formation of personality problems, interpersonal difficulties and psychiatric illness.

The most important factors in the development of a person's self-image are the attitudes parents and other emotionally important persons show toward him during his formative childhood years. The child who is reared by parents who treat him with reasonable love and respect tends to feel that he is a person worthy of love and respect. The child who is reared with coldness and hostility from his parents tends to assume that he is an inadequate person who merits only coldness and hostility from others. Parents who by their words and attitudes show the child that they feel he is a reasonably capable person tend to produce a person who views himself in that light; parents who constantly harangue a child about his alleged inadequacies and failures tend to produce a child who views himself as inferior and inept.

A child has a strong tendency to assume that the parental attitudes expressed toward him during the first 12 years of his life are justified by the nature of his personality. If a child were reared in an environment in which he was told every day that the moon was the center of the universe, and if no one ever informed him to the contrary, he would tend to take for granted the contention that the moon was the center of the universe. He would accept this belief as part of the reality of the universe in which he lived. Similarly, a child who is always treated as a worthwhile, lovable individual tends to assume that his real personality is worthwhile and lovable. A child who is reared in an environment of hostility, criticism and depreciation often tends to assume that this pervasive attitude is realistically based on the inadequacies and shortcomings of his personality.

Identification

An important aspect of personality development lies in the kinds of identification a child makes with important people around him. As the child grows he gradually incorporates into himself qualities of personality and behavior adopted from the significant people in his life. This process is known as identification. The child usually is not articulately aware that he is identifying with certain aspects of the personalities of his mother and father and is taking on some of their personality qualities. Identification is a slow, imperceptible process which goes on largely outside the child's range of conscious awareness.

A child incorporates personality qualities from both his parents, but in a healthy family environment a child incorporates more qualities from the parent of the same sex. Thus, if a boy has a sound, warm relationship with his father, he tends to take on more of the attributes of his father than his mother. Similarly, a girl tends to incorporate into herself many of the personality traits of her mother. Identification is a complex process in which many influences impinge on the child's developing character structure. Other close people in the child's life, such as other relatives or important adult friends, may in this way contribute to the gradual formation of the child's personality. Identification is one of the significant processes by which the child's personality is gradually formed in the matrix of his interpersonal relationships.

Identification is also an important aspect of the process by which a child takes on the moral standards and ideals of his parents. The self-imposed moral restrictions and ideals of a person are much influenced by the process of identification. The child who has a healthy, warm relationship with his parents tends to assume their moral standards. The child who has an unhealthy, traumatic relationship with his parents may rebel and reject their standards, either openly or covertly. The child with a sound identification with his parents also tends to incorporate into his life the concepts they hold regarding educational achievement, economic accomplishment and social adjustment.

An identification may be healthy or unhealthy. Just as a child may incorporate ideals of achievement and integrity from his parents, he may, in unhealthy relationships with them and other close persons, take on qualities of deceit, brutality, dishonesty or moral laxness. When a child has identified with undesirable aspects of his parents' behavior, he is said to have made a corrupt identification.

Identification also plays a significant role in determining a person's sexual orientation. A boy with a sound relationship with his father tends to take on the masculine attitudes of the father, and a girl with a healthy relationship with her mother assumes the feminine qualities that characterize her mother. However, when a boy's relationship with his father is traumatic, distant and unsound, he may fail to identify fully with the masculine role. He may instead develop a confused identification with his mother, resulting in a homosexual pattern of personality structure. A girl who has an unsound, distant relationship with her mother may be unable to adopt a femine identification and may develop a homosexual pattern. A homosexual personality development usually is the result of unhealthy relationships with both parents. The boy, for example, has a distant, hostile relationship with his father and an unhealthy closeness to an overprotective, hovering mother. Out of the matrix of these unhealthy relationships with both parents the homosexual identification takes place, and such an identification becomes deeply rooted and difficult to change later. Unhealthy identifications may also contribute to a certain extent to the formation of other sexual problems.

Later Childhood: From Age Eight to Puberty

In later childhood, from the age of eight to the beginning of puberty, the child is rapidly developing an ever wider circle of friends and activities. Though his home will continue to be the major emotional focus of his life for many years yet, he is taking increasing interest in interpersonal relationships outside the home. He has increasingly important interpersonal activities at school, in the neighborhood, in clubs and scout groups, and in other social areas. His mobility is greater and he is away from home more. During this time the child tends to be interested mainly in friends of his own sex. The boys tend to group together in games and sports, and the girls tend to associate together in their activities. This grouping goes on until puberty and adolescence stirs greater interest in the opposite sex.

Harry Stack Sullivan called this period the juvenile era and felt that it was important in personality development. During these years the child has innumerable opportunities to consolidate healthy personality qualities in new social settings, or to correct previously developed personality warps in the contexts of sounder relationships. For example, the child who has been reared in an irritable, depreciating parental atmosphere, and who finds more warmth and respect in neighborhood associations, school relationships, and interactions in other social groups, may solve some of the emotional problems he has been developing. How successfully this can occur depends on various factors, such as whether the child's home-bred emotional difficulties are mild or major, and whether the social influences outside the home are weakly or strongly helpful, and whether his parents impede his exposure to these influences or leave him free to explore new social groups freely.

For example, a child who emerges from his early, home-bound years with mild personality warps may solve his problems in sound interpersonal relationships during his later childhood period, whereas a badly damaged child is but little affected by healthy extrafamilial influences. Also, the nature and degree of the child's emotional problems affects the extent to which social forces can reach him. Thus, a shy child with low self-esteem may be fairly accessible to warm, encouraging persons who treat him as an esteemed, worthwhile individual; whereas a child who emerges from his early years with feelings of diffuse hostility and rebellion toward people may alienate the very persons who might otherwise exercise a beneficial effect on him. The varieties of intermeshing between developing personality structure and environmental impacts during the juvenile period are legion.

Social influences may also damage personality structure and create emotional problems during later childhood. It is of great importance whether the child who steps outside his parental door finds himself in a violence-ridden, drug-infested ghetto or a secure, gregarious suburban neighborhood. Of course, the strengths or weaknesses he brings out of his parental environment determine to some extent how well he can resist the corrupting influences of a sick neighborhood or benefit from the constructive influences of a healthy one.

Thus, there is a broad middle ground where psychiatry, sociology and economics merge. Psychiatrists and all other mental health specialists encounter these social and economic factors each day in their work with patients. A child guidance clinic which treats a child and his parents for two hours each week has very different problems to overcome, depending on whether, for the other 110 waking hours of the week, the child and his parents are surrounded by brutality and deprivation, or by comfort and affluence.

Possessiveness and Independence in Later Childhood. Throughout the years of later childhood, the parents must gradually allow the child more independence and liberty. As he becomes able, the child must assume responsibilities and privileges consistent with his age group. Some parents have trouble allowing their children to participate in ever wider circles of interpersonal relationships outside the home. Some parents tend to keep their children overly dependent on themselves and the home. Such parental possessiveness and the resultant overdependence of the child may have unfortunate effects upon the child's developing personality structure and may limit his capacity for comfortable interpersonal relationships in broader social groups.

Unhealthy parental posessiveness may arise from a variety of causes. Some parents are unduly fearful of the ordinary risks of interpersonal living; they fear exploitation or corruption of their children outside the home, and they carry their fearfulness into management of their children. Other parents cling to their children because of their own self-centered needs. Such parents may use distorted concepts of filial gratitude to inculcate into the child the feeling that his first responsibility is always to serve their needs. They may be unable to tolerate the idea that he will ever leave their home and establish a family of his own that will occupy most of his attention. Such parents often make a child feel guilty if he makes any move of independence. They are prone to portray themselves in the roles of martyrs who have suffered and sacrificed endlessly for the child's welfare. Such parents constitute, at the most, a minority of several per cent of all parents in the general population, but their children frequently are seen for emotional problems in childhood or adolescence, or for long-standing personality difficulties in their later years.

I recall a young adult patient whose mother used her mild heart disease as an agent to keep her daughter chained to the home. She told her that it was only by virtue of her daily care of her that she was able to continue living and that if the girl were to leave the home the mother would die soon after. Behind these maneuvers was a thinly disguised wish to keep the daughter tied to the home in a dependent relationship. During the girl's earlier years the mother had used a long series of fears and self-centered demands to shut the girl off from interpersonal life outside the home. Although on the surface the girl had become a compliant companion of her aging mother, enormous resentment and anger smoldered beneath her passive, dependent façade. This anger, of which she was largely unaware, threatened chronically to erupt into consciousness, and it filled her with anxiety and guilt. In time her anxiety became so painful that she came for psychiatric help, and the ensuing months of interview treatment not only alleviated her anxiety attacks but also freed her from her unhealthy dependence on her mother.

When a child during his developing years or in his adult life is tied to the parental home by the fearfulness or self-centeredness of his parents, it is an unhealthy interpersonal situation for all concerned. There is usually much underlying bitterness and resentment in the child who finds his capacities for mature interpersonal living curtailed by his parents. In their attempts to hold his wavering allegiance, they often become more demanding and domineering. They may sink into hypochondriacal semi-invalidism in their attempts to hold on to him, and such patterns of unhealthy interpersonal relationships may become ingrained. Such parents may become selfish, irritable autocrats who exploit the timid dependence of the child, with crippling effects on the interpersonal lives of both the child and themselves. In emotionally healthy families, on the other hand, the parents gradually relinquish more freedom in the later years of childhood and encourage the child's early steps to establish wider circles of interpersonal living.

The Expression of Feelings

Reasonable comfort with a broad spectrum of feelings and emotions is an important feature of personality development. The child should be reasonably comfortable with his affectionate feelings, his angry feelings, his dependent yearnings and his aggressive feelings. He should be able to give appropriate, reasonable expression to some of these feelings in socially acceptable ways, and he should be able to suppress the excessive expression of those feelings society requires that he restrain. He should not be terrified of his feelings nor should he feel guilty about them. A healthy comfort with his feelings, coupled with a reasonable capacity to control socially undesirable impulses, can arise only in the context of sound interpersonal relationships throughout childhood.

Emotional health demands that a person should be able to express a certain amount of his feelings. The most common way to express feelings is to put them into words. Children should be encouraged to put their affectionate feelings into words, and they should learn from their parents and from other close persons that it is healthy to be able to discuss their fears, problems and pleasures.

Children who are raised in unaffectionate homes may have much difficulty in developing the capacity for expressing love in comfortable ways. They may feel inhibited and awkward in both the verbal and physical expression of all kinds of affection. On the other hand, children who are reared in homes where there is a give-and-take of love are usually able to form warm interpersonal relationships with friends and to establish sound, close associations in marriage and parenthood. The inability to engage in affectionate interpersonal relationships is a crippling defect in personality development, and it predisposes to various kinds of emotional difficulties in adult life.

Emotional health also requires that a person be able to put at least a certain amount of his assertive feelings into socially acceptable expression. He must be able to stick up for himself against those who would impose on him unduly, and he must be able to be firm with those persons who would exploit him. Occasionally, he should be able to be angry and to express his feelings reasonably.

People who are unable to be reasonably self-assertive often develop emotional symptoms. The pent-up, accumulated hostility that is found behind the passive façade of an unassertive person may contribute to the development of anxiety neuroses, phobias, depressions, some types of psychosomatic disturbances and other psychiatric difficulties. The inability to give reasonable expression to assertive and angry feelings usually arises in the context of interpersonal relationships with parents and other close persons who throughout the child's formative years made him feel overwhelmingly guilty and inadequate whenever he was at all assertive or aggressive. When these patterns of suppression of feelings become deeply rooted in a child's personality during the formative years of his life, they tend to persist throughout his adult years, causing him persistent interpersonal problems. The resolution of psychiatric problems that arise to a certain extent out of the inability of the person to be aware of a wide range of suppressed normal feelings within himself and to give expression to some of them, is a frequent task of psychiatric interview treatment. The unassertive person's passivity is usually so ingrained that he is unaware, or only partially aware, of his problem with the expression of feelings. Even when he is aware of this personality difficulty he usually does not connect it with the emotional symptoms that bring him for psychiatric help.

Awareness and Unawareness

Each person at all moments in his life has varying degrees of awareness about the nature and causes of his feelings, actions and experiences. He can become clearly aware of many things in both his current and past life experiences merely by focusing his attention on them. He can become aware of a wide range of other things only by careful attention and laborious reminiscing. There are other areas of his past and current life of which he cannot become aware by the ordinary methods of self-scrutiny, observation and thought.

For example, a surgeon performing an operation knows, on the most superficial level of his awareness, that he is performing an appendectomy on a patient whose internist or family physician has called him in consultation. He is aware of the details of the operative procedure, his interaction with the other persons in the operating room, and the immediate technical problems with which he is struggling. However, he may be only partially aware of many other things that are going on. He may not be clearly aware of his increasing tenseness and irritability with his assistant and the circulating nurse as he runs into trouble with a ruptured appendix or one that is difficult to locate behind a distended bowel. However, if he is a reasonably well adjusted person, he could become aware of his tenseness and irritability if someone, such as his assistant or the patient's internist who is standing behind him, pointed it out by saying, "Don't get so tense and upset about this; we all know this is a difficult case." If, on the contrary he had various kinds of personality warps, he might attribute all problems to the persons assisting him and state that it was their tenseness and slovenliness which was causing his operative problems. If his personality difficulties were different, he might feel ill-at-ease and guilty about the operative problems, and his duodenal ulcer might begin to pain him as his upper gastrointestinal tract became hypersecretive, hypervascular and hyperactive.

Looking at another aspect—the operation—the surgeon is acutely aware of the maneuvers that he and his assistant are going through to locate and remove a remote, ruptured appendix. However, he is not aware of the rapid motions of his fingers as he ties each knot to stop a bleeding vessel. When he was an intern he carefully thought through each of these finger movements, and was directly aware of them, as he practiced tying knots in his room. Again, he could become aware of these individual finger movements if his attention were directed to them, but this would happen only under unusual circumstances.

In a similar way, he has varying levels of awareness about why he is performing the operation. On the most superficial level he knows that he is doing it because the patient's clinical condition requires it. On a deeper level of awareness, he may be doing it because he is following the life pattern of an admired father who was also a surgeon. In other circumstances, he may be a hard driving surgeon because he was reared in a rejecting parental environment and he is on an endless treadmill to achieve professional and social eminence to prove to both himself and others that he is not the worthless, inept person he inwardly has feared, since childhood, that he is.

As we probe more deeply into these levels of awareness, or unawareness, we find areas of both past and current feelings, attitudes and experiences that are increasingly unavailable to the person. Some of these experiences and feelings are so painful that they can be brought into the focus of his awareness only by detailed interview work with a psychiatrist or other mental health therapist. Others are less painful, and the individual can come to grips with them in varying degrees by careful reflection and self-examination.

In the interpersonal approach to psychiatry the concepts of *aware* and *unaware* experiences are somewhat similar to the Freudian-psychoanalytic concepts of conscious and unconscious experiences. However, the interpersonal approach views the relationship between aware and unaware thoughts and memories in a much more flexible, fluid way than conscious and unconscious thoughts and memories are conceived in Freudian psychoanalysis. The difference may be made clear by a simile. Freudian psychoanalysis, and the neo-Freudian schools of thought that have grown out of it, view unconscious thoughts, feelings and painful memories of past experiences as items firmly padlocked in endless sets of drawers which can be opened only by the therapeutic procedures of Freudian psychoanalysis. Interpersonal theory, on the other hand, views them as things that are carried to and fro on a tide that continually ebbs and flows; thus, interpersonal theory views the unaware feelings, thoughts and experiences (both past and current) of an individual as much more accessible to him by means of either informed, alert experience or professional therapy.

Much of the work of psychiatry is devoted to exploring the unaware roots of emotional functioning and interpersonal relationships, for painful or warped unaware processes have a tendency to produce distortions of interpersonal activity and many kinds of emotional and physical symptoms.

Adolescence

During adolescence an individual undergoes more extensive changes in his interpersonal behavior than at any subsequent time in his life. At the beginning of adolescence, the individual is a child, dependent on his home and on his parents. At its end he is an adult and is either independent of his home or in the process of acquiring the education and the training that will soon make him so. During adolescence, the individual progressively moves toward more emotional, social and economic independence. During a period of such extensive change, there is always a certain amount of emotional turmoil and conflict between the adolescent, who is rapidly developing independence in many areas, and his parents, who must supervise this development.

At the beginning of adolescence, the individual lives in interpersonal circles that have been chosen for him mainly by his parents. His associations at school, in the neighborhood, and in other interpersonal groups have been largely determined by the associations and plans his parents have made for him. The parents have exercised a close jurisdiction over his interpersonal activities and have encouraged certain friendships and have discouraged others. During adolescence, the individual begins to choose his own friends and to enter into interpersonal relationships over which his parents have less supervision. As the years proceed and adulthood approaches, the interpersonal circles of the individual become increasingly divorced from his parents' home.

At the beginning of adolescence, the individual's major emotional investment is still mainly in his parents and in his brothers and sisters. At its end, his investment in his parents and siblings usually has changed a great deal. The well-adjusted adolescent usually has much affection and respect for his parents and feels much comradely friendship for his brothers and sisters. However, he is beginning to make major emotional investments in persons outside the home. The boy is becoming interested in girl friends, and the girl is now devoting much of her emotional energy to her relationships with boy friends.

The progressive interpersonal independence of the individual from his parental home eventually results, as a rule, in marriage and the establishment of a new home during young adulthood. The individual's major emotional investment is then in his wife and children, though his relationship with his parents should be one of deep affection and respect. This radical transition from complete emotional dependence on the parents to the independence involved in setting up a home of one's own is one of the major interpersonal changes that begins during adolescence.

The sexual maturation of the person takes place during adolescence. His interest in adult sexuality is awakened and he must work out socially acceptable ways of channeling his sexual drives. The healthy, socially desirable channeling of sexuality has a major influence in all his subsequent interpersonal life. The success or failure of an adjustment to sexuality has profound effects on the person's social adjustments in adolescence and on his adult ability to enter into a healthy marriage and family life. It also affects his interpersonal stability, or instability, in many other areas, such as work and recreational situations, in which he must deal comfortably and soundly with many new persons of both sexes.

Most psychiatrists feel that throughout childhood there are rudimentary sexual feelings in the child, but that these yearnings express themselves in diffuse ways. They contribute to yearnings for closeness and affection, as well as some conflicts, with parents and other persons. They serve as part of the motivating force that draws the child close to people. (The various interpretations of sexual yearnings that occur before puberty and adolescence are dealt with at length in Chapter 3.) However, sexuality in an adult sense first develops in adolescence, and it remains a significant force in interpersonal life throughout adulthood.

Emotional health and sound personality development require that the individual be reasonably comfortable with his sexuality. He should be neither frightened by it nor driven unrestrainedly by it. A person's capacity to adjust to sexuality in emotionally comfortable and socially acceptable ways is enormously influenced by his interpersonal relationships with his parents and other close persons during the formative years of his life. A boy who has a sound relationship with his mother and a good relationship with his father during his formative years tends to look forward to comfortable relationships with girls in his adolescence and tends to adjust well in marriage. The girl who has sound interpersonal relationships with both her parents tends to accept her mother's feminine orientation and to look for masculine qualities in boys such as the ones she found in her father. On the other hand, children who have traumatic relationships with their parents and who are exposed to turmoil, conflict and unhealthy interactions in their parents' marriage may emerge from childhood with confused, frightened feelings about the ways in which persons of the opposite sex interact in intimate relationships. Such turmoil in the child may grossly affect his later capacity to adjust in marriage and may affect his capacities for a healthy, comfortable sexual relationships. Each person is much influenced by the nature of the marriage of his parents, and what he experienced in being reared in the environment of that marriage has profound influences on his capacities and expectations in the complex adjustments of marriage. Also, the attitudes of the parents toward sexuality and the ways in which the young child's questions about sex were answered or were shunned have much effect on his feelings about sexuality.

Some persons emerge from childhood profoundly frightened of sexuality and marriage. They view marriage with fear and sexuality with anxiety. Their fears may prevent them from forming close relationships with persons of the opposite sex during adolence and young adulthood, or may cause them many problems in sexual relations and marital adjustments if they marry. Impotence and frigidity in the bedroom and turbulence and hostility in the living room often result. On the other hand, a person may emerge from childhood with a lack of socially desirable restraint on his sexuality. Out of his daily exposure for many years to a disturbed parental marriage the child may develop little capacity for basic respect or profound affection for a sexual partner, and marital turmoil and sexual chaos in adult life result. Sometimes hostile feelings and sexual impulses become merged in a person who comes out of a childhood in which parental hostility and neglect left him with a diffuse bitterness toward persons of the opposite sex and unsound feelings about how people interact with each other sexually and in marriage. Many problems of the marriage bed begin in the nursery room, and the bases of many divorces are laid in the turbulence of unhealthy relationships of children with their parents.

In the interpersonal approach to psychiatry, personality development continues actively throughout adolescence, but adolescent experiences exert their impacts on an individual who has already been extensively molded by all his preceding years of interpersonal activity. However, adolescence is also a period in which the previous personality evolution of the person is tested. If his interpersonal development has been sound, he usually adjusts well to the process of gradually taking over emotional, social and economic independence as he moves slowly toward adulthood. If his personality development has been unhealthy, he may react with anxiousness, rebellion or social withdrawal under the stresses of proceeding toward adulthood and channeling his sexual drives. Various kinds of psychiatric illness begin to increase in frequency during adolescence and early adulthood as the individual's emotional soundness and interpersonal capacities are put to the test of mature, independent living.

Intimacy. *Intimacy is a state in which the well-being of another person is as important to an individual as his own welfare.* This is the highest, healthiest level of interpersonal experience. Intimacy may occur in a parent-child relationship, between lovers, in a marital relationship, and in some other kinds of human interactions. Intimacy is akin to, but not necessarily identical with, the broad spectrum of feelings grouped under the term "love." In a sense, and to a limited extent, intimacy may exist in social groups, religious congregations, and even political groups;

people may put the welfare of the group to which they are dedicated on the same level with, or even above, their own well-being.

Intimacy is both the goal and the test of interpersonal life. It can exist only when there is little or no *anxiety* between the persons involved, and when each feels a high, justified degree of security in the relationship. Communication, both verbal and nonverbal, is usually unimpeded in an intimate relationship, and its very nature to a large extent protects the person against emotional stresses in other areas of his life. Thus, a child with a sound, intimate relationship with his parents can better face and master interpersonal conflicts at school and in the neighborhood, and a person with a good, intimate marriage can better adjust to disappointments and problems in his job and social life.

In the various kinds of psychiatric disturbances, intimacy is impaired in different ways. In a neurotic disorder intimacy is limited by the person's internal conflicts and the various ways in which he struggles constantly to quell the rising titers of anxiety within him. In a psychosomatic illness intimacy is impeded by the individual's continual or intermittent physical discomforts. In a personality disorder intimacy is contaminated by the individual's pervasive hostility, or passivity, or social withdrawal, or other warped interpersonal pattern. In a psychotic illness intimacy is disrupted by the patient's flight into a delusional schizophrenic world, or his withdrawal into profound depressiveness, or his slow loss of intellectual and emotional capacities because of organic brain damage, or by some other psychotic process.

From childhood to old age, the emotional health of a person can, to a large extent, be measured by his capcaity to achieve and maintain intimacy in various areas of his life.

Other Aspects of the Interpersonal Approach to Personality Development

Before leaving childhood and adolescence, we shall review a few other concepts in the interpersonal approach to personality development. Although to some extent they overlap parts of our previous discussions, they throw new light on various aspects of emotional growth.

Harry Stack Sullivan divided infancy and childhood into three successive stages of development: (1) *prototaxic*, (2) *parataxic* and (3) *syntaxic*. However, these awkward words have not been widely adopted, though the basic concepts they represent have had much influence on psychiatric thinking. Therefore, we shall designate them by simpler, more descriptive terms as the phases of (1) *crude sensations*, (2) *misconnected experiences* and (3) *realistic appraisals*.

Although these three stages overlap each other widely, they may, quite artificially, be said to occur in the following age brackets: (1) The phase of *crude sensations* (prototaxic phase) occurs during the first year to 18 months of life. (2) The phase of *misconnected experiences* (parataxic phase) occurs from about 19 moths to the age of three or four. (3) The phase of *realistic appraisals* (syntaxic phase) stretches from the age of three or four into middle and late adolescence, though its main function is probably achieved in childhood and early adolescence.

We shall consider these three phases of development in detail.

The Phase of Crude Senastions. During most of the first year or more of life, a child's experience consists of intense, poorly defined, brief sensations unconnected with one another in his consciousness. They are like scenes of unrelated subjects thrown by a slide projector on a screen one after another in a pell-mell manner. For example, the infant feels uncomfortable in a vague manner and he cries. A nipple is thrust into his mouth and he sucks. He feels at ease and is drowsy. He awakes after an indefinite period and stares at meaningless light. However, he has no distinct memories of these events, nor does he have any sense of their relatedness and time sequences.

During this phase of *crude sensations* (or prototaxic phase) the infant has no concepts of himself, other people and his environment, and he does not differentiate what is he from what is not he. This phase has been called the *oceanic stage*, because it is as if one were immersed in, and part of, an endless ocean in which there is a vague ebb and flow of currents but no differentiation of objects. This is the only kind of experience the child has during the first four to six months of life, and it continues in decreasing degrees until the age of three or four years. After that it is present only in sleep, periods of extreme stress and various kinds of psychiatric disorders.

Some persons who have painful interpersonal relationships in childhood and later life have a tendency during periods of marked stress to return to more primitive levels of personality functioning. For example, a child with early infantile autism (a childhood psychosis akin to schizophrenia, discussed in Chapter 14) returns to, or remains fixed at, this primary level of crude sensations. Finding interpersonal life very painful, he unconsciously clings to this oceanic kind of existence in which interpersonal relationships do not exist or are only dimly perceived. The adult who develops catatonic schizophrenia has retreated from the suffering of life with people to this noninterpersonal way of life; however, such a retreat is never complete, for the schizophrenic retains fragments of his interpersonal capacities from the two succeeding levels of development. The severity of a schizophrenic illness depends on how deeply into this phase of crude sensations the patient has retired and how firmly he is tied there. In similar ways, minor degrees of fixation at this level of experience, or brief retreats into it, play roles in some other kinds of psychiatric problems.

The Phase of Misconnected Experiences. During the second half of the first year of life, the child enters the phase of *misconnected experiences*. This phase is dominant until about the age of 3 or so when it gradually is replaced by the stage of realistic appraisals. However, as noted above, there is extensive overlapping, often of several years or more, between each of these phases and the succeeding one. Thus, a child retains elements of crude sensations well into middle childhood, and misconnected experiences continues to a certain degree into late childhood and adolescence. The extent of overlapping between these periods differs much from one person to another.

During the stage of misconnected experiences the child slowly separates from the vast number of stimuli he experiences a concept of himself as something separate from his environment, and he gradually develops concepts of the people and things around him. The first thing that he distinctly separates from himself is the nipple, whether flesh or rubber, from which his food comes. Then he slowly develops a concept of the person who gives him the nipple. Other things slowly loom out of the mist—his crib, the ceiling light, his blankets and the room. During the second year of life the members of his family begin to assume clearer images, and from then on the process of identifying things and people expands rapidly.

However, in his early concepts of things and people, the child does not have valid ideas about relatedness and cause and effect. He does not know that his Teddy bear was given to him by his father who works in an office each day to make money to buy things for him. He knows only that he finds the presence of the familiar Teddy bear reassuring, that his father is somehow different from his mother, and that his father disappears early in the morning on most days and reappears as it is getting dark. He has no concepts of the relatedness of these things, and thus, although his experiences are becoming clearer, they are poorly connected, or in many cases misconnected. They become connected in helter-skelter ways, by chance associations, and by haphazard sequences and incorrect associations. Again, using our previous metaphor, it is as if the child is allowed to study carefully a series of related pictures projected on a screen but is given no clues about the relationships of the scenes to each other; in time he arrives at poor or erroneous connections in his ideas about their relationships. These erroneous connections constitute what Sullivan called parataxic distortions.

The concept of misconnected experiences (parataxic distortions) can be made clearer by a simple example. A one-year-old child observes that in the late afternoon his mother comes less quickly when he cries or calls for her; he also notices that this is about the time his father comes home. Joining the two events by their sequence rather than by realistic appraisal, which is as yet beyond him, he may feel that his father is hostile to him, or to his mother, or is coming between his mother and him in some fearful, malicious way. The truth is that in the late afternoon Mother and Father sink into chairs in the family room or on the patio to exchange news about office and home events. The child has put various experiences together in a misconnected way and has arrived at an unrealistic conclusion about one aspect of his interpersonal life. Beginning in the third or fourth year of life the child begins to correct these misconnections by the final type of experience, realistic appraisals.

The soundness of the child's eventual personality depends to a large extent on how successfully his misconnected experiences are corrected. All misconnected experiences are, of course, to some extent incorrect, and in many cases if not corrected may warp the child's personality and limit his capacities for sound interpersonal relationships. They also are a common cause of anxiety and other forms of emotional distress, and hence may contribute to later neuroses, psychosomatic illnesses, situational maladjustments and, in severe instances, psychotic disorders. Hence, the gradual correction of his misconnected experiences between early childhood and middle adolescence is a central part of personality development.

In some instances several or many misconnected experiences may become ingrained because of unhealthy interpersonal relationships in childhood and adolescence. In a simple example, let us further consider the above-described child who misinterprets the significance of his mother's disappearance when his father comes home and who develops both fearful and hostile feelings toward his father. In a few months he begins to have healthy contacts with his father and slowly corrects these misconceptions, and he also sees his parents living together harmoniously. His misconnected experience (or parataxic distortion) is gradually erased and sound conceptions take its place. However, if his father is chronically irritable toward him, or if his mother, because of her own personality problems, tearfully confides to him, from the age of four or five years onward, how unjustly she feels the often-absent father treats both of them, the child's misconnected experience tends to become fixed. He feels increasingly that his father, and perhaps all fathers, are hostile and malicious, and that he and his mother, and perhaps all children and mothers, are victims of such a man. He draws closer to his mother in a dependent, unwholesome way and has a deep dread and anger toward his father.

In late childhood these concepts, often by this time inarticulate and unconscious, have become deeply embedded, and he then has more than average probability of developing various kinds of personality disorders in adult life. In addition, the misconnected experience (parataxic distortion) limits his interpersonal life in late childhood, adolescence and adulthood and, in a vicious circle, decreases his opportunities for correcting it. Because of his dread and anger toward men and his discomfort with women (for, though close to his mother, he finds her clutching possessiveness uncomfortable), he is unable to have healthy, comfortable relationships with persons of both sexes at school, in the neighborhood and in other social groups. Thus, he is deprived of the close interpersonal contacts that might have enabled him to correct his misconceptions of men and women and the ways they get along with each other and with him.

Misconnected experiences have another clinical significance. A well-adjusted person who is under severe stress may retreat into childhood misconnected experiences which he has largely corrected in his day-to-day life but which, nevertheless, still linger obscurely within him. In the case of the boy discussed above, if his later relationships with his parents and other close persons are healthy, he may to a large extent correct his misconceptions, but deep inside him aspects of this misconnected experience still lurk. Throughout his entire lifetime they may cause him no trouble. However, if in late adolescence or early adulthood he has a disastrous love affair with a domineering, emotionally immature girl who in many ways resembles his mother, he may under this stress return to the ways of feeling and thinking that characterized his childhood misconnected experience, and he is flooded with feelings of dread and hostility toward both men and women. Depending on many factors, which vary much from one person to another, this emotional turmoil may subside in time or it may precipitate a neurosis, a psychosomatic disorder, or some other type of psychiatric difficulty.

Much of the work of psychotherapy is designed to resolve the residues of misconnected experiences, and thus to allow healthy personality development and sound emotional functioning to proceed.

The Phase of Realistic Appraisals. The third and final phase of personality development is that in which the person, from early childhood through adolescence, gradually perceives the relatedness of interpersonal events and grasps the realistic cause and effect connections of the varied happenings in his life. One of the main ways by which this occurs is consensual validation, which we discussed earlier in this chapter.

The other processes which contribute to realistic appraisals have one crucial feature in common: *they occur only in the contexts of healthy interpersonal relationships.* In them the individual suffers pain in misadventures, has pleasure in sound relationships, enlarges his perceptiveness in a wide range of situations, and slowly weaves all these experiences into new ways of feeling, thinking and living with people. He develops a sound grasp on reality and flexible ways of solving each new problem.

The term realistic appraisals perhaps seems to imply that this process is mainly intellectual and conscious. However, the opposite is true. Although conscious and intellectual factors have their roles, emotional and unconscious processes are much more important. Most of what contributes to realistic appraisals (or, in Sullivan's words, the syntaxic mode of emotional functioning) occurs by imperceptible additions and corrections that are never clearly put into words and at no time are sufficiently in the individual's focus of awareness to be called conscious.

Emotional health depends to a large extent on how firmly the individual arrives at this stage of realistic appraisals. Under severe stress a well-adjusted person may waver slightly backward toward the levels of misconnected experiences and crude sensations, but he soon adjusts to the stress and masters the turmoil within him and once more is able to deal with the challenges of his life by realistic appraisals.

The Adult Years and the One-Genus Postulate

Personality structure never becomes a fixed, final thing. It is influenced throughout a person's entire life by his changing interpersonal relationships, by the events of his social, economic and emotional experiences, and his physical health or illnesses. However, by the time a person reaches early adulthood the basic features of his personality structure are established. Subsequent changes tend to modify rather than basically alter personality structure and interpersonal capacities.

The success or failure of the emotional adjustment of each person in adult life depends on the interaction of his basic personality structure with his interpersonal environment and his changing life circumstances. The individual also is affected by the constantly altering social, economic and cultural situations in which he is living. For example, a man may have lurking feelings of inferiority and a strong need for economic and professional achievement to prove constantly to himself and to others that he is truly a worthwhile, capable person. If he is successful in his educational strivings and his later economic or professional ventures, he may adjust reasonably well throughout his adult life. He may have only minimal discomforts arising from the underlying fears of inferiority, which gnaw at him and spur him on. On the other hand, if he fails in his drive for achievement he may be overwhelmed by his fears of inadequacy. His emotional adjustment may deteriorate badly under such adverse circumstances, and he may develop anxiety states, depressive problems, psychosomatic illnesses or other kinds of psychiatric difficulties.

Similarly, if a girl emerges from her childhood with strong needs to control the people around her, she may adjust reasonably well if she marries a passive man who allows her to make the important decisions in their marriage. If she can give warmth and love in such a marriage and does not exploit the passivity of her husband, the marriage may go reasonably well. On the other hand, if she marries a man who does not tolerate her leadership, chronic marital turbulence may ensue. She may find herself failing as a wife and as a mother, and her prolonged emotional distress may precipitate psychiatric problems. The outcome of such a situation depends much on the flexibility or rigidity of her personality structure and on her other personality resources. I have seen women with such personality problems deteriorate into mild depressiveness, alcoholism, psychosomatic illnesses and other psychiatric difficulties. The outcome is also much affected by the husband's flexibility or rigidity in resolving such interpersonal conflicts.

Some persons emerge from their formative years with such unstable personality structures that the normal stresses of daily life precipitate severe psychiatric problems. Other people come out of childhood with relatively stable personalities and develop psychiatric problems only if they are assaulted by prolonged, severe emotional traumas in adult life. The variations of personality structure and environmental stress that combine to produce minor or major emotional problems are endless. In psychiatry each person must be studied as an individual whose personality was formed in a unique set of circumstances and whose life is composed of his own particular world of interpersonal relationships. In a sense, psychiatry does not deal with diseases in the usual medical sense of the word; it deals with sick people, each one of whom has a special set of problems arising out of his past and present interpersonal relationships. Even those psychiatric illnesses caused by organic brain disease are much colored by pre-existing personality structure and interpersonal life.

It was this basic concept that Harry Stack Sullivan, in his somewhat esoteric terminology, was encapsulating in his oft-cited "one-genus postulate"; namely, that *everyone is much more simply human than otherwise.* By this, Sullivan meant that the things we call psychiatric illnesses differ from the state we call normality in *degree* rather than *nature*. For example, the difference between a schizopherenic and a well-adjusted person is the marked exaggeration in the schizophrenic of certain processes which can be found to some extent in the well-adjusted individual. Whereas the well-adjusted individual retreats into daydreams only in a limited way and always retains the capacity to return at once to firm contact with reality, the schizophrenic has fled into a distorted world of inner fantasies and has lost his ability to return to reality at will.

The same difference in degree, rather than nature, exists in all other psychiatric disturbances. The student with a minor, emotionally caused stomach upset before crucial examinations and the patient with a duodenal ulcer are merely at the opposite ends of a continuous spectrum of mild to severe gastrointestinal problems. The irritable, mildly resistant adolescent and the chaotically rebellious teenager differ in the degree of their hostile feelings and behavior, rather than in their basic nature. The person who occasionally feels somewhat tense in crowded places and the individual with a severe phobia of leaving home are suffering from widely varying degrees of the same problem. The patient with organic brain damage is struggling to meet the same challenges as the person with an intact brain, but he is doing it with fewer brain cells at his command, and his behavior consequently deteriorates.

The one-genus postulate has far-reaching implications. It emphasizes the origins of psychiatric problems in warped past and current interpersonal experiences, and it points to their solutions by therapists who employ healthy, new interpersonal relationships in both outpatient and inpatient settings to help patients achieve better levels of emotional functioning. Even when medications and other physical agents are used, their long-term effectiveness is strongly influenced by the interpersonal relationships between the persons who are administering them and the individuals who are receiving them.

The one-genus postulate also removes from psychiatric disturbances all hints of bizarreness or uniqueness. We are all much more simply human than otherwise.

In this chapter we have dealt with only a few of the basic interpersonal forces that affect emotional health and personality development. Our main purpose in tracing this development has been to explain the interpersonal approach to psychiatry; many other aspects of personality development and functioning are covered in later chapters. In a sense, most of the rest of this book is devoted to presenting the interpersonal approach to the full range of psychiatric problems and their treatment.

BIBLIOGRAPHY

Greenbaum, H.: Marriage, family and parenthood. Am. J. Psychiatry, *130*:1262, 1973.
Havens, L. L.: Approaches to the Mind. Boston, Little Brown, 1973.
——— The existential use of the self. Am. J. Psychiatry, *131*:1, 1974.

Hinde, R. A. (ed.): Non-Verbal Communication. New York, Cambridge University Press, 1972.

Lourie, R. S.: The first three years of life. Am. J. Psychiatry, *127*:1457, 1971.

Ruesch, J.: Disturbed Communication, New York, W. W. Norton, 1957.

Ruesch, J., and Bateson, G.: Communication. The Social Matrix of Society. New York, W. W. Norton, 1951.

Sullivan, H. S.: Conceptions of Modern Psychiatry. New York, W. W. Norton, 1953.

——— The Interpersonal Theory of Psychiatry. New York, W. W. Norton, 1953.

——— The Fusion of Psychiatry and Social Science. New York, W. W. Norton, 1964.

2

The Historical Evolution of Modern Psychiatry

Modern psychiatry is the product of a long evolutionary process. In this chapter we shall trace psychiatry from its earliest origins down to the present time. We shall give particular attention to the history of psychiatry in the last 100 years in order to understand how the concepts were developed that we use in clinical psychiatry today.

Knowledge of the history of a medical specialty has practical usefulness. The study of the past evolution of a medical field emphasizes that there must be future evolution. Knowledge of fruitful methods of the past stimulates productive research in the future, and the study of past misconceptions and errors sometimes points out pitfalls to be avoided. The history of a medical specialty stresses that a medical field is never static; it is in a process of continual change. The present is a narrow point which divides a long, instructive past from a broad, hopeful future. So long as our treatment methods need improvement and human suffering remains, the need for constant evolution in a medical specialty presses us on. The past is our teacher, the present is our opportunity and the future is our hope.

Finally, the history of medicine shows the physician where he stands in a long tradition. He has inherited a rich past, and many of the things he does took centuries to develop. For a physician to know the history of his profession gives his work fascination and dignity, and gives him an awesome sense of responsibility.

CONCEPTS OF MENTAL ILLNESS FROM ANCIENT TIMES TO THE RENAISSANCE

The ancient Greeks were the first people who recognized that mental illness is caused by physical or emotional disorders and that its treatment should be included in the practice of medicine. Until that time the mentally ill had been considered to be infested by evil spirits, and treatment consisted of magical or religious incantations and exorcism. The enlightened concepts of Greek medicine were first formulated authoritatively by Hippocrates who lived from about 460 to about 370 B. C. He taught that mental illness is caused by physical disorders of the body, and he accurately described the clinical features of depressions, manic disorders and hysteria.

The concepts of Hippocrates and his followers were absorbed into Roman medicine. The clinicians Caelius, Asclepiades, Celsus, Aratus and Soranus elaborated on the theories of Hippocrates and extended his clinical observations. Greek and Roman physicians felt that mental illness was caused by disturbances in the main physical constituents, or "humors," of the body, and that these distrubances affected the brain, thus producing the various forms of mental illness. Hysteria was felt to be caused by undue mobility of the uterus. Primitive as these concepts were, they constituted an enormous advance over previous demonological concepts of mental illness, and they firmly placed mental illness in the domain of medical practice. Later Roman physicians accurately described febrile delirium and senile organic brain disorders.

The principles of treatment of mental illness in Greek and Roman times were humane and reasonable. They included sedation with opiates, music therapy, good physical hygiene and gentle management of the patient's daily activities. The Greek and Roman achievements in psychiatry, as well as other medical fields, were summarized by Galen, who lived from about 130 to 200 A. D.

It is probable, however, that medical concepts of mental illness and its treatment by physicians, were limited to the educated and propertied classes in Greco-Roman times. Among the vast masses of the illiterate poor, almost half of whom were slaves in many parts of the Greco-Roman world, demonological concepts of mental disorders and treatment by magical exorcism, probably prevailed. However, the available historical and medical records, with a few notable exceptions, tell us mainly about the upper social and intellectual segments of Greek and Roman societies.

The accomplishments of Greek and Roman medicine were virtually abandoned in the decline of learning and science which began with the deterioration of the Roman Empire and lasted, except in a few instances, until the Renaissance. Though the writings of Galen and other Greco-Roman physicians were preserved in Byzantine and monastic libraries, and in the commentaries of Arabic physicians who flourished from the Middle East to Moorish Spain during a significant part of this period, they had little influence on the prevailing concepts of mental illness. It was again believed to be caused by infestations of demons and evil spirits, and the mentally ill often were considered to be in voluntary league with the evil forces inhabiting them. Treatment was by exorcism and magical devices. The mentally ill were neglected, ostracized or occasionally executed as agents of supernatural evil forces.

From the latter part of the 15th Century to the latter part of the 17th Century the mentally ill were legally prosecuted on a vast scale and burned as witches on the grounds that they were in voluntary alliance with the infesting evil spirits, or that they were willing collaborators and agents of Satan. Hundreds of thousands of mentally ill persons, most of whom were women, were cruelly executed in this manner. This movement was given a strong impetus in its early stages by the publication by two theologians of a book *Malleus Maleficarum* (The Witches' Hammer) in which they urged as a moral necessity the prosecution and extirpation of witches; their descriptions of persons who might be identified as witches and infested by evil spirits contain some astonishingly accurate descriptions of psychiatric syndromes. Legal prosecution and execution of the mentally ill declined in the late 17th Century but persisted sporadically for another 100 years. Though the Renaissance had begun and a great revival of scientific medicine had started, psychiatry did not again become a significant field of medical activity until the early part of the 18th Century.

THE BEGINNINGS OF MODERN PSYCHIATRY

The German physician Johann Weyer (1515–1588) is often considered the founder of modern psychiatry and the first true clinical psychiatrist. In 1563 he published his major work, in which he condemned the prosecution and execution of mentally ill persons as witches. He wrote the first comprehensive treatise on psychiatry, and accurately described clinical pictures that we can recognize today as toxic organic brain disorders, hysteria, senile organic brain disorders, depression, paranoid states, schizophrenia and epilepsy, although, of course, he did not use these terms to designate them. He advocated taking careful case histories of the illnesses of mentally ill persons, and he treated some of his patients by sitting and talking with them for long periods of time. He felt that childhood experiences were important in forming personality structure, and he attributed many instances of mental illness to emotional turmoil and interpersonal stress.

Weyer's immediate influence was limited, but his writings mark a turning point in psychiatric history. His concepts had a slow, progressive influence on the psychiatric developments of the 17th and 18th Centuries. The 16th Century physicians Paracelsus and

Agrippa also opposed the persecution of the mentally ill and advocated their treatment by medical means.

During the 17th Century the significant medical advances in anatomy, chemistry and the clinical study of illness were not accompanied by advances in the study and care of the mentally ill. The demonological concepts of mental illness persisted and the execution of the mentally ill continued. At the end of the 17th Century physicians such as Stahl in Germany again urged including the treatment of mentally ill persons in the domain of medical practice, and the distinguished English physician Willis attributed mental illness to physical causes. However, the full influence of these physicians and their predecessors was not felt until the 18th Century.

During the 18th Century the demonological concepts of psychiatric illness were progressively abandoned and mental illness again became recognized as a medical field. The mentally ill were largely neglected, however, or they were incarcerated in prison-like hospitals where they were often put in chains and badly treated. A notable exception was the large colony of mentally ill persons who were allowed to live openly in the community of Gheel, Belgium, the site of the shrine of St. Dymphna, the theological patroness of the mentally ill. (This colony, which began in the 14th Century, still exists and has about 2,000 patients lodged in private homes and other places.) Under the guidance of physicians such as Boerhaave, Reil and Langerman, mental illness became a subject of medical discussion in the 18th Century, although the prevailing theories of mental disorders were little advanced beyond those of rediscovered Greco-Roman authorities.

Toward the end of the 18th Century some great leaders in the development of humane care of the mentally ill began to make reforms whose influence was to have a revolutionary effect on psychiatry in the 19th Century. Probably the most important of these psychiatric pioneers was Phillipe Pinel (1745–1826) who in 1793 was appointed medical director of the Bicêtre and Salpêtrière hospitals in Paris. He there found mentally ill patients chained, brutally treated and kept in filth. He began extensive reforms.

He abandoned the use of chains and organized these hospitals into clean, humanely run institutions. He was the first physician to keep systematic case histories on hospitalized psychiatric patients, and he wrote widely and convincingly about the medical treatment of the mentally ill. He believed many mental illnesses were caused by emotional stress, and he emphasized that many patients had good prognoses when well treated. He urged "moral treatment," in which the interpersonal influence of the physician was a major therapeutic measure.

A similar leader in the late 18th Century was the Philadelphia physician Benjamin Rush (1745–1813), often called the father of American psychiatry; the official seal of The American Psychiatric Association bears his picture. He advocated building hospitals for the care of the mentally ill, and in 1812 he wrote the first American textbook of psychiatry. He was, incidentally, one of the signers of the Declaration of Independence (of the 56 signers, four were physicians).

In 1796 an English lay philanthropist William Tuke (1732–1822) founded the York Retreat as a humanely run institution for the medical care of the mentally ill. He established a family tradition of interest in their care, which persisted for several generations and culminated in the work of his great-grandson, Daniel Hack Tuke (1827–1895), a physician who devoted his medical career to the advancement of psychiatry. The York Retreat, in which the Tuke family played a prominent role, had much influence in diffusing the concept of medical care for the mentally ill in a well-run psychiatric hospital. Vincenzo Chiaruggi (1759–1820) was a similar pioneer in Italy in the medical care of the mentally ill; there is evidence that Pinel may have gotten some of his basic ideas from Chiaruggi's work.

PSYCHIATRIC DEVELOPMENT IN THE NINETEENTH CENTURY

During the 19th Century psychiatry gradually developed into a systematic medical specialty. Large numbers of public and private psychiatric hospitals were built, and the concept became established in Western Europe and America that the medical care of the mentally ill was a responsibility of the whole community. Psychiatric journals and psychiatric medical societies were founded, and much progress was made in differentiating and studying the various types of psychiatric illness.

The French school of psychiatry was predominant during the first three quarters of the 19th Century, with important contributions by such men as Esquirol, Falret, Morel and Baillarger. These physicians carried on in the traditions established by Pinel. They defined most of the organic psychoses and studied their characteristics, courses and prognoses. They described general paresis and the alcoholic psychoses, and they studied the manic and depressive psychoses. Though they paid some attention to the possibility that emotional stress played a role in causing mental illness, they were mainly interested in searching for neurophysiological causes of psychiatric illness.

In the last quarter of the 19th Century the leadership in psychiatric development passed to the German school of psychiatry. Many psychiatric hospitals had been developed in Germany during the 19th Century, and German clinicians emphasized the abandonment of physical restraints, good hygiene, hydrotherapy and medications. They extended the study of the characteristics and prognoses of psychiatric illnesses. Kahlbaum (1828–1899) defined catatonic phenomena and introduced the term cyclothymic. Hecker (1843–1909) described hebephrenia, and other clinicians filled out full range of psychiatric diagnoses.

German psychiatry culminated in the work of Emil Kraepelin (1856–1926), who gathered together all of European psychiatry and, with his own important contributions, organized it into a comprehensive diagnostic system. His distinguished textbooks diffused his system of classification throughout the medical world. He delineated the manic depressive psychoses, involutional psychoses and dementia praecox (later renamed schizophrenia). He incorporated personality disorders and the neuroses into his system. Kraepelin believed that physical constitution was important in the etiology of psychiatric illness and that in time neurophysiological dysfunctions would be discovered to explain most types of psychiatric problems. Kraepelin crystallized psychiatry into a systematic medical specialty, and in him European descriptive psychiatry reached its full development. By the end of the 19th Century the way was prepared for the next stage of development, the exploration of the emotional and interpersonal roots of psychiatric problems.

In England during the 19th Century many psychiatric hospitals were built, and humane care of the mentally ill was established. Two of the most prominent British leaders were Conolly, who stressed the abandonment of all types of restraining devices in psychiatric hospitals, and Daniel Hack Tuke who, working in the York Retreat founded by his lay great-grandfather, had much influence through his writing and his work in reforming the care of psychiatric patients in Britain.

The United States was the scene of similar developments. American psychiatry was characterized by careful case studies, special training of psychiatric nurses and aids, and skillful hospital administration.

In 1841 a Boston spinster, Dorothea Lynde Dix (1802–1887), began a personal crusade lasting four decades to arouse public concern about constructing state psychiatric hospitals, and her work was an important incentive in building many hospitals for the mentally ill.

In 1844 the American psychiatric Association was founded by 13 physicians, among whom were Isaac Ray (1807–1881), who wrote the first American book of medical jurisprudence, and Thomas S. Kirkbride (1807–1883), who pioneered better planning in mental hospital architectural design. The American Journal of Psychiatry, still a leading psychiatric journal, was founded in 1844 with Amariah Brigham (1798–1849) as its first editor. Among the prominent American psychiatric leaders in the late 19th Century and early years of the 20th Century were S. Weir Mitchell (1830–1914), who developed a widely used rest cure for the neuroses, and Morton Prince (1854–1927), who is remembered for his work on multiple personality hysterical dissociative states.

A development of great significance in the 19th Century was the discovery of the neuroses. Their discovery proceeded from hypnosis, which had been introduced in Paris in 1778 by Anton Mesmer under the name of "animal magnetism." Mesmer attributed hypnosis to obscure astrological influences, but he used it to treat disturbances we can recognize today as neurotic. Mesmer's hypnotic technics, called "Mesmerism," remained the subject of fluctuating interest, doubt and reinvestigation during the first half of the 19th Century. In 1843 Baird renamed "animal magnetism" hypnotism, and by this time its therapeutic usefulness in hysteria had been medically noted.

During the 1860's Liébault developed hypnotism into a regular medical treatment in a small clinic in Nancy, France, and out of his work two influential schools of investigation of hypnosis and the neuroses developed.

The most prominent of these schools was under Charcot (1825-1893) who investigated hysteria at the Salpêtrière hospital in Paris. Out of this work, interest spread to other forms of neurotic illnesses. Charcot emphasized the descriptive aspects of hysteria and he inclined toward a neurophysiological explanation. He advanced, however, the concept that hysterical disorders were due to "fixed ideas" in the patient, and he recognized that suggestion could induce hysterical symptoms. Charcot did not proceed further with his concept that hysteria was in some way related to pathological "ideas" in the patients, but this concept made a profound impression on some of his students (one of whom, for six months, was Sigmund Freud), and it was the seed from which major psychiatric developments of the 20th Century grew. It marked the beginning of important investigations of how emotional forces and interpersonal stress cause many forms of psychiatric illness.

The second important school of investigation of hysteria and other neuroses was under Bernheim (1837-1919) in Nancy, France. Bernheim was the first physician to formulate a system of psychotherapy, which he based on hypnosis, and he taught that hysteria is caused by emotional disturbances. He probably was the first physician to use the word psychoneurosis (the preferred form of which is neurosis, since the 1968 revision of psychiatric nomenclature), and to group hysteria and the other neurotic illnesses together under this term. The French psychiatrist Pierre Janet (1857-1947) extended Charcot's work and advanced the concept of subconscious ideas ("fixed ideas" of which the patient was unware) in the etiology of the neuroses. However, he taught that neurophysiological weaknesses made the patient susceptible to the pathological influence of these unconsicous ideas. Nevertheless, he advocated a psychotherapy based on persuasion and environmental influences. Having arrived at the threshold of the emotional and interpersonal understanding of the neuroses, the French psychiatrists who delineated them could go no further. The task of unraveling the interpersonal origins of the neuroses and their treatment by interview technics was to be the task of psychiatrists in the next century.

PSYCHIATRIC DEVELOPMENT IN THE TWENTIETH CENTURY

In the present century extensive psychiatric developments have proceeded along many avenues. The interpersonal causes of many forms of psychiatric illness have been elucidated, and various forms of interview treatment have been evolved. Among the new fields opened and developed are child psychiatry, psychosomatic medicine, public mental hygiene education, the integration of psychiatric concepts into social service case work and social welfare programs, and the building of psychiatric divisions in general medical hospitals. Other advances include the development of clinical psychology as a professional specialty (with its special tests for evaluating personality structure), the evolution of the field of psychiatric nursing, the organization of therapeutic environments for patients in psychiatric hospitals, and the marked expansion of psychiatric teaching in medical schools (until this century psychiatry, when taught at all, was considered a minor branch of neurology). Penicillin has virtually eliminated the once common psychoses due to syphilis of the central nervous system, and the various antibiotics have reduced the incidence of bacterial organic brain disease. The development of the phenothiazine medications, antidepressant medications and electroshock therapy has vastly improved the treatment of psychotic illnesses. Psychiatric concepts have found wide acceptance among the lay public, and psychiatry has affected educational technics, child-rearing customs, counseling on sexual problems, marital counseling and many other areas of human activity. The number of physicians who devote themselves exclusively to psychiatry has increased greatly during the present century.

THE DEVELOPMENT OF EMOTIONAL CONCEPTS OF PSYCHIATRIC ILLNESS

The exploration of the emotional causes of psychiatric illness proceeded along two important channels. The first channel consisted of the development of an interpersonal understanding of psychiatric illness in American psychiatry under the leadership of Adolph Meyer (1866–1950). His views were expanded by a large number of psychiatric teachers and writers, among whom Harry Stack Sullivan (1892–1949) was the most prominent. The other channel was the development of the Freudian-psychoanalytic approach to psychiatric illness by the Austrian psychiatrist Sigmund Freud (1856–1939), whose views were expanded by a large number of later psychoanalytic investigators. In American psychiatry these two currents of development often have intermingled and have had much influence on each other, though both developments are sufficiently recent to make objective historical evaluation difficult.

In addition to these two main channels, a wide variety of other psychiatric approaches have been proposed, but their effects on psychiatric practice in the non-Communist world have been inconstant and relatively minor. We shall briefly discuss these other approaches later in this chapter.

The Development of the Interpersonal Approach

Adolph Meyer was professor of psychiatry at Cornell from 1904 to 1909, and headed the department of psychiatry at Johns Hopkins from 1910 to 1941. He was a stimulating teacher, and he trained many of the men who later headed medical school psychiatric departments. His great influence rested as much on his personal teaching as on his writing. Meyer advocated the comprehensive study of the patient's emotional, interpersonal, social and physical life history in the study of a psychiatric illness. He felt that every aspect of the patient's past and current life must be inventoried to understand his psychiatric problems. He taught that most forms of psychiatric illness, including schizophrenia and the other psychoses, arise from emotional turmoil and interpersonal trauma, and he advocated flexible interview treatment to help the patient resolve his conflicts and understand how his illness had arisen out of past and current interpersonal disturbances. He felt that the therapist-patient relationship was an important aspect of psychiatric treatment. He urged, however, that the psychiatrist should never lose sight of the fact that the emotional life of the patient is intimately woven into his biological functioning. Meyer taught that each patient must be understood as an individual person with a unique set of problems that caused his psychiatric illness. He shunned formulations postulating identical kinds of traumatic life experiences in patients who had the same clinical picture.

Meyer called his concepts the "psychobiological" approach to psychiatric illness and he termed his psychotherapy "distributive analysis and synthesis." His terminology never gained wide acceptance, but his basic teachings had enormous influence in the United States and other English-speaking countries. He had much influence in directing American psychiatry into channels of interpersonal and emotional understanding of psychiatric disorders, as opposed to the preoccupation with neurophysiological concepts of mental illness that has predominated to this day in continental Europe and many other parts of the world. Meyer advocated the acceptance of some aspects of the Freudian-psychoanalytic approach, but he felt that a comprehensive understanding of psychiatric illness necessitated a flexible approach to each patient, and that the emotional causes of a psychiatric illness varied much from patient to patient, depending on his life circumstances.

The interpersonal concept of personality development and psychiatric illness was further crystallized by the work of the American psychiatrist, Harry Stack Sullivan. Sullivan was a stimulating teacher and writer who focused attention on how the various aspects of the person's interpersonal relationships in childhood and adolescence contributed to personality development, and how the patient's painful interpersonal relationships both in his past and current life situations produced psychiatric illness. Sullivan's teachings were summarized in his books, *Conceptions of Modern Psychiatry*, published in 1940, and *The Interpersonal Theory of Psychiatry* and several other books, drawn mainly from his recorded lectures and seminars (published since his death in 1949).

Many other psychiatric writers have contributed to the development of the interpersonal approach to psychiatric illness. Many of them have integrated selected aspects of the Freudian-psychoanalytic viewpoint into the structure of interpersonal psychiatry. The historical development of the interpersonal approach to psychiatry is like a house whose design gradually evolved through the work of many collaborating architects, and whose structure has been erected by many workers. In contrast, the basic structure of the Freudian-psychoanlytic approach is largely the work of Sigmund Freud, though his followers have modified and extended some of its features.

Many of the basic principles of the interpersonal approach are outlined in the first chapter of this book, and they are further developed and applied to the full range of psychiatric disorders in the following chapters.

The Development of the Freudian-Psychoanalytic Approach

The other major current in the development of the emotional concept of psychiatric illness proceeded from the work of Sigmund Freud (1856–1939). In 1885 Freud, a young neurologist in Vienna, studied for six months at the clinics of Charcot in Paris and Bernheim in Nancy. He returned to Vienna greatly impressed with the concept that hysteria and other neuroses were caused by subconscious pathological ideas, and that eradication of these ideas through hypnosis was a fruitful method of treatment. Freud soon abandoned hypnosis, however, and used the technic of having the patient talk freely about whatever came to mind as a means of discovering the pathological ideas and emotions that were locked within him and were causing his illness.

After a short association with Joseph Breuer, Freud carried on his work alone. In 1900 he published his influential book, *The Interpretation of Dreams*, in which he laid down many of the basic principles that were to characterize his work. In this book and in his subsequent writings, Freud advanced the thesis that most psychiatric illness was caused by painful conflicts repressed in the patient's unconscious mind. He felt that the most important emotional conflicts causing later psychiatric illness occurred during the first seven years of life, and that, although subsequent experiences might be precipitants of psychiatric problems, they were not basic causes. Freud attributed much importance to a broad concept of sexual experiences during the first seven years, and felt that most psychiatric illness in adults had its roots in the inadequate resolution of problems that had occurred during the child's psychosexual development. By means of spontaneous, uninhibited talking, which he called "free association," Freud felt that these pathological conflicts could be brought out of the patient's unconscious mind and into his awareness, and that when relieved of these painful internal pressures the patient would recover from his illness. Among other methods, Freud felt that the analysis of the latent meaning of dreams and of the complex feelings the patient developed toward the therapist were fruitful means to uncovering unconscious conflicts.

From this basis Freud went on in his further writings during the first three decades of this century to evolve the comprehensive theory of personality development and psychiatric illness that he termed psychoanalysis. He also applied this term to the type of interview treatment he developed. (These concepts are outlined at length in Chapter 3.)

At first Freud worked in isolation and his publications were largely ignored, but by 1910 his work had begun to attract attention. Some of his early followers, including Carl G. Jung (1875–1961), Alfred Adler (1870–1937) and Otto Rank (1884–1939), deviated from Freud's leadership and developed divergent opinions; however, with the exception of Jung, about whom a significant reawakening of interest occurred in the 1970's, their influence was small and has waned with time. Others of Freud's followers, including Sandor Ferenczi and Karl Abraham, expanded and diffused psychoanalytic viewpoints.

Psychoanalytic concepts were introduced into the United States by A. A. Brill (1874–1948), who translated many of Freud's works into English, and by others, such as William Alanson White (1870–1937). Freud's teachings were advanced in England by Ernest Jones (1879–1958), who became Freud's foremost biographer.

The Freudian-psychoanalytic approach has had a profound effect on American psychiatry. Freud's viewpoints on the importance of unconscious feelings and thoughts in human behavior, and his emphasis on the importance of childhood experiences in forming personality structure, have been widely accepted. Aspects of his technic of interview treatment have been modified and incorporated into many forms of psychotherapy for a wide range of emotional problems. His theories about the emotional causes of the neuroses, the psychoses and the personality disorders have influenced the thinking of a majority of modern American psychiatrists. However, many psychiatrists feel that extensive modifications must be made to adjust Freudian psychoanalytic doctrines to the realities of psychiatric pathology and treatment, and a minority of American psychiatrists accept Freud's teachings completely; fewer still devote themselves exclusively to psychoanalytic therapy. In actual practice, there has been much crossfertilization between the Freudian-psychoanalytic approach and the broad interpersonal approach to psychiatry that grew out of the work of such men as Adolph Meyer and Harry Stack Sullivan.

The influence of Freudian psychoanalysis is mainly restricted to the English speaking countries, especially the United States. However, even in Great Britain Freud's influence has been quite limited; for example, in its distinguished series entitled *Twentieth Century Thinkers*, the British Broadcasting Corporation chose Jung as a more important thinker than Freud. Freudian psychoanalysis is forbidden in the Communist countries, and it has never gained wide acceptance on the continent of Europe, or in Asia and South America. Freud's thought has attracted much interest in American lay circles, especially in artistic and literary groups.

THE EXPANSION OF PSYCHIATRIC ACTIVITIES

Since 1900 the range of psychiatric activities has expanded widely. Psychiatry has grown beyond its conventional domain of the psychoses and the neuroses into new fields such as child psychiatry, psychosomatic medicine, psychiatric services in general hospitals and many other areas.

The Development of Child Psychiatry. Psychiatric interest in children had been slight prior to the present century. Between 1900 and 1920 a few investigators began to explore the emotional problems of children. In the early 1920's a major stimulus to the development of child psychiatry came from the Commonwealth Fund, a private philanthropic foundation, which financed the creation of child guidance clinics in many large American cities. Moreover, the interpersonal approach to psychiatry and Freudian-psychoanalytic theory both emphasized childhood experiences in the formation of personality structure and the production of psychiatric illness; thus, they strongly directed interest toward the emotional problems of children. Physicians, parents, educators, social workers, psychiatric nurses, juvenile court authorities and others began to take increased interest in treatment facilities for children and adolescents. During the first four decades of the 20th Century, child psychiatrists continued to study the psychiatric difficulties of children and to develop special treatment methods of child psychiatry (outlined in Chapter 24). Since the late 1940's the number of psychiatrists and other mental health professional workers engaged in child psychiatry and the number of outpatient and inpatient child psychiatric treatment facilities has expanded immensely.

The Development of Clinical Psychology. In 1905 the French psychologist Binet, and his colleague Simon, a psychiatrist, developed the first test for intelligence. Their work marks the beginning of the evolution of the various intelligence tests that have become a basic tool in the study of intellectual functioning and mental retardation. In 1921 the Swiss psychiatrist Hermann Rorschach published his classical work on the ink blot test, which has since then born his name, and in 1935 Murray introduced the Thematic Apperception test. (These tests are described in detail in Chapter 5.) The modern profession of clinical psychology developed gradually out of the study of the application and interpretation of these tests and the many other personality tests that have been developed. From the late 1940's onward clinical psychologists have been trained in psychotherapy; from a medical point of view, interview treatment by clinical psychologists is most soundly conducted in collaborative teams that include psychiatrists and other mental health professionals, as in child guidance clinics and other multidisciplinary outpatient and inpatient settings.

The Development of Psychiatric Social Work and Psychiatric Nursing. During the 1920's and 1930's it became clear to many workers in the developing field of social service casework that many of the economic and social problems they were attempting to deal with arose out of, or were interwoven with, emotional difficulties in their clients. Advice, financial aid and job opportunities solved few problems if many of the recipients were crippled by personality difficulties which prevented them from benefiting from the social workers' assistance. For example, it was of little use to arrange a job for a rebellious adolescent who could not stick to it, or an alcoholic who would be frequently absent from it, or a person with a phobia of leaving home unaccompanied. Thus, the new insights into personality problems and emotional functioning which were developing in psychiatry became gradually incorporated into social service casework. The counseling technics of social workers were widened to include various modifications of psychotherapy that were suited to their settings. The specialty of *psychiatric* social service work has thus developed as a separate profession, with education and training through the doctorate level. Most psychiatrists feel that psychiatric social service work is best done in collaboration with psychiatrists, or with psychiatric consultation services available, in both outpatient and inpatient settings.

Similarly, the profession of psychiatric nursing has evolved. The first formally trained American nurse was Linda Richards, who graduated from the newly organized Nursing School of the New England Hospital for Women and Children in 1873. After further education at the original Nightingale school of nursing at St. Thomas Hospital in London, she spent much of her long career reforming nursing services in American psychiatric hospitals, in addition to founding 12 schools of nursing in various American cities. She may justly be considered the first American psychiatric nurse.

During the 20th Century, and especially since the 1930's, psychiatric nursing has developed into a separate professional discipline, with degrees through the doctorate level. Nurses with advanced training now do both group and individual psychotherapy in collaboration with psychiatrists and other mental health professionals. Instruction in psychiatry has been much increased in all fields of nursing to enrich the work of nurses in pediatric nursing, medical and surgical services, public health work and other fields.

The Integration of Psychiatry Into General Medicine. Until the 20th Century psychiatry was isolated from the general body of medical practice. Most psychiatrists worked in psychiatric hospitals that had only loose associations with other medical fields. However, during the 20th Century psychiatry gradually has become integrated into the main currents of medical practice.

The study of psychosomatic medicine has contributed to the integration of psychiatry and general medicine. Though perceptive physicians had known for many centuries that the emotional state of the patient played a large role in causing many kinds of illness, it was not until the 1920's and 1930's that psychiatrists began to explore systematically the ways in which emotional states caused various kinds of physical illnesses. By doing so they formulated the basic concepts of psychosomatic medicine. These studies did much to draw psychiatry closer to other medical specialties in medical school hospitals and clinics, and this closer collaboration of psychiatry and general medicine spread gradually into the general body of medical practice.

The development of interview treatment in the 20th Century gradually changed psychiatry from a specialty attached almost entirely to mental hospitals, often located in towns remote from large cities, into a specialty that became oriented also toward office treatment. In the development of psychotherapy, psychiatrists acquired a technic by which they could help office patients who were suffering from neuroses, personality disorders, emotionally caused physical problems and other types of difficulties. Increasing numbers of psychiatrists entered private practice as the century progressed, and psychiatry gradually took on the professional characteristics of the other medical specialites. Since the late 1940's there has been a widespread movement to build psychiatric divisions in private and public general medical hospitals. This development has brought psychiatrists onto the staffs of general medical hospitals, and has further integrated psychiatry into the mainstream of medical practice.

These developments have been accompanied by a marked expansion of psychiatric teaching in medical schools. Before the 20th Century psychiatry occupied little space in the medical school curriculum, and until the 1930's neurology and psychiatry were often combined in one medical school department, in which neurology often dominated. Since then psychiatry has been split off from neurology and has acquired a prominent independent status. In well-staffed psychiatric services medical students now receive training in both inpatient and outpatient settings, in addition to instruction in the principles of personality development, psychosomatic medicine, counseling with patients in various kinds of medical situations, and other areas. The percentage of physicians who devote themselves to psychiatry has increased immensely.

Other Psychiatric Activities. Prior to the 20th Century the general public was apathetic to psychiatry and uninterested in conditions in psychiatric hospitals. Psychiatric progress had not come as the result of public interest; it had come as the result of the action of interested physicians and a few humanitarian lay persons. Their efforts were carried on against the background of public indifference about the care of the emotionally ill. However, in the present century the general public has begun to take increasing interest in psychiatric services and in the reform of psychiatric institutions.

A strong stimulus to such public interest in America came from the work of Clifford W. Beers (1876–1943). As a young man Beers underwent a psychotic illness from which he recovered after an extensive period of hospitalization. He wrote an account of his illness in his book *A Mind That Found Itself*, and in 1909 he founded the National Association for Mental Health. To a large extent through Beers's lifelong work, the National Association of Mental Health grew into a organization of laymen interested in arousing public interest in mental health education and reform of psychiatric institutions. Many other lay groups also have taken interest in psychiatric progress, and special groups devote themselves to the development of better facilities for the mentally retarded and other types of patients.

Psychiatric hospitals have been reorganized to offer their patients therapeutic environments which play significant roles in their recovery; the terms *milieu therapy, therapeutic community* and *therapeutic hospital environment* are applied to these hospital programs (which are covered in Chapter 21). This has been accompanied by systematic psychiatric training of hospital aids and the introduction of occupational therapists, recreational therapists and other special personnel into psychiatric hospital services.

The use of psychiatric concepts and psychiatric consultation services in many kinds of social welfare programs is another significant development of this century. Psychiatric viewpoints have had a profound effect on rehabilitation programs for the physically handicapped, social welfare planning for socially and economically deprived groups, criminology and many other fields. Although psychiatric concepts have not always prevailed, they have markedly affected attitudes toward drug abuse, juvenile delinquency, homosexuality and many other diverse problems.

In recent decades there has also been increased interest in the ways in which cultural, social and economic forces are related to psychiatric disturbances. This is particularly so in the delivery of psychiatric services to culturally deprived groups in slums, impoverished rural areas and other neglected situations. For example, the relapse rate of recovered schizophrenics who return to chaotic family situations in violence-ridden, drug-filled slums is much greater than in recovered schizophrenics who are discharged to more privileged environments. Hence, some psychiatrists have begun to emphasize the need for various kinds of social and economic reforms on the basis of public mental health as well as humanitarian grounds.

Developments in Pharmacological Physical Therapies

Since the early 1930's pharmacological and physical treatment methods have been developed that much improve the prognoses of various psychotic illnesses. We shall outline these developments in chronological order. (The details of most of these treatments are discussed in Chapters 22 and 23.)

In 1933 Sakel described insulin coma therapy in Austria, and three years later he introduced it in the United States. It remained a widely used treatment for schizophrenia until it was largely replaced in the mid-1950's by long-term phenothiazine therapy. A few psychiatrists, however, still advocate insulin coma therapy for selected schizophrenic patients.

Sakel's discovery of insulin coma therapy stimulated the search for other methods of physical treatment of the psychoses, and in 1938 Cerletti and Bini in Italy reported the technic of electroshock therapy. During the early 1940's electroshock therapy became widely used in the treatment of depressive psychoses, schizophrenic illnesses and manic psychoses, but its use has decreased markedly since the development of the phenothiazine and antidepressant medications.

Important advances in the pharmacologic treatment of the psychoses have occurred since 1940. Penicillin's effectiveness against all forms of central nervous system syphilis has made luetic psychoses rare in American psychiatric hospitals; prior to the introduction of penicillin, general paresis and other luetic brain disorders were responsible for from several to 10 per cent of the first admissions to psychiatric hospitals. Penicillin and the other antibiotics also have sharply cut the incidence of psychiatric disorders caused by bacterial intracranial infections.

In the middle 1950's the phenothiazine medications were introduced into clinical psychiatry and their usefulness in schizophrenia soon became clear. Chlorpromazine was the first phenothiazine to be clinically tested, and it probably is still the most widely used drug of the phenothiazine group, though many other phenothiazines and related compounds are extensively employed. Phenothiazine therapy has markedly improved the prognosis of schizophrenia; it also is useful in manic psychoses and some agitated states. In the middle and late 1950's two new groups of antidepressant drugs were developed, and for the first time effective drugs for depression were available. The monoamine oxidase inhibiting drugs were used first; soon afterward the imipramine tricyclic medications, which were to prove much more valuable, were discovered. The development of these medications has stimulated much research for further pharmacologic agents in the treatment of the psychoses.

These medications have had so striking an impact on the treatment and prognoses of psychotic illnesses that their effects are sometimes referred to as the "pharmacologic revolution" of the 1950's and 1960's. Despite rising admission rates to psychiatric hospitals and the constantly increasing national population, the number of patients in American psychiatric hospitals has steadily decreased since 1955. This decrease is undoubtedly due to many factors, but the new medications probably constitute the most important one.

Other Psychiatric Developments

The study of schizophrenia published in 1912 by the Swiss psychiatrist Eugen Bleuler (1857–1939) was a further notable achievement of 20th Century psychiatry. Bleuler ascribed schizophrenia to three basic dysfunctions: (a) the fragmentation of logical thinking processes, (b) disturbances of affects, with a strong tendency toward diffuse ambivalence, and (c) autistic withdrawal into fantasy and away from reality. He felt that the delusions, hallucinations, catatonic phenomena and other features of schizophrenia occurred secondarily to these three basic dysfunctions.

He introduced the term schizophrenia, which gradually replaced the older term dementia praecox. Although Bleuler felt that the three basic dysfunctions in schizophrenia were due to an undiscovered neurophysiological defect, his brilliant study of schizophrenia stimulated much research on its interpersonal and emotional causes.

During the 20th Century several schools of psychological thought and psychiatric practice have been derived from Pavlov's extensive work on conditioned reflex behavior in animals. Of these schools of thought, the most sophisticated and clinically applicable is the one now designated by the terms *behavior theory* and *behavior therapy*. This body of psychiatric concepts (which we shall discuss in more detail in Chapter 3) has to a large extent been evolved by numerous American and British psychiatrists and psychologists since 1950, but its antecedents go back earlier. It is too early to evaluate the long-term importance and clinical usefulness of behavior theory, but it seems likely that it will become an established part of the psychiatric scene. (Behavior theory and therapy are discussed in more detail in Chapter 3.)

Also, the 20th Century has seen the first truly scientific studies of human sexuality. Freud, of course, was a significant force in directing attention to this field, even among those who did not accept his viewpoints. The work of the American biologist Alfred C. Kinsey (1894–1956) to discover the range and nature of human sexual behavior on a broad statistical basis was, from a psychiatric point of view, superficial and perhaps in many respects misleading, but it has historical importance. Numerous other psychiatrists, mental health professionals and nonpsychiatric physcians contributed to a better understanding of both normal and maladjusted sexual functioning. Since the 1950's the American investigators William H. Masters and Virginia E. Johnson (a gynecologist and a psychologist working, with others, in a clinical team) have made detailed psychological and physiological studies of human sexual activity and have evolved useful methods for treating impotence, frigidity and other sexual dysfunctions. Despite what many psychiatrists view as the naiveness of their psychiatric theories, their pioneering physiological studies are sound and their treatment approaches give much better results than previous types of therapy. (This subject is discussed in Chapter 25.)

During the 20th Century, and especially since 1950, much progress has been made in understanding the biochemical functioning of the central nervous system and the chromosomal determinants of human physical development. Extensive research, moreover, has been done in both Europe and America to discover biochemical correlates, or perhaps causes, of various kinds of psychiatric disorders. So far, the results of all studies in this complex field are highly controversial, and little of clinical applicability has been found. However, it seems likely that future decades will see vast progress in this area, and it is possible that it will in time affect our treatment methods and concepts. Until now, the medications we use have all been discovered empirically; that is, they have been developed by trial and error experiences in pharmacological laboratories or have evolved out of chance observations in clinical practice. The theories to explain how medications and other physical measures work in psychiatry have invariably come after the clinical usefulness of the treatment was demonstrated. There is now some reason to expect that pharmacological agents and biological manipulation technics may be evolved in time on the basis of increased understanding of biochemical, chromosomal and other features of human body functioning and structure. This does not mean that our present psychological viewpoints and treatment technics will then be any less valid; it merely emphasizes that, in the final analysis, the things we call anxiety, guilt, awareness and interpersonal relationships cannot go on unless very intricate chemical reactions occur constantly in central nervous system tissue. As Freud pointed out, behind us always stands the man with the syringe. However, despite the large amount of work that has been done on the biochemical and physiologic correlates of psychiatric disorders, there is among workers in this field so little general agreement, and opinions are in such constant change, that summary of its results is not easily given in a textbook of this kind; at various points in this book, nevertheless, some of the more widely held views will be pointed out.

Through the work of many psychiatrists in this century, the psychosomatic illnesses, personality pattern disorders and other emotional disturbances gradually have been added to the full range of psychiatric diagnoses. In 1952, after several years of work, a committee of the American Psychiatric Association introduced an improved, simplified, comprehensive system of psychiatric nomenclature, which gained immediate general acceptance; prior to 1952 at least three nomenclatures were in widespread use, and none of them complied with the International Statistical Classification. In 1968 the 1952 system was modified in various ways to make it conform to a new international nomenclature of psychiatric disorders.

Continental European Psychiatry

Continental European psychiatry has remained, on the whole, oriented toward a neurophysiological view of psychiatric illness. Most such illness is seen as determined by as yet undiscovered neurophysiological dysfunctions in persons who have constitutional central nervous system predispositions to psychiatric disorders. According to this view, the chromosomally controlled constitution of the person strongly predisposes him to specific kinds of psychiatric illness, and interpersonal factors are precipitants rather than causes of emotional disorders; obviously, this implies hereditary tendencies in many instances.

The interpersonal approach to psychiatry has had a limited influence on continental European psychiatry; it has had a somewhat greater influence on child psychiatry. The Freudian-psychoanalytic viewpoint has received limited support on the Continent. Many of the medications and physical methods of treatment outlined earlier in this chapter were developed in continental European centers in their continuing search for neurophysiological explanations of psychiatric illness and for physical methods of treatment. Though a certain amount of counseling and brief psychotherapy is done in Europe, it is a limited aspect of psychiatric activity. The discovery in 1959 of chromosomal abnormalities as the causes of Down's syndrome, the disorder long called mongolism, and the elucidation of various kinds of metabolic disorders as the causes of several per cent of cases of mental retardation, has stimulated renewed efforts in European psychiatry to find chromosomal or metabolic abnormalities to explain psychotic illnesses, neurotic reactions and personality disorders.

An exception to the neurophysiological orientation of continental European psychiatry is the development of existential psychiatry. This approach was stimulated by the existential philosophies of Kierkegaard, Heidegger, Sartre and many others. Many European psychiatrists have contributed to the development of existential psychiatry: among them, Binswanger, Kuhn and Boss have been prominent. Existential psychiatry is based on the premise that each patient must be studied and understood in terms of his own perceptions, ideas and experiences, and that general formulations about the specific causes of a psychiatric illness cannot be carried from one patient to another, even though they may have similar clinical pictures. For example, the existential psychiatrist feels that the kinds of traumatic experiences that lead to schizophrenia vary so much from one patient to another that generalizations cannot be made about its interpersonal causes; each patient must be studied as a unique case, and in treatment the patient's perceptions, feelings and experiences must be understood from that point of view. In psychotherapy the patient and the therapist seek the roots of the patient's illnesses in his unhealthy experiences, perceptions, feelings and ideas. However, only a small percentage of European psychiatrists devote themselves to existential psychiatry, and it has not had a marked impact in the United States.

Psychiatry in the Communist Countries. One third of the world's population now lives under communist governments; therefore in a comprehensive survey of the history of modern psychiatry, we should briefly review psychiatric practice in the Soviet Union and its allied nations. Psychiatry in these nations has followed a different course from that in the rest of the world. The following discussion applies to the Soviet Union and its dependent states in Eastern Europe; a clear picture of psychiatric theory and practice in communist China is not now available.

Communist psychiatry has retained to some extent the neurophysiological orientation of continental European psychiatry toward the psychoses, and this viewpoint also influences somewhat the communist approach toward the neuroses. Freudian-psychoanalytic theories are forbidden in communist countries, and the interpersonal approach to psychiatry also is rejected. The official Soviet approach is based on a mixture of Pavlovian neurophysiology and the communist political doctrines of economic determinism and intellectual materialism.

The work of the Russian neurophysiologist Ivan P. Pavlov (1849–1936) on conditioned reflexes in animals has been extended into an elaborate system which attempts to explain all human behavior in terms of complex systems of neurophysiologic conditioning. For example, whereas in dogs the stimuli for neurophysiologic conditioning may consist of food and accompanying visual or auditory signals, human neurophysiologic conditioning is determined by the words and actions of other people. This concept is elaborated in complex ways and is applied to all aspects of human intellectual and emotional functioning. The communist doctrine of intellectual materialism is applied by insisting that all psychiatric concepts must be firmly tied to neurophysiologic experiments that can be clearly demonstrated. In their efforts to substitute state-sponsored social groups for family life, the communist theoreticians reject interpersonal relationships in the family as factors in personality development. From the Western point of view, communist psychiatry uses concepts determined mainly by political theories that do not have roots in the clinical observation of patients.

The second Marxist doctrine upon which Soviet psychiatry is based is the theory of economic determinism, which proposes that all human behavior, feeling and thinking are determined by economic circumstances. Hence, the elimination of economic problems in a society theoretically would eliminate psychiatric problems. The unsoundness of this point of view is demonstrated by the failure of the communist economic system to influence the incidence of psychiatric disorders in the communist nations. Communist psychiatry has evolved a type of psychotherapy that relies heavily on exhortation, persuasion and occasional changes in the patient's environment. A Soviet psychiatrist is expected to see between six and eight outpatients in each hour of office practice.

The communist system of psychiatry has aroused little interest outside the communist countries. Any valid approach to psychiatry must begin with careful clinical study of patients, and psychiatric theory and treatment procedures must evolve from clinical experience. The Soviet system of psychiatry, on the other hand, is determined mainly by political and economic doctrines, and it must conform to the prevailing views of a totalitarian government.

Epilogue to the History of Psychiatry

Psychiatry has entered the last quarter of the 20th Century as a full-fledged medical specialty, after its slow evolution over several centuries. Psychiatry now has the tools to aid large numbers of emotionally ill patients, and the future holds much hope for further advances to enlarge the scope of its therapeutic effectiveness and its comprehensive understanding of interpersonal problems.

BIBLIOGRAPHY

Brozek, J., and Slobin, D. I.: Psychology in the USSR: An Historical Perspective. White Plains. N. Y., International Arts and Sciences Press, 1972.

Dain, N.: Disordered Minds: The First Century of the Eastern State Hospital in Williamsburg, Virginia, 1766–1866. Charlottesville, Virginia, University Press of Virginia, 1971.

Ellenberger, H. F.: The Discovery of the Unconscious: The History and Evolution of Dynamic Psychiatry. New York, Basic Books, 1970.

Grob, G. N.: Mental Institutions in America: Social Policy to 1875. New York, Free Press, 1973.

Hale, N. G., Jr.: Freud and the Americans: The Beginnings of Psychoanalysis in the United States, 1876–1917. New York, Oxford University Press, 1971.

Jones, E.: The Life and Work of Sigmund Freud 3 vols. New York, Basic Books, 1953–1957.

Jones, K.: A History of the Mental Health Services. Boston, Routledge and Kegan Paul, 1972.

Kors, A. C.: and Peters, E.: Witchcraft in Europe, 1100–1700. Philadelphia, University of Pennsylvania Press, 1972.

Sullivan, H. S.: Conceptions of Modern Psychiatry. New York, W. W. Norton, 1953.

Zilboorg, G., and Henry, G. W.: A History of Medical Psychology. New York, W. W. Norton, 1941.

3

Various Concepts of Emotional Functioning

Many concepts and terms are used in modern psychiatry to describe various aspects of healthy and unhealthy emotional functioning. Many psychiatrists feel that the profusion of these concepts and terms is more likely to confuse the student or the physician than to enlighten him. However, a textbook of psychiatry should survey these concepts and terms since they are an established feature of the specialty. We shall do so in this chapter. Some of these concepts and terms are basic tools in psychiatry, and are used many times during later chapters of this book; others, less commonly used, are covered only in this chapter.*

---

*My prejudices in psychiatric writing run strongly in favor of using simple words and concepts whose meanings are clear and stick closely to what the words usually mean in general usage. Dr. John M. Davis and Ms. Elza M. Almeida, in the sections they have contributed, have attempted to follow the same rule, though Dr. Davis must, of course, use a wide variety of biochemical terms. With the exception of this present chapter, I have therefore tried wherever possible to use clear, simple words and concepts rather than complex terms. For example, I prefer to say that a person is comfortable with his anger rather than to say that his anger is "ego-syntonic," and I prefer to say that an individual has mixed feelings of both affection and hostility toward another person than to say that he is "ambivalent" toward him. Nevertheless, technical terminology has its usefulness, and a book of this sort should at some point lay such terms before the student. The dangers of technical terminology in psychiatry are that it often deteriorates into obscure jargon, which alienates and confuses the reader. Students and physicians who are reading this book for pleasure, or who are not taking a systematic course in psychiatry, should feel free to skim through some parts of this chapter lightly.

GENERAL TERMS AND CONCEPTS

Instinct, Drive and Heredity

Instinct. An instinct is an inborn biological tendency for a specific kind of activity; it is inherited and not dependent on the individual's previous experience. In human beings, the influence of interpersonal relationships on behavior and personality structure is so great from the earliest months onward that it is difficult to define the instincts that lie hidden in the basic levels of a person's behavior. Hence, psychiatrists differ much about what instincts are in man and how they work. We can talk about the instinct of birds to build nests, but we cannot speak of the instinct of a young couple to go house hunting, and we can talk of the instinct of an animal to seek food, but we cannot speak of the instinct of a child to open a refrigerator to get a snack or of a person to go to a supermarket.

Psychiatrists agree most readily about instinctive behavior in the first year or so of life. The newborn infant instinctively seeks food from a nipple, cries when he is hungry or has other discomforts and relaxes when his biological needs are met. However, as the first two or three years of life pass, these inborn instinctual patterns begin to be extensively modified by the interpersonal relationships of the child with his parents and other persons in his environment. He learns to limit his eating to certain times of the day when the family eats, and he begins to master the rudiments of table manners. He no longer cries each time he is uncomfortable, but he often goes to his parents and tells them about his needs. He learns to control his defecation and urination. During his early years his environment so drastically modifies his instinctual behavior that in late childhood his instincts can be discerned only dimly through the enormous changes his interpersonal environment has placed on him. Hence, there is little general agreement among psychiatrists about the role of instinctual behavior in man after the first year or two of life.

The instincts most commonly described in man are those of self-preservation, sexuality and aggression. Some writers also describe a social, or herd, instinct.

The self-preservative instinct includes those inborn forces that cause the person to seek satisfaction of the needs necessary for his physical survival and personal welfare. In the infant, these needs are relatively easy to define. They include instinctual seeking for food, and crying when physical needs are not met. However, to extend the concept of self-preservation instincts into modern adult life is complex and controversial. Modern civilized society rarely places a person bluntly in the position of struggling crudely for his physical survival. His desires for economic security and social advancement are greatly affected by environmental forces, and to say that they are motivated by self-preservative instincts is to hazard a gross confusion between interpersonal experience and inborn instinct; for example, we cannot say that a man's struggle for promotion in his company or admission into a prestigious country club are evidences of instinctive behavior. On the whole, the self-preservative instinct is much less important than the total of the influences of interpersonal experiences and social environment.

Psychiatrists recognize sexuality as an important instinctual force, but they differ much about the nature of sexual instincts and how they operate in human behavior. Freudian-psychoanalytic writers recognize sexuality, in various forms, as the broad basis for all forces that draw people together in intimate relationships and social groups. They also ascribe much importance to sexuality in the various stages of childhood personality development, and trace its ramifications into many areas of human life. (These concepts are outlined more fully in a later part of this chapter.) Many other psychiatrists define sexuality in a more restricted way, and apply the term mainly to all the facets of human behavior that have as their direct, indirect or possible goal the satisfaction of yearnings for physical sexual contact with a sexual partner.

The overt expression of sexual instinct, in any sense, is greatly influenced by the individual's life-long experiences in his interpersonal environment. The person modifies or restrains his sexual expressions because of his interpersonal experiences, moral ideas and social concepts. Most psychiatrists agree, however, that sexual instincts restrained due to social and moral concepts often furnish some of the unconscious basic forces that motivate men in many nonsexual activities—activities in which they serve generously the needs and interests of family, friends and the broader social community. Psychiatrists believe that many of the affectionate acts and generous deeds of people are, at least in part, sublimated expressions of the large amount of restrained sexuality required by modern social life. Most psychiatrists feel that interpersonal experience is more important than inborn instinct in determining man's sexual behavior, even in the broadest sense of the term.

A few writers have speculated that man has an inborn instinct of aggression. They feel it is controlled in varying degrees by the overlying personality structure formed by a person's environment, but that it finds expression in many kinds of aggressive and destructive acts. Most mental health professionals, however, feel that aggression is produced by traumatic and frustrating interpersonal experiences rather than by an inborn instinct. The concept of an instinct of aggression is speculative and is not generally accepted.

Other psychiatrists feel that man has an instinctual yearning to be a member of social groups and to shun solitary living. This is sometimes called the herd instinct. Most psychiatrists, however, feel that man's desire to live in social groups is produced by his interpersonal environment rather than by an inborn instinct.

In recent times the concept of instinctual

behavior has been somewhat refined by Lorenz and others in the concept of "imprinting." In imprinting, a young animal adopts a certain type of behavior at a particular time in its development because (a) it observes this type of behavior in older animals of its group and (b) is genetically ready at that time to take over the behavioral pattern. As applied to psychiatry (if indeed it can be validly applied to man), this concept does not change any of the above statements; it merely emphasizes more strongly the impacts of environment on the instinctual substrata of behavior.

Drive. The word drive is employed to indicate a strong motivation determined by both instinct and environment. Because of the difficulties in separating the components of inborn instinct and interpersonal experience in many human actions, drive is more commonly used in modern psychiatry than instinct. For example, one may speak of a man's drive for achievement or a woman's drive to establish a sound marriage and rear a family. In both instances, the word is easily applied since it combines the mixture of instinctual forces and interpersonal experiences that have combined to produce the motivation.

Depending on their concepts of psychiatry, different psychiatrists may use the word drive with different weights assigned to the roles of instinct and environment. Some would use it to indicate the instinctual forces that are lightly covered with a veneer of interpersonal experience. Most, however, use the word in the more flexible sense outlined above.

Heredity. Heredity in human beings is difficult to study because the life span of the research worker is the same as the life span of his subjects. It is much easier to study heredity in rats, which reproduce every few months, than in human beings. To attempt to study heredity from family histories is a difficult process. Hence we do not know much about human heredity as it applies to personality development, emotional functioning and psychiatric disturbances. The consensus of opinion among psychiatrists at present, however, is that the influence of heredity on emotional functioning and psychiatric illness is much less than the influence of environment.

The influence of heredity on personality structure probably has been much overestimated in the past. Such qualities as a good disposition, a hot temper, or an outgoing personality are not much affected by heredity. They are produced by the day-to-day family environment in which the child is reared and by the social and cultural environment which lies immediately outside the family structure. If a boy has a hot temper like his father's, he did not inherit it; he probably acquired it through living intimately with his father.

When emotional illnesses occur in two or three successive generations of a family, psychiatrists feel it is probable that environment played a much larger role than heredity. Emotionally unstable parents often provide an emotionally unhealthy family environment for the children they rear. Their children have a greater than average chance of having personality disturbances in adult life, and their problems may in turn cripple them in their child-rearing capacities. Hence, a web of emotional illness may sometimes be spun from one generation to the next. From a precise scientific point of view, it is not possible to be dogmatic about the roles of environment and heredity in such instances, but most psychiatrists think that disturbed interpersonal environments are much more important than heredity in the transmission of any emotional disturbance from one generation to the next.

In the last two decades a great deal has been learned about heredity from the viewpoint of the chemical and biophysical structures of chromosomes and genes, but as yet this knowledge has given no insights into personality development and emotional functioning. With the exception of Down's syndrome (mongolism) and some very rare conditions such as Klinefelter's syndrome, Turner's syndrome, phenylketonuria and others in which there are gross physical abnormalities as well as psychiatric ones, this new information has shed no light on any kind of psychiatric disturbance.

We shall deal further with the subject of heredity in later chapters of this book when we discuss a few specific types of psychiatric illness in which some investigators have raised the question of a possible hereditory factor, or in which chromosomal defects have been demonstrated, as in Down's syndrome (mongolism).

Psychology, Psychodynamics and Psychopathology

Psychology. The term psychology usually is employed by psychiatrists to refer to the study of mental, emotional and interpersonal functioning in a non-medical setting. For example, in the non-medical divisions of colleges and universities, the activities of teaching, research and writing about mental and emotional functioning fall under the category of psychology. Psychology often is divided into animal psychology dealing with the behavior of animals, and human psychology, dealing with emotional and interpersonal features in man. Psychology in this way is distinguished from the medical specialty of psychiatry. Of course, the word psychology is sometimes used in a less specific sense to indicate all kinds of normal mental and emotional functioning; thus we may speak of the psychological development of children or the psychology of middle-aged persons.

Psychology is sometimes divided into normal psychology and abnormal psychology; abnormal psychology usually refers to psychiatric problems when they are discussed in non-medical settings. Psychologists are often, quite artificially, divided into three groups: (1) Academic psychologists, who devote themselves mainly to teaching in colleges and universities; (2) research psychologists, who do research in animal or human psychology; and (3) clinical psychologists, who do diagnostic and therapeutic work with patients (desirably in a multidisciplinary setting with psychiatrists and other mental health professionals). Many psychologists work in two of these fields, or even in all three.

The boundaries and the professions of psychology and psychiatry merge at many points, just as the boundaries between biochemistry and internal medicine often merge. Similarly, psychologists have developed a group of procedures and skills important to clinical psychiatrists, just as biochemists have produced a wide variety of laboratory procedures and chemical analyses which are now an integral part of internal medicine.

Psychodynamics. Psychodynamics is the study of the emotional and interpersonal causes of human behavior and psychiatric problems. It stresses that the past and current interpersonal relationships of the individual are the most important factors in determining his personality structure, emotional functioning and psychiatric disturbances.

In the historical evolution of modern psychiatry, *psychodynamic* psychiatry developed in opposition to *descriptive* psychiatry, which merely described the symptoms and course of a psychiatric illness without attention to the person's emotional life and interpersonal experiences. Psychodynamic psychiatry also evolved in opposition to *organic* psychiatry, which postulated the eventual discovery of physiological disturbances in the brain or elsewhere as the causes of most psychiatric illnesses and attributed little etiologic importance to the life experiences of the individual. (In Chapter 2 we traced the development of modern psychodynamic psychiatry and its differentiation from descriptive and organic psychiatry.) A majority of psychiatrists today accept the psychodynamic point of view, although they hold various opinions about the nature and relative importance of the different emotional and interpersonal factors. The word *dynamic* is most commonly used in psychiatry as a synonym of psychodynamic, and psychiatrists and other mental health professionals often speak of the "psychodynamics," or the "dynamics," of a patient's problem. A psychodynamic, or dynamic, psychiatrist is one whose main interests are in the emotional and interpersonal causes of patients' difficulties.

Psychopathology. Psychopathology is the study of the characteristics (both mental and behavioral), emotional aspects, and interpersonal causes of psychiatric illnesses and personality abnormalities. Interpersonal and emotional causes, as opposed to organic or physical causes, are studied. In actual practice, psychiatrists often use "psychopathology" and "psychodynamics" interchangeably, though some writers draw distinctions between the two terms.

Conscious and Unconscious

Consciousness. The term "consciousness" is used two ways in psychiatry. Firstly, it refers to a person's usual state of alert awareness of himself and his environment during his waking hours. Consciousness in this sense is opposed to the loss of this alert awareness that occurs normally during sleep, or abnormally in the stupor or coma produced by organic brain disease. The moment-to-moment flow of a person's perceptions, thoughts and feelings is sometimes called the "stream of consciousness." (The various disturbances of this type of consciousness, such as delirium and stupor, are described in a later part of this chapter.)

Secondly, "conscious" is used to refer to all the thoughts, feelings and memories of past experiences and information an individual can recall by intentional efforts. At any particular moment, of course, a person's consciousness is restricted to a limited sphere of thoughts and feelings, and he is drawing on only a small part of his total conscious life experiences. For instance, a physician interpreting an electrocardiogram is conscious mainly of the electrocardiographic tracings and the immediate needs of his patient, and many aspects of his medical training and experience. However, each person has a vast fund of other experience and information that he can recall under other circumstances, stimuli or necessities. For example, the physician at other times can recall many of the interpersonal experiences, feelings and emotions of his boyhood, though he is not aware of them at the time he is interpreting the electrocardiogram. Thus, psychiatrists use "consciousness" to refer to the immediate alert awareness of the person and also to the total amount of life experience and information he can recall at various times and under various circumstances.

Unconscious. The term "unconscious" is used in psychiatry to describe those feelings, urges, thoughts and residues of past or present experiences that are so painful or unacceptable to a person that he cannot easily summon them into conscious awareness and therefore remains unaware of them.

Many painful emotional conflicts and socially unacceptable urges from a person's past life are lodged in his unconscious mind. Although the patient is unaware of them, these unconscious forces may have much influence on his behavior. For example, a man who during his childhood had a hostile, traumatic relationship with his father may have no recollection or awareness of this unhealthy facet of his past interpersonal life. These painful experiences have been repressed into the unconscious areas of his mind. However, the lurking energy of these repressed experiences influences his behavior toward male authoritative figures in later life. He finds himself chronically rebelling and quarreling with teachers in college and with his superiors at work. Unconsciously, he is carrying his old, unresolved conflicts with his father into current situations with authoritative male superiors. He may find many rationalizations for his behavior, or he may in time realize that this behavior constitutes a problem whose roots he cannot find. Many psychiatrists today attribute an important role to unconscious thoughts, feelings and experiences in the production of psychiatric disturbances. (The concept of the unconscious mind is discussed in more detail in later parts of this chapter.)

The term "preconscious" is sometimes used to designate those thoughts, feelings and memories that at a particular time are not in the focus of a person's awareness, but can be brought into consciousness by an effort to recall them.

Intelligence

Intelligence is composed of complex capacities enabling a person to acquire knowledge and to use the lessons of his past experience in coping with new situations. Intelligence enables a man to engage in many kinds of mechanical and creative activities and to acquire large amounts of education from his fellow men and from the recorded experience of his predecessors in past centuries. Intelligence helps a man to some extent in solving his interpersonal, economic and cultural problems.

The capacity of a person to use his intelligence, however, is much influenced by his personality stability and his interpersonal soundness. The practical day-to-day intelligence of a person is determined by a complex fusion of his reasoning abilities and his emotional state. High intelligence may be crippled by marked personality problems, and average intelligence may be much aided by a sound personality structure.

Both psychiatrists and psychologists differ much on the precise determinants and components of intelligence, and they find it easier to give a superficial description of intelligence than to define the particular functions that go into its making. (We shall further discuss the nature and measurement of intelligence in Chapter 5.)

Intelligence plays a much lesser role than emotions and interpersonal experiences in determining the soundness of a person's personality structure. Also, the individual's past and current interpersonal relationships are much more important than intelligence in determining whether or not he develops psychiatric problems.

Emotion, Conation and Cognition

Emotion. An "emotion" is any one of a number of feelings such as anger, grief, fear, joy or affectionate yearning. Many psychiatrists further define emotions as having physiological concomitants in response to the person's feelings. Thus, anger often results in slight increases of cardiac rate and blood sugar level, and grief may cause decreased gastrointestinal activity and loss of appetite. In this way, some psychiatrists differentiate between "emotion" and "affect" (covered in the following division of this chapter).

In actual practice psychiatrists often use the words "emotion" and "emotional" in a much broader sense. They use them to refer to all the complex feelings and attitudes a person has in his interpersonal relationships. Moreover, the term "emotional disturbance" is commonly employed to designate all psychiatric problems not primarily caused by organic brain disease or defective intelligence. Thus, most psychiatrists speak of a phobia as an "emotional" disturbance, and many of them would call an abrupt schizophrenic disorder an acute "emotional" illness. In the last few decades the general psychiatric use of "emotion" has undergone a transition from its narrower sense to its much broader meaning.

Conation and Cognition. The word "conation" is rarely used today by clinical psychiatrists in speaking of patients. However, it is used by some psychological writers to indicate all the forces of the person contributing to his strivings and urges. Conation involves the concepts of will and impulse to action. "Cognition," on the other hand, designates the reflective thoughts, knowledge and reasoning processes of the person. Cognition also involves the concept of an alert perception of the individual's environment as part of his reflective thinking process.

AFFECTS AND THEIR DISTURBANCES

The term "affect" is used in psychiatry to designate a person's feeling tone or prolonged emotional feeling state. Depressiveness, exhilaration or prolonged anxiousness are examples of affects, or affective states. Most psychiatrists use the words "affect" and "emotion" somewhat interchangeably. Others, however, draw a distinction between them. They define "affect" as a prolonged feeling tone, and "emotion" as a shorter state of strong feeling accompanied by physiological concomitants. For example, they would say that a state of depressiveness lasting several weeks is an "affective" disturbance, and that strong anger during a brief marital spat is an "emotion." (The other, broader senses of the word "emotion" in common usage are discussed in the preceding section of this chapter.)

Disorders of affect constitute a large group of psychiatric problems. They may vary from mild disturbances to serve psychotic processes. (The various types of affective disorders are extensively covered in Chapters 10, 15 and 16.) We shall here describe briefly the different kinds of disturbances of affect.

Depressive and Manic Affects

Depression. Depression is a state of sadness in which the person views himself and the world about him with pervasive melancholy pessimism. Depression may be so mild that it causes only a slight disturbance in feeling tone, or it may be so severe that it becomes an incapacitating illness. Extreme states of depression may endanger the patient's life by the possibility of suicide.

The depressed patient views himself and the world around him through gray-colored glasses. He feels that he is inadequate, incapable, worthless and defeated. He often has profound feelings of guilt over his minor failings and small misdeeds. In severe depressions, the patient's guilty or inadequate feelings may reach delusional proportions. I recall a depressed patient who felt that she was mentally retarded with an I. Q. of 60, despite the fact that she held a doctorate from a leading university and had done outstanding professional work in her field.

The depressed person is slowed down in his physical and mental alertness. He feels tired, sleeps poorly, loses interest in his usual activities and may lose weight. His depressiveness usually is evident to his family and friends, though an occasional depressed person may hide his depression behind a façade of forced normal behavior. He often becomes preoccupied with body sensations and may complain of upper and lower gastrointestinal difficulties or vague discomforts in various parts of his body.

A depression may be precipitated by discouraging or saddening life circumstances, and in such cases is sometimes called a "reactive" or "situational" depression. Other depressions are caused by deeply rooted, unresolved conflicts within the person arising from traumatic interpersonal relationships in the past. The depressed patient often suffered much emotional rejection and hostile coldness during his early years, which left him with profound, underlying feelings of worthlessness and isolation. He often has much hostility and resentment stored within him, but he feels guilty when these angry feelings erupt into expression. (The causes of depressions are discussed further in Chapters 10 and 15.)

Manic Affects. The manic affects are the opposite of the depressive affects. In the manic affects the individual has exhilarated optimism, enthusiastic joyfulness, buoyant self-confidence and physical overactivity. The various degrees of manic affects, in order of increasing severity are *euphoria, hypomania* and *mania*.

In *euphoria* the patient radiates a feeling of exuberant well-being. He is excessively jovial and self-confident, and he can see only the optimistic side of things. He brushes caution and prudence aside and feels assured of success in whatever he may attempt. Euphoria may be the initial affect during the development of a hypomanic or manic reaction. It also occurs in some of the organic brain disorders.

In *hypomania* the patient's joyful overactivity and grandiose self-confidence are more pronounced, and his behavior becomes disorganized as he flits from one activity to another without completing any task. He often has elaborate schemes for personal achievement, and he talks a great deal, passing rapidly from one subject to another. In his exhilaration he ignores the realities of his life and he brushes aside any unhappy circumstances.

In a *manic* disorder the patient's exhilarated overactivity and grandiose thinking reach psychotic proportions and his behavior deteriorates into a chaotic series of uncompleted plans and acts. He sleeps little and he talks and moves incessantly. All the features of hypomanic affect are augmented, and grandiose delusions often are present.

Hypomanic and manic reactions are defenses against depressiveness. The patient unconsciously flees into the hollow gaiety and exaggerated self-confidence of manic affectivity to ward off depressive rumblings within himself. Hence, manic and depressive episodes sometimes alternate in the same patient, and even in the midst of a manic state a patient may for a few minutes break into tears and despair. (The nature and causes of manic disorders are covered at greater length in Chapter 16.)

Anxiety, Tension and Panic

In Chapter 1 we discussed anxiety, and its opposite, security, in the context of personality development. We shall here consider it from other points of view, and shall cover the related terms of tension and panic.

Anxiety. Anxiety is an apprehensive uneasiness in which the person has a sense of vague impending danger. The anxious person is unquiet and distressed, and he often has physical concomitants of his anxiousness such as muscular tenseness and cardiac palpitation.

Often the patient cannot attach his anxiety to any idea or object and his distress may then be called "free-floating" anxiety. At other times he may attribute his anxiety to a rapidly shifting series of worries and possible misfortunes. Anxiety is very common. All people probably experience at least minimal amounts of anxiety from time to time. It is the most common manifestation of emotional distress and psychiatric illness, and it occurs in all variations from barely noticed discomfort to disorganizing panic.

The concept of anxiety is basic in psychiatry. Anxiety often is the first reaction to painful interpersonal conflicts. Also, the forces of old, unconscious, unresolved emotional problems often shower the person with anxiety as they threaten to erupt into his awareness. Anxiety is so painful that the individual tends to mobilize many kinds of unhealthy defenses against it, and these unhealthy defenses and their consequences constitute many of the forms of psychiatric illness. For example, free-floating anxiety may become bound into the dread of specific objects such as elevators or automobiles, producing a phobia. The person is then free from his anxiety except when he must come into contact with the object of his phobia. He has, in a sense, found an unhealthy way of freeing himself from much of his anxiety at the cost of developing a specific neurotic difficulty. (The role of anxiety in many forms of psychiatric difficulty is covered in later chapters.)

Tension and Panic. Tension is a state of prolonged anxiousness accompanied by muscular tautness and restlessness. In modern psychiatric usage, the word "tension" is loosely employed to designate mild or moderate prolonged anxiety states. The extreme degree of anxiety is "panic." The patient in panic is devastated by overwhelming anxiety. His behavior and thinking become disorganized as he crumbles in sheer terror. Panic is occasionally the preliminary phase of a schizophrenic illness, or it may occur in acute organic brain disorders such as delirium tremens. As a state of panic disintegrates into a psychotic reaction the patient may have persecutory delusions, hallucinations and physical combativeness. In contradistinction to the terms anxiety, tension and panic, psychiatrists use the word "fear" to designate the normal reaction of alarm and dread to realistic danger in life.

Flatness of Affect, Inappropriate Affect and Depersonalization

Flatness of Affect. The absence of apparent feeling tones in response to interpersonal relationships is called "flatness of affect." Neither distressing events nor pleasant occurrences elicit reactions, and the person seems emotionally oblivious to his interpersonal environment. Flatness of affect is often a feature of schizophrenic illnesses. In a sense, the schizophrenic patient has retreated from interpersonal contacts into an inner world of fantasies, delusions and hallucinations. His flatness of affect is both a product of his retreat from reality and a defense against involvement in an interpersonal world he has found emotionally painful. Flatness of affect occasionally occurs in other psychiatric disorders.

Inappropriate Affect. Inappropriate affect occurs when the patient's affect is at variance with his apparent thought processes and actions. For example, the patient may laugh while telling of the death of a relative or giggle while discussing a painful illness he had. Inappropriate affect is common in schizophrenia, but it also occurs occasionally in other psychiatric disorders.

Depersonalization. Depersonalization is an affective state in which the person has an eerie, persistent feeling that his personality and the world around him have undergone a profound change. The person cannot specify what the change is and he does not feel that he is someone else, but he feels that he is not the same person that he was and that his environment is strange and unreal. His emotions, thoughts and actions seem alien and unreal to him. Depersonalization may occur in early schizophrenic reactions, depressions, dissociative disorders and other psychiatric disturbances.

In the 1968 revision of the American standard psychiatric nomenclature the diagnosis *depersonalization neurosis* (or depersonalization syndrome) was introduced as a specific type of neurotic disorder. This was done, along with a number of other changes, to make the American system of psychiatric diagnoses consistent with the International

Classification of Diseases, which contains a number of terms used mainly in continental European countries and in the Soviet Union and its dependent nations. Very few American psychiatrists employ the term *depersonalization neurosis*, since it raises a single, somewhat infrequent symptom, which may be present in various kinds of psychiatric disorders, to the status of an independent disorder. It is as if the standard medical nomenclature contained diagnoses such as "cough" and "fever." (The term depersonalization neurosis is discussed at somewhat greater length in Chapter 10.)

DISTURBANCES OF THOUGHT PROCESSES

Delusions. A delusion is an unrealistic, false belief, usually involving the person himself, which is caused by an emotional disturbance or an organic brain disorder. It is out of keeping with the person's educational level and realistic life experiences. The delusional person usually has strong feelings about his false convictions and persists in his delusional beliefs despite all kinds of logical, objective evidence that they are untrue.

Delusions may occur in schizophrenia, paranoid disorders, depressions and some other kinds of emotionally caused illnesses. They also may occur in various types of organic brain disease. Delusions may be divided into (a) *persecutory* delusions, (b) *grandiose* delusions, and (c) *self-accusative* and *self-depreciative delusions*.

Persecutory Delusions. The person with persecutory delusions believes that various persons or vague forces are attempting to harm, deceive or manipulate him in hostile ways. Persecutory delusions are the most common kind of delusions seen in clinical practice. They may occur in schizophrenia, paranoid disorders, depressions and other types of emotionally caused illnesses. They may also be present in some types of organic brain disturbances, such as those associated with alcoholism, cerebral arteriosclerosis and senile brain deterioration.

Persons with persecutory delusions may feel that they are being persecuted by high governmental officials, leaders of political parties, notorious criminals, agents of foreign governments, their families, their acquaintances or the people with whom they work. They often feel that they are being poisoned or "doped" by substances put in their food or water, that their houses are "wired" by spying enemies, or that secret messages about them are being sent on their television sets and radios. They may believe that people are attempting to control their thoughts or destroy their minds by x-rays, electronic devices or less clearly defined means. They may feel that their persecutors are attempting to rob them, kill them, alienate their families from them, or dominate them for use in vile or immoral ways. The person may feel that his spouse is maritally unfaithful with hostile, exploitive intentions; he may believe that his spouse is in league with his persecutors against him.

Persecutory beliefs may be vague, poorly organized and fluctuating. In other instances, they become fixed into *systematized delusions*, in which an elaborate framework of false beliefs is built with apparent logic on the foundation of a few basic, deeply rooted delusional ideas. A man may believe, for example, that his employers are hostile to him and are attempting to exploit him. On this basis he may gradually evolve a network of systematized delusions in which he feels that his ideas and achievements have been stolen from him at work, that everyone at work is involved in the conspiracy against him, and that they have corrupted his wife to turn against him.

Persecutory ideas may occur briefly, as in some acute schizophrenic illnesses and acute alcoholic psychoses, or they may become ingrained and last for decades, as in some chronic schizophrenic illnesses and paranoid reactions. Psychiatric theory holds that persecutory delusions occur when the individual projects his own unacceptable feelings onto other people. Thus, for example, persecutory delusions can occur when a person cannot come to grips consciously with his powerful hostile urges, and he therefore projects them onto others whom he then perceives as hostile to himself. He thus finds an unhealthy release for his hostile impulses and for the emotional impulses associated with them. (The emotional forces producing persecutory delusions are discussed in greater detail under the illnesses in which they occur.)

The term "paranoid" delusion is loosely used as synonymous with "persecutory" delusion. However, the word "paranoid" is also used by some psychiatrists to cover both persecutory and grandiose delusions. Paranoid schizophrenia is the type of schizophrenia in which delusions and hallucinations are prominent features.

Ideas of Reference. These are false interpretations that events around the person are specially related to him. The individual may feel, for example, that many remarks and actions of people around him are accusatory, ridiculing or depreciatory to him. Ideas of reference sometimes occur in unduly sensitive, insecure people, or they may coexist with persecutory delusions in various types of psychiatric illness.

Grandiose Delusions. The patient with grandiose delusions feels that he has exalted power, significance or identity. Thus, for example, he may feel that he controls the destinies of nations, or that his thoughts manipulate large groups of people, or that he is a divine religious leader. Delusions that the individual is a sublime religious figure or that he has extraordinary religious feelings and attributes constitute the most common type of grandiose delusions seen in clinical practice. Grandiose delusions may occur in schizophrenic illnesses, manic reactions and some organic brain disorders.

In grandiose delusions, strong, underlying feelings of worthlessness, inadequacy and insecurity find a psychotic resolution in beliefs that the person is important, exalted and powerful; by his delusions the individual reassures himself that he is not inferior and despised. The terms "megalomanic delusions" and "delusions of grandeur" are commonly employed as synonymous with "grandiose delusions."

Self-Accusative and Self-Depreciative Delusions. Self-accusative and self-depreciative delusions may occur in psychiatric illnesses with strong depressive features. They are most common in severe depressions, but also may occur in schizophrenic illnesses and organic brain disorders that have marked depressive coloring.

The patient with self-accusative and self-depreciative delusions feels that he is overwhelmingly worthless, inadequate and guilty. He may believe that in various ways he has harmed people, killed members of his family and others, or that he has robbed his employers and friends. He may feel that he has committed heinous sexual crimes and vile sex acts, or that he is responsible for widespread destruction. I recall a 20-year-old schizophrenic patient with strong depressive features who stood for hours at the window of his hospital room surveying what he felt were the ruins of the city outside which he said he had destroyed by bombs and fire. Suicidal urges are a common problem in patients with self-accusatory and self-depreciative delusions; the patient feels that he is so worthless and guilty that suicide is the only possible course.

Other depressed patients believe they have loathsome diseases and body deformities. They may feel that they have gruesome dysfunctions due to cancer, syphilis or gonorrhea, or infestations with repulsive insects and worms. I recall a patient who complained bitterly of the small white worms he said were covering delusional sores on his legs and trunk. Some patients believe they are dead, or that a part of the body is dead, or that they are dying or being physically destroyed in some way; these sometimes are called "nihilistic delusions." Other depressed patients have false beliefs that they are impoverished and economically destitute.

Self-accusative and self-depreciative delusions are produced by profound feelings of guilt arising from old, unresolved interpersonal conflicts. These conflicts often occurred in the patient's childhood, but they usually have been augmented by further emotional trauma in the patient's adult life. Deeply rooted feelings of inadequacy and inferiority may break through in bizarre exaggeration during a depressive illness and contribute to self-accusative and self-depreciative delusions. Self-accusative and self-depreciative delusions are often a response to strong unconscious hostile or sexual urges that arise within the person and mobilize much guilt and turmoil. (We shall consider the ways in which emotional forces produce self-accusative and self-depreciative delusions in more detail in the chapters dealing with the psychiatric illnesses in which they occur.)

OTHER DISTURBANCES OF THOUGHT PROCESSES

Blocking. In blocking, the patient abruptly stops in his train of thought and speech. He becomes suddenly silent and seems distracted from his flow of thought into some unrelated preoccupation. He may sit in silence briefly or for a long time. Blocking occurs most often in schizophrenics and is due to the fragmentation of thought processes and a broken flow of conflictual thoughts and feelings, which are prominent features of schizophrenia. Blocking may occur when strong unconscious feelings or unacceptable thoughts flood the person and temporarily paralyze overt speech and articulate thought progression.

Retardation. In retardation, the patient feels that his thought processes are slowed down. He speaks slowly and feels that all kinds of physical and mental exertion are painful burdens. He may sit wearily for hours at a time and he walks in a slow, shuffling manner. Retardation occurs in many depressed patients, and in some patients with other types of psychiatric difficulties that have depressive coloring. Retardation of thought processes in this sense is not to be confused with the term "mental retardation," or "mental deficiency," which refers to those persons who have defective intelligence dating from birth or early childhood.

Flight of Ideas. Flight of ideas is the opposite of retardation. The patient with a flight of ideas flits rapidly from topic to topic as his ideas crowd swiftly to the surface one after another. He does not complete any train of thought and cannot follow any idea to a logical conclusion. He chatters rapidly and continuously, and the casual observer often cannot follow his helter-skelter thread of discourse. His succeeding ideas often have no logical connection with one another, but are connected by the similar sounds of words, puns of one word with another, or chance associations. For example, I recall a manic patient who noticed a small crack in the wall of her hospital room and said, "The foundation of this building is settling. My ancestors were early settlers in this community. Now, let's settle down and settle my situation once and for all." Behind the rapid flow of apparently unrelated ideas, an experienced psychiatrist may be able to discern basic emotional themes disturbing the patient. Flight of ideas occurs in manic psychoses and in some schizophrenic disorders with manic features.

Perseveration. In perseveration the patient makes the same reply to several succeeding different questions. Sometimes the reply is appropriate to the first question but the patient applies the same answer to all succeeding questions. I recall a patient who replied "seventy-six" to all questions involving arithmetic or numbers, and another who answered, "No, darn it" to all questions asked. Perseveration is most common in organic brain disease, but may also occur in schizophrenia.

Fragmentation of Thought Processes. In fragmentation of thought processes, which is a basic feature of schizophrenia, the logical, rational connection of one thought to another is impaired. Instead, the thought sequences of the patient are determined by strong, conflicting urges and emotions which cast the patient's speech into a chaotic jumble. The schizophrenic patient has retreated from logical, rational thought processes back to the more primitive, archaic forms of thought that occur in dreams and in very early childhood. His thoughts are strung together by conflicting emotional forces rather than by logical bonds. Also, the schizophrenic patient uses words in ways that have special meanings for him, he coins new words called "neologisms," and he condenses various meanings into particular words and symbolic phrases. I recall a schizophrenic patient who wrote in a note to me, "The atomic radiation of the dementalized systems has come to me. Impotentialized forces draw me closer to your television and spiritual forces from the universalized are spreading. Benjamin knows of this and will arrive in the morning-glory."

Fragmentation of thought processes may produce a flow of incomprehensible speech to which the term "word salad" is sometimes applied. At times the patient may repeat the same apparently meaningless words or sentences over and over; this is called "verbigeration." The fragmentation of thought processes that occurs in schizophrenia is sometimes called "autistic" thought or "dereistic" thought, and it is also labeled by some psychiatrists as one form of "primary process" thinking. (We shall cover fragmentation of thought processes more extensively in our discussion of schizophrenia in Chapter 14.)

Deterioration of Thought Processes Due to Organic Brain Disease. Destruction of brain tissue often causes a deterioration of thought processes. The patient wanders from topic to topic in a drifting way. Some patients start out toward a goal in their thinking, but arrive there only after long, rambling detours on unrelated topics; this is called "circumstantiality." Many patients with organic brain deterioration stray aimlessly from item to item in their speech, forgetting the thread of their discourse and picking up new, unrelated themes every minute or two. In advanced stages, their speech may become so disconnected that it is completely incoherent. Aphasic disturbances in organic brain disease produce a futile grasping for words and names that cannot be found, or which are found only after trial and error. (The various kinds of deterioration of thought processes in organic brain disease are discussed at greater length in Chapters 18 and 19.)

DISTURBANCES OF PERCEPTION

Perception is the process by which the person becomes aware of the stimuli in his environment through the activities of his sensory systems and their ramifications. As used by psychiatrists, perception includes the emotional and intellectual interpretation of these sensations in the context of the past experience of the person and his current life circumstances. Thus, for example, when a person sees a German shepherd dog he fondly recognizes it as the kind of animal he had for a pet in his childhood. (The overlapping term "apperception" is discussed later in this section.) The main avenues of perception are sight, hearing, touch, smell and taste. The major disturbances of perception are illusions and hallucinations.

Illusions

An illusion is a misinterpretation of an actual sound, sight or other sensation. For example, a woman who is anxiously awaiting her husband's return home late at night may misinterpret the noise of the wind as the distant sound of his automobile. Illusions are common in normal people who are under emotional strain.

The content of the illusion usually expresses the underlying emotional tension of the person. For example, the fearful person may interpret minor sounds in the house at night as the possible footsteps of a burglar. The girl who is awaiting a visit from her boy friend repeatedly interprets small noises as the ringing of the doorbell. An individual who is anxiously awaiting a message often mistakes a casual noise as the sound of his name being called. Other illusions may express more deeply rooted emotional turmoil in the person. Illusions also may occur in acute organic brain disorders associated with infection, chronic alcoholism, intoxication, head trauma and other causes. They may occur occasionally in other psychiatric disturbances.

Hallucinations

A hallucination is a false perception for which there is no actual sensory basis. For example, a schizophrenic patient may hear voices in the ceiling talking to him or he may see people entering into, and emerging from, the walls of his room. The content of hallucinations is not haphazard; it is determined by the nature of the emotional turbulence within the patient. For example, the patient with strong feelings of guilt may hear accusatory voices denouncing him for alleged misdeeds. The patient who is seeking release from feelings of inferiority may see exalted religious figures who by their actions indicate their esteem for him. Even in hallucinations occurring in patients with organic brain disease, the hallucinations reveal underlying conflicts and strong feelings which have been unleashed from previous controls by the impairment or destruction of brain tissue.

Hallucinations of Hearing. Auditory hallucinations are the most common form of hallucination. They occur at some time in the course of the majority of schizophrenic illnesses, and may also occur occasionally in severe depressions, acute and chronic organic brain reactions, manic psychoses, hysterical disorders and other psychiatric illnesses. In the most common types of auditory hallucinations the patient hears voices speaking to him or about him. He may describe the voices as coming from the walls, from outside his window, from ventilation or heating ducts, or from other sources. At times the patient may state that the voices are inside his head, but he hears them as loudly as he hears usual sounds. The voices may criticize the patient and condemn him, or praise him and promise him extravagant things. At other times the patient may hear the voices talking about him, other people or other topics. Some patients consistently hear only one voice, which may be male or female, and other patients hear many voices talking clearly or confusedly at the same time.

The patient may be upset about the voices or he may hear them placidly. He usually believes the voices are real, but at other times the question of their authenticity may puzzle him. Some patients have partial insight and know that the voices are a symptom of psychiatric illness. I recall a schizophrenic patient who worked for four years as a nurse while hearing auditory hallucinations daily; none of her associates knew of her disorder. At times she knew the voices were symptoms of psychiatric illness, and at other times she would inquire, "Do you really think that I'm just imagining them? They seem so real, How can you be sure, doctor?" The voices sometimes may command the patient to say things, to make trips, to commit violence, to commit suicide or to do many other things. The patient also may hear other sounds such as music, horns, bells and the noise of machinery, but voices are a much more common form of auditory hallucination.

Hallucinations of Sight. Visual hallucinations are common in acute organic brain disorders. For example, a lady with acute bromide intoxication complained about the small green boys riding bicycles in her hospital room. Visual hallucinations of small animals, snakes, insects and threatening people are characteristic of acute organic brain disorders associated with alcohol; they also occur in chronic organic brain syndromes. An elderly lady with cerebral arteriosclerosis complained for years of a small animal "like a basketball with feathers on it" running around her room. Visual hallucinations also occur in a minority of patients with schizophrenia. They often are menacing and frightening to the patient, especially when they occur in acute organic brain disorders. Visual hallucinations occur characteristically in persons taking lysergic acid diethylamide (LSD) and related substances, and they are common in individuals who use cocaine heavily. They may occur in other forms of drug abuse.

Hallucinations of Taste. Hallucinations of taste are uncommon. They occur mainly in schizophrenic patients who believe they taste poisons, sedatives or "dope" in their food and drink. Hallucinations of taste occur occasionally in other kinds of psychiatric illness.

Hallucinations of Smell. Olfactory hallucinations occur occasionally in schizophrenia. The patient may smell gases or other noxious odors, which he feels his persecutors are piping into his room. Olfactory hallucinations usually involve disagreeable odors, but the patient occasionally may smell fragrant aromas. Olfactory hallucinations occur rarely in other forms of psychiatric illness.

Hallucinations of Touch. Tactile hallucinations occur occasionally in some acute organic brain disorders and in schizophrenia. For example, the patient with an acute organic brain syndrome associated with alcohol or other toxic substances may feel insects crawling on his skin. Schizophrenics also may feel insects crawling on them, and they may have bizarre tactile hallucinations in the genital, perineal and rectal regions. Persons who use cocaine heavily often have hallucinations that ants or other insects are crawling beneath their skin.

OTHER ASPECTS OF PERCEPTION

Orientation. Orientation is the process by which an individual maintains alert awareness of himself with reference to time, place and identity of persons. Orientation in time involves knowing the approximate time of day, the date and the year. By orientation in place the person knows where he is, and by orientation for persons he knows who he is and who the people around him are.

Orientation involves various activities of perception, memory and knowledge. Acute and chronic organic brain disorders are the most common causes of disorders of orientation, though occasionally a patient in an acute schizophrenic disorder may be disoriented. It may be present in hysterical amnesias, fugue states and related disorders. Disorientation may be partial or complete and occasionally it may also occur in other psychiatric conditions in which the patient has great emotional distress or self-preoccupation.

Attention. Attention is the process by which the person focuses his alert awareness on specific aspects of his environment. For example, he gives attention to something he is reading or to a piece of work he is doing. Attention involves perception, memory and knowledge, and the capacity to associate them with previous experience and to focus them on the object at hand.

Organic brain impairment, defective intelligence, emotional turmoil, distressing thoughts, fatigue or conflicting feelings about the task at hand may all interfere with attention.

Distractibility is the inability to maintain attention on any object for a significant period of time. The person with distractibility moves his attention from object to object rapidly without sufficient attention on any task to comprehend it well or execute it fully. The length of time a person can concentrate on a particular object or task is sometimes called his "span of attention" or "attention span."

Apperception. Apperception is the complex process by which new perceptions are interpreted and integrated by the person in the context of his previous life experiences and knowledge. Apperception also includes focusing these new perceptions and their correlated emotions and ideas into at least a certain degree of articulate awareness. Apperception involves so many intricate emotional and ideational activities that it is a difficult concept to use in clinical psychiatry, and it is now employed much less commonly than formerly. Its most frequent use in modern psychiatry is in the interpretation of certain psychological tests, such as the Rorschach Test and the Thematic Apperception Test (which are discussed further in Chapter 5).

Hypnagogic and Hypnopompic Hallucinations. Hypnagogic hallucinations are auditory or visual hallucinations that occur while the patient is falling asleep. They last only a few minutes and disappear as the patient enters deeper sleep. For example, I had a patient who often heard her long-deceased mother calling her name during such hallucinations; I had another who sat up in bed each night while going to sleep and arranged the "thick, blue drapes" that she felt were enclosing her. Hypnopompic hallucinations occur during the process of awakening. These two types of hallucinations may occur occasionally in people who have no significant emotional problems. When they occur frequently they may be symptoms of underlying emotional turmoil that seeks a hallucinatory release when the censoring powers of consciousness are in abeyance in the twilight zone between sleeping and waking. In my opinion, they are not forerunners or indications of psychotic tendencies.

Extrasensory Perception. Extrasensory perception is a concept which postulates the transmission of thoughts and feelings from one person to another without the use of physical sensory perception. The ways by which such thoughts and feelings might be transmitted from one mind to another are unknown. However, since these means must lie outside the usual physical senses of sight, hearing and touch, they are termed "extrasensory." The word "telepathy" is commonly used by the lay public to describe such communication, and the initials ESP are often employed as an abbreviation for extrasensory perception. The study of extrasensory perception and related phenomena is called "parapsychology." Only a minority of psychiatrists and psychologists accept extrasensory perception as a valid concept, but the subject has aroused much interest. The experiments and writings of the psychologist J. B. Rhine have given much impetus to this field.

Many psychiatrists who do not accept the concept of extrasensory perception have, however, an open mind on the subject. Events occur from time to time in clinical pratice which awaken interest in the possiblity of its validity. I recall a patient who awoke at four o'clock in the morning and in great agitation announced to her family that her husband had just died of a great pain in the chest in a distant state in which he was traveling. On the following day they learned that about the time the patient said this her husband died in an automobile accident in which the steering wheel of his car crushed his chest and upper abdomen. This patient developed a prolonged manic psychosis which began the morning she announced her husband's death. Such experiences suggest to some psychiatrists that by electromagnetic means or other processes some people can perceive events and thoughts in extrasensory ways. I cannot accept extrasensory perception, but I have seen enough such experiences in practice to prevent me from being dogmatic in my rejection of it.

DISTURBANCES OF MEMORY

Memory is the process of registration, retention and recall of experience. It is crucial to interpersonal relationships of all kinds; without intact memory interpersonal relationships deteriorate quickly. Memory may be conscious or unconscious, and it is much influenced by emotions and personality structure.

Registration is the process by which experience and knowledge are perceived by a person and transmitted to the diffuse systems of the brain where they are stored.

Retention is the process of storing and preserving experience and knowledge. The person may not direct his attention to vast amounts of his experience and knowledge for long periods of time. Nevertheless, it may affect his intellectual and emotional functioning in ways of which he is articulately unaware. For example, in rapidly tying his shoelaces a person does not think through the successive motions of his fingers, but his memory nevertheless guides his hands in this task.

Recall is the process by which a person summons past experience and previously acquired knowledge into his conscious, articulate focus of attention. Recall may be disturbed or delayed by emotions, fatigue and many other factors, and it may be partial or complete for a specific thing at a particular time.

The concept of memory has been extended in modern psychiatry to include the registration and retention of much experience which can be recalled only with great difficulty or which cannot be recalled at all. This is called "unconscious memory," and it may strongly affect the individual's interpersonal life in ways of which he is unaware. Thus, a man in his childhood may have had a prolonged traumatic relationship with his mother, but the experience was so emotionally painful that he cannot recall it. Nevertheless, it may contribute to make him somewhat shy and ill at ease with women in his adult life. The subject of unconscious memory is covered further later in this chapter.

In recent years much laboratory research has led to suggestions that memories are stored in brain cells through changes in ribonucleic acid molecules and other molecules; the recall of such memories presumably would require exceedingly intricate chemical reactions involving many cells and circuits of nerve fibers. However, as is often the case in psychiatry, the gap between laboratory findings and clinical work with patients is so wide that there are no therapeutic or diagnostic applications of this information at this time.

Amnesia. Amnesia is the loss of memory; it may be caused by emotional factors or organic brain disease. Amnesia caused by emotional factors usually affects only the ability to recall experience and knowledge; registration and retention as a rule are unaffected. Amnesia due to organic brain dysfunction usually involves retention and registration as well as recall.

Amnesia may be anterograde or retrograde. Both anterograde and retrograde amnesia may be caused by either organic brain disease or emotional factors.

Anterograde amnesia extends forward in time from the moment of onset of the etiologic process. For example, following a blow on the head a person may have amnesia for all or most events that occur in the next few hours, or the next several weeks, or longer. During a brief anterograde amnesic episode, especially if it is of hysterical nature, the patient may or may not be recognized as abnormal by casual observers.

Retrograde amnesia covers the period of time before the onset of the causative process. For example, a patient with an emotionally caused retrograde amnesia may have a memory defect for the events of many days, weeks or years prior to the moment when the amnesia began. In many instances of both organically caused and emotionally caused amnesias, the defects of memory are both anterograde and retrograde.

Emotionally caused amnesia may occur in hysterical dissociative disorders and in other psychiatric disturbances in which emotional turmoil deprives the patient of his capacity to recall past experiences. If the person is under great emotional stress his capacity to perceive and register experience may also be impaired by his lack of attention to events in his environment. In hysterical dissociative states, amnesia often begins abruptly and ends abruptly. In time, the patient often regains his memory, partially or entirely. Emotionally caused amnesia is an unconscious way in which the person protects himself from painful memories, emotions, ideas and circumstances. (Emotionally caused amnesic states and their differential diagnosis from organically caused loss of memory are covered in Chapter 9.)

Organically caused amnesia may be reversible or irreversible, depending on the acuteness or chronicity of the causative process. It tends to affect recent events more than events in the distant past. For example, the patient cannot remember the happenings of the past few days, but he can remember things that happened several years ago. Upon recovery from his illness the patient with amnesia due to an acute organic brain disorder usually regains his normal memory for events of the period before and after his illness, but he often has a persistent memory defect for events that occurred while he was ill.

Sometimes the patient with an organic brain disorder fills in his memory gaps with elaborate fabricated stories which may at first seem plausible to the hearer; this is called "confabulation."

In modern psychiatry the term "dementia" is mainly used to designate states of marked deterioration of memory, personality and behavior caused by organic brain disorders. The most common causes of organic dementia are cerebral arteriosclerosis and senile brain deterioration in the aged. (The memory disturbances that occur in organic brain disease are further covered in Chapters 18 and 19.)

Hypermnesia. Hypermnesia is exceptionally acute memory; the individual with hypermnesia has an extraordinary capacity to remember minute details of his experiences. It occurs mainly in paranoid patients who observe each event with alert, watchful suspiciousness. It may also occur in other emotionally caused disturbances in which the patient undergoes experiences which have strong emotional significances for him.

Paramnesia. Under the term paramnesia are grouped various kinds of memory distortions, of which the commonest are *déjà vu, jamais vu* and *retrospective falsification.*

Déjà vu is the eerie feeling of having lived through a current experience before, when in fact one has not. For example, a person enters a room in which he has never been before, yet he has the feeling that he has been in this room before and has gone through the same actions he is currently carrying out. Déjà vu is common in late adolescence and young adulthood. It is less common during middle age and afterwards. It frequently occurs in normal people and is usually not a sign of emotional illness. On rare occasions it occurs in association with organic brain lesions of the temporal lobes or in acute organic brain disorders. Many theories have been offered to explain déjà vu. Some psychiatrists have suggested that déjà vu occurs when a person is going through an experience of which he has previously daydreamed or about which he dreamed in his sleep. Other writers have suggested that déjà vu is produced by the similarity of the experience to previous emotionally charged experiences which the person cannot recall and correlate with the current one.

Jamais vu is a related but much less common experience in which the individual feels unfamiliarity with a situation which he has actually experienced before. It is probably a limited type of amnesia caused by emotionally painful associations to the particular situation.

Retrospective falsification occurs when the person unconsciously distorts his memories of past life experiences to meet his current emotional needs. For example, a person who had a traumatic relationship with cold, rejecting parents in his childhood may in later life be unable to remember how his parents failed him emotionally and may view them as having been affectionate. To a certain extent, everyone views his past life experiences in the light of his emotional needs. However, when the person has had prolonged emotionally painful past experiences, or when he has marked unhealthy personality needs, his views of past experiences may become very distorted. Retrospective falsification occurs to some extent in most emotionally caused psychiatric illnesses. One of the tasks of interview treatment in psychiatry is to help the patient unravel the twisted strains of his retrospective falsification and to come to grips with many of his life experiences in more realistic and healthier ways.

DISTURBANCES OF CONSCIOUSNESS

Earlier in this chapter we indicated that the word consciousness is used in two ways in psychiatry. In the first of these two ways, consciousness is defined as the person's usual state of alert awareness of himself and his environment during his waking hours. We shall now examine the various clinical disturbances of this form of consciousness. In order of increasing severity, the states of impaired consciousness are *confusion, clouding of consciousness, stupor* and *coma*.

Confusion. Confusion is a state of mild to moderate impairment of the person's alert awareness of himself and his environment. The confused patient is perplexed and bewildered. He grasps in a puzzled way for fragments of information to try to orient himself in time and place, and to try to understand what he is doing and what is going on around him. His span of attention is poor and his capacities for perception, memory and orientation are defective. Confusion occurs most often in acute or chronic organic brain disorders. For example, it is common in organic brain dysfunctions due to head injury, drug intoxication or impaired cerebral oxygenation in congestive heart failure. Most psychiatric writers restrict the technical use of the word "confusion" to organic brain disorders.

Clouding of Consciousness and Stupor. In clouding of consciousness there is a severe impairment of the patient's awareness of himself and his environment. He is unresponsive to stimuli and his capacity for perception of his environment is diminished. He may appear drowsy or he may sit and stare blankly at his surroundings. Often an examiner must speak loudly in the patient's ear, shake him slightly or make elaborate gestures to gain his attention. Communication with the patient is very difficult or impossible, depending on the degree to which his consciousness is clouded. Clouding of consciousness is also called "clouding of the sensorium" by some psychiatrists, and an extreme clouding of consciousness may be termed a "stupor."

Clouding of consciousness may be due to organic brain disease or severe emotional disorders. The degree of clouding of consciousness in a patient with organic brain disease often fluctuates somewhat, and the patient emerges from it only by slow degrees.

Clouding of consciousness may occur in various emotionally caused disorders such as hysterical dissociative reactions, schizophrenic states and severe depressions in which the patient is so immersed in his inner turmoil that he becomes oblivious to his environment; the terms "catatonic stupor" and "stuporous depression" are sometimes used to describe severe impairment of awareness of the environment in these two types of disorders. However, the apparent lack of contact with the environment in an emotionally caused stupor is sometimes a façade for more awareness than is evident. This is often true in catatonic schizophrenic stupor. The patient in an emotionally caused stupor sometimes emerges from it rapidly, and a schizophrenic may go from catatonic stupor to marked excitation in a short time.

Coma. In a coma a patient has such severe impairment of consciousness that he cannot be aroused by any kind of stimulation, such as shouting at him, shaking him, or squeezing his Achilles tendon; he is entirely unaware of events in his environment and has no self-awareness. At most, in lighter coma states, the patient makes slight physical movements or low moans when attempts are made to arouse him. This term is used only in talking about patients with severe organic brain disorders.

Delirium. A delirium is an organically caused clouding of consciousness associated with disorientation, illusions or hallucinations, delusions, panic and agitation. A delirium may be caused by high fever, inadequate oxygenation of the brain in pneumonia or congestive heart failure, prolonged alcoholic excess, uremia, head trauma or many other disease processes.

The classic and most common type of delirium is alcoholic *delirium tremens*. The term "delirium" usually implies that the disorder is due to an acute organic brain dysfunction and is reversible. However, some acute deliriums go on to become chronic psychotic states; for example, an alcoholic delirium tremens may lengthen into a chronic organic brain syndrome strongly colored with delusions and hallucinations. (The clinical characteristics of the various types of deliriums are covered in detail in the discussions of organic brain disorders in Chapters 18 and 19.)

CONCEPTS OF BODY CONSTITUTION AND PERSONALITY STRUCTURE

Some psychiatrists have attempted to find correlations between body constitutional types and personality structure. Most American psychiatrists now devote little attention to this subject, but it continues to interest some European psychiatrists, and the terminology used in defining the various body constitutional types is still employed occasionally in American psychiatry. Those who advocate classification of body constitution and personality structure in a single system of terminology feel that through the endocrine glands, the central nervous system and other physiological pathways, the same forces that determine the individual's body structure have a profound effect on his personality type. In recent years there has been a slight increase of interest in this point of view because of advances in understanding the structures of chromosomes and the ways in which genes influence body structure and functioning. Also, the development of the field of ethology, which has demonstrated in lower animals an intimate correlation between genetic structure and behavior, has caused some psychiatrists, mainly in Europe, to give more attention to the concept that body form and total emotional and behavioral functioning in humans may be interwoven in ways that are as yet undecipherable.

The two systems of body constitutional classification that have attracted the widest attention are those of Kretschmer and Sheldon.

Kretschmer divided body constitutional types into four groups and described the personality characteristics accompanying them. His four constitutional types are *pyknic, leptosomic, athletic* and *dysplastic*.

The person with a *pyknic* body constitution has a short, stocky, rounded figure, and he is described as energetic, gregarious and outgoing. Kretschmer felt that manic and depressive disorders are more common in pyknic individuals.

The *leptosomic* person is thin, long-limbed and flat-chested; secondary sexual characteristics are not prominently developed. Kretschmer felt that leptosomic persons are socially retiring and do not engage comfortably in interpersonal relationships. Some psychiatrists prefer the term "asthenic" to "leptosomic" in this scheme of classification.

The *athletic* person has prominent skeletal and muscular development of the body and limbs.

The *dysplastic* individual has physical abnormalities which are caused by defective functioning of the endocrine glands or other body regulative organs. Kretschmer felt that schizophrenia occurred mainly in persons with leptosomic, athletic and dysplastic body constitutions.

In a similar way Sheldon divided constitutional types into *ectomorphic, mesomorphic* and *endomorphic* depending on the prominence of the various body structures developed from ectoderm, mesoderm and endoderm of the embryonic cellular structure. Sheldon also attempted to correlate body constitutional types with personality structures and with proclivities to develop specific kinds of psychiatric illness. For example, he felt that persons of ectomorphic body type are prone to develop schizophrenia.

Most American psychiatrists think that personality structure and psychiatric illness are mainly the result of past and current interpersonal relationships and life experiences. They think that there is no consistent correlation between body type, personality structure and incidence of psychiatric illness.

VARIOUS CONCEPTS OF PERSONALITY FUNCTIONING

In Chapter 1 the *interpersonal approach to psychiatry* was discussed in detail. Throughout this book the interpersonal approach will remain the basic point of view we shall use in discussing the causes and treatment of the full range of psychiatric illness.

In modern American psychiatry, however, the *Freudian-psychoanalytic approach* has many adherents, and in recent years *behavior therapy* has attracted much attention. We therefore shall cover Freudian-psychoanalytic concepts in detail (along with some of its outgrowths, such as the approaches of Jung and Adler), and shall outline salient aspects of behavior therapy.

Actually, many aspects of the Freudian-psychoanalytic point of view have been modified and incorporated into the interpersonal approach to psychiatry, and it is probable that some features of behavior therapy will in time acquire a secure place in the wide spectrum of psychiatric therapies. Thus, the student of psychiatry should be familiar with Freudian-psychoanalytic theory and the main principles of behavior theorapy.

FREUDIAN-PSYCHOANALYTIC CONCEPTS

The Freudian-psychoanalytic approach to personality structure and psychiatric illness was developed by the Austrian psychiatrist Sigmund Freud, who published his major works in the first three decades of the 20th Century. Though later psychoanalytic writers have extended and modified some of Freud's concepts, the basic structure of psychoanalytic theory and practice remain essentially as Freud developed them. The term "psychoanalysis" was introduced by Freud to designate his comprehensive theories of personality development and his methods of investigating and treating psychiatric disorders. (The place of Freud's work in the historical development of modern psychiatry is outlined in Chapter 2.)

The Freudian-psychoanalytic system of treatment is taught in psychoanalytic institutes in various cities. The psychiatrist who wishes to devote himself exclusively to Freudian-psychoanalytic practice undergoes several years of extra education after he has completed the customary residency training required for psychiatric specialization. His education includes a personal therapeutic analysis, which aims at freeing him of whatever personality problems he may have that may be obstacles to his psychoanalytic work. Besides seminars and supervised treatment of patients, he often undergoes a training analysis in which he learns the Freudian-psychoanalytic technic by further direct personal involvement in it. Some Freudian-psychoanalytic psychiatrists have modified the treatment technics and theories of Freud in various ways, and they are sometimes said to practice modified psychoanalysis.

Freudian-psychoanalytic theory proposes that the most important events in determining personality structure and psychiatric illness occur during the first seven years of the person's life. The events which occur after the age of seven are viewed as possible precipitants of psychiatric illness but not as basic determinants. An essential feature of Freudian-psychoanalytic theory is the use of a very broad concept of sexuality in tracing the development of the person during his first seven years. This concept of sexuality includes all the passionate yearnings that the child has for the significant people in his environment and the physical sensations accompanying these feelings. The main source of these strong affectionate feelings is an inborn instinctual force called "libido." Libido, in this sense, is the motivating instinctual force that is the basis of most affectionate and achieving drives throughout his life.

Psychosexual Development

In Freudian-psychoanalytic terminology, a large part of the child's personality development during his formative years is called his "psychosexual development." Psychosexual development is divided into a series of successive periods, which occur in all human beings. The impact of each period upon the child varies depending on his interpersonal environment and his biological constitution. During each period, a particular part of the body is more important than any other in the child's intense libidinal relationships with the significant people around him. These particular parts of the body are called the *erogenous zones*. For example, during the first year the mouth is the most important erogenous zone, because the sucking activities of the child constitute his first essential contact with people. Hence, this stage is called the *oral stage*.

The broad Freudian concept of sexuality may at first be difficult to grasp, but it becomes easier to understand when one recollects that the mouth and the other erogenous zones are used in sexual fondness in adults. Though Freudian psychoanalysis uses the term "sexuality" in a very wide sense, it means basically what sexuality implies: the passionate yearnings of a person for other people and the physical sensations that may accompany such yearnings.

Oral Stage. In Freudian-psychoanalytic terminology, the first year of life is called the "oral stage" because the most crucial contact the infant has with people is through receiving food by sucking. The most intense perceptions he has of the world are his oral sensations during the feeding process; his main erogenous zone is the mouth.

In this process the child forms a strong libidinal attachment with his mother, his first *love object*. The oral stage is a time of complete dependency of the child on others, and the ways in which the child's dependent needs are met or not met have profound effects on his later personality structure. The child whose needs for satisfaction of his oral needs are not met may in later life have persistent difficulty in giving and accepting affection. His lifelong sense of well-being is affected by how much secure affection he gets at this time. The child whose oral needs are not adequately met may emerge with unfulfilled needs for affection and deep yearnings to be dependent on other people. He is said to have an "oral personality," and such persons are prone to have passive personality problems, depressions, various psychosomatic illnesses and other psychiatric difficulties. Some Freudian-psychoanalytic writers feel that in the latter half of the oral stage the child also has aggressive biting urges, and that the ways in which these urges are handled or frustrated affects the amount of aggressiveness or passivity the individual has in later years.

Anal Stage. The second and third years of life form the anal stage, because during this period the main erogenous zone is the anal mucosa. The child passes through an initial phase of interest in his feces and pleasure in alternately retaining them and excreting them. The parents, however, begin to toilet train the child and require him to control his feces in an orderly manner. Hence, much of the mother-child relationship in the second and third years centers on the toilet training process. If the mother-child relationship is sound and if the toilet training proceeds without hostile coercion, the child passes through this period without emotional trauma. However, if the mother-child relationship is characterized by hostility and coldness, the child often reacts with obstinate resistance and anger to toilet training.

Various persistent personality problems may arise out of the emotional traumas of a prolonged struggle over toilet training. When for an extended period of time the child obstinately refuses to defecate and holds back his feces in a toilet training struggle with his mother, he may be inclined to be excessively obstinate and frugal in later life. Excessive preoccupation with cleanliness during the anal period may lead the individual to be intensely preoccupied with order and meticulous neatness. Such a person may emerge from the anal period so concerned with order, precision, cleanliness, and the meticulous accumulation of material things that he has little capacity for warm relationships with people. He is mechanical and cold in his interpersonal relationships. Such a person is said to have an "anal personality."

Various kinds of psychiatric difficulties in later life may have their origins in emotional trauma in the anal period. Trauma during this period may contribute to obsessive compulsive neuroses, compulsive personality disorders, male homosexuality, unhealthy aggressiveness and various other emotional disorders.

Phallic Stage and the Oedipus Complex. Freudian-psychoanalytic theory proposes that between the ages of three and seven the child goes through an important period of development called the phallic stage. At this time the main erogenous zone moves to the genitals, and the child goes through a period of passionate attachment to the parent of the opposite sex and competitive hostility toward the parent of the same sex. Thus, the boy develops a passionate sexual fondness for his mother and hostile, competitive feelings toward his father. The girl develops passionate yearnings for her father and hostility toward her mother. This is viewed as a developmental phase through which every human being passes. It is called the "Oedipus" complex, after the Greek legendary figure Oedipus who slew his father and married his mother.

Because the child cannot in reality satisfy either his passionate yearnings or his hostile feelings during the Oedipal period, he experiences much emotional conflict. In addition, he fears hostile retaliation by the parent of the same sex. Thus, a boy fears retaliation from his father, with whom he feels he is competing for possession of the mother. In healthy personality development, after many vicissitudes the child resolves his Oedipal conflict by identifying with the parent of the same sex and preserves in a more moderate form his basic affectionate inclinations toward the parent of the opposite sex. Thus, a boy—in a sense—unconsciously resolves to be like his father since he cannot replace him, and the boy maintains his affection for his mother. The girl in a similar way identifies with her mother's role since she cannot displace the mother, and she maintains an affectionate orientation toward her father.

As Sir Carl Popper, the eminent British philosopher of science has pointed out, the Oedipus theory, along with almost all Freudian-psychoanalytic theories, is so set up that it can neither be proved nor disproved, and must forever remain a matter of faith. As Popper makes clear, there may be much or little truth in the Oedipus concept, but it cannot be considered scientific, nor can any therapy based on it be scientific. The matter is not settled by therapeutic results, since, as a number of impartial studies have shown, the percentage of patients who recover under Freudian-psychoanalytic therapy is no greater than the percentage who recover spontaneously.

Freudian-psychoanalytic theory proposes that out of the healthy resolution of his Oedipus conflict a boy assumes the masculine attitudes, orientations, standards and ideals of his father, and a girl in the resolution of her Oedipal complex takes on the feminine qualities, aspirations and ideals of her mother. All this development is largely unconscious in the child, who has little articulate awareness of any of the psychosexual development of his first seven years despite the strong passions involved.

Sometimes the child cannot resolve his Oedipal conflict in a healthy way. This may occur when the child's relationship with his parents is distorted by hostility, rejection, inadequate affection or various personality problems of the parents. Freudian-psychoanalytic theory hypothesizes that much of the anxiety of adult life is derived from unresolved Oedipal conflicts, and that this anxiety and the unhealthy methods of attempting to control it are at the root of a wide spectrum of psychiatric problems. Moreover, since the development of the superego (which is discussed later in this chapter and which is somewhat analogous to the lay term conscience) occurs in the latter part of the Oedipus period, Oedipal conflicts may contribute to a wide variety of neurotic, psychotic and personality problems. Hence, the incomplete or unhealthy resolution of the Oedipal period contributes heavily to a wide variety of later psychiatric difficulties.

If a child undergoes much emotional trauma at the oral, anal or Oedipal periods he may be crippled to some extent in his further psychosexual development. He ceases to mature in some areas of his personality development and maintains some of his childhood personality characteristics into adult life. This process is called *fixation*. For example, a dependent, clinging person who never progressed in some respects beyond the dependent phase of his oral period is said to have an *oral personality,* and he is said to be partially fixed at the oral stage of his development. Similarly, a person who is pathologically meticulous, orderly and frugal and who has excessive preoccupation with material things and has impaired capacity for warm relationships with people is said to have an *anal personality*. The term "narcissism" is applied to persons whose personality development is partially arrested at an infantile level in which the infant's chief concern is with the satisfaction of his own body needs and has little capacity for perceiving the needs of others. The narcissistic person in adult life is self-concerned, with little capacity for giving affection to other people, and he views other people only as objects to satisfy his needs and demands.

Latency Period. After the age of seven, and until puberty, the child goes through a period of relative quiescence in his psychosexual development; this stage is termed the "latency period" in Freudian-psychoanalytic theory.

At puberty and during adolescence the individual begins the development of his adult sexual maturation; this phase and the succeeding adult life of the person are called the *genital period*. By the time the genital period is reached, the person's basic personality structure and patterns of emotional functioning have been established, and subsequent changes are minor. The stresses of adult life may act as precipitants of emotional illness, but they are not true causes.

The Unconscious Mind

The Freudian-psychoanalytic approach places great importance in the concept of the unconscious mind. In the unconscious mind are locked the basic instinctual strivings, repressed urges, unresolved conflicts and many painful emotional experiences. The person is not aware of the restless turmoil in his unconscious mind, and its forces are unavailable to his conscious scrutiny by all the usual means of self-examination, thought and introspection.

Most of the contents of the unconscious mind are so emotionally painful and socially unacceptable to the person that they are actively prevented from reaching conscious awareness. Repressive, censoring mental forces keep them locked in the unconscious mind. Psychoanalytic theory maintains that the major means by which unconscious feelings and ideas may reach articulate awareness is by the technics of psychoanalytic interview treatment. This treatment seeks (by technics outlined later in this chapter) to resolve the stresses caused by unconscious turmoil by bringing them into awareness and helping the individual to achieve comfortable resolution of them.

The painful conflicts of the unresolved traumas of the oral, anal and Oedipal period become locked in the unconscious mind. Each trauma is organized into a group of unresolved basic urges, feelings and ideas called a *complex*. For example, the persistent traumas of the Oedipal period may persist as an Oedipal *complex*. During his Oedipal period a boy may fear that his father will retaliate against him because of his hostile feelings toward the father in competition for the mother's affection. The boy's apprehension may be focused on fear of retaliative damage to his genitals— a *castration complex*. These complexes continue to have effect on the person's emotional life so long as they are unsolved.

Freudian-psychoanalytic thought defines *repression* as an important mechanism by which painful emotional experiences are submerged into the unconscious mind during the child's psychosexual development. Repression is an unconscious process, and after repression of a painful conflict all conscious memory of it is removed. Sometimes the individual substitutes a false, pleasant memory to cover up a true, painful memory; the false memory serves to hide the painful event from the person's awareness and is called a "screen" memory.

However, the power of the repressive and censoring part of the mind is sometimes insufficient to keep the tumultuous contents of the unconscious mind submerged. The simmering, unresolved conflicts push to the surface; this is called *the return of the repressed*. As the repressed material impinges on the limits of conscious awareness, much painful distress floods the person; this painful distress is *anxiety*. Anxiety plays an important role in setting in motion chains of events which produce psychiatric symptoms.

A person may experience anxiety directly, producing the clinical picture of an anxiety neurosis. However, various mental mechanisms often operate to prevent the person from experiencing the pain of anxiousness. These unconscious mechanisms for deviating anxiety into other less painful channels are called *defense mechanisms*. Repression is one of the most important defense mechanisms. The ways in which the defense mechanisms operate produce a wide spectrum of psychiatric symptoms. In the following section we shall describe how Freudian-psychoanalytic theory suggests that some of the other defense mechanisms work.

Defense Mechanisms

Displacement. This is a defense mechanism in which the basic emotion causing anxiety is transferred from its original object to a new one. By its nature, the new object helps to prevent the person from coming to grips with his true, prohibitively painful conflict. For example, a boy may have a profound fear of his father, and this fear presses for some sort of expression. To come to grips with his fear and his conjoined hostility to his father would be devastating for the boy. Therefore, his fear is displaced to another object. It might be displaced to dogs, or automobiles, or the dark, and the child develops a conscious strong fear of dogs, or automobiles, or the dark. He is aware of his fear of dogs, but he unaware that it is a displaced fear of his father. Hence, in an unhealthy way and at the expense of developing a pathological fear, he resolves his unconscious conflict. In this way, displacement produces phobias and may contribute to other forms of psychiatric illness.

Conversion. Conversion is a defense mechanism in which unacceptable, unconscious emotions and conflicts are converted into specific types of physical symptoms. The resultant clinical picture is called a "conversion reaction." Conversion reactions and "dissociative reactions" (discussed in the following paragraph) constitute the disorders termed "hysterical neuroses" in the current standard nomenclature; they are termed "hysterical neurosis, conversion type" and "hysterical neurosis, dissociative type."

The nature of the particular hysterical conversion symptom usually has symbolic ties to the type of conflict which produced it. For example, a law student who had a long-standing hostile relationship with his father was attending law school largely because of his father's insistence. During the first year of law school he developed a hysterical conversion paralysis of his right hand which made writing impossible and greatly interfered with his legal studies.

Dissociation. In dissociation the painful conflict and its attendant anxiety produce an altered state of consciousness which impairs memory and in many cases allows some of the underlying turmoil to take over the person's actions and achieve release. Dissociation produces such symptoms as hysterical amnesias, amnesic fugue states, multiple personalities and other similar disorders (covered in Chapter 9).

Denial. In the defense mechanism of denial, the person denies the existence of emotions, thoughts, or whole areas of feeling and knowledge; in this way, denial prevents painful conflicts from producing overt anxiety. I recall, for example, a 42-year-old single woman who had spent her life living with her mother. She was emotionally dependent on her mother, but behind her dependence lurked much hostility against the mother who had selfishly kept her chained. When the mother died suddenly the patient was grieved to lose her lifelong companion and at the same time unconsciously relieved at her abrupt release from her domination. In the conflictual turbulence of the first week of her grieving period, she at times denied that her mother was dead. For periods of half a day at a time she behaved as if her mother were still alive. In Freudian-psychoanalytic terms, her reaction would be called a "denial mechanism."

Reaction Formation. A reaction formation is a type of defense mechanism in which the person unconsciously takes on attitudes and behavior which are the opposite of his painful feelings. He adopts opposite behavior to hide from himself his emotionally unacceptable urges. For example, a mother may have strong feelings of hostility and rejection toward an unwanted child. She unconsciously finds these feelings so unacceptable and painful that, to hide these feelings from herself, she adopts an overly solicitous, overprotective, hovering behavior toward the child.

Regression. In regression a person unconsciously seeks to avoid anxiety by a return to an immature stage of his life. For example, a woman who finds the problems of marriage and child rearing too stressful may regress into the immature role of a dependent child. She may flee into psychogenic physical symptoms that allow her to become a dependent, childlike invalid, and she thus frees herself of the complex responsibilities of marriage and child rearing which she finds overwhelming. Regression in a wide variety of degrees is a a common defense mechanism. Minor instances of regression occur occasionally in most people under stress; in painful circumstances they may regress for a short time to childish levels of behavior. Overwhelming regression plays a large role in schizophrenic illnesses and other psychiatric disorders (which are covered in later chapters).

Projection. Projection is a defense mechanism in which a person unconsciously rejects emotionally unacceptable features of himself and attributes them to other people. For example, an individual with strong hostile feelings may reject these feelings as existing within himself and attribute them instead to various people around him. In a sense, he unconsciously says, "I am not the hostile one. It is the people around me who are hostile to me, do not like me and persecute me." Projection in minor degrees is common. It is common knowledge that some people tend to see their own faults in others; a dishonest man often suspects others of trickery. Severe degrees of projection, however, play an important role in paranoid schizophrenia and other psychiatric illnesses. Freudian-psychoanalytic theory proposes that many delusions and hallucinations are projections of the individual's inner tumult and unacceptable urges onto the outside world

Sublimation. Sublimation is the healthiest mechanism of defense. In sublimation the repressed instinctual forces and unacceptable feelings of the person are channeled into socially acceptable activities. Through sublimation instinctual drives and other powerful feelings provide the energy for many creative activities. For example, repressed aggressive forces may be channeled into energetic activity in business and professional life, and repressed sexuality finds diluted, diffuse expression in broad social activities, in helping others, and in affectionate acts in friendships and community life. Freudian-psychoanalytic theory suggests that a major cohesive force in uniting social groups is a diffuse sublimation of sexual drives, and that most of the creative, artistic and scientific activities of people are produced by sublimation of basic instinctual forces.

Rationalization. This is a defense mechanism in which a person unconsciously finds seemingly plausible reasons to justify actions caused by repressed unacceptable feelings. For example, I recall a father who had much hostility toward his 15-year-old son who had been an unwanted child at birth and a persistent inconvenience to the father since then. The father could not consciously come to grips with the true reasons for his persistent hostile, rejecting feelings toward the boy. Instead, he rationalized his continual harsh criticism and depreciation of his son by saying that the boy was lazy, disobedient and malicious. In actuality, the boy had none of the defects of which his father accused him. However, by his chronic depreciation of his son the father rationalized his profound hostility toward him. Most persons rationalize some of their acts to a limited extent, but many times rationalization becomes an unhealthy method for justifying unacceptable urges, feelings and actions.

Introjection. In Freudian-psychoanalytic terminology, introjection is a defense mechanism in which the person turns inward upon himself feelings that he has toward other people, but that he cannot comfortably express toward them. For example, a person may be so uncomfortable with his hostile feelings toward his father that he cannot become aware of them; instead, he turns his hostile feelings inward upon himself. He then becomes very critical and depreciating of himself, venting upon himself the hostility he unconsciously feels toward his father. In this manner, introjection is an important mechanism in causing depressions. The ultimate in inwardly directed hostility toward oneself is self-destruction.

In Freudian-psychoanalytic theory, *incorporation* is a defense mechanism closely allied to introjection. In incorporation the person symbolically takes another person inside himself and vents toward himself the feelings he has toward that person. Incorporation is viewed as a primitive, infantile mechanism in which the infant in his fantasies orally swallows up the other person. The mechanism of incorporation may persist into adult life.

Introjection and incorporation are the opposite of the previously discussed defense mechanism of projection, in which the person's unacceptable feelings are cast out of himself onto other people.

Identification. Identification is used in Freudian-psychoanalytic terminology to designate a defense mechanism in which the individual resolves painful feelings about an important person in his life by unconsciously taking on the personality characteristics of that person. In a sense, the individual unconsciously resolves to be like the person about whom he is in conflict, since he cannot in any other way resolve his mixed attitudes toward him. As pointed out earlier in this chapter, identification is the method by which the child resolves his Oedipal conflict. Since in his Oedipal conflict a boy cannot effectively compete with his father for the possession of his mother, he unconsciously decides to be like his father. An oversimplified version of identification is found in the old adage, "If you can't beat 'em, join 'em." Many psychiatrists use the term identification in a broader sense than the Freudian-psychoanalytic sense. (Its broader use is employed in Chapter 1 and in later sections of this text.)

Other Mechanisms. Various Freudian-psychoanalytic writers describe other mechanisms of defense. These to a certain extent overlap the defense mechanisms we have described above.

Compensation is a mechanism in which the individual unconsciously attempts to ward off anxious doubts about his capabilities and attributes by reassuring behavior. Thus, a man with fears of physical inadequancy and weakness may act the role of a blustering bully to hide his fears from himself.

In the defense mechanism of *intellectualization* the individual uses elaborate ideas and reasons to deny the existence of unconscious feelings and to avoid recognition of them. Thus, a person with pathological aggressiveness may intellectualize that he is legitimately defending his natural rights against large numbers of people who would exploit and dominate him if he did not fight back so forcefully.

Isolation is a defense mechanism in which painful thoughts, feelings and memories are emotionally separated from the experiences to which they rightfully belong. For example, a man who had a conflictual relationship with his parents may talk of their deaths in an unemotional, impersonal way. His tumultuous feelings attached to their deaths are isolated, and may find separate expression later in an unrelated context. He may break down crying at a later time without apparent reason. The event and the emotions have been isolated from each other.

In *symbolization*, an emotionally painful object, idea or person is blotted from awareness and another object is put in its place. The second object is the symbol of the first. Symbolization occurs frequently in emotional processes, but one of the clearest examples is in dreams. For example, a child who has much dread of his father may not be consciously aware of this fear, but in his dreams he sees himself threatened by masked assailants who are symbols of his father.

Some psychiatrists use the term *substitution* to designate a defense mechanism in which emotionally painful objects or experiences are replaced by other objects or experiences that can be achieved and comfortably enjoyed. Substitution is closely allied to other defense mechanisms and overlaps them.

In *undoing* the patient carries out a physical act by which he symbolically tries to cancel out a previous act that has much anxiety or guilt attached to it. The compulsive handwashing common in compulsive neuroses is usually an attempt to undo previous guilt-ridden acts, such as masturbation, by symbolically washing the guilt away; undoing is common in compulsive neuroses.

Personality Structure

Id. Freud developed a three-layer concept of personality structure. At the bottom is the id, a turbulent mass of instinctual forces. The contents of the id are entirely unconscious, and the person becomes aware of them only through their disguised, indirect products. Many unconscious, repressed conflicts and complexes also are lodged in the id.

Freud described two basic instincts in the id. The first is libido (discussed earlier), the basis of all the person's sexual, social and creative strivings. In later writings Freud redefined libido as part of a broader life instinct, *Eros,* which contains all the instinctual forces that preserve life and impel the person to seek emotional closeness with others.

Late in his life Freud also defined a second basic instinct, *Thanatos,* the death instinct. Thanatos was viewed as the opposite of Eros, or libido. It impelled the person to aggressiveness, destructive actions and, in its final stages and in unclear ways, to his own death and dissolution. However, the concept of the death instinct has not been widely accepted among Freudian psychoanalysts and is not an established feature of psychoanalytic theory.

Ego. The ego is superimposed on the id and is the part of the personality structure dealing directly with the environment of the person. The ego has three main functions: (1) It must modify and channel the instinctual drives of the id in socially and emotionally acceptable ways. (2) It must perceive and interpret the environment of the person, and carry out his actions in relation to his environment. (3) It must also correlate and moderate the impact of the superego (discussed in the next section) with the id and with the external environment. In addition, the mechanisms of defense discussed in the preceding section are all functions of the ego in protecting the person from the impact of painful anxiety. The ego is not present at birth. It gradually forms as the person experiences contact with his environment during his formative years.

The concept of the ego is closely involved with the concepts of the *pleasure principle* and the *reality principle.* Freudian-psychoanalytic theory holds that the instinctual (and other) forces of the id are under constant tension for expression and release. Man continually seeks to avoid discomfort and to find release for his basic needs and drives. This constitutes the "pleasure principle." However, the realities of the social and cultural environment of man require that his instinctual forces be modified and harnessed in many ways. This is termed the "reality principle." A large part of the ego's work is in moderating the demands of the pleasure principle to conform with the requirements of the reality principle.

In Freudian-psychoanalytic terminology those experiences or forces that are harmonious with the aims and comfort of the ego are called *ego-syntonic.* Those experiences and forces that are painful to the ego are called *ego-dystonic.*

Modern psychoanalysts give much attention to *ego psychology,* which is the study of the structure of the ego and its many functions. The analysis of the structure and functions of the ego in psychoanalytic treatment is called *ego analysis.* As psychoanalysis reached the middle of the 20th Century, analysts were faced with two basic problems: (1) the need to bring psychoanalytic theory into harmony with the concepts of extrafamilial social and cultural influences which obviously affect personality development and emotional functioning, and (2) the need to divorce some aspects of psychoanalysis from Freud's biologically oriented concepts of crude id urges producing conflicts with ego and superego forces. Hartmann and other American analysts have attempted to achieve these goals on a theoretical level by hypothesizing that there are areas of the ego that are autonomous of the id, and that there are ego urges which operate as independent motivating sources. These highly abstract proposals have caused much controversy among psychoanalysts, and coverage of them obviously lies beyond the scope of this book.

Superego. The third of the three parts of the personality structure (the first two being the id and the ego) is the superego, which lies above the ego and contains the moral restrictions and ideals of the person. The superego contains those features that in lay language are attributed to conscience. When the person contemplates or carries out actions contrary to the principles contained in the superego, the superego inflicts pain on the ego. This pain is *guilt,* a feeling which has wide implications in normal and abnormal emotional functioning. By use of guilt, the superego works to keep the person within the bounds of moral restrictions.

According to Freudian-psychoanalytic

theory, the major part of the superego is formed in the resolution of the Oedipal conflict. As described earlier in the chapter, during the resolution of his Oedipus complex the child takes on the moral standards, ideals and restrictions of the parent of the same sex. Freudian-psychoanalytic theory holds that the child incorporates into himself symbolic images of his parents, and that these images are woven into the structure of the superego. Thus, the superego contains the admonishing, correcting forces of the parents. A small child does not do morally reprehensible things because he fears censure and punishment from his parents. The adult does not do morally reprehensible things because he fears the painful censure and admonishment of his superego, which contains the incorporated images of his parents. Though other cultural and social forces may contribute to superego formation, the influence of parents is much greater.

A superego may be unduly harsh or unduly lax. If the child had harsh, unhealthy relationships with parents who made him feel guilty and inadequate, his superego, which incorporates the parental images, may be overly harsh and punishing. The superego may then flood the ego with pathological guilt and depreciation. Thus, a punitive superego plays a significant role in producing depressions, obsessive compulsive neuroses and various other psychiatric difficulties. On the other hand, the superego may be unduly lax. It may not inflict enough guilt on the ego to keep the person from committing morally and socially prohibited acts. A lax superego contributes heavily to the formation of antisocial and dyssocial personality disorders and other personality problems.

In the Freudian-psychoanalytic approach, many psychiatric disturbances are described as due to imbalances in the forces of the id, the ego and the superego with each other. Thus, an anxiety neurosis is produced when the forces of the id overpower the ego and threaten to push painful instinctual urges into the person's awareness. A depression results when an overly punitive superego inflicts painful guilt on a weakened ego. These are simplified examples of the actually complex interactions of the id, the ego and the superego. Every psychiatric disturbance involves complex interactions of all three sections of the personality. Also, concomitant interactions of the ego with the interpersonal environment of the person often play a significant role.

Emotional conflicts are sometimes divided into *intrapsychic conflicts* and *extrapsychic conflicts*. An intrapsychic conflict is a disturbance of the relationships of the id, the ego and the superego. It is caused by unresolved stresses in the person's past life and is not significantly related to current problems with people in his environment. An extrapsychic conflict is a disturbance between the person and current people in his environment. It operates largely through the ego, but is always influenced as well by the contents of the id and the superego.

The Concepts and Terminology of Freudian-Psychoanalytic Therapy

In completing our coverage of Freudian psychoanalysis, it is necessary to give a brief summary of the basic concepts and terminology used in Freudian-psychoanalytic therapy. Our primary concern here is to define the terms used in that therapy and to list the concepts it employs. (In Chapter 21 on psychotherapy, we shall further discuss psychotherapy from the Freudian-psychoanalytic point of view and compare it with other forms of psychotherapy.)

Freud developed a system of treatment technics designed to resolve the unconscious conflicts of the patient and free him of his emotional difficulties. The psychiatrists who adhere closely to Freud's concepts of treatment are called *psychoanalysts*.

Free Association. In Freudian-psychoanalytic therapy the patient is required to follow the *basic rule* of spontaneously putting into words without hesitation or interruption all the thoughts and feelings that come to mind during each treatment session. In classical Freudian-psychoanalytic technic the patient does this while lying on a couch. The sessions last 50 minutes each, and occur three to five times each week; the total treatment lasts from three to five years. The process of verbalizing unreservedly all one's thoughts and feelings is called *free association*.

Freudian-psychoanalytic theory holds that

through the process of free association the unconscious urges, thoughts, feelings and repressed conflicts of the person gradually come to the surface. By his *interpretations* the psychiatrist helps bring the pathological unconscious forces within the patient to conscious awareness, and he helps the patient to resolve his repressed conflicts and to find healthy, socially acceptable expression for his instinctive drives. In practice, the work of analysis is more complex than this simple model indicates, but these are the essential principles.

Transference. Transference is an important concept in Freudian-psychoanalytic therapy. In transference the patient casts upon the therapist his unresolved feelings such as hate, love or dependent yearning, which are attached to the patient's unresolved conflicts; these unresolved feelings arose originally in traumatic relationships with close people during the patient's childhood. Thus, a person who has strong repressed hostility to his father may go through a period of much antagonism to the analyst while working out his unresolved conflicts about his father.

Transference may be positive or negative. In a *positive* transference, the patient has affectionate, admiring feelings toward the psychoanalyst. In a *negative* transference, the patient has antagonistic, hostile feelings toward the analyst. Transference occurs in the context of a *transference neurosis*, in which the patient emotionally repeats with the psychoanalyst the original traumatic conflicts he experienced in childhood with his parents. The strong feelings, such as anger or dependent clinging, that the patient develops in transference may evoke feelings in the therapist are called *countertransference*. Desirably, the analyst has much self-knowledge and a sound personality structure which reduces countertransference feelings to a minimum and prevents them from obscuring the therapist's objective view of the patient's problems. By analysis of the transference situation the patient gains an intense insight into his repressed conflicts. In the transference relationship with the therapist the patient resolves unconscious emotional problems that he was not able to work out with his parents.

Through the therapist's interpretations the patient gains *insight*. He achieves *intellecutal* insight as he gains an articulate awareness of his conflicts and feelings. He gains *emotional* insight as he works out his unconscious conflicts in the emotional turmoil of resolving his transference feelings about the therapist. When the therapy is successful, the patient gradually resolves his emotional problems through intellectual and emotional insight and resolution of transference.

However, Freudian-psychoanalytic theory proposes that the emergence into consciousness of the patient's emotional conflicts and painful memories is opposed by mental forces that strive to keep them out of his awareness. These mental forces are called *resistances*. Much of the therapist's work consists in identifying and removing these resistances, most of which are unconscious. Resistances may take many forms. For example, the patient may stop talking, or he may talk profusely about trivial things to deflect attention from the crucial issues of the analysis. Some of the defense mechanisms, such as rationalization and intellectualization (discussed earlier in this chapter), may occur as unconscious resistances to the therapeutic process. Resistances appear in all phases of the treatment, and dealing with them is one of the psychoanalyst's major tasks.

Character Analysis. The patient often must become aware of many aspects of his character structure obstructing the work of the analysis; this is called *character analysis*. For example, a very dependent patient with a strong need to please everyone may be unwilling to say anything he fears might annoy the therapist. Such a patient must become aware that this part of his character structure is obstructing effective treatment. Also, as mentioned earlier, analysis of ego functions occupies a prominent place in modern psychoanalytic procedure and is called *ego analysis*.

The unconscious mind sometimes reveals itself in slips of the tongue and similar errors of actions and words. For example, the patient in treatment may accidentally call the therapist "father," revealing a facet of his transference feelings at the time. In another instance, the patient during a period of hostile transference may mistake the hour of his appointment and come too late to see the therapist. Freud termed such errors the *psychopathology of everyday life.* They reveal unconscious feelings and thoughts both in everyday life and in psychoanalytic treatment, and they can be used in interpretations during therapy.

Interpretation of Dreams. Freudian-psychoanalytic treatment puts much emphasis on the *interpretation of dreams.* Freud called dream analysis "the royal road to the unconscious." Freudian-psychoanalytic theory holds that in dreams the unconscious feelings, urges and conflicts of the person find expression. However, to protect the person from crude awareness of his painful conflicts, which would frequently awaken him from sleep, the material of the dream is disguised and camouflaged by elaborate mental processes. Thus, the dream has a *manifest* content, which the person perceives in his dream. Behind the manifest content is the *latent* content, which contains the true, undisguised unconscious conflicts and urges. Between the latent content and the manifest content stands the *censor,* a force which prevents the painful latent conflicts from intruding unchanged into the dream. The process of changing the conflicts of the latent content into the narrative pictures of the manifest content is called the *dream work.* By the spontaneous, uninhibited flow of his free associations, the patient traces the various parts of the dream, or the dream as a whole, back to its unconscious meanings. Thus, in a simplified example, a person who had a hostile relationship with his brother may dream of two savage animals fighting each other; through his free associations he discovers that the two animals symbolize his brother and himself, and by further analyzing the dream he may discover various aspects of the unconscious fears and hostilities that existed in his relationship with his brother.

The dream work of camouflaging the unconscious content of the dream consists of several mental operations. They are: (a) *symbolization,* in which a new object, person or action is substituted for the true object, person or action; the symbol usually has some characteristics in common with the object it represents; (b) *condensation,* in which two or more persons or concepts are fused into a single item in the dream, which represents all the contributing sources; (c) *elaboration,* in which disguising features are added to the details of the dream; (d) *overdetermination,* in which two or more emotions or unconscious conflicts are represented by one feeling or event in the dream narrative; and (e) *displacement,* in which meanings and feelings are displaced from the true source to a disguising object in the dream.

The mental operations of dreams are also characteristic of the primitive thinking processes of infants. In Freudian-psychoanalytic terminology this primitive type of mental activity is called *primary process* thinking. In adults, primary process thinking persists in dreams, in the unconscious mind and in some psychiatric disturbances. During childhood, primary process thinking is gradually succeeded by *secondary process* thinking, which is the rational, logical thinking needed for the daily dealings of the person with his realistic environment.

CONCEPTS FROM SYSTEMS THAT WERE OUTGROWTHS FROM THE FREUDIAN-PSYCHOANALYTIC APPROACH

Several of Freud's early followers formed divergent schools of thought. They included Jung, Adler and Rank (whose positions in the history of the development of modern psychiatry are noted in Chapter 2). Adler and Rank never achieved a wide following among psychiatrists, and their influence has tended to fade with time; however, a few of their concepts have achieved a permanent niche in modern psychiatric terminology.

Jung, on the other hand, has always had a small but dedicated following among psychiatrists, psychologists and other behavioral and social scientists, and this following has increased perceptibly in the 1970's; his influence in Europe is decidedly greater than in the United States. The amount of literature about Jung and his concepts has grown markedly in recent years, in both the United States and Europe.

Concepts from Jung

Jung developed a complex system of theories about personality structure and emotional functioning. He called his system *analytic psychology*. His concepts that have attracted the most attention are *extraversion, introversion,* the *personal unconscious,* the *collective unconscious, archetypes,* and the existence in man of inborn, unconscious needs and capacities for certain basic beliefs that can be termed spiritual, or philosophical.

Extraversion and Introversion. Jung divided personality structures into two main groups, depending on whether the emotional orientation of the person was mainly in other people or in himself.

The emotional energy of the extravert is directed mainly toward other people. He is gregarious, active and outgoing, and he is more inclined to vigorous action than to quiet contemplation. The introvert, on the other hand, directs most of his emotional energy inward toward himself and is less involved in close relationships with people. He tends to be quiet, studious, contemplative and socially solitary. Jung further divided extraverts and introverts into various subgroups.

Most psychiatrists have found this type of classification of people inadequate to describe the full range of variations in personality structure, but the terms extravert and introvert have become established in popular lay usage and find occasional employment in psychiatric terminology.

The Personal Unconscious and the Collective Unconscious. Jung divided the unconscious into two major divisions, the "personal" unconscious and the "collective" unconscious. The personal unconscious contains the unconscious feelings, thoughts and memories which have been repressed during the individual's lifetime. They can be recovered in analytic therapy.

The collective unconscious, on the other hand, is the same in all humans. It contains inborn tendencies, or capacities, for thinking and feeling in various specific ways; it includes various images, crude beliefs and basic ways of conceiving things. The collective unconscious is passed hereditarily from one generation to the next, presumably in the chromosomal structures of cerebral cortical brain cells. It is not directly discoverable or recoverable by the individual, since he has never directly experienced it. It is only indirectly discernible in widespread myths, legends, ideas and ways of conceiving things that are found in some form in all cultures and civilizations. Much of the material of the collective unconscious is organized around *archetypes*, which are discussed below. For many years most psychiatrists and other behavioral scientists considered the concepts of the collective unconscious and archetypes outlandish, but recent advances in understanding chromosomal structures and the ways in which inborn tendencies for specific behavior are made manifest in lower animals (the work of Lorenz and others) have caused some psychiatrists and behavioral scientists to take a more tolerant view of these subjects.

Archetypes. In Jungian psychology, an archetype is a basic tendency to think, to visualize and to act in fairly specific ways, and it is inherited. These tendencies, or capacities, become manifest in ways of thinking, visual images and narrative accounts; the experiences of the individual give form and substance to them. Archetypes include such prototypal concepts as the all-giving Mother, the rescuing Hero, the all-knowing Helper, the utopian Paradise, the all-creating Godhead, and others. The specific idea, image, or way of feeling is not inherited in an archetype; only the capacity for such a development is inherited, and its particular form is determined by the culture in which the person is reared.

It is obvious from examination of the archetypes listed above that Jungian psychology can easily be made consonant with a religious (or other spiritual) approach to life. Indeed, Jung stated that in many of his patients, especially those in middle age, a common problem was the inadequate realization and development of those archetypes which had spiritual possibilities. Jung seems to imply, though he never clearly states, that total human development requires coming to grips with the derivatives of such archetypes as the all-creating Godhead. In this he is in marked contrast to Freud, who was an uncompromising atheist and whose attitude toward religion is reflected in both the title and the content of his book "The Future of an Illusion." It is, perhaps, this capacity of Jungian psychology to include in its framework the added dimension of religious experience that has caused a marked growth in interest in it during the 1970's, when disillusionment with materialism has become widespread in Europe and America.

Concepts of Adler

Adler's concept of the *inferiority complex* has achieved a persistent position in modern psychiatric thinking, though often it is cast in different terms. Adler felt that emotional problems frequently were caused by a sense of inferiority regardless of whether the feeling was partially justified or not. The individual reacts against his fears of inferiority with aggressive strivings to demonstrate to himself and others that his fears of inferiority are not valid. Out of the tumult of such feelings and their inadequate resolution, many psychiatric problems arise. Though the concept of the inferiority complex, often under other terms, has been widely used in psychiatry, most psychiatrists feel that it explains only a small part of the emotional turbulence which causes psychiatric disorders. Adler called his system *individual psychology*.

Concepts of Rank

Rank developed a complex system of theories concerning personality development, psychiatric illness and psychotherapy. Although his concepts never achieved widespread acceptance, two of his ideas have had some influence on a small number of psychiatrists. These are his concepts of the *birth trauma* and *individuation*.

Rank felt that the experience of birth, in which the person leaves the protective security of the maternal body and enters a world of difficult physical and emotional adjustments, is an emotionally traumatic event that leads to much anxiety in later life. He also felt that most human beings preserve an unconscious wish to flee the stresses of life and seek some kind of sheltering substitute for the maternal uterus. Rank viewed personality development as a long struggle to achieve full, separate individuality from the mother and to achieve complete comfort as an autonomous person. He called this process "individuation" and viewed it as the fundamental process in personality development. He felt that much psychiatric illness was due to the inabilities of persons to conquer the impact of the birth trauma and to achieve full individuation. The concept of individuation, usually separated from the concept of the birth trauma, has been employed by some child psychiatrists as a useful theoretical framework.

BEHAVIOR THEORY AND BEHAVIOR THERAPY

Various schools of psychologic thought and psychiatric practice have evolved out of the work of the Russian neurophysiologist Ivan P. Pavlov, who received a Nobel Prize in 1904 for his studies of conditioned reflexes in dogs and other animals. Pavlov and his collaborators also developed an elaborate system of human psychology in which the conditioning stimuli were the words and actions of people and broader social forces. As mentioned in Chapter 2, psychiatry in the Soviet Union and its dependent nations has adopted this body of theory as the basis for its standard psychologic viewpoints and modes of psychiatric practice.

However, in the United States and Western Europe a number of schools of psychology and psychiatry (independent of the Soviet system and differing from it in many ways) have grown out of Pavlov's work. In the 1920's the American psychologist J. B. Watson elaborated a conditioned reflex concept of human behavior which he termed "behaviorism"; for 10 or 15 years it attracted much attention, but interest in it then subsided. Since then, other schools of thought based to some extent on Pavlovian principles have arisen and have enjoyed varying degrees of popularity; they include the theoretical systems called "learning theory," "operant conditioning," behavior theory," "behavior therapy," and others. Workers prominent in these schools include Skinner, Eysenck, Mowrer, Hunt, Dollard, Neal, Wolpe, Lazarus and many others. Since the concepts of these writers overlap so extensively it would be tedious and confusing to trace the development of their various points of view.

At the present time, *in psychiatry* the most widely discussed and clinically practiced form of Pavlovian-derived work is designated by the terms "behavior theory" and "behavior therapy." We shall outline its central themes, but in doing so we shall also be sketching the main features of its predecessors and less prominent contemporaries.

Pavlov found that in a lower animal, such as a dog, a repetitive stimulus such as a bell would cause a predictable response of salivation if each ringing of the bell was followed by offering the dog food. Thereafter, for a limited time, the dog would salivate every time the bell was rung, even if food was not offered. This was called a *conditioned reflex*. This reflex could be *reinforced* by repeating the bell-food sequence periodically, or it could become *extinct* if repeated ringing of the bell was not followed by offers of food. Also, the conditioned reflex could be more quickly extinguished if the dog was given short, painful electric shocks after each ringing of the bell, instead of food. Pavlov and his colleagues went on from these simple experiments into complex sets of experiments and theories that sought to explain all animal and human behavior in related neurophysiological ways.

Behavior theory proposes that human personality characteristics and modes of emotional functioning are molded by the rewards or pain that the growing infant, child and adolescent receives for various kinds of behavior throughout his formative years. He tends to adopt those types of behavior, thinking and feeling which bring gratifying responses (rewards) from his parents, other close persons and the social environment; he tends to desist from behavior that causes discomfort and pain. In man, rewards and pain are mainly interpersonal; the rewards consist of love, approval and acceptance, and the pain includes loss of love, disapproval and lack of acceptance (or outright hostility) from both familial persons and broader social groups.

Behavior theory looks on personality characteristics and emotional functioning as fluid, ongoing processes that are constantly reinforced or extinguished by the kinds of responses (rewards or pain) that the individual meets in his environment. Thus, a pattern of behavior (such as marital affection or job enthusiasm) may become extinct if an individual does not receive rewarding, pleasurable responses from the persons (marital partner or work associates, in the simple cases cited here) in his particular environment; also, more general factors, such as economic stresses in the marriage or severe tensions in the job situation, may affect the individual's patterns of behavior. Behavior is therefore subject to constant change depending on how the environment reacts to reinforce (by pleasure and rewards) or extinguish (by pain and lack of rewards) it. Of course, in its full development behavior theory is much more complex than this; behavior, which includes patterns of thinking and feeling as well as overt action, is affected by processes termed desensitization, reinforcement, reciprocal inhibition, extinction, conditioned avoidance, negative reinforcement and others (which we shall discuss when we cover the therapeutic applications of behavior theory in Chapter 21).

Since the 1960's behavior therapy, the term commonly applied to therapeutic technics based on behavior theory, has enjoyed a marked increase in interest, and a small but growing percentage of American and British psychiatrists and clinical psychologists now use it as their main method of treatment. Although we shall give more detailed consideration to behavior therapy in the chapter on psychotherapeutic technics, we shall here sketch an instance of its application to clarify the clinical possibilities of behavior theory.

Behavior theory proposes that a phobia is, in somewhat oversimplified terms, a conditioned reflex of alarm and anxiety to a particular type of objects or situations. For example, a child with a phobia of cats has developed a conditioned reflex of apprehension and revulsion to cats because of repetitive anxious or painful experiences with them in his past life. Treatment therefore may focus on progressively desensitizing the child to cats in small increments. In a number of therapeutic sessions the therapist talks reassuringly to the child about cats, shows him pictures of cats and praises him for his lack of alarm about them, has him touch pictures of cats, instructs him to draw outlines of cats and gives him candy or other rewards for this performance, lets him play with toy cats, permits him to see cats at a distance, urges him to come close to cats and gives him praise and small presents when he does so, and finally succeeds in having him fondle cats. Thus the child is desensitized to cats and loses his phobia of them.

Although the behavior therapist investigates his patient's past to determine how he developed his problem, his treatment concentrates more on *present* stimuli and responses, and their *future* consequences. This separates behavior therapy markedly from other psychotherapeutic approaches (such as the interpersonal approach and the Freudian-psychoanalytic approach) which emphasize exploration and resolution of past etiologic experiences. Psychiatrists of other theoretical persuasions sometimes criticize behavior therapy as oversimplified and rooted in animal experiments that are not relevant to man, but impartial investigations have repeatedly shown that in some types of psychiatric problems, such as phobias, behavior therapy gives better results than other forms of psychotherapy and that removal of symptoms by behavior therapy is rarely followed by the development of other symptoms in their places.

Our opinion is that behavior theory cannot explain the full range of personality development, interpersonal relationships and emotional functioning, and that behavior therapy is limited in its clinical applicability. However, behavior theory does have a contribution to make in understanding some aspects of man's psychology and behavior therapy will probably achieve in time a secure place in the treatment of some kinds of psychiatric problems. Its usefulness in phobias is clear and its value in other kinds of disorders is under evaluation. Some behavior therapists advocate use of a combination of behavior therapy technics and other psychotherapeutic methods; there is ample room for such fusion. Even Sigmund Freud over half a century ago said that at some point in the psychoanalysis of a phobic patient, the therapist must sternly insist that the patient begin to face his phobia in increasing degrees if treatment is to be successful.

VARIOUS OTHER CONCEPTS CONCERNING EMOTIONAL FUNCTIONING

In this chapter we have surveyed a broad spectrum of concepts and terms which are used in psychiatry. In this final section we shall define some miscellaneous concepts which have not been covered elsewhere.

Ambivalence. The simultaneous existence in a person of two opposing emotions, drives or attitudes regarding another person, or regarding a specific object or situation, is called ambivalence. For example, a person may simultaneously have feelings of affection and anger toward the same individual, or he may yearn for a specific situation and yet fear it.

Ambivalence is universal in emotional functioning. If his feelings are analyzed fully, a person rarely has a completely pure feeling toward any situation or person. However, ambivalence occurs with special intensity in many psychiatric problems. The coexistence of love and hate, or of yearning and fear, toward important persons in the patient's life often excites strong feelings of guilt and anxiety. The patient may or may not be aware of his ambivalence. Often he knows of only one aspect of his feelings. For example, he may be aware only of his affectionate and dependant yearnings, and he may be unaware of his coexistent hostility or fear. Hence, ambivalence is a frequent cause of emotional distress and a common contributant to psychiatric difficulties.

Fantasy. In fantasy a person envisions actions, circumstances and events in which he sees himself and others playing emotionally significant roles. Conscious, well-organized fantasy is popularly called "day-dreaming." Fantasy, in its broadest psychiatric sense, may be conscious or unconscious and it plays a large role in emotional life. Most fantasies are wish fulfilling and pleasant, but some of them express fears, ruminative worries and painful personality problems.

Fantasy can be constructive. The individual can work out plans for his social and vocational life in fantasies he judiciously moderates for execution in day-to-day life. Artists, writers and many business and professional people use well-organized fantasies to develop their concepts for creative activities. In the same way, everyone uses fantasy for future hopes and plans.

However, fantasy also may be a means of substitute gratification for wishes and needs the person cannot fulfill in daily life. Fantasies of economic advancement, political prominence, athletic achievement, sexual gratification and social prominence fill the hungry gap left by the difference between the person's desires and his actual circumstances. Elaborate, wish-fulfilling fantasies are profuse in childhood and adolescense. Much of the play of children is the open expression of fantasies in which children act out admired adult roles. In adult life fantasy continues to play an active part in emotional life, but in general it is harnessed more closely to realistic considerations and day-to-day life circumstances.

In both childhood and adult life, fantasy can become an unhealthy refuge for persons with emotional problems. It can become an attractive sanctuary drawing the individual away from confronting and solving his daily problems. Fantasy may occupy an unhealthy dominance in the emotional life of withdrawn and insecure persons.

Many psychiatrists feel that fantasies may be unconscious. In some instances, an unconscious fantasy was conscious at one time and later was repressed. In other instances, the unconscious fantasy was never conscious, or was only partly conscious. In either case, an unconscious fantasy may exert a marked force in a person's life. To cite a simple example, an officious, self-important person who acts in a commanding, authoritative manner may be living out a fantasy that he is a powerful figure whose destiny is to direct the actions of everyone around him. The fantasy that controls so much of his behavior may be an unconscious residue of a once conscious childhood fantasy, or it may never have been clearly present in his consciousness.

Nonverbal Communication and Empathy. Nonverbal communication consists of the transmission of feelings and ideas from one person to another without the use of words. It includes facial expressions, gestures, body positions and movements, body-to-body contacts, inarticulate voice noises (sobs, groans), body noises (hand-clapping, finger-snapping), gait (slow shuffle, brisk approach), body smells, dress (slovenly or neat), ornaments (headband, Rotary Club pin in lapel), physical settings (chairs arranged for intimate chat, or no convenient places to sit), and many other wordless ways in which people convey information, attitudes and feelings. Some psychiatrists feel that nonverbal communication is more important than spoken communication in determining the nature of interpersonal relationships.

People who live intimately with one another often become aware of the attitudes and feelings of each other by the accumulative effects of minor actions and small behavior characteristics they cannot consciously identify. Nonverbal communication is particularly strong in child-parent relationships. Children often are more sensitive to nonverbal cues than adults, and the sensitivity of adults to nonverbal communication varies much from person to person. The acute ability of some schizophrenics to perceive nonverbal clues sometimes is uncanny. Many psychiatrists pay much attention to how nonverbal communication affects the individual both in emotional health and illness. The analysis of nonverbal communication in the patient's life situations and also in his inteview relationship with the psychiatrist plays an important part in the treatment technics of many psychiatrists.

Empathy is a frequent form of nonverbal communication. In empathy one individual has a special intuitive awareness of the needs, feelings and problems of another person. Such insight usually establishes a bond between the two people, and this bond may enable the person who has the empathic insight to help the other person with his problems. The roots of empathy lie in nonverbal communication, but it later may be put into words between the two people involved. In other instances, as in some aspects of parent-child relationships, neither person may be able to express the empathy articulately; it may nevertheless be a powerful tie between them. Many psychiatrists become skilled in combining empathy with clinical objectivity in understanding patients and in helping patients to understand themselves.

General Systems Theory. General systems theory (or, more simply, systems theory) represents an attempt to reduce all human functioning to a set of basic processes and principles; it has been developed by Miller, Gerard and others since 1950. It tries to apply these simple principles to all human functions, from intracellular biochemistry to the working of large social groups. It uses analogies drawn from mechanics, computers, and thermodynamics.

General systems theory essays to reduce cellular, physiological, emotional, interpersonal and social phenomena to processes of (1) input, coding and output of information (2) intake, transformation and discharge of energy, and (3) incorporation, assimilation and either breakdown or buildup of matter. All these processes are viewed as occuring in various levels, or hierarchies, of complexity and significance.

To date, general systems theory must be regarded as a laudable but inadequate effort to construct a comprehensive concept of human life. It has not achieved widespread acceptance and has not led to clinically useful technics. Its heavy reliance on mechanical and electronic analogies (vector arrows and computer technology) does not seem appropriate for understanding people and their emotional problems.

Communication Theory. Partially based on initial concepts advanced by the mathematician Norbert Wiener (who coined the term *cybernetics* to designate systems in which the to-and-fro flow of information is subject to predictable rules), the psychiatrist Jurgen Ruesch and other behavioral scientists have, since the late 1940's, developed communication theory. Communication theory embraces psychiatric and social phenomena, and seeks to explain them in terms of the flow of ideas, feelings, attitudes and other information between people. It uses concepts of input, codification, feedback and output, among others. Undistorted, unobstructed communication leads to healthy personality development and sound emotional functioning, and blocked or disturbed communication leads to personality problems and emotional disorders.

Communication is both verbal and nonverbal; nonverbal communication is often more significant than verbal exchanges. All human interaction, from a two-person marital couple to a national group encompassing millions of people, is seen in terms of complex transmissions of information and feelings.

Communication theory is a helpful and enlightening adjunct to both interpersonal theory and Freudian-psychoanalytic theory. It focuses attention on the unhealthy verbal and nonverbal interchanges between the patient and the significant people about him in past and present life experiences that have produced his problems, and points toward healthy verbal and nonverbal interactions between the therapist (or therapeutic groups and environments) and the patient in treatment.

Unfortunately, communication theory does not adequately explain many kinds of psychiatric disturbances; this may be due to insufficient work by its proponents or to limitations in communication theory itself. For example, it is difficult to explain phobias, compulsive neuroses, depressions and manic disorders by communication theory. However, it can explain schizophrenia (a distortion or breakdown in meaningful interpersonal communication), organic brain disturbances (communication defects due to impaired brain cells), some personality disorders and some other conditions. Also, though it gives new perspectives on psychotherapy, communication theory has not led to the development of new psychotherapeutic technics.

At present, therefore, communication theory offers new perspectives about other psychiatric approaches, but it does not constitute a comprehensive system in itself. Its development seems to have slowed down in recent years.

Symbiotic and Anaclitic Relationships. In symbiosis two persons with unhealthy emotional needs find limited gratification in their interpersonal relationship with one another. For example, a person with unhealthy needs for clinging to another person may form a close relationship with an individual who has strong unhealthy needs to dominate others. In another example, an insecure child may form an unhealthy closeness to a self-centered parent who has a strong need to keep the child tied to him emotionally in an immature role. Unhealthy symbiotic relationships are damaging to both persons involved, for the symbiosis makes the problems of each one more inflexible. Moreover, a longstanding symbiosis tends to make the personality problems of each one more difficult to modify, because both persons often resist any change in the behavior of either one.

In an *anaclitic* relationship one person is

very dependent emotionally upon another. The term "anaclitic" is usually employed in referring to the dependence of an infant or young child on his mother. In infancy and early childhood, an anaclitic relationship of the child on his parents is normal; if the anaclitic relationship persists into later life it becomes unhealthy. If an infant or young child is suddenly separated from his mother, he may become depressed and withdrawn; this disturbance is called an anaclitic depression.

Primary and Secondary Gains. When an emotional symptom is formed it frequently results in a decrease of anxiety or guilt. This decrease in anxiety or guilt is called the "primary gain" of a psychiatric symptom. For example, a small child with much anxiety in his relationship with his father may unconsciously transfer his strong anxiety to the dark or to dogs. Thus, by developing a fear of the dark or of dogs, he gets a release from the more painful, persistent anxiety in his relationship with his father. This is the primary gain of the symptom.

However, once a symptom is established the patient may obtain special gratifications from the people around him because of it. For example, a patient with a hysterical conversion paralysis of the legs may find gratifying the attention he receives as an invalid. This gratification that the symptom obtains for the patient is called a "secondary gain." A secondary gain may be minor or it may become an entrenched obstacle making removal of the psychiatric symptom more difficult. Primary and secondary gains of symptoms receive further attention in later chapters.

BIBLIOGRAPHY

Barbizet, J.: Human Memory and Its Pathology. San Francisco, W. H. Freeman, 1970.

Birk, L., and Brinkley-Birk, L. W.: Psychoanalysis and behavior therapy. Am. J. Psychiatry, *131*: 499, 1974.

Fancher, R. E.: Psychoanalytic Psychology: The Development of Freud's Thought. New York, W. W. Norton, 1973.

Freedman, D. A., Canady, C., and Robinson, J. S.: Speech and psychiatric structure: a reconsideration of their relation. J. Am. Psychonal. Ass., *19*:705, 1971.

Gelder, M. G., et al.: Specific and nonspecific factors in behavior therapy. Brit. J. Psychiatry, *123*:445, 1973.

Goodwin, D. W., Alderson, P., and Rosenthal, R.: Clinical significance of hallucinations in psychiatric disorders. Arch. Gen. Psychiatry, *24*:76, 1971.

Jones, W. L.: Manifest dream content, an aid to communication during analysis. Am. J. Psychother., *25*:284, 1971.

Lazarus, A. A. (ed.): Clinical Behavior Therapy. New York, Brunner Mazel, 1972.

Levinson, E. A.: The Fallacy of Understanding: An Inquiry Into the Changing Structure of Psychoanalysis. New York, Basic Books, 1972.

McDonald, C.: A clinical study of hypnagogic hallucinations. Brit. J. Psychiatry, *118*:543, 1974.

Meir, A. Z.: General systems theory. Developments and perspectives for medicine and psychiatry. Arch. Gen. Psychiatry, *21*:302, 1969.

Meissner, W. W.: Correlative aspects of introjective and projective mechanisms. Am. J. Psychiatry, *131*:176, 1974.

Misak, H., and Sexton, V. S.: Phenomenological, Existential and Humanistic Psychologies. New York, Grune & Stratton, 1973.

Mosak, H. H. (ed.): Alfred Adler: His Influence on Psychology Today. Park Ridge, N. J., Noyes Press, 1974.

Nemiah, J. C.: Foundations of Psychopathology. New York, Jason Aronson, 1973.

Piaget, J., and Inhelder, B.: Memory and Intelligence. New York, Basic Books, 1974.

Ruesch, J., and Bateson, G.: Communication. The Social Matrix of Psychiatry. New York, W. W. Norton, 1951.

Stoller, R. J.: Overview: the impact of new advances in sex research on psychoanalytic theory. Am. J. Psychiatry, *130*:241, 1973.

Storr, A.: C. G. Jung. New York, Viking Press, 1973.

Sullivan, H. S.: Clinical Studies in Psychiatry. New York, W. W. Norton, 1956.

Part Two

Psychiatric Evaluation of the Patient

In this section we shall discuss all aspects of the psychiatric evaluation of the patient. In Chapter 4 we shall cover the psychiatric interview examination, the basic method of psychiatric evaluation. We shall outline in detail the technics for interviewing the patient and his relatives. Emphasis will be placed on the interviewer as a participant-observer who uses his personality resources and interpersonal relationships with patients as diagnostic tools.

In Chapter 5 we shall discuss further examination procedures that may be employed in psychiatric evaluation. These include the personality examination technics used by clinical psychologists, special interview technics such as interview after barbiturate injection, and aspects of the physical evaluation of the patient. We shall conclude with a discussion of the process of formulating a psychiatric diagnosis and a brief survey of the standard classification of psychiatric disorders.

4

The Psychiatric Examination

The main method of conducting a psychiatric evaluation of a person is to interview him. When the patient is well motivated for psychiatric examination, this interview usually takes place in a face-to-face position in which the examiner asks questions and the patient answers with reasonable spontaneity. When the patient is not motivated for a psychiatric evaluation, or is unable to understand the nature and purposes of it, the examiner modifies his approach. In many cases the examiner gets supplementary information about the patient's problems and personality characteristics from his family; the examiner may interview members of the family himself, or in many clinics and hospitals a psychiatric social worker interviews the family. Further information often is obtained from testing by a clincial psychologist. In many instances, particularly when there is a question of organic brain involvement, the examiner reviews the results of previous or subsequent physical and neurological evaluation of the patient.

A thorough psychiatric evaluation includes a comprehensive survey of the patient's life history and current personality status. The examiner gradually outlines the significant current interpersonal relationships in the patient's life, and he traces the patient's lifelong history of emotional functioning and interpersonal adjustment. The examiner seeks to understand how the patient's current problems have arisen in the context of his past and current interpersonal relationships.

We shall discuss the psychiatric examination under the headings of (a) *interview examination of the patient,* (b) *obtaining information from the patient's family,* and (c) *examination of the unmotivated patient.* (The special examination procedures, such as psychological testing by a clinical psychologist, are covered in Chapter 5. The psychiatric examination of children and adolescents involves special technics which are outlined in Chapter 24.)

The Interviewer's Role as a Participant-Observer. Harry Stack Sullivan described the role of a psychiatric examiner as that of a *participant-observer*. The interviewer uses his personality resources, special information and interpersonal relationship with the patient as both diagnostic and therapeutic tools in helping the patient to achieve a better level of living. The examiner and the patient deal with three general kinds of data: (1) all the past and present experiences of the patient, (2) new insights into the patient's life which are designed to help him solve his emotional difficulties, and (3) the interpersonal relationship between the examiner and the patient, often the only sample of the patient's interpersonal functioning available for direct scruitny.

Sullivan states that for this task the examiner must have three special attitudes: (1) He must give the patient a high degree of respect as an individual whose personality characteristics and emotional problems merit expert evaluation, and, perhaps, treatment. (2) The interviewer must keenly and intently focus his attention on what the patient says and does. (3) He must have information and attitudes which qualify him to assume the role of an expert on interpersonal relationships and the emotional distresses they can produce. Such expertness may vary from that of the novice examiner to that of the experienced clinician, but it is the element of some degree of expertness that gives psychiatric interviewing its particular value.

The interviewer is a participant-observer. He is constantly observing and analyzing what goes on in the interview. However, he is also a participant. Though he holds his emotional reactions in check he is inescapably forming an interpersonal relationship of a very special sort with the patient. In many cases he notes his reactions to the patient in order to understand better the feelings the patient often arouses in others and his customary ways of interacting with people. Regardless of whether the patient is facing the examiner in a chair, or lying on a couch without direct view of the interviewer, or walking down a hospital corridor with him as they talk, an interpersonal relationship has been set up. The examiner is an alert *observer* of this relationship, in which he takes advantage of his *participation* to broaden his understanding of the patient and his capacity to help him.

The following outline of a psychiatric evaluation follows the main lines laid down by Harry Stack Sullivan in his classic book "The Psychiatric Interview." We shall not use Sullivan's four-part scheme (the inception, the reconnaissance, the detailed inquiry, and the termination, or interruption), but we shall employ the broad principles and general sequences he suggests.

INTERVIEW EXAMINATION OF THE PATIENT

As we outline step by step an initial psychiatric interview, it should be kept in mind that the skillfulness of examiners and the accessibility of patients produce endless variations. The material outlined in this section occasionally can be covered in one interview, but in other instances it requires several sessions. Moreover, this interview outline should not be viewed as a rigid procedure. The experienced examiner condenses and modifies sections of it; his experience and training enable him to sort through unimportant material and to focus his attention on the most important aspects of the patient's problems and life experiences. However, the student or inexperienced examiner should follow a fairly systematic outline in performing a psychiatric examination, in order to survey thoroughly the patient's difficulties and life history.

The Examiner's Behavior and Attitudes

I feel that the examiner should greet a new patient in a pleasant professional manner. I often shake hands with patients, but opinions differ on this matter. Sigmund Freud is reported to have shaken hands with each patient as he met him at the door of his consultation room at each session. Other psychiatrists feel that any physical contact may be misinterpreted by some patients as unduly familiar or solicitous. The examiner should probably do what seems comfortable and natural to him. If the examiner is ill at ease in shaking hands with patients, he should not do it; if he feels more comfortable greeting each patient with a handshake, it is an acceptable procedure.

In his role as a professional participant-observer, the examiner should not be overly solicitous nor should he be aloof. Some psychiatrists feel that the examiner should maintain a reserved, neutral attitude to allow the patient to use him as an objective sounding board. If, by such "neutrality" the physician means detached coldness, he is likely to frighten many patients or to give them the impression that he does not have a professional interest in helping them and is merely going through a perfunctory routine.

On the other hand, the examiner should not be overly solicitous. He should give the patient the impression that he is keenly alert and willing to help, but he should not leave him feeling that he is overly anxious to aid him. Many patients are tense and insecure; they feel most comfortable with an examiner who is helpful, but who has calm, professional objectivity. Moreover, a patient sometimes interprets undue solicitousness as a special personal interest the examiner is showing to him, and he infers that the examiner's interest goes beyond strict professional bounds. In such cases the patient may quickly develop a strong emotional attachment to the examiner, and the patient's feelings usually become an obstacle rather than an aid to treatment.

Despite what Sullivan called the interviewer's "inescapable, inextricable involvement" in the patient-therapist relatinship, the examiner should work to keep his emotional reactions to the patient to a minimum. For example, if the patient is so depressed that suicide seems an imminent threat, the examiner should not become frightened and overtly alarmed. Such an emotional reaction creates an uncomfortable breach in the patient's relationship with the examiner and may partially paralyze the interviewer in his efforts to make effective plans to deal with the problem. On the other hand, if the patient is hostile and critical, the examiner does not argue and bicker with him. He merely listens and notes the patient's behavior as part of the data of the interview. If the patient flatters the examiner and asks personal questions, the examiner does not allow these actions to sway him, but he deflects such comments and directs the interview into other channels. He notes such behavior as a way in which the patient probably approaches many people in his attempts to manipulate them.

Thus, although the examiner carries out his role as a participant-observer, he does not become emotionally entangled. To the extent that he becomes so entangled, his professional objectivity is decreased and his ability to help the patient is impaired.

However, all examiners have feelings and sensitivities in all interpersonal relationships, and emotional reactions in psychiatric interviewing can be reduced but not abolished. The behavior of the patient inevitably arouses some feelings and attitudes in the examiner. But, by his professional orientation and alert awareness of his reactions to patients, the examiner reduces his feelings and attitudes to a minimum. Moreover, the interviewer can note his reactions and they may help him to evaluate the patient. For example, if the examiner finds himself on the defensive and a little cowed by the blustering hostility of a patient, he may understand better how this patient makes many people around him feel and how the patient attempts to dominate the close people in his life. A weeping, complaining patient who incriminates all her previous doctors for not having helped her in many years of difficulty with multiple psychogenic symptoms may make the examiner feel impatient and irritable toward her; he may then feel somewhat guilty about his irritability. If the examiner is aware of these feelings within himself, they may help him understand why the patient's relatives treat her with exasperated irritation and yet are dominated by her in her role of a complaining invalid.

In each of these situations, as Sullivan points out, the patient is treating the interviewer as if he were someone who he really is not. For example, the patient described above is treating the examiner as if he were a person (or persons) in his past life whom he could browbeat or mainpulate by guilt; the examiner's interest is to find out who that person (or persons) was, and what kinds of unhealthy interpersonal relationships produced these warped patterns of living.

The psychiatric examination is the only interpersonal relationship in which a person may discuss freely his problems, his feelings and his interpersonal dilemmas without emotional reactions, moral advice or censure from the listener. Elsewhere in life the person who discusses his problems at length with people arouses sympathy, solicitous overconcern, irritability, disgust, perplexed indifference, moral censure, or other reactions. These reactions do not help the patient and often upset him more. Only in the psychiatric interview does the patient have the opportunity to lay out his problems and examine them with the professional cooperation of a keenly interested but emotionally unentangled person. This is the special quality of the psychiatric examination which makes it a unique type of interpersonal undertaking.

Note Taking. After greeting the patient, the examiner can indicate a comfortable chair for him to sit in while the examiner takes another chair. I never put a desk between the patient and myself. I arrange my office so that my desk is at my left hand and the patient is on my right about six to eight feet away from me. Psychiatrists disagree on the advisability of taking notes during the interview. Some psychiatrists feel that note taking distracts the examiner's attention from the patient and obscures his alert awareness of the patient's behavior. They feel that it also tends to inhibit the patient by making him self-conscious of what he is saying and concerned about what use his words will be put to. Thus, they feel that note taking diminishes the spontaneity of the interpersonal relationship by its effect on both the patient and the interviewer.

On the other hand, many other psychiatrists feel that note taking is a practical necessity for the vast majority of examiners. They simply cannot remember and organize the material of the interview without it. I agree with this point of view. However, skilled interviewers with much experience sometimes can dispense with notes during the interview, and summarize their material after the interview is over; Harry Stack Sullivan and Sigmund Freud followed this latter course.

A simple way for the average interviewer to handle note taking is to make notes on conventional medical record paper firmly attached to a clipboard. Most patients have no objections to note taking. Often they respect an examiner who seems careful, systematic and interested. Some patients are puzzled when the examiner does not take notes, for they wonder how he can possibly keep the facts of his cases clear when he sees patient after patient all day long. Of course, note taking is suspended or abandoned when circumstances require it. The examiner should not go on methodically taking notes while a patient is sobbing; he should suspend note taking until the patient is less upset. If a paranoid patient becomes agitated because "my words are being written down," the examiner quietly abandons note taking with a mild, brief reassurance. Children and adolescents react poorly to note taking and often become uncommunicative; so in my opinion, it is best not to take notes when interviewing them. A few psychotic patients become uncommunicative when they see the interviewer taking notes, but the majority accept it well.

As a rule, I take notes only during the first two or three interviews; after that I usually have enough basic data to abandon note taking while I am with the patient. Thereafter, I write or dictate brief summaries of each session and return to note taking during interviews only at special times, such as when I am recording the details of a long dream or other intricate data.

Interview Length. The conventional length of a psychiatric interview is 50 minutes. Less time usually does not permit effective work, and a longer time may tire and distract both the patient and the examiner. However, the inexperienced interviewer often can spend up to two hours in his initial interview with a new patient in getting enough information to grasp the essential outlines of the patient's problems and his background.

Opening the Interview

The examiner may open the interview by asking a broad, general question that invites the patient to discuss his problems. The interviewer may say, "Mr. Gibbons, perhaps you might begin wherever seems comfortable and tell me about the problem or difficulties that bring you to see me." With a hospitalized patient, the question is altered to inquire about "the problems or circumstances that brought you to the hospital." This question is broad enough to allow the patient to begin to talk in whatever way he can about his problems.

The patient may start to discuss his difficulties in a fairly direct manner. Other patients wander confusedly from topic to topic or may drift off into unrelated details. The interviewer may let the patient talk at will for a short time to observe how his flow of thought and feelings proceeds when uninfluenced by further questions. If the patient narrates the history of his problems with reasonable directness, the examiner may listen attentively with only occasional comments or brief questions. However, when the patient drifts aimlessly, the examiner after a short period should begin to ask specific questions to elicit the information he must obtain to outline the patient's problems and background. Some psychiatrists ask very few questions and allow the patient to talk with unobstructed spontaneity, feeling that in this way the essential information will in time come forth and that it will be uncolored by the questions of the examiner. Such an approach, however, often requires several or more interviews to get a clear history, and even then large gaps may remain. The less experienced examiner working in a clinic, a hospital or his office usually finds that he must follow an organized outline of pertinent questions in order to grasp the patient's needs and life history.

The Presenting Problem

I favor following a modified form of conventional medical history taking; this follows, in general, the outline recommended by Harry Stack Sullivan. Thus, the examiner first records the presenting problem and then follows with the history of the present illness. He then obtains the patient's past history, surveys his past and current interpersonal relationships and so forth (as outlined in the succeeding pages).

The patient's initial statement of his problem may be briefly recorded as his presenting problem. Nevertheless, in psychiatry the patient's chief complaint may disclose more of his attitudes and personality than his true problems. The chief complaint often is revealing, even when it is not the central problem or even related to it. For example, the patient with paranoid delusions may state that he is coming only because his relatives feel he is "a little nervous due to trouble with the neighbors." A depressed patient may state that he comes because of profound fatigue for which his family doctor could not find a physical cause. He may be unable to describe his depression because of his concern with physical sensations accompanying it. An alcoholic may state that his only problem is a "nervous wife," and a patient with an anxiety neurosis may indicate that his trouble consists of episodes of palpitation and shortness of breath. Other patients define their chief problems clearly and promptly.

The Present Difficulty

After noting the chief complaint, the examiner proceeds to trace the history of the present illness. Some patients unfold this history fairly well with only a few questions, whereas others require many inquiries to enable the interviewer to get a coherent concept of the evolution of the problem. For example, a patient with a phobia or a psychosomatic illness often can describe the history of his disorder clearly, whereas a schizophrenic or a patient with an organic brain disorder cannot give a coherent history. In some cases the examiner gets his most relevant history data later from the relatives or other informants. In hospital cases, the nurses on the floor, through their contacts with the patient and his visiting relatives, may be able to orient the examiner on general points that the patient cannot describe.

In the present illness, the examiner should establish when and how the difficulty began. The duration and the mode of onset of a psychiatric disorder are important in determining treatment plans and prognostic hopes. Problems that have been present a few months or a year or two are usually much more amenable to treatment than those of many years' duration. Sometimes a patient states that his difficulty began recently, but a detailed history reveals that in various forms it trails back many years. For example, a patient may say that his anxiety states began four months previously when he first noted episodes of palpitation and "dizziness," but further history reveals that his anxiety attacks, accompanied by other types of physical symptoms, acutally began several years before.

The onset of a psychiatric illness may be abrupt or insidious. For example, a schizophrenic disorder may begin so abruptly that its date of onset can be pinpointed to a specific two- or three-day period, or it may develop so insidiously over a period of many years that it is arbitrary to say at what point the illness really began. The examiner should learn what the initial symptoms or behavior disturbances were and the circumstances in which they arose. He should inquire about any interpersonal stresses the patient feels may have been relevant to the onset.

The concepts the patient has about causative factors may be obviously irrelevant or profoundly significant. For example, the patient may attribute his anxiety states to an inconsequential blow on the head that occurred months or years before the symptoms began, or he may identify a crucial interpersonal crisis that played a large role in causing his difficulty.

The examiner inquires how the present disorder evolved and traces its fluctuations or steady progression. He asks how previous treatment procedures or other measures have affected it. He inquires what things make it better or worse and the effects of various interpersonal relationships. He seeks to discover how stresses in the various past or current interpersonal relationships of the patient's life affect the problem, and he inquires about the reactions of the patient's family, friends and work associates. The examiner wants to know if new symptoms and disturbances have arisen in the course of the illness, and whether the original ones have changed. He asks if the patient has ever had similar trouble before. The interviewer seeks any evidences of changes in behavior and interpersonal adjustments at home, at work, or in the neighborhood. He wants to know if there have been changes in the patient's memory, mood, thinking processes or daily habits. (Further information about ways in which the examiner searches for evidence of hallucinations, delusions, organic brain changes and other changes in the patient's intellectual and emotional functioning are covered later in this chapter.)

The interviewer then inventories the present state of the problem and inquires if some recent event precipitated psychiatric consultation at this particular time. For example, a patient may have had a problem for a long time but did not seek aid until his superiors at work urged he do something about it. This information may reveal much about the patient's motivation for the consultation and the effects of the problem on the patient's social and vocational adjustment.

As the patient discusses his condition, the interviewer gradually may become aware that the patient's true problems are very different from the ones he is describing. Some patients are unable to see their problems clearly, or they describe irrelevant difficulties as their central problems. In such cases the examiner sketches briefly the patient's concepts of his difficulties, which may have significance in his emotional functioning even when they are not the main issues. The examiner's picture is filled out by the information he later gets from the relatives and the clinical psychologist's examination as well as further direct observation of the patient. Other important data may come from reports of previous physicians or clinics where he has been seen.

Some patients, particularly reluctant ones who are brought by relatives, evade their problems. For example, alcoholics and persons who are misusing drugs often describe an array of small symptoms and deny the misuse of alcohol or drugs. The true story often comes only from the relatives and is later begrudgingly admitted by the patient.

The specific content of the present illness narrative varies much with the nature of the problem. However, the examiner should keep in mind that the present illness includes not only the history of the particular difficulty, but it also embraces information on how the patient's personality structure and interpersonal relationships have contributed to the illness and are woven into it. The interviewer also seeks to know what roles the patient's vocational, social and marital activities have played in his problems. As in all medical history taking, the more the examiner knows of a field the more skillful he is in taking the history of a disorder in it. In a sense, most of the subsequent chapters of this book are pertinent to background for history taking.

Past History

The survey of the patient's past history may be considered under four broad headings: (1) *the history of any psychiatric difficulties prior to the onset of the present illness*, (2) *the patient's personality development and his interpersonal relationships from childhood to the present*, (3) *the history of the patient's adjustment in school, work, social groups and recreational groups*, and (4) *a brief outline of the patient's significant medical illnesses and major medical treatments*.

The experienced examiner usually merges these four aspects into a single, skillfully directed past history. The beginning examiner should inventory these four categories separately to get a comprehensive past history.

Past Psychiatric Difficulties

The interviewer inquires if the patient has had any previous emotional troubles. He asks if the patient has ever seen a psychiatrist before or has consulted physicians about tension problems or personality difficulties. A brief letter, with the patient's signed authorization to release information, should be sent to any physicians or hospitals from whom the patient previously has had psychiatric care. The information received from such inquiries often reveals important data which the patient and his family were unable or unwilling to give.

Failure to send out such routine inquiries is one of the most common omissions in a psychiatric workup. I use a routine printed letter with an authorization for release of information at the bottom. I have the patient sign the authorization to release information, and I fill in the doctor's name and address and the patient's full name, age and date of consultation at the previous facility (if the psychiatrist is in a distant city his address may be readily found in the American Psychiatric Association's annually issued membership directory). Such a form takes two or three minutes to execute and to mail. I often append a two- or three-sentence explanatory note at the end of the letter and sign it personally. This takes some of the coldness out of a printed form. The use of printed form letters is somewhat impersonal and has its disadvantages, but I have found that in clinics and hospitals where a form letter is not used, the burden of writing many personal letters is so great that after a few months such inquiries are frequently omitted. These inquiries should be routine. It is better to benefit from the mistakes of your predecessors than to repeat them.

The examiner inquires about any emotional upsets during the patient's childhood, adolescence, college life, military service or adult life. He asks if the patient has ever seen a marriage counselor, or consulted a clergyman or any other kind of counselor about personal problems. He may inquire if any relatives or close friends have ever suggested psychiatric consultation or if the patient has considered it before in his life but did not act upon it. Such questions usually lead to discussion of any previous psychiatric problems.

Past and Current Interpersonal Relationships and Personality Development

The interviewer next traces the patient's interpersonal relationships and personality development from childhood to the present. He begins by asking about the patient's mother's personality and her relationship with the patient during his formative years. He also inquires about the father's personality and his relationship with the patient. The nature of the parents' relationship with each other is investigated, and the examiner asks about the present circumstances of the parents, if they are still living, and the patient's current relationship with them. The examiner outlines the patient's relationships with his siblings and finds out if any other persons played a significant role in his family life during the formative years. He asks if any other relatives, such as grandparents, lived with the family while he was growing up.

The examiner inquires about any rivalries, hostilities, especially close and helpful relationships, or distant and traumatic relationships during the patient's childhood. In tracing the family structure, I use the brief diagram shown in Figure 4-1. This helps to keep the family structure clear, and aids in a quick review of the chart prior to subsequent interviews. From these questions the interviewer sketches the main close interpersonal relationships of the patient's early life. He pays careful attention to the qualities of love or coldness, acceptance or rejection, domination or passivity, and emotional comfort or stressfulness that characterized all these relationships. Any stressful relationships or personality problems in childhood are investigated, and the examiner tries to visualize the patient's personality development in the context of these relationships. He inquires how the patient handled his affection, his anger, his dependent yearnings, and other needs during his formative years.

The interviewer inquires about the patient's relationship with his family during adolescence and asks about any adjustment problems at that time. He asks about the patient's education and how he adjusted in college or any type of vocational training. He traces the patient's comfort or problems in forming close relationships with persons of the opposite sex during adolescence and he follows these currents of development into early adulthood. At this point the examiner can inquire about the patient's sexual development, his sexual experience to the present and any problems in his sexual adjustment.

I feel that an examiner can ask easily about sexual development in a patient of his own sex, but that an inexperienced interviewer should be cautious in asking questions about sexual development and experience in patients of the opposite sex. For example, many women feel uncomfortable if a male inter-

86   *The Psychiatric Examination*

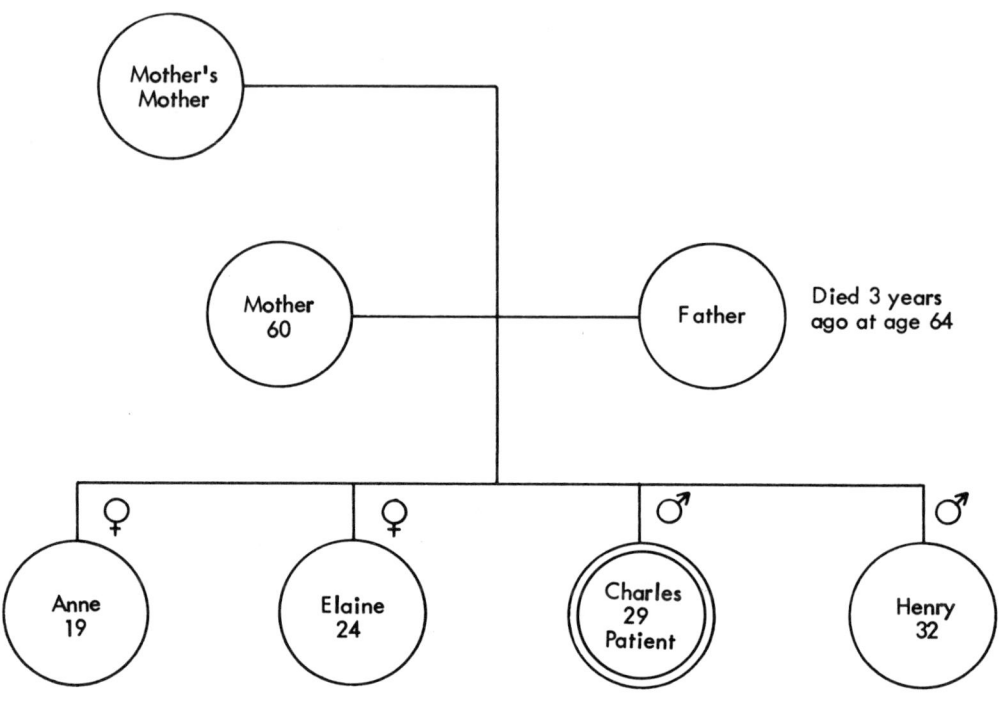

Fig. 4–1.

viewer in the initial interview asks questions about sexual activity, unless the patient's major reason for consultation is a sexual maladjustment. Although an interviewer may ask a person of the opposite sex if he or she has any significant problems in sexual functioning, other probings into sexual behavior should be left until later interviews and should come up spontaneously in the context of related emotional problems. If the interviewer proceeds with methodical questions about sexual behavior with patients of the opposite sex (or, occasionally, even with patients of the same sex), some patients feel that the examiner's preoccupation with the subject goes beyond the bounds of professional concern and indicates special interest in them. Some patients are frightened by such questions, and in others they awaken feelings of attraction toward the examiner. The precipitation of either type of attitude becomes an obstacle to useful interviewing.

The examiner proceeds to outline the patient's adult interpersonal relationships. An adult's close interpersonal relationships can be summarized visually in the type of diagram shown in Figure 4–2 (in conjunction with the material already included in Figure 4–1). The interviewer asks about the patient's relationship in his marriage, and he inquires about the relationships of both the patient and his marital partner with their children and with members of the marital partner's family. He inquires about any past marriages and divorces.

The comprehensive outline of the patient's past and current close interpersonal relationships is in time filled in with details, and special emphasis is given to any areas in which stresses or conflicts existed or persist. The complete exploration of the details of this interpersonal outline may constitute a significant part of the treatment process of many personality problems, neurotic distur-

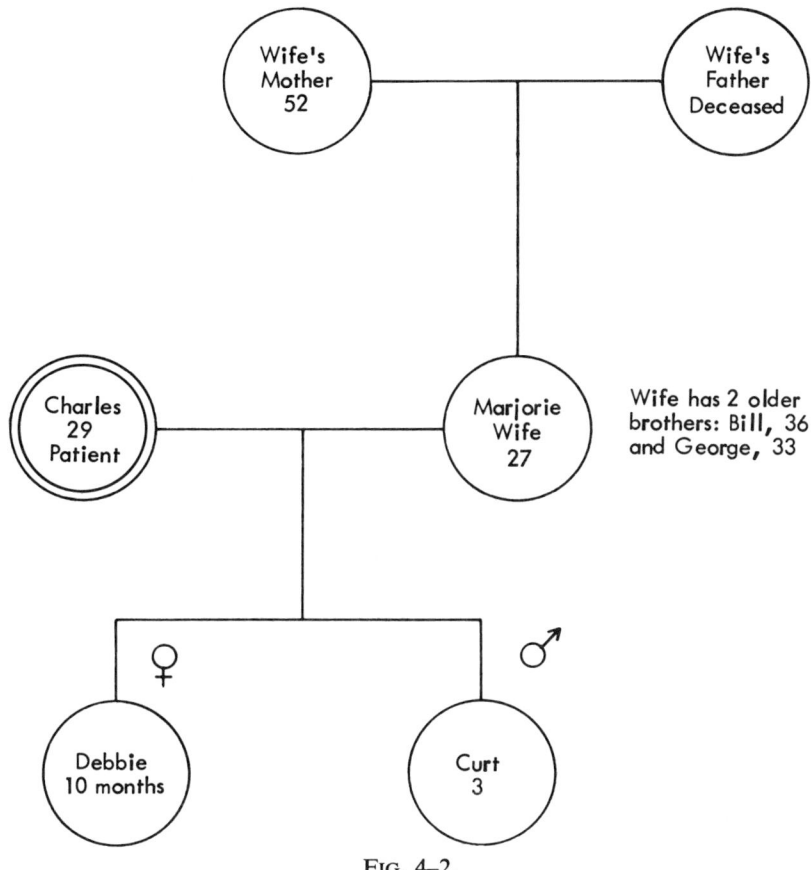

FIG. 4-2.

bances, psychosomatic illnesses and other difficulties. However, in the first interview or two, only the broad general outlines of the patient's past and current interpersonal relationships can be surveyed to give the interviewer a comprehensive picture of all possible areas of interpersonal stress.

Adjustment in Broader Social Groups

Having traced the patient's development in close interpersonal relationships, the examiner seeks information about his adjustment in social groups outside his home. The first major, long-term social adventure of a person outside his home is school. The interviewer inquires about the patient's interpersonal adjustment in his school years and asks how well he did in his studies. The examiner surveys his adjustment in neighborhood groups and social groups outside of school and inquires if there were any problems in adjusting comfortably to people in these areas.

Careful attention is given to the patient's adjustment to the stresses of adolescence, because adolescence in addition to being a period of further emotional maturation, is a testing time of the soundness of prior personality development, and it often contains forewarnings of problems in adulthood. If the patient had military service his adjustment in it is outlined, with inquiry into any associated emotional problems. If the patient was not accepted for military service or if his term of duty was ended because of medical reasons, the interviewer should find out the details. Work adjustment is traced with note of any interpersonal problems there, and the interviewer inquires about the patient's adjustment in social and neighborhood groups.

Past Medical History

The interviewer makes at least a brief inquiry into the patient's history of major medical illnesses, accidents and medical treatments. This inquiry may be more detailed for a patient whose long history of many medical consultations for many poorly defined dysfunctions suggests strong emotional factors in his complaints. The medical history also is more detailed in patients with organic brain syndromes and psychosomatic illnesses. The examiner should discover what medications have been taken lately. This is often a point at which discrete questions about any problems with alcohol or illicit drugs may be inserted, and followed up if the patient has had such difficulties. The interviewer should ascertain also if the patient has been taking proprietary medications containing such compounds as bromides and chloral hydrate, which can produce toxic reactions mimicking other types of psychiatric illness.

CURRENT INTERPERSONAL FUNCTIONING

The examiner next surveys the patient's current interpersonal functioning in day-to-day activities. He investigates how the patient handles his feelings. Can he express affection easily or does he inhibit his affectionate feelings? Does he get somewhat angry occasionally and can he defend his rights, or does he usually suppress his assertive feelings and let people dominate him? Is he comfortable with moderate amounts of aggressive feelings or do they make him feel guilty? Does he meet people easily and get along with them comfortably or is he ill at ease in social groups? Is he outgoing and gregarious or shy and retiring? Are his needs for affection met in his current family life? Does he feel secure in his family, his work situation and his social relationships, or is he apprehensive about any of these areas? Does he worry about his marriage, his children, his job, his financial status, his health or the health of members of his family?

What does the patient do for recreation and how much time does he spend in it? What does he do on his vacations? It is useful to inquire at least briefly about how the patient spends his time. What is his usual routine on weekdays and how does he spend his weekends? How much time does he spend with his marital partner and what do they do together? The interviewer asks a mother how much time each week she spends away from her home and children and what she does then. The examiner asks an unmarried patient how much he or she dates and what the patient likes to do on dates. The interviewer asks if the patient is interested in clubs, social organizations, church groups, religious activities, civic activities, work groups, professional societies or recreational groups.

MENTAL STATUS EXAMINATION

While exploring the patient's present illness and the various aspects of his life history, the examiner has had the opportunity of observing many of the patient's emotional reactions and intellectual processes. He has observed the patient's general behavior, his emotional reactions to the topics discussed, his memory capacities and many other things. In the psychiatric workup these direct observations of the patient's behavior are traditionally grouped together under the heading of the *mental status examination*.

There is a tendency in some psychiatric training centers today to overlook or abandon the performance of mental status examinations, and to concentrate solely on exploration of personality development and emotional functioning. This is a mistake. In the course of a long, active consultative and therapeutic practice I have seen a sizable number of patients who had elaborate workups in outstanding psychiatric facilities without the detection of subtle organic brain disorders, petit mal epilepsy, borderline mental retardation, neurological disease and other conditions, because systematic mental status examinations were not done—or at least thought through—by the patients' examiners.

We shall now consider the details of a mental status examination. In actual practice, the interviewer usually observes most of these details while discussing the patient's problems and life history, and later asks specific questions which complete the mental status examination.

General Appearance and Behavior. The details of the patient's dress and grooming are sometimes significant. A deterioration of personal cleanliness and attire may be an early sign of chronic organic brain disease. I recall an elderly attorney whose family first became aware of his beginning senile deterioration when they noted coffee stains and butter grease on his neckties and suit coats. The depressed patient or the withdrawn schizophrenic may be unaware of gross neglect of grooming, whereas patients with some types of personality disorders dress fashionably and elaborately to impress the examiner.

The interviewer notes the patient's general behavior. He observes whether the patient is matter-of-fact, or uncooperative, or anxious to please, or indifferent during the interview. He notes the patient's manners, his politeness or rudeness, and whether there are any discrepancies between his situation in life and his behavior. For example, if a person of good education and upbringing behaves in crude, offensive ways it may indicate a recent deterioration of his emotional and social adjustment.

Affect and Emotional Reactions. The examiner pays careful attention to the affect of the patient. He notes whether his affect is alert or flat, appropriate or inappropriate, depressed or exhilarated. He observes whether he is anxious or comfortably at ease. The patient's affective state often is not clear, and the interviewer should ask specific questions. For example, he may ask a patient in whom he suspects depression, "How have you been feeling lately? Have you felt depressed, melancholy and blue, as if you lost your last friend? Have you felt worthless and guilty?" He should inquire carefully about states of prolonged anxiousness or joyful exhilaration.

The interviewer notes the patient's emotional reactions. He observes during the interview if the patient shows anger, fear, joy, acute grief or other emotions. He notes whether he is easily moved emotionally or seems emotionally unresponsive to both pleasant and painful topics.

Physical Actions. The examiner observes physical actions. The anxious patient may sit tensely on the edge of his chair, twist his handkerchief tightly between his hands or fidget restlessly with the arms of the chair or whatever minor objects lie within reach. The depressed patient may move in slow, dragging steps and gestures, or he may sit enveloped in gloomy withdrawal. Other depressed patients are agitated and move distractedly whether sitting or standing. A catatonic schizophrenic may sit mute and motionless for long periods; he may have repetitive mannerisms or leave his arms and hands for some time in whatever position the examiner places them. The paranoid patient may glance suspiciously about the room, and the hallucinating patient may cock his head and listen carefully for voices. The manic patient is overactive; he is in continual rapid movement as he flits from item to item, concentrating on none of them. The patient with organic brain disease often is restless in an aimless way; children with organic brain disease may be hyperactive and carelessly destructive, and adults with organic brain syndromes sometimes pick at their clothing and other minor objects in ceaseless agitation. The examiner notes any tremors, tics, grimaces, mannerisms, or aimless aggressiveness.

Thought Processes and Thought Content. While talking with the patient the examiner has made many observations about his thought processes. He has noticed the slowed, painfully dragging thought processes of the deeply depressed patient, or the rapid, helter-skelter flight of ideas of the hypomanic or manic patient. The schizophrenic often has abrupt blocking in his flow of thoughts, and his thinking frequently shows evidence of fragmentation of thought processes which makes it difficult to follow the thread of his discourse from one topic to the next; the employment of coined words, obscure symbolic phrases and words with unusual, special meanings may produce the confused speech sometimes called a "word salad." The patient with organic brain disease often wanders from topic to topic vainly trying to remember the links in the narrative he has begun. He may eventually arrive at the goal of his discourse after long, detailed detours on unrelated topics. In advanced organic brain disease the patient's thought processes and speech may deteriorate into incoherent ramblings. The examiner notices any abnormalities such as perseveration, in which the patient responds repeatedly with the same answer to various questions, or echolalia, in which the patient parrots back whatever is said to him. Major abnormalities of thought content, such as obsessions and compulsive thoughts, have become evident while the patient was revealing the details of his present disorder and past history.

During a detailed interview the patient usually reveals any delusions he has. Persecutory delusions, grandiose delusions or self-accusatory and self-depreciatory delusions are discovered as the patient tells about his past and current life situations. However, at times the patient evades areas in which he has delusions unless the interviewer asks specific questions. The examiner may ask a patient in whom he suspects persecutory delusions, "How have people been treating you lately? Do you feel you have any special problems with people who do not like you or who are against you?" If the patient answers affirmatively the interviewer pursues the subject further. To the patient in whom he suspects grandiose delusions, the examiner may ask, "Do you have any large projects going on or any plans for special achievements and important goals? What are your most important responsibilities at the present time?"

The evaluation of suicidal risk is a common problem in psychiatric evaluation, and exploring it is sometimes a difficult matter. If the interviewer bluntly asks the patient if he has any suicidal urges he may be very frightened. He may feel that the examiner thinks he is in a desperate psychiatric state and that an impulsive suicidal step may erupt unexpectedly at any time. I usually phrase this difficult question in the following manner: "Do you ever get so discouraged about all this trouble that you feel that maybe life isn't worth living?" If the patient answers affirmatively, I proceed to inquire, "Well, do you sometimes feel so bad that the idea of doing away with yourself even flits through your mind?" If the patient answers affirmatively, I then ask, "Do you mean that you sometimes think of suicide, or even consider how you might do it? How strong are these feelings and thoughts?" (The problem of suicidal risk and the ways of evaluating it are covered at length in Chapter 15.)

Memory. As the patient has discussed his past and current life situations the examiner usually has developed a clear impression about his memory. If the examiner wishes to explore the patient's memory further, he may test his distant memory by asking detailed questions about events in his past, and he may test recent memory by asking the patient when or by what means he came to the hospital or office, what he ate during his last two meals, and so forth. Often it is useful to inquire if the patient can remember acquaintances, physicians, or hospital personnel whom he has first met in the preceding week or two. Any tendency to confabulate is noted.

Current memory can be evaluated by several conventional tests. In one such test the examiner names three objects, such as a pencil, a tree and a shoe; the interviewer tells the patient that he will ask him later to repeat these items. After five minutes or longer, the examiner asks what the three items were.

Another conventional test is to tell a two-minute story of commonplace events, such as a person's trip to a supermarket with a brief listing of things he bought; the examiner immediately afterwards asks the patient to repeat the story. In another test, the patient repeats a series of four, five or six digits (such as 6, 4, 7, 8, 1) in the same order, or reverse order, after the examiner gives them.

These memory tests should be interpreted with caution, for patients who are emotionally upset often do not concentrate well on such routine tests. In my opinion, memory is best evaluated by discussing events of the patient's past and current life, with supplementary questions about his actions during the preceding 48 hours.

Orientation and Consciousness. During the interview it usually has become clear whether the patient is well oriented as to the time, the place, and the identity of himself and other persons. Occasionally, however, the examiner wishes to check these points carefully, and he can inquire if the patient knows the date, the year and the name and location of the hospital or clinic in which he is being examined. The interviewer can ask the patient to state his name, vocation and usual activities and to state the names and functions of some of the personnel in the hospital or other current surroundings. As a rule, such questions are asked only to pinpoint the amount of disorientation in a patient who has shown some degree of disorientation in previous parts of the interview.

During the session the examiner has become aware of any disturbances of consciousness. He has noted any evidence of confusion, clouding of consciousness or delirium.

Disturbances of Perception. During the examination the interviewer may become aware that the patient is having hallucinations. The patient may describe them while talking about his problems and life history. A patient with auditory hallucinations may refer to them in a matter-of-fact way, or he may complain that the voices are saying depreciating or obscene things to him. Sometimes the patient cocks his head and listens for them, thus giving the examiner his first hint that he is hallucinating. In other instances, he does not discuss his hallucinations unless the examiner inquires.

The examiner should approach the question of auditory hallucinations gently, for if he asks the patient bluntly if he is hallucinating the patient may become very frightened. He may fear that the examiner feels he is severely ill psychiatrically or in imminent danger of becoming so, and he may leave the session more anxious than he entered it. However, the presence or absence of auditory hallucinations sometimes is an importnat diagnostic point and should be ascertained. I approach the problem by first asking, "Have you been troubled by noises lately?" I then proceed to feel my way by asking such questions as, "Have the noises which bother you any special characteristics? Are they like humming sounds, or like the noises of machinery, or like the rumbling of muffled voices?" If the patient answers affirmatively or if he hesitates and has a troubled facial expression, I next inquire, "Do the rumbling sounds of voices at times become clear?" If the patient discloses that he is having auditory hallucinations, the examiner should find out more about them by asking, "Are the voices male or female? Are they familiar voices? What do they say to you?"

Visual hallucinations are much less common than auditory hallucinations, but they occur in some acute organic brain disorders and in a small percentage of schizophrenic patients. Patients with visual hallucinations may talk about them openly; this is especially true in acute and chronic organic brain disorders. However, in some instances the patient may not mention them if the examiner does not ask, and an occasional patient hides them from the examiner. I recall an ambulatory schizophrenic whom I saw each week for two years in posthospitalization outpatient interviews before he disclosed that he often had visual hallucinations. I first suspected it when I noticed that he sometimes looked out of the corner of his eye in a frightened way at one wall of my office. He finally disclosed that he sometimes saw his long-deceased father standing there in a threatening attitude.

In asking about visual hallucinations, the examiner may inquire, "Have you seen any puzzling or frightening things lately?" When the patient hesitates and looks troubled, or answers affirmatively, the interviewer may ask, "Do you sometimes mistake things for other things than what they are? For example, do you sometimes see a shadow moving and mistake it for someone entering your room?" If the patient indicates that he has such illusions, the examiner may ask about hallucinations more directly by saying, "Does this sort of thing happen when nothing may really be there? What unusual things or people have you seen here in the hospital, or elsewhere lately?"

The examiner may inquire about the less common hallucinations of smell, taste and touch by asking, "Have you noticed any strong or unusual odors lately?" "Have you had any unusual tastes in the last few weeks, or has your food or water tasted different lately?" "Have you had any unusual feelings on the skin of any part of your body recently?"

Fund of Information and Judgement. The patient's general level of information usually has become evident during the course of the examination, but in some cases the interviewer should explore it further. In patients in whom the examiner suspects mental retardation or organic brain damage, exploration of the patient's fund of information may give diagnostic clues and help to evaluate the degree of intellectual defect or deterioration. Evaluation of the patient's fund of information is occasionally relevant in other types of psychiatric problems.

The patient's fund of information must be interpreted in relation to his life experience and his education. A farmer knows little about finding his way around the city on subways, and a city dweller knows little about caring for cattle. A person with an eighth grade education may not know the capital of France, but an individual with a high school education or better should know this fact. Common questions used in testing the fund of information are to ask the names of the current president and vice president of the United States, the names of the three preceding presidents, the names of the largest cities in some of the more populous states and their approximate populations, and central facts about recent important events in national and world news.

Judgement is a complex function in which personality stability, experience, knowledge and reasoning all play roles; it consists of the ability to evaluate facts, ideas and circumstances and to draw reasonable, proper conclusions from them. (The relationship between intelligence and judgement is dealt with in Chapter 20.) Defects of judgement usually become apparent as the patient discusses his current and past circumstances.

When the examiner wishes to evaluate judgement objectively, various traditional test questions are used in a psychiatric examination. Two such questions are: What would you do if you found a fully addressed, stamped, sealed letter on the sidewalk, and what would be the reasons for what you did? What would you do if you were sitting in a theater and noticed that a small fire had broken out? However, a survey of how the patient has been handling his recent interpersonal, economic and vocational activities gives a sounder concept of his judgement.

Insight. In a mental status examination, insight is defined as awareness by the patient that he has psychiatric difficulties and that he needs treatment. In a broader sense, the term insight is employed to designate awareness of the emotional causes of his illness and how past experiences have led to his present difficulties.

While the patient discusses his problems and his past and current life circumstances, the examiner usually learns the extent to which he understands his disorder, the causes of it and the need for treatment. Some patients do not have any insight and are puzzled or indignant that they are being examined psychiatrically. Others, such as those with organic brain disease, may not understand the nature of their surroundings or realize that they are undergoing psychiatric evaluation. Some patients with personality disorders, such as aggressive or antisocial personality problems, may feel that they do not have emotional difficulties and that their problems arise entirely from the inadequacies and maliciousness of the people in their various life situations. Others patients are aware that they are ill and may be able to identify some of the factors that have led to their troubles. In some instances the patient's insight varies much from day to day or from week to week. For example, a hallucinating schizophrenic may sometimes know that the voices he hears are symptoms of an illness, and at other times he may feel that the voices come from people hidden outside his room or elsewhere. When the examiner wishes to pinpoint the patient's degree of insight he may inquire directly about how the patient views his illness and its causes and how he feels about treatment plans.

Ending the Interview

At the end of the first interview most examiners make at least a few observations, tentative formulations, or simple recommendations to the patient. Harry Stack Sullivan, for example, felt that the patient should leave with the feeling that he "got something out of the interview"; he should not go away empty-handed, so to speak. Sophisticated patients who know a good deal about psychiatry (particularly from the Freudian-psychoanalytic point of view) may feel comfortable and satisfied with no more than a return appointment date and a formal farewell, but the vast majority of patients need more than this, and expect more.

In my opinion, the interviewer should make at least brief statements (which he may label somewhat speculative, if he wishes) about what he feels the patient's problems are and how they may be helped. The examiner who terminates the interview without comments of this kind often sends the patient away puzzled, disappointed and, perhaps, frightened. A patient who is puzzled, disappointed and frightened by the first session has a much diminished probability of returning for a second one.

For example, in ending the first interview the examiner may say, "Mrs. Williams, I think we have outlined fairly well these periods of acute anxiousness that you have several times a week. This is a common kind of emotional problem that we see in patients, and by talking about what has gone on, and is going on, in their lives, we often can help them." To another patient the interviewer might say, "Mr. Harris, we have defined your phobias today and we have begun to discuss various aspects of your life. Exploring your past experiences, your current stresses, and how you handle many kinds of feelings and situations is the way we work to resolve these difficulties." The examiner sometimes may feel that he has learned enough to make some limited interpretations to the patient about the causes of his difficulties. In some instances hospitalization is a necessary recommendation or medication may be useful while the patient is working on his problems in further sessions.

The inexperienced interviewer sometimes is at a loss for a comfortable way to terminate the session without seeming to reject the patient bruskly. I often end an interview by saying, "Well, I think we are going to have to stop now and go on next time." This terminates the interview but indicates a forward-looking continuity toward the next session.

OBTAINING INFORMATION FROM THE PATIENT'S FAMILY

A psychiatric work-up should in most instances include an interview with a close relative of the patient. If he does not get information from a relative as part of the total data from which he forms his conclusions, the examiner occasionally may make serious errors in his diagnostic formulation and treatment plans. Some patients are unable to give important diagnostic information and others fearfully hide essential material. For example, a patient may not disclose recent suicidal attempts or suicidal feelings which he has told to relatives. A patient may hide paranoid delusions or hallucinations from an examiner for fear that disclosure of them might lead to a recommendation of hospitalization. Alcoholism, drug abuse, recent assaultiveness, serious criminal legal problems, previous psychiatric hospitalizations, sexual offenses and many other significant things often are not disclosed by patients during diagnostic interviews and may be hidden for long periods of time after the patient enters interview treatment. In my opinion, physicians who do not interview relatives often end up treating the wrong problems or irrelveant ones, and the consequences range from ridiculous to tragic.

I recall a businessman whom I saw for 14 months in psychotherapy for personality problems that were gravely affecting his family relationships and business activities. His wife requested an interview and revealed that his main adjustment problem was severe chronic alcoholism, of which I had been unaware and which he had denied in the routine life survey of the initial interviews. I also recall a painful episode early in my practice in which I did not learn of a patient's recent suicidal episodes until I met her relatives in a hospital emergency room after she made an almost fatal suicidal attempt with medication I had prescribed. Psychiatrists who do not interview relatives are either treating people with relatively minor problems or are due for some distressing surprises.

An interview with a close relative often gives the examiner a more comprehensive view of the patient's problems, or at least puts him on a sounder footing in making his diagnostic formulations and treatment plans. There are, of course, exceptions to this rule, as in the case of a homosexual patient who does not want his relatives to know of his problem or to arouse suspicion of it by the knowledge that he is seeing a psychiatrist. Other similar examples are the patient who lives alone and has no close relatives available, the single male with sexual impotence or premature ejaculation, the married patient who comes because of emotional turmoil precipitated by discontinuing an extramarital affair, and others is whom clinical judgement indicates that seeing a close relative is impractical or unwise.

Some psychiatrists feel that interviewing a relative causes a hindrance in the patient's subsequent flow of confidential communication to the interviewer. There is some justification for this point of view, but it varies much depending on the type of patient and his problems. For example, an adolescent often becomes less communicative if he knows that his parents have seen the interviewer. A person with a marital problem may feel that if the interviewer sees his marital partner, the marital partner will prejudice the therapist against him. A patient may fear that the examiner will have further interviews with the relative and may inadvertently reveal confidences the patient does not want the relative to know, and the patient may tend to become less communicative.

Despite such possible problems, I feel that there is greater risk in not interviewing a relative in the majority of cases. The examiner should always assure the patient of the confidential nature of the interview, and this usually helps to assuage any misgivings the patient has.

Some psychiatrists delegate the responsibility for interviewing relatives to psychiatric social workers who work in close association with the psychiatrists. This is common practice in child guidance clinics and also in many clinics and hospitals for adults. This may help relieve apprehension in the patient about the interviewer seeing a relative, but it does not resolve the problem entirely, for the patient may fear that communication between the psychiatrist and the social worker opens possibilities of disclosures of the patient's confidences to his relatives. Moreover, in my opinion, the examiner has a much firmer understanding of the patient's relationships with his family when he has talked directly with a relative.

The interviewer should always see the patient first, even when he expects to get only limited information from him, as in the case of a severely psychotic patient or one with advanced organic brain disease. Preliminary interviewing is a courtesy to him and also is clinically sound. The examiner can interpret the information of the relatives better after he has seen the patient and has a better idea about what kind of information will be most helpful.

During his interview with the relative the examiner follows the same general outline that he used in his examination of the patient. He may let the relative speak spontaneously for a while in response to his initial question, but he wants at least partial information about the parent's present difficulty, past psychiatric problems, current and past interpersonal relationships, childhood and adolescent experiences, adjustments in social groups and at work, medical history and current emotional functioning. In actual practice, the examiner tends to focus his attention on whatever areas he feels are most relevant and revealing. At the end of the interview the examiner should ask, "Is there anything else you feel you would like to tell me which you feel might be important or useful in helping the patient?" Some relatives do not discuss important points unless a broad invitation to do so is given to them.

EXAMINATION OF THE UNCOMMUNICATIVE PATIENT

The examiner occasionally must perform a psychiatric evaluation on an uncommunicative patient. He may be a mute catatonic schizophrenic, or a severely depressed patient who does not respond to questions, or an incoherent patient with organic brain deterioration, or a patient with one of various other types of psychiatric problems. In such instances the observer relies heavily on history data from the patient's relatives and the referring physician. When the patient is hospitalized the examiner also seeks information about his behavior from the nurses and aides on the ward. However, the examiner can also make observations of the patient that help in arriving at a diagnostic formulation. Many of the following points were also covered earlier in this chapter in our discussion of the mental status examination, but we shall list them briefly here for convenient use in making a systematic evaluation of an uncommunicative patient.

General Appearance and Behavior. The examiner notes the patient's state of cleanliness and grooming. He notes whether the patient appears cooperative or uncooperative, or whether he is apparently detached from emotional and intellectual contact with the people and things in his environment. Does the patient make any sounds, and does he respond in any way to noises and voices? Does he speak, and is his speech comprehensible? If he does not speak, will he write or will he respond to written questions and suggestions? Does he seem to understand gestures and can he be requested by gestures to do simple things? What are his eating habits and does he take care of his excretory needs in socially acceptable ways?

Affect and Emotions. By careful observation of the patient the examiner may get some clues about the patient's affect and his emotional reactions. He watches the patient's facial expressions in particular, but he also notes movements of the hands and body. He notes if the patient's affect seems depressed or exhilarated, appropriate or inappropriate, flat or alert, anxious or placid. Does he seem frightened, perplexed, angry, defiant or joyful? Does he smile, cry, or stare vacantly? Does he clench his fists in anger or tension, or does he twist his handkerchief ceaselessly in anxious agitation? Does he seem emotionally moved by events in his environment or emotionally detached? By his smiles or frightened glances, does he seem to be responding to emotional turmoil and vivid fantasies within himself? Does he react emotionally to visits from relatives or to particular physicians, nurses or aides on the ward?

Physical Actions. The examiner observes whether the patient is motionless, slow moving, restless or hyperactive. Does he wander aimlessly about the ward or stay quietly in one place? Does he show tendencies toward combativeness and destructiveness, or do the nurses and aides report such tendencies at other times? Does the patient have unusual mannerisms, repetitive gestures, facial grimaces, tremors or tics? Does he sit tensely on the edge of his chair and clutch its arms tightly? Does he pick pointlessly at his clothing and small objects around him? Can his limbs be placed in various positions and does the patient then maintain them in these positions, or does he rigidly resist efforts to have him change position?

Disturbances of Perception. By observing the uncommunicative patient carefully the examiner may get some useful clues about whether delusions and hallucinations are present. The delusional patient may appear suspicious and tensely on guard. He may glance fearfully about the room or cast anxious looks at the doors and windows. He may shun food and drink, or taste it cautiously, as if he fears it may contain harmful drugs or poisons. He may hide things in his room, as if to deceive those who would rob him. The delusional patient sometimes explores the corners of his room, carefully looking for electronic devices he feels are being used to spy on him. Many of these actions are more marked when the patient feels he is not being observed. The patient with grandiose delusions may walk about in an officious manner and look at people with a condescending smile or an arrogant stare. He may stand or kneel in poses of religious devotion or prayer if he feels he is a divine person or in communication with divine persons.

The hallucinating patient may nod and smile in ways that suggest he is hearing voices. He may cock his head as if to hear them better, and he responds with gestures or words to the voices. He may watch the ceiling attentively or stare out the windows for long periods, quietly moving his lips as if responding to voices. Sometimes an uncommunicative patient reveals his delusions or hallucinations only in written notes. I recall a patient who had remained mute for several years on a psychiatric ward. He revealed his delusions only in brief notes he occasionally wrote; they contained messages "to the troops on the front line" and were signed with the name of a well known general.

Other Observations. At times the examiner notes apparent clouding of consciousness or delirium in the uncommunicative patient, and he can speculate on how well oriented the patient is for time, place and identity of persons. To a limited extent the examiner also can speculate on whether the patient has any insight into his condition.

Further Steps in the Psychiatric Work-Up

Before making his diagnostic formulation in a psychiatric work-up, the examiner often wants other data from special examination procedures; consequently, our discussion of the process of making a psychiatric diagnosis is deferred until the last part of Chapter 5, where such procedures are discussed.

BIBLIOGRAPHY

Chapman, A. H.: The Physician's Guide to Managing Emotional Problems. Philadelphia, J. B. Lippincott, 1969.

Enelow, A. J., and Swisher, S. N.: Interviewing and Patient Care. New York, Oxford University Press, 1972.

Group for the Advancement of Psychiatry: Assessment of Sexual Function: A Guide to Interviewing. New York, Group for the Advancement of Psychiatry, 1973.

Mackinnon, R. A., and Michels, R.: The Psychiatric Interview in Clinical Practice. Philadelphia, W. B. Saunders, 1971.

Mendel, W. M., and Solomon, P. (eds.): The Psychiatric Consultation. New York, Grune and Stratton, 1968.

Novey, S.: The Second Look. Baltimore, Johns Hopkins Press, 1968.

Stevenson, I.: The Psychiatric Interview. Boston, Little Brown, 1969.

Sullivan, H. S.: The Psychiatric Interview. New York, W. W. Norton, 1954.

5

Further Examination Procedures

In this chapter we shall consider all procedures—aside from the interview examination technics discussed in Chapter 4—that may be part of a psychiatric work-up. We shall consider these procedures under three headings: (1) psychological testing by a clinical psychologist, (2) special interview technics, such as examination after barbiturate injection, and (3) physical evaluation of the patient.

At the end of the chapter we shall discuss the process of formulating a psychiatric diagnosis. We shall also consider the problem of handling psychiatric material in psychiatric hospital and clinic records, general hospital records (as in psychiatric consultations on nonpsychiatric floors and in psychiatric divisions of general medical hospitals), abstracts, insurance reports and other kinds of records.

PSYCHOLOGICAL TESTING

A wide variety of psychological tests are used to evaluate personality structure. These tests are usually administered and interpreted by clinical psychologists who work in close collaboration with physicians in the care of emotionally disturbed patients. We shall first describe some of the tests used for personality evaluation; these often are called *projective tests*, because they are designed in such a manner that the patient projects many features of his emotional functioning into them as he gives his responses. After considering the personality tests we shall discuss some of the tests employed to evaluate intelligence.

Personality Tests

While administering tests the clinical psychologist observes the patient's attitudes and emotional reactions. He often precedes testing by a brief period of discussion to put the patient at ease, to explain the testing procedures and to observe his behavior. There is much art, as well as science, in administering and interpreting psychological tests, and the patient who is at ease and establishes a comfortable relationship with the psychologist gives a more valid picture of his emotional functioning on the psychological tests. Some psychologists spend a full session with the patient discussing his difficulties before focusing on selected problems with tests.

The Rorschach Test

The Rorschach test was developed by the Swiss psychiatrist Hermann Rorschach, who published his major work on it in 1921. The Rorschach test is one of the oldest and most reliable psychological tests used for personality evaluation. The psychologist shows the patient 10 cards, one at a time. Each card contains a standardized, printed ink blot, and the patient tells the impressions, thoughts and associations that come to his mind as he looks at it. He may see persons, animals, parts of human anatomy, man-made objects, objects from nature and other types of things. The patient usually gives two to five responses to each card and the psychologist writes down the responses verbatim. The Rorschach test is based on the principle that since the cards contain only ink blots, the patient's responses come mainly from within himself.

The psychologist later scores each response according to (1) what part of the ink blot the patient uses in the response, (2) the nature of the object seen, and (3) the features of the particular ink blot, such as form or color, which evoked the response. For example, the response "a butterfly" to card number 5 would be scored as (1) located in the entire ink blot, (2) of animal content, and (3) determined mainly by the form of the ink blot. Other responses might include only small parts of ink blots and might be determined by the texture, the color or the shading of the card.

Long experience with the Rorschach has led to well-established correlations between the various types of responses and personality features. For example, the ways in which the patient uses the colored parts of the cards and the amount of color he uses reveal much about how he handles his emotions. The patient who does not give any responses involving the colored parts of the cards tends to inhibit expression of his emotions and is uncomfortable with them. The person who uses the colored parts of the cards in well-organized, well thought out ways tends to be a person who is comfortable with his emotions and expresses them in healthy ways. The person who uses the colored parts of the card in crudely constructed responses or merely names the colors and points them out tends to have poor control of his emotions and expresses them in impulsive or chaotic ways.

Many other aspects of the Rorschach reveal symptoms, personality features and facets of the individual's emotional functioning. For example, the person with much preoccupation with diseases usually gives many responses involving parts of the body, x-rays and internal body organs. The overly neat, compulsive person tends to use small details of the cards in meticulous, precise ways. Insecure, anxious people tend to see three-dimensional scenes such as landscapes with lakes and mountains in the background or geographical formations as seen from an airplane. These are only a few examples of the ways in which the Rorschach responses are interpreted. The Rorschach is the most highly developed of all psychological tests used in personality evaluation, and there is a large literature on its administration and interpretation. Learning to administer and interpret the Rorschach requires much training and experience.

The Thematic Apperception Test

In the Thematic Apperception Test, often called the TAT, the psychologist shows the patient a standard series of cards one at a time with pictures of people in various emotionally significant situations. He asks the patient to describe what is going on in the picture and perhaps to tell a story centered on it. The details of the pictures are vague enough to allow the patient a wide range of choice in the stories he weaves into them.

The Thematic Apperception Test is based on the principle that the patient tends to project his emotional turmoil, interpersonal problems and daydreams into the stories he tells. The pictures on the cards are drawn in ways which make it easy for the patient to identify himself with a central figure in the picture. In describing the activities, interpersonal problems, emotional reactions and hopes of the person in the picture, the patient reveals much of his own emotional life. The scoring of the Thematic Apperception Test is not as precise as that of the Rorschach, but it offers a standardized set of stimuli for exploring emotional life. The psychologist is particularly interested in themes and interpersonal problems that appear in the responses to several cards. Special adaptations of the Thematic Apperception Test have been designed for children; in them the central figure in each card is a child. One adaptation uses cartoons of animals in various situations similar to those which children may experience, since small children often can make warm identifications with animals.

The Minnesota Multiphasic Personality Inventory

The Minnesota Multiphasic Personality Inventory, often called the MMPI, consists of 550 statements which cover a wide range of personality features and emotional functioning. To each statement the patient must respond "true," or "false," or "cannot say." These responses are then scored in various categories, and from them a clinical profile of the patient's personality structure is drawn. This profile is sketched in the form of a line connecting nine points of varying altitude on a piece of graph paper. The nine different points vary in height depending on whether the patient shows strong or weak tendencies toward different personality problems, and the fluctuations of the line that connects these points show the areas of personality difficulty and their respective severity. Thus, the test scores the patient's tendencies toward (1) body preoccupation about diseases, (2) depression, (3) hysteria, (4) antisocial personality, (5) masculine or feminine features, (6) paranoid qualities, (7) anxiety, phobias and psychogenic fatigue states, (8) schizophrenic features, and (9) manic features. The test also can be interpreted in further ways to elucidate other aspects of the person's emotional and intellectual functioning.

The proponents of the MMPI point out that it gives a broad examination of personality functioning with a minimum of professional time involved in its administration and interpretation, since it is largely self-administered by the patient and lends itself easily to statistical interpretation. In recent years there has been much interest in the MMPI as a personality inventory tool that can be given easily to large numbers of people and can be scored quickly on computers. Hence, some writers have advocated its use for screening people in colleges, industries, business organizations, government agencies and many other settings.

Many psychiatrists and clinical psychologists object to such mass inventories of people by computer technics. They feel that people are so varied and complex that such screening has limited validity and that each person should have the benefit of an individual evaluation. The MMPI has value when administered by an individual clinical psychologist who uses it as one of several tests in evaluating a person. Its mass application to serve the purposes of industry and other large groups causes many psychiatrists to cringe. I am one of them. A basic principle of psychiatry is that each person is a separate individual with his unique problems, requiring separate, careful scrutiny.

Other Personality Tests

Many other psychological tests have been devised for personality evaluation, but many of them are of more recent origin, and less well validated than the Rorschach and the Thematic Apperception Test. They are useful, but they must be interpreted with caution. We shall discuss a few of those most commonly used.

The Sentence Completion Test. This test consists of an extensive number of incomplete sentences the patient completes in a spontaneous manner with the thoughts that first come to mind as he reads them. The sentences are constructed to explore the fears, daydreams, identifications, aspirations and preferences of the patient as well as other aspects of his emotional functioning.

The Bender-Gestalt Test. A series of nine geometric designs are printed on separate cards. The psychologist presents the cards one at a time to the patient, and requests that he draw the designs as well as he can on a separate sheet of paper. In some instances, the examiner shows the patient the design for a brief time, then takes the card away and asks the patient to draw the design from memory. This test is useful in evaluating the level of maturation in the coordination of visual, muscular and intellectual functions in children. It is also used in evaluating personality structure and emotional problems in both children and adults. However, many psychologists feel that the Bender-Gestalt test is most useful in detecting organic brain damage in persons of all ages.

Draw-A-Person Test. In the Draw-A-Person test the psychologist requests the patient to draw a human figure. The patient is allowed to draw a person of either sex, and some psychologists then ask the patient to draw a figure of the sex opposite to the first one. In children these figures give some information about the child's level of intelligence, because the ability of a child to draw a human figure correctly progresses with his age level in fairly reliable increments. Thus, at various age levels the child begins to include more lifelike facial features, better formed limbs, a well-proportioned trunk, and so forth. The age level of expression in the drawing can be compared with the age level of the child, and a rough approximation of the child's intelligence is obtained.

However, many clinical psychologists use the drawings to analyze the feelings of both child and adult patients about themselves and other people. A patient may reveal his concepts of his own body and his personality structure in the kind of figure he draws of a person of his own sex. For example, a passive, insecure man with strong feelings of inferiority may draw a small, weak looking male figure. The man who in his two figures draws a large, aggressive woman and a smaller, inactive man often is projecting his views of the roles of men and women in marriage and life. The patient's drawings also may reflect some of his basic feelings about his parents. Thus, a skillful interpreter of these drawings sometimes elicits useful clues about the patient's emotional conflicts. The terms Goodenough test and Machover test are sometimes applied to various versions of the Draw-A-Person test.

This type of test may be enlarged by asking the testee also to draw a house and a tree, in addition to a person, and it is then called the House-Tree-Person (HTP) test.

Intelligence Tests

The clinical psychologist includes an intelligence test in his battery of examinations for comprehensive evaluation of a person. Intelligence testing is, of course, particularly important when mental retardation is suspected or when a more accurate appraisal of the degree of mental retardation is needed. However, the level of intelligence is useful information in a throrough psychological evaluation, though in most instances the psychologist's study of personality structure is much more important in helping to understand the patient's problems. (The limitations of intelligence tests in predicting and evaluating an individual's total life adaptation are discussed in Chapter 20. We also consider there the distinction, and only limited correlation, between intelligence and judgement.)

The Stanford-Binet Test. This is a widely used intelligence test for children; there are many modifications of it bearing somewhat varied names. It consists of a graded series of tasks, each set of which is more difficult than its predecessor. Each set of tasks is designed to correlate with the abilities of children of a particular age group. For example, one of the sets of tasks is designed for accomplishment by 7-year-old children and the next highest level of tasks is adjusted to the abilities of 8-year-olds. The 7-year-old child should be able to do all the tasks of the test up through those for his own age level, and the 8-year-old child should be able to do all the tests up through those for 8-year-olds. In actual practice, most children of normal intelligence do some tests beyond their age level and fail a few at their age level and below it. The child with average intelligence, however, averages out at about the level of his age group. Children of superior intelligence perform the tasks appropriate for their age level, and are able to do many tasks at levels beyond it.

Children with low intelligence can do the tasks only up to a level one or more years behind their age group. The tasks are divided into different groupings which test such functions as comprehension, ability to solve problems and so forth. The tasks stop at about the level of 15 years, since it is felt that after that age the child does not increase in his basic intellectual capacities. Some I. Q. tests are based on the assumption that the individual reaches his full intellectual potential at the age of 15 and others place this point at 16.

The intellectual quotient, or I. Q., of the child is calculated by making a fraction by placing the mental age derived from the test over the child's age in years and multiplying this fraction by 100. Thus, an 8-year-old child with a mental age of 8 years on the test would have an I. Q. of $8/8 \times 100 = 100$. An I. Q. of 100 is the theoretical average figure for a child of normal intelligence. A 10-year-old child whose mental age on the test is 12 would have an I. Q. of $12/10 = 120$. An I. Q. of 120 places the child in the range of superior intelligence. The normal range of intelligence, in terms of I. Q. numbers, is between 83 and 115. By the standards of the official American (and World) medical nomenclature, a person with an. I. Q. below 83 falls in the mentally retarded group. However, some psychiatrists place lower levels of normal intelligence at 80 or 85. A person with an I. Q. of 115 (or 120, in some classifications), or above, is in the range of superior intelligence.

An I. Q. test, in the final analysis, compares a person with other people on a standard set of various performances. Though each section of an I. Q. test is designed to test a particular intellectual function, such as comprehension or reasoning ability, it basically compares a person with many thousands of others who have taken the test.

An I. Q. test should be given by a well-trained clinical psychologist. If the examiner does not get the testee's full cooperation, or if the testee has emotional tensions that inhibit him, he may do less well on the test than he would do otherwise. I have seen persons whose I. Q. scores came up as much as 30 points over a period of several years because they resolved emotional problems and were able to give better cooperation in testing. An adequately administered and scored I. Q. test cannot be falsely high; a person cannot do better on the test than his intellectual level merits. However, a frightened or uncooperative person may score at a lower I. Q. figure than he would attain if he were better relaxed. When an examiner administers and interprets an I. Q. test, he should take this possibility into account.

The Wechsler Adult Intelligence Scale. Sometimes called the WAIS, this is designed for testing intelligence in adolescents and adults, whereas the Stanford-Binet is structured for testing children. The Wechsler test evaluates the person on a performance scale involving such features as picture completion and block design, and a verbal scale covering subjects such as general comprehension and identification of similarties. The is widely used and it gives reliable I. Q. scores. It also gives separate ratings for the patient's performance scale and verbal scale. Examination of these scales and the proficiency of the patient on their various subgroups gives added information about the patient's personality structure and intellectual functioning.

The Wechsler Intelligence Scale for Children. This test is sometimes called the WISC, and is organized along lines similar to the Wechsler test for adults. It gives reliable results, with a performance scale, a verbal scale and ratings in the various subgroups. The study of these scales and ratings may give clues about personality structure and possible organic brain damage as well as I. Q. evaluation.

Other Tests. In the *Gesell Developmental Schedules* and the *Vineland Social Maturity Scale* small children may be rated on scales that inventory their muscular skills and social development. These scales have some usefulness in estimating the intelligence of children who are too young or unable to cooperate in other types of tests. (The clinical application of intelligence testing is covered further in Chapter 20 on mental retardation.)

The Psychologist's Formulation

Our discussion of the examiner as a *participant-observer* at the beginning of Chapter 4 applies equally to the clinical psychologist. A psychological testing session is merely a special kind of interpersonal relationship in which the psychologist makes general observations of the patient's emotional state and employs various tests to deepen his understanding of him. The psychologist's skill as a participant in this relationship affects both his degree of success with the patient and the accuracy of his observations.

The psychologist uses a battery of several tests which he feels will be most useful in evaluating the patient's personality and problems. The administration of the tests requires one or two sessions of about two hours each, and the psychologist spends an equal amount of time scoring the tests and drawing up his report. The report deals with the patient's diagonsis, his personality structure, his emotional functioning and his capacity for interpersonal relationships. The report may give suggestions about areas of emotional conflict that can be explored in interview treatment, and it also may speculate on the patient's prognosis.

SPECIAL INTERVIEW TECHNICS

Psychiatrists occasionally use special interview technics to uncover material that could not be obtained in conventional interview procedures. These special technics are of limited value and have certain dangers, and hence most psychiatrists use them sparingly. However, they have an established place in psychiatry and we shall discuss them briefly.

Examination Under Barbiturate Sedation

Although barbiturate interviews are much less employed than formerly, some psychiatrists feel that they still have a place in the diagnostic evaluation of some types of psychiatric problems. The terms *narcoanalysis* and *narcosynthesis* are sometimes used in referring to barbiturate interviews.

In an examination under barbiturate sedation, a 10 per cent solution of amobarbital (Amytal), thiopental (Pentothal), or some other short-acting barbiturate is injected intravenously very slowly while the patient is reclining on his hospital bed or on a couch. As the barbiturate is injected during a period of several minutes, the examiner talks with the patient on neutral topics to determine when he is sedated enough to talk with fewer inhibitions, but not so sedated that he cannot articulate well. Some psychiatrists have the patient count backwards slowly from 100 and stop the injection when the patient first begins to have difficulty in counting. The amount of barbiturate injected usually is about 0.2 Gm. (3 gr.), but may be somewhat higher or lower. When the patient is in a lightly drowsy state, the examiner begins to question him about emotionally significant experiences.

An interview under barbiturate sedation must be conducted and interpreted with skill, for although the sedation diminishes some of the patient's inhibitions and resistances it does not eliminate them. Moreover, the things the patient says under barbiturate sedation are not always factually true. He may relate his daydreams and unconscious wishes as if they were factual events that had occurred. Hence, these interviews are not the "truth serum" examinations they have been purported to be by some lay publications. Moreover, some patients talk less openly under barbiturate sedation than in a regular interview.

Barbiturate interviews may be useful in evaluating and treating patients with hysterical mutism. Also, they sometimes can clarify whether amnesia is due to organic brain dysfunction or emotional factors; the patient with organic brain dysfunction cannot recover his lost memories under barbiturate sedation, whereas the patient with amnesia due to emotional factors (mainly hysterical) sometimes can do so. Barbiturate interviews occasionally may be useful in differentiating prolonged psychomotor epilepsy states from hysterical seizures, because the hysterical patient sometimes can recall under barbiturate sedation what he did during his seizure, whereas the epileptic patient cannot.

Barbiturate interviews have certain dangers. A patient occasionally has an adverse reaction such as laryngospasm, hypotension or idiosyncrasy to the drug. Moreover, if the patient is emotionally quite disturbed beneath a façade of seemingly well-organized behavior, the weakening of his defenses by a barbiturate interview may make him worse. Severe anxiety reactions, depressions and schizophrenic psychoses have been precipitated by barbiturate interviews. Hence, a patient should be carefully evaluated before submitting him to a barbiturate examination.

Interview Under Hypnoisis

A few psychiatrists employ hypnosis as a diagnostic interview technic. They base its use on the principle that by hypnosis they can reduce the patient's inhibitions against freely discussing emotionally important material. (The technic for inducing hypnosis is outlined in Chapter 21.)

Diagnostic interviewing under hypnosis sometimes is useful in distinguishing organically caused amnesia from emotionally caused (usually hysterical) amnesia, and in distinguishing prolonged psychomotor epileptic states from hysterical seizures (for the same reasons outlined concerning these conditions in the preceding section on barbiturate interviews). In addition, some psychiatrists feel they are able to probe more quickly into the patient's emotional problems when his inhibitions are diminished by hypnosis.

Most psychiatrists, however, feel that the problems involved in hypnotic interviews outweigh their usefulness in most instances. The examiner who employs hypnosis must have considerable experience with it to employ it efficiently and safely. Often several sessions must be spent gradually training the patient to undergo hypnosis before a trance of satisfactory depth can be induced, and some patients cannot be hypnotized at all. The material obtained under hypnosis must be carefully integrated with what is known of the patient from previous interviewing, for the patient may describe daydreams and unconscious wishes as actual past events in his life. Moreover, as in the case of barbiturate interviews, a patient with much underlying emotional tumult covered by a thin veneer of seemingly well-integrated behavior may be precipitated into a severe neurotic or psychotic state by hypnosis. (Other possible dangers of hypnosis are outlined in Chapter 21.) Hence, hypnosis is employed as a diagnostic technic only by a small number of psychiatrists who have much experience in its use and are cautious about its possible dangers. (*Special diagnostic interview technics for children* are discussed in Chapter 24.)

PHYSICAL EVALUATION

Psychiatry is a medical specialty, and the psychiatrist who neglects physical evaluation of his patients is in for some unpleasant surprises. I recall a 58-year-old woman who had lived with her mother all her life and whom I first saw four months after her mother's sudden death, after which she had developed anxiety attacks, severe phobias, headaches and fatigue. After evaluation by her internist, who found no physical pathology, I saw her for four months in weekly interview treatment sessions. She became steadily worse. At her family's insistence, she was hospitalized by her internist who examined her again and found a glioblastoma multiforme of the right frontal lobe from which she died six weeks later.

I recall a 46-year-old woman who had interview treatment sessions three times each week for eight months for what were believed to be emotionally caused physical symptoms and anxiety attacks. Autopsy thereafter revealed widespread collagen disease. I remember a patient who for two and one-half years was in intensive inpatient psychotherapy for personality problems in a well-known private psychiatric center. Subsequent neurological and electroencephalographic evaluation elsewhere revealed classical petit mal epilepsy with 20 to 30 seizures each day; these had previously been diagnosed as emotional blocking. I recall a 52-year-old woman who had profound personality change with apathy and depression following her mother's death. Fortunately, I ordered skull films as part of her hospital work-up before beginning treatment, and I was spared the chagrin of having given extensive psychiatric treatment to a patient who had a large parasagittal meningioma. I have seen patients with carcinoma of the pancreas who were treated for psychosomatic gastrointestinal pain, and I have seen persons who after years of intermittent psychiatric treatment turned out to have porphyria. This melancholy recitation of the errors of my colleagues and myself could be extended considerably, but I feel I have made my point.

Most psychiatrists feel that the physical evaluation of office patients should be done by the patient's family physician or internist. They feel that the intimacy of physical examination, especially of patients of the opposite sex, may introduce subsequent problems in the interview relationship. In many cases the patient is referred for psychiatric consultation by the family physician and the physical examination thus has been done prior to the first psychiatric interview. In the outpatient psychiatric clinics of medical centers the physical examination may be done by the medical clinic prior to referring the patient for psychiatric evaluation, or the patient may be referred to the medical clinic from the psychiatric clinic for this purpose. Some psychiatrists perform the physical evaluation, or at least the neurological part of it, on hospitalized psychotic patients; other psychiatrists place this responsibility in the hands of internists who act as consultants. A neurological examination should be part of the physical examination. The patient whose psychiatric problems are due to acute or chronic organic brain disease may require further neurological study using such procedures as an electroencephalogram, a lumbar puncture, a brain scan, skull films or other tests.

There are, of course, many cases in which physical examination is usually omitted. These cases include most marriage counseling problems, many child guidance cases and adolescent difficulties, problems of clear (for example, vocational or cultural) situational adjustments, long-standing personality disorders (such as a passive personality disorder), and others. The examiner uses clinical judgement and common sense to pick the cases in which physical evaluation is felt to be unnecessary.

When a psychiatric interviewer refers a patient for a physical examination as part of his psychiatric work-up, he should tell the patient that his tentative impression is that the patient's symptoms are caused by emotional tension, but that to be entirely sure he is requesting a routine physical examination. If the examiner does not make this point clear, the patient with physical symptoms accompanying an anxiety neurosis or other emotional disorders may conclude that the examiner feels his symptoms are due to some physical disease that has not yet been elucidated. This idea may become more firmly fixed in the patient's mind as he goes through the physical checkup, and subsequently the examiner may have increased difficulty convincing the patient that his symptoms are due to emotional factors. The examiner should say, "Mr. Monroe, having discussed your problems in our first interview, I feel 95 per cent certain that your physical symptoms are caused by tension and emotional stress. However, since you have not had a physical checkup for some time, as part of your psychiatric work-up we will have you checked over physically to rule out the very unlikely possibility of any physical trouble. When you've had your physical checkup you can then settle down to work on your emotional problems with complete confidence that your physical symptoms are due to emotional tensions."

The physical evaluation should be competent, but not needlessly meticulous. The patient should have the minimal number of necessary laboratory examinations; he should not be subjected to prolonged evaluation with many tests to rule out obscure, highly unlikely diseases. Every patient with fatigue should not be thoroughly evaluated for chronic adrenal cortical insufficiency, and very few patients with headaches require lumbar punctures. When a patient with psychogenic physical symptoms is subjected to unduly thorough physical evaluation, or makes prolonged odysseys through medical clinics, the probability of help from psychiatric treatment is diminished, because he frequently becomes convinced that his trouble is due to undiscovered physical disease. Hence, the physical checkup should be adequate but not exhaustive, and the patient should be reassured at various points that the purpose of the examination is simply to rule out the unlikely chance that he has physical difficulties in addition to his emotional problems.

FORMULATION OF THE PSYCHIATRIC DIAGNOSIS

The everyday necessities of medical practice require on many occasions a diagnosis for each patient who has been examined or who is under treatment. Diagnoses are required for hospital charts, hospital admission forms, discharge summaries, insurance forms, statistical recording purposes, communication with other doctors and many other purposes. Hence, in most instances a psychiatric patient must be given a diagnosis.

However, psychiatry differs from other medical specialties in that the physician often is not dealing with a specific disease in the usual sense of the word. He is dealing with the emotional turmoil of a particular person enmeshed in unhealthy interpersonal relationships, and with that person's personality structure, which has been produced by a continual chain of interpersonal relationships stretching back over the patient's entire lifetime. As a result, a simple psychiatric diagnosis often gives little idea of what is really wrong.

For example, the diagnosis *anxiety neurosis* may refer to a temporary, mild discomfort precipitated by recent unusual stresses, or it may indicate a severe process with lifelong incapacitation due to overwhelming emotional trauma in childhood. In contrast, diagnoses in other fields of medicine convey much more information. Most physicians have a fairly accurate concept of the clinical picture when they hear that the patient has acute appendicitis, steptococcal tonsillitis or a fractured left clavicle. A psychiatric diagnosis conveys less information, and often, in itself, does not make the picture clear. A major reason for this difficulty is that appendicitis, tonsillitis and a fractured left clavicle involve only small parts of the body which are essentially the same in most people; a psychiatric diagnosis sums up a lifetime history of interpersonal relationships, and the life histories of people are radically different from one another.

In attempting to deal with this problem, the psychiatrist may think of each patient's diagnosis in two ways: (1) a *descriptive diagnosis*, which uses an appropriate term from the standard medical nomenclature, and (2) an *interpersonal diagnosis*, which presents a brief summary of the unhealthy interpersonal relationships and emotional turmoil that have produced the condition.

The *descriptive* diagnosis is amplified and completed by the *interpersonal* diagnosis. The former gives a surface, cross-sectional designation to the patient's condition, whereas the interpersonal diagnosis gives an etiologic explanation which traces the patient's problem back into his life history and relationships with people.

In actual practice, the descriptive diagnosis, such as anxiety neurosis or phobic neurosis, is used for administrative purposes on hospital charts, outpatient records, insurance forms and similar purposes. The interpersonal diagnosis appears as a narrative paragraph at the conclusion of a psychiatric work-up and in other places in the patient's private file. The interpersonal diagnosis contains confidental information about the patient and is available only to the psychiatrists and allied professional persons, such as clinical psychologists and psychiatric social workers, who may play a role in the patient's care.

For example, the following diagnosis might appear at the end of a patient's outpatient work-up, in which the *descriptive diagnosis* is given on the first line and the *interpersonal diagnosis* begins in paragraph form on the line below:

Anxiety neurosis.
Acute anxiety attacks with palpitation and hyperventilation have occurred about twice each week for the past 3 months in this 32-year-old married woman. She is a passive person with strong feelings of personal inadequacy and she rarely expresses anger or asserts herself. Her personality problems arose in a loveless childhood in which her critical, domineering parents made her feel inadequate. Her present symptoms seem related to recent stresses with her husband and problems in coping with the aggressiveness of her 3 children who range in age from 3 to 7 years.

The following is an example of the use of the descriptive diagnosis and the interpersonal diagnosis in a patient with an organic brain disorder.

Psychosis associated with bromide intoxication.
Intellectual confusion, disorientation and visual hallucinations have been present for 10 days in this 47-year-old man with a blood bromide level of 410 mg. per 100 cc of blood serum. He has been taking a proprietary sedative containing bromides for the past 3 months to assuage anxiety which seems related to stresses on his job and with his aged mother who came to live with him and his family 6 months ago. The patient had many conflicts with his dependent, clinging mother during his childhood and adolescence, and her presence in his home has reawakened many old feelings of hostility and guilt. The whining dependency of his semi-invalid mother has also caused trouble about her between the patient and his wife. The patient's emotional distress has caused his job performance to deteriorate and has led to conflicts with his supervisor and his coworkers.

The *interpersonal* diagnosis is a very simplified sketch of a few prominent points of the patient's emotional difficulties and interpersonal background, but it amplifies the *descriptive* diagnosis. The full picture of the patient's problems can be found only by surveying his entire case history. Nevertheless, the interpersonal diagnosis has much usefulness and gives much more meaning to the descriptive diagnosis.

THE STANDARD OFFICIAL CLASSIFICATION OF PSYCHIATRIC DISORDERS

The descriptive diagnosis of the patient is drawn from the standard official classification of psychiatric disorders. This classification was instituted in 1968 after several years of work by the Committee on Nomenclature and Statistics of the American Psychiatric Association. It is published, with extensive explanations and commentaries, in the widely used booklet "Diagnostic and Statistical

Manual of Mental Disorders," commonly referred to by the abbreviation DSM-II. This nomenclature also forms the psychiatric part of the comprehensive system of diagnoses of the American Medical Association, which is employed in almost all American hospitals and clinics.

The 1968 DSM-II nomenclature was designed to make American psychiatric diagnoses consonant with the worldwide nomenclature set up by the World Health Organization; this is called the International Classification of Diseases (ICD-8). In order to do this, a number of features of continental European and Soviet psychiatry had to be incorporated. Most American psychiatrists, including myself, do not employ some of these terms; they include such diagnoses as "explosive personality," "depersonalization neurosis," "asthenic personality" and "involutional paranoid state." Many American psychiatrists also deplore the division of organic brain disorders into psychotic and non-psychotic (difficult terms to define) instead of the previously employed designations of acute and chronic (easily defined). In addition, the use of such numbers as 52 and 67 (in referring to intelligence quotients) as dividing lines for the various degrees of mental retardation seems oddly bureaucratic, as opposed to the previously employed round numbers such as 50 and 70; this is particularly so after decades of emphasizing to the professions and the public that they ought not to pay too close attention to I. Q. numbers in the total evaluation of mentally retarded persons.

In this book we shall define all terms of the DSM-II 1968 standard classification and use them wherever they seem consonant with clinical soundness and general American practice. In some places, however, we shall modify this system to conform with terms and concepts in general use by American psychiatrists and other mental health professionals.

The current, standard (DSM-II 1968) system of psychiatric diagnoses divides psychiatric disorders into 10 general groups:

I. *Mental retardation*, in which low intelligence states of known and unknown etiology are divided into borderline, mild, moderate, severe and profound on the basis of I. Q. numbers and other factors.

II. *Organic brain syndromes*, which are divided into psycotic and non-psychotic, and may be caused by senile dementia, intracranial infections, brain trauma, intracranial neoplasms and many other conditions.

III. *Psychoses not attributed to physical conditions*, which contains schizophrenia, manic disorders, severe depressions, paranoid states and other disorders.

IV. *Neuroses*, which contains anxiety neurosis, the conversion and dissociative forms of hysterical neurosis, phobic neurosis, obsessive compulsive neurosis and other neurotic conditions. The term neurosis is the preferred synonym for psychoneurosis in this classification.

V. *Personality disorders*, which embraces paranoid personality, schizoid personality, obsessive compulsive personality and other disorders in which the main difficulty consists of ingrained patterns of interpersonal relationships and emotional functioning.

VI. *Psychophysiologic disorders*, which encompasses all the psychosomatic disorders. They are divided according to the organ system involved, such as psychophysiologic gastro-intestinal disorder, psychophysiologic cardiovascular disorders, and so forth.

VII. *Special symptoms*, in which such particular problems as speech disturbances, sleep disorders, enuresis, and various others are placed.

VIII. *Transient situational disturbances*, which includes adjustment reactions of infancy, childhood, adolescence, adult life and late life. These are brief upsets caused by strong environmental (usually interpersonal) stress.

IX. *Behavior disorders of childhood and adolescence*, which includes overanxious reaction of childhood or adolescence, hyperkinetic reaction of childhood or adolescence, group delinquent reaction of childhood or adolescence, and others.

X. *Conditions without manifest psychiatric disorder and non-specific conditions*, which provides a category for marital maladjustments, occupational maladjustments, social maladjustments, and other maladjustments in persons who are defined as "psychiatrically normal" but who nevertheless have sufficient interpersonal difficulties in these areas to merit psychiatric attention.

The psychiatric work-up and diagnostic formulation prepare the way for treatment of the patient. They are not ends in themselves, but steps toward the goal of helping the patient. Subsequent chapters deal with various types of psychiatric disorders and their treatment.

SPECIAL PROBLEMS IN HANDLING PSYCHIATRIC DIAGNOSES AND RECORDS

The first rule of Hippocrates, which was *primum non nocere*—first of all, do no harm—has special relevance to the handling of psychiatric records and diagnoses. A classical example occurred in the 1972 presidential elections, in which the previous psychiatric records and diagnoses of a vice-presidential candidate were brought to public attention in a most unfortunate manner that had widespread repercussions.

Long-standing problems in handling psychiatric diagnoses and records have been made more difficult by the widespread use of photocopying and computerized information. I know cases in which, in reply to routine requests for psychiatric information from nonmedical bodies (insurance companies, prospective employers, government agencies, and others), record room clerks have photocopied several pages of highly confidential, potentially damaging psychiatric information and have sent them off; the requests were accompanied by release-of-information forms signed by the patients, and these protected the senders but did not protect the patients. Psychiatric diagnoses concerning alcoholism, drug abuse, exhibitionism, pedophilia, schizoid personality, paranoid personality and others can be fed into computers, which often are linked to other computers in distant states, with grave consequences for patients; they may be denied jobs, driver's licenses, bank loans, home mortgages and many other things because of material that was entered into computers years previously and is no longer relevant to the patient's life adjustment. Two dangerous features are that once such information gets into computer banks it is very difficult to get out, and that the patient usually does not know what is being reported about him and hence cannot take steps to refute it.

The following recommendations, therefore, merit close attention by all persons engaged in mental health work. There are, of course, exceptions to them, but they are infrequent.

1. Each psychiatric clinic, ward or diagnostic service should have a private file which is available only to mental health professionals (psychiatrists, clinical psychologists, psychiatric social workers, psychiatric nurses and, occasionally, other professional persons) who are working with the patient. Material from this file should never be photocopied or directly released to any other source. It should *not* be available to insurance company investigators and others who have permission forms signed by patients giving them the right to inspect the patient's hospital or outpatient records. It should be prominently stamped on many of its pages: "Not to be photocopied or released in this form under any circumstances. For use only by mental health professionals working directly with the patient."

2. Each case file should contain a brief but ample summary and a diagnosis (or diagnoses) which is sent to the hospital or clinic general record room. This can be released to requesting persons or organizations when written permission by the patient or his guardians is given. This should be stamped: "This data may be photocopied or abstracted for release to persons or institutions, when the patient's written permission is given." This summary is drawn up by the psychiatrist in charge of the patient, or by an experienced mental health professional whom he designates, and all material which may damage the patient or be erroneously interpreted by lay persons is excluded; drawing up such a summary obviously requires good judgement and ample clinical experience, and the guiding rule should be: when in doubt, leave it out. The report should end with the sentence: "Physicians and other mental health professional workers who are directly treating or evaluating the patient may write the psychiatric service for any further necessary data." Replies to such inquiries should give only the information requested and should vary depending on who the inquirer is and what his purposes are. More extensive reports which are sent to professional persons should be stamped: "Confidential, Not to be Released," since it often goes into folders which are available to secretaries, typists, clerical assistants and others.

3. A carbon copy of any special report is always kept in the patient's confidential file. It is stamped with a notation that it is not to be photocopied or released at any future

time without the initialed permission of the person who drew it up or the person who now holds that position and reads the report.

4. Give the inquiring party only the information it requests. This refers mainly to nonmedical inquiries. For example, an insurance company often wants only dates of hospitalization or outpatient visits, the final diagnosis, and the last date on which the patient was seen. Such material should be easily available on a "flow sheet" which lists such information at the beginning of the patient's record.

5. Use diagnostic terms that will not damage the patient. For example, we usually employ the diagnosis *anxiety reaction* (from the DSM-I 1952 classification) in place of *anxiety neurosis* (from the DSM-II 1968 classification) since the word *neurosis,* and its adjective *neurotic,* often prejudice nonmedical inquirers (prospective employers, government agencies and others) against the patient. If a patient had a 3-month period of alcoholism while going through a depression, we treat the alcoholism as a symptom and put only the term *depression* in the diagnostic phrase. We completely avoid some vaguely defined, highly controversial terms such as "explosive personality," "asthenic personality," and "depersonalization neurosis."

6. Material written by patients to psychiatric examiners and therapists (letters, suicide notes, autobiographical sketches) should never be photocopied, should rarely be quoted, and should only occasionally be referred to in reports.

7. Always keep in mind the legal aspects of this subject (which are covered in Chapter 26).

BIBLIOGRAPHY

Bates, L. A., Metraux, R. W., Rodell, J. L., and Walker, R. N.: Child Rorschach Responses. New York, Brunner Mazel, 1974.

Bellak, L.: The Thematic Apperception Test and the Children's Apperception Test in Clinical Use. New York, Grune & Stratton, 1971.

Committee on Nomenclature and Statistics of the American Psychiatric Association: DSM-II, Diagnostic and Statistical Manual of Mental Disorders. ed. 2. Washington, D. C., American Psychiatric Association, 1968.

Fitzgibbons, D. J., and Hokanson, D. T.: The diagnostic decision-making process. Am. J. Psychiatry, *130*:972, 1973.

Goldfried, M. R., Stricher, G., and Weiner, I. B.: Rorschach Handbook of Clinical and Research Applications. Englewood Hills, N. J., Prentice-Hall, 1971.

Goodstein, L. D., and Lanyon, R. I.: Readings in Personality Assessment. New York, John Wiley, 1971.

Lanyon, R. I., and Goodstein, L. D.: Personality Assessment. New York, John Wiley, 1971.

Lerner, E. A.: The Projective Use of the Bender Gestalt. Springfield, Ill., Charles C Thomas, 1972.

Matarazzo, J. D.: Wechsler's Measurement and Appraisal of Adult Intelligence. Baltimore, Williams & Wilkins, 1972.

Sarbin, T. R., and Coe, W. C.: Hypnosis: A Social Psychological Analysis of Influence Communication. New York, Holt, Rinehart & Winston, 1972.

Spitzer, R. L., and Endicott, J.: Can the computer assist clinicians in psychiatric diagnosis? Am. J. Psychiatry, *131*:523, 1974.

Stahl, M. O., and Lewis, N. D. C. (eds.): Differential Diagnosis in Clinical Psychiatry (Lectures of Paul H. Hoch). New York, Science House, 1972.

Sullivan, H. S.: The Psychiatric Interview. New York, W. W. Norton 1954.

Part Three

The Interpersonally Caused Disorders

In this section we shall cover the main psychiatric disorders caused by unhealthy interpersonal relationships. These disorders usually arise as the result of various traumatic interpersonal relationships in both the past and current life situations of the patient, though the relative importance of past and current emotional trauma varies much from patient to patient.

The main interpersonally caused disorders fall into four broad groups. They are (1) the neuroses, (2) the psychosomatic illnesses, (3) the personality disorders, and (4) the interpersonally caused psychoses. We shall consider in detail the various disorders included in each of these four groups.

(Other interpersonally caused disorders, which do not fall in these four categories, are covered in Chapter 25 of Part VII where we discuss special problems of adjustment in children, special problems of situational adjustment in adulthood, and special problems of sexual adjustment.)

Section One

The Neuroses

The term "neurosis" designates a group of emotional disorders which may be divided into the following categories.

1. *Anxiety neurosis,* in which the patient experiences much tension, varying from mild restlessness to sheer panic. Anxiety neuroses may be acute or chronic.

2. *Phobic neurosis,* in which the patient has one or more abnormal fears of specific things or situations.

3. *Obsessive compulsive neurosis.* In an obsessive neurosis the patient is afflicted with persistent, distressing ideas of which he cannot rid himself, and in a compulsive neurosis he feels strong urges to perform repeated physical acts to relieve tension. A patient may have a purely obsessive neurosis or a purely compulsive one, but since in many instances a patient has both kinds of difficulties these two neuroses are usually discussed together.

4. *Hysterical neurosis,* which may be of either *conversion* or *dissociative* type. In a conversion type of hysterical neurosis the patient has some kind of emotionally caused disorder of sensation, or movement, or special sensory perception. In a dissociative type of hysterical neurosis the patient has some kind of emotionally caused disturbance of awareness or memory, as in psychogenic amnesias.

5. *Other neurotic syndromes,* which embrace the dysfunctions which in the current standard nomenclature are termed depressive neurosis, neurasthenic neurosis, depersonalization neurosis, and hypochondriacal neurosis. American psychi-

atrists differ much in opinion about the nature of these neuroses and, with the exception of depressive neurosis, many psychiatrists do not use these terms.

The words "neurosis" and "psychoneurosis" are synonyms. Although "neurosis" is the official term in the standard nomenclature, these words are interchangeably used by most mental health professional workers.

To define the term "neurosis" in a simple one-sentence formulation is difficult. Neuroses are best defined by discussing some of the general features that bind these disorders together in traditional psychiatric thinking.

All neuroses are of emotional origin. They are caused by the interpersonal stresses and unresolved conflicts in the patient's life. Both past and current interpersonal conflicts play their roles. In general, the person who has a neurotic disturbance is not incapacitated by it, though occasionally the difficulty becomes so severe that he is interpersonally disabled. The patient has distressing symptoms which he can feel and describe to at least a certain extent, but there is no loss of contact with reality in almost all cases. The various kinds of neurotic disturbances may be barely noticeable or overwhelming, and they exist in all the intervening gradations of severity. In the final analysis, neurotic difficulties are best explained by describing in detail their clinical characteristics, causes, general courses and treatment. (We shall proceed to do this in Chapters 6 through 10.)

6

Anxiety Neurosis

Anxiety is a state of apprehensive discomfort which may vary in severity from mild restlessness to overwhelming panic. Anxiety, with its accompanying physical distresses, such as palpitation, muscle tension, upper gastrointestinal discomforts and many other body sensations, is the most common problem for which people consult physicians. Anxiety presents itself as the restlessness, the tension, the fearfulness, the panic or the vague malaise of many persons who come to physicians' offices. Everyone has at least a touch of anxiety now and then.

In Chapter 1 we discussed the role of fluctuating amounts of *subclinical* anxiety in molding personality structure; by *subclinical* anxiety we mean anxiety of which the person does not become articulately aware in either emotional or physical ways, but which nevertheless, as an indistinct, uncomfortable force, influences his emotional functioning. In this present chapter we are considering patients in whom the usual safeguards against perceiving strong anxiety have broken down, and clearly recognizable anxiousness is evident as a painful dysfunction over periods of weeks, months or years; in other words, an anxiety neurosis is present.

Anxiety neuroses customarily are divided into *acute* and *chronic* states. Though these two states often shade into each other and frequently occur in the same patient, this classification offers a simple way of approaching the clinical manifestations of anxiety.

CLINICAL CHARACTERISTICS OF ANXIETY NEUROSES

Acute Anxiety States

The patient with an acute anxiety state feels a sudden wave of panic and tension come over him. He may have his episode of acute anxiety at any time; he may be engaged in any type of work, recreation or social activity. It may occur while he is alone or with others; sometimes he may awake from sleep in a state of frightened distress.

The patient often cannot describe easily what he feels, but he is sure that some physical or mental calamity is overtaking him. He is terrified, and thoughts of sudden illness such as heart disease, stroke, insanity or less clearly defined but equally dreaded, things race through his mind. He describes himself as "dizzy," "light-headed" and "fainty;" he fears he will collapse or "black out." He feels his pulse racing and his heart pounding heavily in his chest. He may feel nauseated and may feel pain in his epigastrium as the wave of dread passes through him. Muscle tension pains in the head, neck, upper back and chest wall are common. He may pant rapidly in shallow, gasping respirations. On occasion he may be slightly tremulous, and he may sit in tight rigidity, or fidget restlessly, or pace in agitation. His face and palms may break out in perspiration. He may feel in desperate need of medical help, though he does not know what is wrong with him and fears the medical verdict.

The patient with an acute anxiety state frequently calls his physician or goes to the emergency room of a hospital. If this is the patient's first anxiety attack, his relatives are equally alarmed and may take him promptly for medical attention. An acute anxiety state may last a few minutes, or it may stretch out to several hours or a full day. It may subside slowly or rapidly, but it usually leaves the patient shaken and worried about himself.

He and his family may or may not recognize that it is an emotional state. They may label it "an attack of nerves" or "nervousness," but their concepts about "nerves" often involve vague notions of emotional stress mixed with ominous dysfunctions of the central nervous system. However, both the patient and his family often feel that an alarming disturbance of such abrupt onset must indicate a physical illness of some sort, and they reason that the patient's fearfulness is a legitimate reaction to the sudden onset of the physical disorder.

Acute anxiety states may be occasional or frequent. A patient may have them several times a day, or once every several months, or at any frequency between these extremes. They may occur from puberty onwards, but they are not common until after middle adolescence. When acute anxiety states occur in children they usually become attached to a specific object or situation, producing fears of animals, or automobiles, or leaving the house, or other things or situations, and they acquire the clinical characteristics of phobias (which are described in Chapter 7).

Some acute anxiety states are milder than those we have described above, but an acute anxiety state usually is sudden, severe and very distressing to the patient and the people around him. When the patient has had many previous acute anxiety episodes, his relatives and close friends sometimes are not alarmed at the appearance of a new period of anxiety; nevertheless, the alarm of the patient himself is undiminished. Acute anxiety states often occur in patients who also have varying amounts of chronic anxiousness in the intervals between the acute anxiety attacks. However, in other instances the patient with acute anxiety states may be relatively free of anxiety between his acute episodes.

Acute anxiety states are common. Though there are no reliable statistics, perhaps as high as 25 per cent of people have at least a few episodes of acute anxiety at some time during their lives. Often they interpret their anxiety attacks as manifestations of a physical disorder such as "dizzy spells," "racing heart spells," "stomach cramps," "nausea attacks" and many other camouflaging physical complaints. Careful evaluation of the patient reveals the acute anxiety that lies beneath his physical complaint.

Chronic Anxiety States

The patient with a chronic anxiety state suffers from prolonged, intermittent, fluctuating anxiousness. The intensity of his discomfort usually is less than that of the patient with an acute anxiety attack, but the degree of his anxiousness may at times approximate the panic of the acutely anxious patient. A chronic anxiety reaction may extend over a period of days, months or years. It may, with fluctuations, stretch out over decades.

The chronically anxious patient experiences varying amounts of dread, restlessness and tension. He may be free of it for periods of several hours at a time, but usually it is always hovering in the background and splatters his day with periods of anxious distress. Often he is visibly tense, and his family and friends state that he is "nervous," "jumpy" or "on edge" a good deal of the time. He may have persistent anxious worries that preoccupy him much of the time. He looks forward to new, unfamiliar experiences with floating fearfulness. He frequently sleeps poorly, awakes fatigued in the morning after a restless night, and complains of tiredness during the day.

The patient with a chronic anxiety state usually has physical discomforts caused by his chronic tension. Upper gastrointestinal complaints such as epigastric pain, nausea, and vague dyspepsias such as "heartburn" are common complaints which may be present intermittently for months or years. Tension headaches in the back of the neck, over the cranium or in the temples are common. The patient may describe his tension headache as feeling like a tight, painful band encircling his forehead, temples and base of the occiput. Tension backaches in the upper or lower back, intermittent diarrhea, palpitation, feelings of tightness in the thorax, and panting shallow respirations, are all common physical concomitants of chronic anxiety states. They are produced through muscle tension, antonomic nervous system discharges and other physiologic pathways that receive their stimuli from the emotional distress of the patient.

Fatigue is a common complaint of patients with chronic anxiety; persistent muscle tension is physically tiring. If one wishes to demonstrate this to himself, he has but to grasp the arms of his chair tightly for five minutes; at the end of that time he will find himself exhausted. The diffuse, subtle muscle tension of the chronically anxious patient similarly tires him.

Persons with chronic anxiety crowd the waiting rooms of physicians and frequently are evaluated in hospitals to rule out possible physical diseases as causes of their chronic physical complaints. Often they deceive themselves, and occasionally their doctors, into the belief that they have pseudodiseases such as a "nervous stomach," many kinds of headaches, and a host of other syndromes that are merely the superficial symptoms of emotional distress. Small physical dysfunctions such as mild anemias, minor allergies, minor orthopedic anomalies of the back, and so forth, are sometimes blamed as causes of symptoms that actually are produced by chronic anxiety; the physical abnormality is an unrelated finding. Sometimes the patient labels his trouble as "nervousness." He attacks that vague catchall with pills and other measures that help little and tend to confirm in his mind the conviction that he suffers from some occult metabolic or central nervous system disorder.

To diagnose chronic anxiety states promptly and to treat them appropriately is one of the physician's most common challenges.

INTERPERSONAL CAUSES OF ANXIETY NEUROSES

As Harry Stack Sullivan emphasized, the basic cause of anxiety is a strong threat to the emotional balance and well-being of the individual—that is, a threat to his integrity as a person. Such a threat is the result of emotional turmoil, both inside the person and in his relationships with people; this turmoil is caused by traumatic interpersonal relationships in both past and present life situations. As the individual senses that his emotional stability is being menaced, or even crumbling, he is flooded by the profound feeling of dread and apprehension we call anxiety.

However, once anxiety is present, in either acute or chronic forms, it has further unhealthy consequences. It hinders the person from entering comfortably into constructive new interpersonal relationships which he needs and which might offer him ways of solving his emotional difficulties. A person in an acute or chronic anxiety state is partially crippled in his dealings with people; he cannot communicate as freely and interact as well as if he were free of his anxiousness.

In addition, anxiety states constrict the person's awareness; his attention and emotional energy are so riveted on his anxiousness and its physical concomitants that he cannot examine his past and current life situations as well as if he were rid of his anguish. Also, anxiety impairs a person's capacity to form intimate relationships with the close persons in his life——his marital partner, children, parents, close friends and others—at a time when he needs strong, healthy bonds with people in order to achieve new levels of interpersonal effectiveness and to reestablish his emotional balance and well-being.

The forces that threaten the patient's emotional stability and well-being, and thus produce anxiety, arise from his past and present interpersonal life, and the insecurities, conflicts, unresolved stresses and other things that have damaged him. Usually, an anxiety neurosis does not have a single cause; it has multiple causes. Some causes are large, others are small, but they all blend together to produce the disturbance of the patient.

Some of the causes of anxiety neuroses may date from traumatic childhood experiences. The lovelessness, fearfulness, insecurities and conflicts of childhood may lay the bases for anxiety neuroses. The resulting clinical anxiety may begin to be manifest to some extent in childhood or adolescence, but often the emotional traumas lie simmering until they are agitated by further precipitating stresses in adult life and then erupt as marked anxiety states. On the other hand, overwhelming interpersonal anguish of adult life may precipitate an anxiety neurosis in a person who had relatively little trauma in childhood. For example, the massive emotional traumas experienced in civil disasters or in war may flood a person with emotional stresses which cause anxiety states. In all these cases, the patient may have acute or chronic anxiety states, or both.

Another way of viewing anxiety neuroses is

to liken their causes to the various layers of an onion. Some layers are superficial, others are of moderate depth and still others are deeply buried. In a typical anxiety neurosis, there are superficial precipitants in the person's daily life; these agitate deeper, older conflicts and insecurities buried more profoundly, and rooted in experiences of childhood and adolescence. For example, an adult may develop an anxiety neurosis when he feels threatened in his job; he fears he will be demoted, or displaced by someone, or discharged from his employment. However, this vocational fear is merely the superficial cause of his anxiety state. The patient is particularly sensitive to threats of this kind because of previous job failures in early adulthood which aroused feelings of personal inadequacy and inferiority. He dreads another experience that would seem to confirm previously instilled feelings of inadequacy. Furthermore, these experiences may have a special impact for him because he came out of a loveless childhood in which his parents and other close persons gave him little affection and much irritable criticism, berating him for alleged inadequacies, shortcomings and personal worthlessness. Thus, when these three levels of interpersonal, stress—from a current interpersonal situation, from previous stresses in his early adult life, and from great doubts about his worth and ability arising from a traumatic childhood—are combined, they will produce an anxiety neurosis. In this way, interpersonal stresses from various levels of the onion, from various periods of the patient's life, from various levels of his emotional structure, combine to produce the clinical picture of acute or chronic anxiety states.

Obviously, the importance of different types of stresses differs immensely in the causes of anxiety neuroses in various patients. In some patients the painful interpersonal traumas of an emotionally disastrous childhood leave the patient's personality structure so shaken that even minor day-to-day events precipitate an anxiety neurosis. Other persons have much healthier basic personality structures formed in sounder childhood interpersonal relationships, and it requires extraordinarily painful stresses in adult life to produce anxiety. No two patients are the same; the combinations of current and past stresses are different to at least some degree in all patients. This fact emphasizes a basic tenet of the interpersonal approach to psychiatric disorders; each patient must be studied and treated as a special individual with a unique combination of interpersonal problems.

In order to outline the interpersonal causes of anxiety neuroses with systematic ease, we shall discuss them under two general headings: (1) *contributing causes originating in childhood*, and (2) *contributing causes originating in adult life*. Obviously, these two categories overlap and intertwine; a person properly should be regarded as an indivisible whole, but studying him often requires that we consder his life and and emotional functioning in various parts in order to keep our concepts clear.

Contributing Causes Originating in Childhood Experiences

Some children emerge from the first 12 years of life with profound inner turmoil generated from unhealthy interpersonal relationships. These damaging interpersonal stresses may lead to anxiousness, or other emotional symptoms, during childhood, or they may lie smoldering deep within the person and erupt as an anxiety neurosis in adult life. They may not erupt as anxiety states in adult life until new upsetting interpersonal stresses stir up old conflicts. At other times the suppressed turbulence of childhood conflicts rises to the surface despite a relatively sound adult interpersonal life. The nature of the hidden turmoil, its intensity and its proclivity to be rekindled by specific types of adult interpersonal stresses, determine whether childhood traumas will in time lead to adult anxiety states.

For example, a patient may have experienced during childhood much emotional rejection from his parents and other close persons, and this may have left deep emotional scars. As a consequence, he may have underlying feelings of worthlessness and little self-esteem. The patient may have no awareness of these lurking conflicts within him, but as he watches the gradual emotional development of his own children and deals with the day-to-day problems of rearing them, the old conflicts from his own childhood may be reawakened. He may be dimly aware of these connections, or not aware of them at all. However, as his old problems rise to the surface he is flooded with much anxiety that takes the form of acute or chronic anxiety states. As a rule, the patient is only aware of his symptoms and cannot correlate his distress with the chain of interpersonal events that caused it.

We shall now proceed to discuss some of the more common traumatic interpersonal relationships of childhood which may lay the ground for later anxiety neuroses. Of course, several of these causes may be present in any particular patient; the traumas of childhood that lie behind an adult anxiety state usually are multiple, not single.

Inadequate affection and emotional security. Parental coldness, neglect and deficient affection throughout a child's formative years leave the child with a profound sense of emotional insecurity. He feels worthless, inadequate and neither loved nor lovable. His self-esteem and self-confidence are eroded; he is unsure of himself in his interpersonal relationships both in and outside the home.

The parents' lack of affection for the child may be caused by various factors. Some parents are unaffectionate and hostile in most of their interpersonal dealings, and offer their children the same coldness that characterizes their interpersonal relationships with people in general. In other instances the child is born at a time when he is unwanted, or he is the least favored of two or three siblings, or he is caught up as a pawn in the marital battles of his parents, or he is left to drift aimlessly through his formative years by parents who are absorbed in their jobs and social life, or he is battered by other kinds of difficulties. The child never understands why he is neglected, or chronically criticized, or brutally rejected. However, whatever its determinants, prolonged parental rejection and inadequate affection lay the ground for fears, insecurities, resentments and self-doubts which often contribute to anxiety states in later years.

Threats to the self-esteem of the child. Some parents, in floundering attempts to control their children, deluge the child with depreciation and criticism which make the child feel guilty and worthless. Some parents plague their children daily with such harangues as: "Why can't you ever do anything right? You're always causing trouble and you never do anything the way you're supposed to." "You're driving me to sickness and an early grave by your badness and disobedience." "You're causing your mother and me nothing but grief, shame and sickness by the way you behave." An immense amount of such parental guilt-slinging and martyr-playing goes on in some homes; it rains on the child in a daily acid drizzle. It slowly soaks into him, and the guilt-slinging and martyr-playing of the parents create in the child a view of himself as an inferior, malicious person. He is both crushed and resentful. Guilt and anxiety corrode the fabric of his personality structure, contributing to future anxiety. Of course, a small amount of guilt-slinging and martyr-playing occurs in most homes, and if it is only occasional it does no harm. However, when these unhealthy interpersonal technics dominate the parent-child relationship, there may be many ominous warps in the child's personality structure.

Hostile, competitive relationships within the family. Hostile, competitive conflicts may arise in a family, and when they are severe and prolonged they may leave in their wake much anxiety, guilt and insecurity in a child. For example, he may be the protected favorite of one parent and the resented enemy of the other. This may occur with the parent of the same sex as the protector (a mother sheltering and favoring her daughter against a hostile father), or a mother similarly treating a son, or a father playing such roles with a son or daughter. In such situations the child may have deep-seated fears of retaliation from the parent with whom he is in conflict. Hostile competition among siblings is common, and occasionally such rivalry may achieve sufficient bitterness to leave much anxiety and guilt in its wake.

Death wishes may creep into the hostile, competitive relationships within a family; the child fantasies that his closeness to the mother or the father would be complete if the antagonistic, competing parent or siblings were dead. The child recoils from such fleeting death wishes in guilt and terror, but their uneasy residuals may lurk as a later cause of anxiety states. If a member of the family actually is seriously injured in an automobile accident, or becomes gravely ill, or dies during such a hostile period in the family, devastating feelings of guilt and terror may occur in the child, for he feels that in some strange way his hostile feelings and wishes have caused this calamity. Such combinations of events may lead to severe anxiety states that do not erupt until adult life.

Undue suppression of feelings. Emotional health requires that a person have a reasonable capacity for expressing his feelings. Rigid suppression of feelings in childhood leads to pent-up reservoirs of emotion which may later emerge as symptoms. Moreover, the capacity for expression of feelings, or the lack of it, which is laid down in the first 12 years of life tends to persist into adolescence and adulthood. Children should be allowed to express their affectionate feelings, dependent yearnings and assertive urges in reasonable, socially acceptable ways. Some parents make their children feel inadequate and guilty if they express any or all of these feelings. Such children often become emotionally rigid, while a mass of confused, painful feelings simmers within them. Such inner turmoil may contribute to anxiety states in adolescence and adulthood. Moreover, once anxiety states are present in adolescence or adulthood, they tend to further inhibit the expression of feelings; Harry Stack Sullivan labeled anxiety "the chief handicap to communication."

Sexual traumas. Various types of sexual traumas may leave gnawing problems in a child. There is some evidence that exposure to sexual intercourse of his parents, especially if such exposure continues over a long period of time and is interpreted by the child as some kind of aggressive struggle, both stimulates and frightens a small child. The sexual seduction of young children, particularly girls, by adults and older children similarly leaves in its wake anguish and guiltiness which may contribute to later anxiety reactions; such sexual exploitation is more common than is generally recognized.

Inadequate interpersonal limitations on the child. A person's capacity for self-restraint is, to a large extent, laid down in the first 12 years of his life, as his parents gradually impose limitations on him. These restraints, if imposed against a background of deep parental love, lay the basis for the self-discipline the individual incorporates into himself in later years when parental authority no longer holds sway. For example, a small child does not smash furniture because of the limitations and discipline of his parents; an adult does not smash furniture because he has internalized the restraints and discipline of his parents into himself, and thus has developed capacities for self-restraint.

However, when throughout his formative years a child's behavior is uncontrolled, the necessary self-restraints for successful social living may not be developed. A person who cannot put reasonable limits on his behavior often is chronically uneasy; he is dimly aware that he cannot grasp where the limits of his actions are and the rights of others begin. The frustrations and tedious chores of life frustrate and frighten him. He often alternates between states of arrogant self-assurance when things go well and panic when they do not. Such problems, especially as the individual arrives into middle adulthood, may lead to anxiety states which in many cases are camouflaged by alcoholism or impulsive, self-defeating behavior.

Other contributing childhood causes of anxiety states. In some instances, chronic instability of the parental home throughout the child's formative years because of severe marital problems of his parents, may leave lingering uneasiness which contributes to later anxiety neuroses. This is particularly apt to occur when the parents use the children as weapons and shields in their unending antagonism.

Open fearfulness in the parental home may add to the turmoil that produces anxiety. Fearful parents who worry endlessly about possible, but improbable, misfortunes sometimes pass on a feeling of apprehension and vague anxiety to their children. Phobic parents who fear to leave the house, or obsessive parents who dread many diseases and are engaged in daily cleansing rituals, or timid parents who view the world as a hostile, threatening place, may inculcate anxiousness into their children. Each person gets his initial impressions of the safety or perilousness of life from the attitudes of his home. An apprehensive view of life may be a contributant to a later anxiety neurosis.

Repeated, extraordinary, frightening experiences, especially if prolonged over extensive periods of time, also may add to the emotional tumult that predisposes a person to later anxiety states. For example, repeated hospitalizations in early childhood, especially if they involve abrupt, long-lasting separations from parents, may leave emotional scars. Despite decades of parental education to the contrary, psychiatrists still see patients who were threatened with deformities of the genitals if they continued to masturbate, and such threats may leave enduring doubts and fearful speculations in the person. In other instances, the death, prolonged illness or severe psychiatric illness of a parent may produce gnawing insecurities in a child. Parental brutality, abandonment or gross neglect may contribute to the personality warps that predispose a person to a later anxiety neurosis.

In the final analysis, the combinations and varieties of traumatic interpersonal experiences of childhood that may contribute to later anxiety states are as innumerable as the patients who suffer from these disorders. Each patient's past life must be evaluated as a unique sequence of events and relationships in order to understand how early experiences have laid the ground for present anxiety.

Contributing Causes in Adult Experiences

Traumatic experiences of adult life usually play significant roles in the etiology of anxiety neuroses. In some instances, the personality structure of the patient is so riddled with insecurity and anxiety bred from childhood traumas that the events of adult life act only as precipitants and play a small role in the combination of causes that produces anxiety. At other times, the basic personality of the patient is relatively stable, and severe stress in adult life is required to precipitate anxiety. Usually, an anxiety neurosis is the result of the intermingling of childhood and adult problems; the stresses of adult life rekindle the insecurities and anxieties long dormant from traumatic childhood interpersonal relationships. We shall now discuss some of the more common adult emotional stresses and interpersonal traumas which may contribute to anxiety neuroses.

Pressures of repressed experiences, feelings and conflicts. Within each person are many repressed experiences, feelings, and conflicts that are emotionally painful and unacceptable to him. These forces often lie entirely beneath the surface of his awareness; at other times, they may be partially or dimly perceived. For example, a person may have repressed the painful memories of traumatic childhood experiences, or he may have had fleeting wishes for the death of someone who obstructed his way to a goal, or there may have been hidden hatreds lurking within a family circle. These repressed feelings and thoughts may from time to time threaten to erupt fully into consciousness, and at such times they flood the individual with panic. Much acute and chronic anxiety arises from such unconscious forces. The painful pressures of old unresolved experiences and past or present interpersonal conflicts which are repressed in the person mobilize anxiety as they crowd to the surface to seek expression.

Problems in important interpersonal relationships. The tasks of being an effective parent, of getting along well with relatives, and of smooth relationships with close friends and work associates often present problems that stir anxieties. The interactions of a parent with his children in meeting their needs for love, for realistic limitations and for guidance in all the dilemmas of child rearing, are particularly apt to arouse old conflicts from the childhood of the parent himself. Stressful relationships with other close persons also may contribute to anxiety neuroses.

Vocational insecurities and failures. Much of a person's life revolves around how he makes his living and how good he is at it. His capacities for getting along well with the people with whom he must deal in his job are equally important. Failure in his work, or gnawing insecurities about his work situation, have a large impact on his emotional ease or unrest. Major problems in his work and in the associated interpersonal environment often play a part in the causes of an anxiety neurosis. They may (1) directly disturb the person, or (2) stir up old doubts and feelings of insecurity about his adequacy as a person.

Social assaults on the self-esteem of the individual. Repeated failures in various kinds of social relationships and enterprises may shake the self-regard of an individual. Open hostility between people, especially if prolonged and severe, can lead to anxiousness. Failures to resolve interpersonal problems, and ruptures of relationships with significant people may act similarly. Harry Stack Sullivan felt that assaults on the self-esteem and feelings of personal adequacy of a person in both childhood and adulthood, constituted the single most important contributant to anxiety neuroses.

Marital problems and failures. Marriage is the most intimate interpersonal relationship of adult life, and in it many interpersonal strengths and capacities of two people are tested. The stresses of marriage, particularly when they resemble the individual's stresses of childhood (unmet needs for affection, conflicts of dominance and passivity, unmet yearnings for dependency, and others) may play significant roles in the etiology of anxiety states.

Other adult interpersonal contributants to anxiety states. The undue suppression of assertive, angry feelings, which often is the continuation of a similar pattern in childhood, leads to the accumulation of much pent-up hostility. The individual may fear, consciously or unconsciously, that this pent-up hostility will erupt in a wild loss of control in which he will become antisocially vicious. As his pent-up feelings crowd to the surface seeking some kind of expression, they may flood him with profound anxiety.

Similarly, a person may fear that he will not be able to control or channel his sexual urges in socially acceptable ways. This is particularly so in adolescents who are struggling to adjust to their burgeoning sexuality. Moreover, unacceptable sexual feelings, such as homosexual ones, may panic adolescents and young adults as they nudge toward the surface and begin to crowd into awareness.

In other instances, massive, prolonged situational stresses in military warfare or in civil disasters such as floods and fires may batter the person with much more emotional turmoil than he can adjust, to, and anxiety becomes manifest as his personality defenses break down. The ability of people to adjust to massive situational stress varies greatly from one person to the next, and is influenced by such factors as the morale of the group he is in, his understanding of the situation, and many other things.

Organic disease. A severe physical illness (such as heart or lung disease), or prolonged disability due to injury (as after automobile or industrial accidents) may contribute to anxiety states. This is particulary apt to occur if the individual does not have much emotional support from others during his period of physical diability, or if the physical incapacitation threatens to destroy an already unstable marital or vocational adjustment. In such cases, realistic apprehensiveness may be linked to old insecurities and anxieties from the patient's childhood and adolescence.

An occasional contributant to anxiety, most commonly in elderly persons, is subtle, progressive organic brain disease. If brain substance is being impaired by degenerative, vascular, or other disease processes, the individual must struggle to adjust to his environment and to interact with people with less brain tissue at his command; often he is vaguely aware that he is losing control of both himself and his interactions with people, and he is flooded with panic. Even minimal stresses and adjustment problems may precipitate acute anxiety.

Many other kinds of experiences in adult life may contribute to anxiety neuroses. However, these are among the more common ones. To understand all the roots of an anxiety neurosis, the entire life of each patient must be searched in detail.

THE CLINICAL COURSE OF ANXIETY NEUROSES

The clinical courses of anxiety neuroses, acute and chronic, vary immesely from patient to patient. Some patients have anxiety states for only a few weeks and recover without specific treatment. Other patients have fluctuating courses with exacerbations and remissions over periods of many months or years. Some patients remain persistently afflicted with anxiety neuroses for decades. The interposition of treatment, however, can alter markedly the course of anxiety neuroses.

The course and prognosis of a patient with an anxiety neurosis is much influenced by the following factors: (1) the duration and severity of the interpersonal causes of the anxiety neurosis, (2) the basic personality strengths and weaknesses of the patient, (3) the length of time the anxiety neurosis has been present, and the time of life, whether in childhood, adolescence or adulthood, in which the anxiety states began, (4) the current stresses in the patient's interpersonal life and the ease or difficulty in resolving them, and (5) the nature, timeliness and duration of treatment.

Obviously, these factors vary much from patient to patient. We shall consider briefly each of these variables.

The duration and severity of the interpersonal causes of an anxiety neurosis. In general, anxiety neuroses which are the results of mild interpersonal stresses are brief and respond easily to treatment. On the other hand, those produced by years or decades of severe interpersonal trauma are more peristent and more difficult to treat. Stressful intimate relationships, as in the immediate family group, have a much greater impact than stresses in less intimate relationships, as in work situations.

The basic personality strengths and weaknesses of the patient. Some patients have sufficient personality resources to gain insight into their problems easily and to make significant changes in their interpersonal relationships that lessen the severity of their anxiety states. For example, when anxiety forces them to focus their attention on what is unhealthy in their lives, they may improve marital situations, or leave stressful jobs and get less traumatic ones, or lessen tensions in other areas of their life situations. They may do this on their own or in treatment. Other patients are overwhelmed and interpersonally paralyzed by their anxiety neuroses, and resist all attempts to deal with the emotional origins of their symptoms. Some patients carry on in their jobs despite much anxiousness, whereas others sink into semi-invalidism. For example, a passive, dependent, shy person with an anxiety neurosis is more likely to be socially hampered by it than an outgoing, aggressive, independent individual.

The length of time the anxiety neurosis has been present, and the time of life, whether in childhood, adolescence or adulthood, in which the anxiety neurosis began. The patient who has had his anxiety neurosis for a few weeks or a few months is much more likely to respond to treatment than a patient whose anxiety neurosis has been present for years or decades. The patient who has had many years of medical physical treatment for the physiologic concomitants of anxiety, such as upper gastrointestinal complaints or cardiac palpitation, is less likely to accept and to work wholeheartedly on an emotional etiology for his trouble. Anxiety states that begin in late childhood and adolescence and have been continuously present for many years are particularly difficult to treat. On the other hand, patients who were free of symptoms and functioned well until recently in adult life often have a good prognosis and do well in treatment.

The current stresses in the patient's interpersonal life and the ease or difficulty in resolving them. A passive woman with an anxiety neurosis who is trapped with several children in a painful marriage with a hostile husband, has a poorer outlook than a person whose contemporary family setting is constructuve, helpful and relatively free of stress. After the onset of anxiety states, the increase or the removal of interpersonal stresses by changing events in a patient's life may greatly affect the course of his anxiety neurosis.

The nature, timeliness and duration of treatment. The ways of treating anxiety states form the subject of the following section of this chapter.

TREATMENT OF ANXIETY NEUROSES

Suggestions for the family physician or internist in dealing with patients with anxiety states. The first professional person whom an anxious patient consults is usually his family physician or internist. How the family physician or internist handles the problem often has a significant effect on its long-term course.

When the family physician or the internist is consulted by a patient with anxiety states, he should make the correct diagnosis promptly and should inform the patient of it in as reassuring a manner as possible. He should emphasize that anxiety states are caused by stressful interpersonal relationships in current and past life situations. The physician should explain clearly that the physical sensations accompanying the anxiety state, such as cardiac palpitation or upper gastrointestinal symptoms, are not diseases in themselves, but the physical concomitants of intense anxiety. He should reassure an acutely anxious patient that his fears of impending disaster, such as heart attack, "stroke" or "nervous breakdown" are unjustified. The doctor also may indicate that anxiety, masquerading in the garb of its many physical symptoms, is the most common difficulty that brings patients to doctors. Prompt reassurance and explanation often diminish the impact of an anxiety state. If it is mild, and if its interpersonal determinants are superficial, these prompt reassurances and explanations occasionally may allow the anxiety to resolve.

Above all, the family physician or internist should not be led into treating the physical comcomitants of an anxiety neurosis, such as a "nervous stomach" or "idiopathic tachycardia," as disease entities in themselves. Such treatment, ignoring the true emotional causes of these symptoms, tends to make the anxiety neurosis ingrained. After many months or several years of such management, an anxiety neurosis often becomes impervious to correct interpretation and exploratory interview work.

If the family physician feels he must do a few laboratory tests or have a brief hospital work-up in evaluating a patient with an anxiety reaction, he should tell the patient clearly at the outset that he feels that the problem is most probably due to emotional stresses and that the physical work-up is merely to rule out less likely possibilities. If the physician does not make such explanations at the beginning of a physical work-up, he leaves the patient in anxious turmoil incubating a host of new fears while the outpatient or inpatient work-up proceeds.

A physician should never use the word "nervous" to describe anxiety states. A large number of patients assume that "nervous" means that there is some vague biochemical or anatomical problem of the central nervous system causing the trouble, or at least playing a large part in its etiology. Also, despite the fact that the term "anxiety neurosis" is now the official designation for this condition in the standard nomenclature, I feel that the word "neurosis" should never be used in talking with patients and their families. It frightens, discourages, or infuriates them, and relatives later may, in moments of irritability or despair, call the patients "neurotic." In talking with patients I still use the older nomencluature term "anxiety reaction," or "anxiety state." The family physician or internist should also use terms such as "emotional stress," "tension," and "anxiousness due to past or present tensions between you and other people," in explaining anxiety states to patients.

In mild anxiety states, the family physician or internist may take a brief inventory of possible relevant stresses in the patient's family life, job situation or other interpersonal areas. He may also inquire whether the patient can be comfortably assertive of his angry feelings and other feelings to a reasonable extent, or whether he bottles up these feelings too tightly. Beyond a superficial inventory of possible interpersonal stresses in the patient's life, the family physician or the internist usually has neither the time nor the special experience for detailed interview work. Hence, the family physician should limit such exploratory work to a brief survey, which will perhaps open the patient's eyes to some relevant stresses in his life or at least make clearer to him what the doctor means by "interpersonal stress" and "emotional factors."

Interview Treatment

The main method of treating acute and chronic anxiety neuroses is interview treatment, the technical term of which is psychotherapy. The nature and depth of the psychotherapy depend on the severity of the anxiety neurosis and the orientation of the psychiatrist from whom the patient seeks help. The psychiatrist usually works by detailed interview technics, often over a period of several months to a year and a half, or longer, to help the patient resolve his emotional turmoil and to dimish the stresses of the causative interpersonal relationships in both his past and current life situations.

The task of such psychotherapy is to help the patient understand how his anxiety neurosis has arisen out of disturbed interpersonal relationships, and to resolve his emotional problems in the context of the patient-therapist relationship. The patient explores his experiences, feelings, fears and personality problems. The resolution of an anxiety neurosis, often requires much skill in interview technics and much earnest work by both the patient and his psychiatrist.

(The details of psychotherapy are covered at length in Chapter 21. The most widely employed psychiatric approaches—the interpersonal approach, the Freudian-psychoanalytic approach, behavior therapy, and others—have been sketched in Chapters 1 and 3. In addition, detailed case histories illustrating technics of psychotherapy in neuroses are given in Chapters 7 and 9.)

Pharmacological measures, which we shall discuss in the two following paragraphs, are quite secondary in importance in the management of anxiety states.

Pharmacologic Measures

Many sedatives and minor tranquilizers (often called antianxiety medications) are used in lessening the symptoms of anxiety neuroses. These medications, when properly used, can abort or lessen many acute anxiety attacks and can ameliorate chronic anxiousness to a certain extent. Though the pharmacologic methods of treating psychiatric disorders receive detailed attention in Chapter 22, a few points about their use in anxiety neuroses are in order here.

The physician, whether he is the family doctor or a psychiatrist, should emphasize to the patient that sedatives and tranquilizers do not cure anxiety neuroses. The cure lies in the resolution of the emotional turmoil within the patient and the interpersonal stresses in his life. The physician should point out that an antianxiety medication merely takes the edge off painful anxiousness while the patient is making progress in understanding the roots of his trouble and solving his problems. The patient should not expect more from an antianxiety medication than it can do. He should understand that, at best, sedatives and tranquilizers can lessen his anxiousness 25 or 30 per cent. (The pharmacology, uses, limitations and risks of many medications used for anxiety are discussed in detail in Chapter 22.)

THE ROLE OF ANXIETY IN OTHER KINDS OF NEUROSES

Anxiety is a basic force in the production of the other neurotic disorders (discussed in Chapters 7 through 10). In the initial stages of the development of a phobic neurosis, or an obsessive compulsive neurosis, or a hysterical neurosis of either conversion or dissociative type, or one of the other neurotic disorders, anxiety floods the person and then becomes secondarily encapsulated in one of these other neurotic disturbances. In a sense, the other neurotic disorders are sick ways of attempting to deal with the pain of anxiety.

For example, in a phobia the initial anxiety that rises in the patient becomes attached to specific kinds of objects or situations, such as automobiles or enclosed spaces; the individual then has profound anxiety only when in contact with automobiles, or when in small, enclosed spaces. He unconsciously has found an unhealthy solution for the pain of anxiety by developing another kind of neurotic symptom. His anxiety has become localized and encapsulated in a phobia of a particular type of object or situation. Somewhat similar basic processes occur in obsessive compulsive neuroses, conversion and dissociative types of hysterical neuroses, and other kinds of neurotic difficulties.

Hence, much of what we have said in this chapter about the interpersonal causes of anxiety neuroses also has bearing on the etiology of the other neurotic disorders (discussed in Chapters 7 through 10). For this reason, the anxiety neurosis is sometimes called "the basic neurosis," and anxiety is sometimes designated "the basic process" in all neuroses. Some psychiatrists have likened anxiety in the neuroses to inflammation in infectious pathology; it is the basic pathologic process from which various clinical pictures arise.

The patient who develops a phobic neurosis, or one of the other neurotic disturbances, may go through a brief phase of clinical anxiety while developing the phobia or other neurotic picture. Frequently the period of frank anxiety is so brief that the patient appears to develop his phobia or other neurosis directly. However, in many cases the patient's neurosis does not control his anxiety entirely, and acute or chronic anxiety accompanies the other neurotic symptoms. For example, much acute and chronic anxiety often accompanies a phobic neurosis or an obsessive compulsive disorder.

(From time to time in Chapters 7 through 10 we shall refer back to this chapter on anxiety neuroses, since its contents are basic to understanding the other types of neuroses.)

BIBLIOGRAPHY

Chapman, A. H.: The problem of prognosis in psychoneurotic illness. Am. J. Psychiatry, *119*: 768, 1963.

Friedman, D. E.: A synthetic approach to the treatment of anxiety. Psychiatry, *35*:336, 1972.

Kuiper, P. C.: The Neuroses: A Psychoanalytic Survey. New York, International Universities Press, 1972.

Lader, M., and Marks, I.: Clinical Anxiety. New York, Grune & Stratton, 1972.

Lesse, S.: Anxiety. Its Components, Development and Treatment. New York, Grune & Stratton, 1971.

Martin, B.: Anxiety and Neurotic Disorders. New York, John Wiley, 1971.

Ruesch, J.: Disturbed Communication. New York, W. W. Norton, 1961.

Shipman, W. G., Oken, D., and Heath, H. A.: Muscle tension and effort at self-control during anxiety. Arch. Gen. Psychiatry, 23:359, 1970.

Sullivan, H. S.: Clinical Studies in Psychiatry. New York, W. W. Norton, 1956.

———: The meaning of anxiety in psychiatry and in life. In Fusion of Psychiatry and Social Science. New York, W. W. Norton, 1964.

Woodruff, R. A., Guze, S. B., and Clayton, P. J.: Anxiety neurosis among psychiatric outpatients. Compr. Psychiatry, *13*:165, 1972.

7

Phobic Neurosis

In a phobic neurosis the patient has an abnormal fear of a specific object or type of situation. The person with a phobic neurosis may have a single phobia or he may have many of them, and a phobia may be so mild as to be barely noticed or so severe as to be incapacitating. Phobias constitute the most common neurotic disorder of childhood, and they are frequently encountered in adults.

CLINICAL CHARACTERISTICS OF PHOBIC NEUROSES

Some phobias consist of marked anxiety when the individual enters a specific type of situation. For example, the person may have a marked feeling of anxiousness when he enters any type of small enclosed place such as an elevator, a telephone booth, a small room, or any situation where a quick, easy exit is not possible. He may fear high places, open spaces, or dark places. Fear of leaving home is a frequently encountered phobia; the individual fears all places except his home. The fear of leaving home to attend school, the so-called school phobia, is common in children.

In the second category of phobias, the individual fears specific types of objects. For example, individuals may fear cats, or dogs, or insects, or storms, or automobiles, or airplanes, or many other kinds of objects. I recall a 23-year-old patient who had such a marked phobia of rats and mice that for several weeks she could not enter a building in which she had seen a rat or a mouse, or in which she had been told that someone else had seen one. Fears of minor medical procedures, such as intramuscular or intravenous injections, or routine dental examinations, are sometimes so marked that they constitute phobias.

We can better understand the nature of a phobia if we imagine what our feelings would be if we were chained in the middle of a busy automobile intersection during rush-hour traffic. We would be very anxious. The feelings of the phobic patient are similar when he encounters his phobic situation or object. The only difference is that the anxiety of the phobic patient is unjustified in terms of what he fears, but his terror is just as great as if it were justified. Often the phobic adult can see the unjustified nature of his fear, but this does not diminish its intensity. A small child, however, frequently feels that his fear is justified ("dogs can bite"), though in many cases he cannot explain why. The phobic adult occasionally offers superficial rationalizations for his fear ("automobile accidents are common"), but these rationalizations vary from time to time and are trimmings of the phobia rather than its substance.

In some instances the patient can avoid the phobic object or situation (bodies of water, airplanes, and others) easily and he may be able to regulate his life in such a way as rarely to come in contact with it. At other times the phobic object or situation is difficult to avoid (automobiles, small rooms, the dark, and others), and the pain caused by the phobia may be marked. Sometimes the patient curtails his activities in socially restricting ways to avoid contact with the phobic object. I have seen housewives who had such strong phobias about leaving the house that for many years they left their homes only once every several months, and some adolescents have school phobias of such severity that they terminate their education. Some phobic patients go to elaborate extents to avoid their phobic situations. I recall a businessman who planned all his appointments, business meetings and professional luncheons carefully to avoid ever entering a small room.

In traditional psychiatric terminology the common phobias have complex specific names derived from Greek roots. Thus, an "acrophobia" is a fear of heights, an "ailurophobia" is a fear of cats, a "panphobia" is a diffuse fearfulness of many things, and so forth; there are over 200 such terms. However, in modern clinical practice only two of these specific terms are widely used. They are "claustrophobia," the fear of enclosure in small places, and "agoraphobia," the fear of open spaces. The term "agoraphobia" often is applied to persons who fear to leave their homes. The other phobias today are called simply by the names of the feared object or situation, such as a fear of automobiles, a fear of water, and a fear of the dark.

Mild phobias are common and at times occur in persons who do not seem to have significant personality problems other than a single, minor phobia. Mild fears of high places, as when near an open window in a high office building, of insects, of high bridges and of other things, are so common that they often are accepted by the general public as being within normal limits. The unreasonable fear that many women have of mice is a culturally accepted phobia. Fears of the dark are so common in children that if they are transient and mild most parents pay little attention to them. Regional and cultural factors influence some phobias. For example, in areas where tornadoes occasionally occur in the spring, there is a significant incidence of unreasonable fears of tornadoes, strong winds and rainstorms.

When the phobic person confronts his phobic object or situation he has the experience described in our discussion of acute anxiety attacks in Chapter 6. His anxiety may vary from mild discomfort to disorganizing panic. If he remains in contact with the phobic object for a period of from several minutes to several hours, his anxiety often tends to diminish somewhat, though in some cases it may not.

Some psychiatrists state that phobias are more common in women than in men, but in my experience they occur with equal frequency in both sexes. Phobias may be single or multiple. When the patient has a single phobia he may be able to arrange his life so that he rarely encounters the phobic object. I recall a patient who had a marked phobia of touching cigarette lighters and matches, but he easily arranged his life so that he never touched them. In other instances, the patient has many phobias with which he cannot avoid contact, and his emotional suffering may be great. When the patient has multiple phobias, they frequently do not encapsulate all his anxiety, and he also has acute or chronic anxiety symptoms in addition to his phobias. The severity of a phobia and the number of them in a patient indicates the severity of their interpersonal causes. The patient with multiple, severe phobias has undergone much interpersonal trauma, whereas the patient with a single, mild phobia may have a relatively stable personality structure and has undergone fewer interpersonally damaging experiences.

Special Characteristics of Phobias in Children

Phobias in children have particular characteristics meriting special discussion. Phobias constitute the most common type of neurosis in children under the age of puberty; they are particularly common between the ages of three and seven. Fears of the dark, dogs, birds, insects, moving vehicles, bodies of water and many other objects and situations are frequently seen in children. The majority of minor phobias in children last from a few weeks to several months or more, and then subside. If the phobia is produced mainly by immediate interpersonal stresses in the child's life and the stresses are resolved, the child may develop no further phobias. However, if there is much continuing interpersonal turmoil, he may lose one phobia only to develop another one, or he may develop multiple phobias.

The phobias of a child often are caused by current or very recent interpersonal trauma, as opposed to phobias in adults, which often are related to interpersonal trauma in the distant past. Even the severe phobias of children usually disappear at puberty, but if there has been severe interpersonal turmoil in the child's life, the smoldering residuals of his emotional damage often lead to the production of other phobias or other types of neurotic difficulties in adolescence or later. Phobias in adolescence often are more persistent and may extend into adulthood. In general, adolescent phobias have the clinical characteristics of adult phobias.

School phobias constitute a frequent type of phobia in children. The child with a school phobia has profound anxiety whenever the time approaches to leave home to go to school. If the child is forced to go to school, he may remain very frightened and he may cry for several hours during the school day. He frequently complains of the physical sensations that accompany his anxiety, such as epigastric discomfort, nausea and vomiting. The school phobia sometimes escapes clinical recognition because of the camouflage of physical distresses which accompany it. I have seen children in the fourth grade who had missed half the school days of their entire school careers because of gastrointestinal or upper respiratory tract complaints that were actually the physical concomitants of the severe anxiety of a school phobia.

School phobias are common up to the age of 9, and phobias in this age group have an excellent prognosis. School phobias that occur between the age of 9 and puberty are more difficult to treat, but the vast majority of them can be resolved with psychiatric management. School phobias in adolescents have a more serious prognosis. They may be the initial symptoms of depressive or schizophrenic illnesses, and half the adolescents who develop school phobias never return to school. In discussing adolescent school phobias, we are not referring to adolescents who are defiant and rebellious against attending school; we are referring to the adolescent who is overwhelmed with panic at the prospect of leaving home and attending school.

A school phobia is actually a fear of leaving home. The child fears that something catastrophic will happen to his parents or to his home while he is away from home, and he feels an urgent necessity to remain at home where he can reassure himself constantly that everything is all right. The phobia centers on school, since school is the main place to which a child goes for long periods of time each day and from which he cannot at will return home. While at school the child is separated from his parents for six or seven hours without the ability to communicate with them. Some children with school phobias fear to go to other places besides school, but frequently the school phobia remains restricted to the school situation.

INTERPERSONAL CAUSES OF PHOBIAS

A phobia is a fear that arises in painful interpersonal conflicts and is displaced onto a phobic object or situation. In ways of which he is unaware, the patient has profound anxieties arising from past and current interpersonal situations, but these situations are too painful for him to recognize consciously. Hence, the patient's emotional turbulence and anxiety are displaced onto some type of object or situation, and the patient develops marked anxiety when he comes in contact with that object or situation. For example, a patient may have marked anxieties that arise from past experiences with his parents and other close persons, and have been rekindled by current interpersonal stresses in his marriage and in his job. However, these anxieties are too painful to recognize consciously, and they are displaced onto a phobia of closed spaces, such as elevators and small rooms. The patient is unaware of the connection of his interpersonal distress and his symptom. He merely knows that he dreads the particular type of situation of which he has a phobia.

Many psychiatrists feel that the phobia the patient develops often has a symbolic connection with the type of interpersonal stress that caused it. For example, the patient who has a fear of elevators and small spaces often has a basic fear of being trapped in painful interpersonal situations. He felt trapped in painful relationships with his parents or other close persons from which he could find no release, and he may find himself similarly trapped in a difficult marriage. He is not able to come to grips consciously with his dread of being trapped in interpersonally painful situations, but his phobia of being enclosed in small spaces such as elevators is a thinly disguised symbol of his basic fear of interpersonal confinement in emotionally painful situations from which he can find no release. In the same manner, a child who fears the dark actually may fear that he may be attacked by unknown assailants in the dark or during his sleep. His basic fears may arise out of hostility and rejection by one or both parents, which produce anxiety. However, these interpersonal conflicts are too painful for the child to face consciously, and his marked anxiety and turmoil are displaced onto a fear of the dark; the unknown assailants he fears are thinly disguised symbols of the parents he dreads.

I recall a 30-year-old married woman who for four months had had a severe phobia of leaving home; for several weeks at a time she did not depart from her house. Like many phobic patients, she felt somewhat more comfortable if another person accompanied her on occasions when leaving the home was absolutely necessary. With such a chaperone, she could go on important errands outside the home, but she still was uncomfortable.

The patient was the second of two children. The first child, a brother three years older than her, had been wanted and he was given much affection and attention. After his birth, the patient's parents had wanted no further children, for they were both working to build up a small family business and more children would present economic problems and vocational obstacles. Hence, when the patient was born, she was from the first treated with rejection and irritability. Throughout her childhood she was criticized and depreciated by her parents, who rationalized their treatment of her by complaining that she was an awkward, difficult, unlovable child. The emotional pain of these daily experiences in the patient's childhood was made bitterer by the open favoritism the parents showed the older brother. In the context of this interpersonal environment, the patient became a shy, passive person who kept all her anger pent up inside her, and she had profound feelings of worthlessness and inadequacy. Beneath her passive, quiet façade simmered much unconscious anger and turbulence about the way she had been treated by her family throughout her formative years.

When she was 18 years old, her parents pushed her toward marriage with a man who was eight years older than her. Eager to be free of the emotional pain of her parents' home, she married this man after knowing him only five months. Her husband was a domineering, self-centered person who dominated the patient callously and criticized her endlessly. The patient's feelings of inadequacy were accentuated when her second child was born with a congenital deformity of his left arm. When this child was two years old, the patient had the abrupt onset of her severe phobia of leaving home.

In 18 months of psychotherapy she gradually came to grips with the painful interpersonal relationships that characterized her childhood. Prior to entering interview treatment she had only dim awareness of how the rejection and hostility of her parents had warped her personality structure, and she had been unaware of the hatred pent up within her. She gradually became aware of how her upbringing had molded her into a passive person with profound feelings of inadequacy. She was able to develop a more realistic concept of herself and acquired more self-confidence. She developed the ability to be more assertive and to express some of the anger that she formerly stored up within herself. She no longer allowed other people to dominate her and to exploit her. She developed a realistic view of her husband and of the unhealthy interactions in her marriage.

At the end of her psychotherapy, her phobia had been resolved and she functioned emotionally and socially in much more adequate ways. Her husband refused interview treatment or marriage counseling to work on their marital problems, but the patient felt that she now had the emotional strength to deal with this problem and to seek marital separation and independent living if her marriage did not improve in time. This patient demonstrates how adult interpersonal stresses are frequently added to childhood interpersonal trauma to produce a phobic disorder.

Role of Anxiety in Causing Phobias

All of the traumatic interpersonal experiences of childhood and adult life we discussed as possible contributants to anxiety in Chapter 6 on anxiety neuroses may also play roles in the production of phobic neuroses. Since a phobia is essentially an anxiety reaction that becomes particularly restricted to a special type of object or situation, any type of interpersonal trauma causing anxiety may also operate in the production of a phobia.

For example, sexual trauma during childhood may be an important contributant to a phobic neurosis in adult life. I recall a 33-year-old married woman with multiple severe phobias, among which were marked fears of automobiles, darkness and being alone. Her parents had been divorced when she was two years old and she had been reared from the age of 3 to 11 by her mother and a stepfather whom the mother married when the patient was three. Beginning when the patient was five years old, her stepfather sexually molested her occasionally by having her engage in mutual masturbation with him. This continued until the patient was 11 years old. The patient was both frightened and sexually stimulated by these experiences, and she had much guilt and anxiety about them. Her feelings toward her stepfather were a confused mixture of fear, hatred and fondness. When the patient was 11 her mother and the stepfather were divorced and she saw him only infrequently after that. However, during the early years of her adolescence she continued to have much lingering emotional turmoil about these sexual experiences, though she never told anyone about them. During middle adolescence, these experiences were repressed from her conscious memory; in time she remembered only the more acceptable aspects of her stepfather's behavior.

She married at 22 and during the next five years had two children. Her marital adjustment was poor, and her feelings toward her husband were a mixture of sporadic affection which alternated with bickering irritability and vague fearfulness. Her husband was very attached to their children, both of whom were girls. As the patient observed the paternal affection of her husband for their daughters, set against the background of the marital problems between herself and her husband, she began to experience much anxiety. The repressed memories of her sexual exploitation by her stepfather and the chaotic emotional distress associated with these experiences began to press toward the surface of her awareness. They flooded her with panic which quickly became encapsulated in a variety of severe phobias. However, these memories and old conflicts were too devastating for conscious recognition. She was aware only of the painful phobias they precipitated.

During 16 months of twice-weekly interview treatment she gradually recalled the long-continued sexual trauma of her childhood and resolved the guilt, terror and anger she had felt about it. In psychotherapy she was able to express the chaotic mixture of anger, fear and sexual attraction she had felt toward her stepfather, and she could see how she had carried these feelings unconsciously into her marital relationship with her husband, and how most of her marital problems arose from them. She also gained insight into how observing her husband's paternal affection for their daughters had caused her childhood experiences to surge upward from the forgotten past and had precipitated her phobias. At the end of treatment her phobias were resolved and her capacities as a wife and mother were improved.

Psychotherapy of phobias is not always as successful as it was in the two cases cited above (and also in other cases cited in this section on neuroses), but for illustrative purposes I have chosen cases with favorable outcomes.

A phobia may arise out of interpersonal conflicts in which the patient has much repressed hostility toward an emotionally close person in his life. Accompanying the hostility is much dread of retaliation by the hated person. These feelings are too painful for conscious recognition, and the turmoil and fear are displaced onto a phobic object or situation. The patient then feels a profound dread of the phobic object, which is a symbol of the person with whom he is in emotional conflict. This mechanism is common in the phobias of children.

For example, I recall a passive 6-year-old boy with a school phobia who rarely expressed any assertive or hostile feelings toward his controlling, domineering mother. His mother made him feel guilty and inadequate if he ever expressed any aggressive feelings of any kind. He stored up his angry feelings and felt guilty if he expressed them in even minor ways. He was a meticulously dressed, polite boy without a spot on his well-creased clothing. When I suggested to his mother that it would be emotionally healthier if he were somewhat assertive at times, she received this opinion with open skepticism.

The severity of the phobia, however, caused the mother to bring the boy for weekly play therapy sessions. During our initial sessions we constructed buildings of blocks and destroyed them by bombardment from toy rocket launchers and airplanes. I accompanied this aggressive, destructive play with many interpretations about how necessary and acceptable it is for people to get angry at times and to blow off steam. We discussed how boys should engage in some rough and tumble play and should not behave like spotless china dolls. We discussed how he should not let other children boss him and how he should stick up for his rights at home, at school and in the neighborhood. I also had conferences with the parents in which I urged that they accept the emerging assertiveness of their son as an emotionally healthy development and that they should not do anything to stifle it. Because of the severity of the phobia, the mother gave lukewarm cooperation in these measures, and the boy's father, a passive henpecked man, was delighted to see his son develop the assertiveness he himself lacked. In time the boy became a a more assertive, aggressive child and he resolved his phobia. However, his mother expressed her frank regret that he no longer was "the sweet, obedient little gentleman he used to be before he had all this psychiatric treatment."

All the interpersonal causes of anxiety outlined in Chapter 6, arising from both childhood and adult experiences, may contribute to produce the anxiety that becomes encapsulated in phobias. The interpersonal approach to psychiatry emphasizes that each patient with a neurotic disorder must be studied as an individual to determine the unique combination of interpersonal traumas that have led to his emotional disorder. No single formula, or type of formula, can explain all cases of any type of neurotic illness. The causes of each patient's illness need careful exploration to unravel the particular chain of causative interpersonal stresses.

CLINICAL COURSE OF PHOBIC NEUROSES

The mild phobias of childhood may last from a few weeks to six months or a year. They often disappear spontaneously, and if the interpersonal problems of the child are minor he may not develop more phobias. The more severe phobias of childhood may last several years or may persist until puberty if the child does not have psychotherapy. However, even without treatment the severe childhood phobias usually disappear at puberty, but if the underlying emotional turmoil of the child is unresolved he may develop new phobias or other types of neurotic disturbances in adolescence or adulthood.

The phobias of adolescence and adulthood, unless favorably influenced by psychiatric treatment, tend to be much more persistent than those of childhood. Adult phobias often undergo periodic fluctuations in severity, depending on the varying interpersonal circumstances of the person. Mild or moderate adult phobias sometimes disappear after lasting from several months to several years. However, it is common in psychiatric practice to encounter adult patients who have had phobias for many years or even for several decades. Some phobias begin in early adulthood and last during the rest of the patient's life.

Some phobic patients develop a way of life that lessens exposure to their phobias, and they develop methods for diminishing the pain of them. For example, persons with severe phobias of crowds and public places may find they can tolerate these situations better if they are always accompanied by a close friend or a relative who acts as a psychological "chaperone," and they arrange their lives so that they never enter a public place without such a companion. Ingrained phobias as a rule do not become more severe as the years or decades go by; they remain the same or may decrease somewhat in severity, but they rarely disappear completely. However, exacerbations of life situational stresses can cause some phobias to become more severe for a time. All these statements refer to the clinical courses of phobias not treated with psychotherapy. Interview treatment may resolve phobias, or at least decrease their severity.

The same kinds of factors (discussed in Chapter 6) that influence the course and prognosis of anxiety neuroses apply equally to the course and prognosis of phobic neuroses. They are (1) the duration and severity of the interpersonal causes of the phobic neurosis, (2) the basic personality strengths and weaknesses of the patient, (3) the length of time the phobia has been present, and the time of life, whether in childhood, adolescence or adulthood, in which it began, (4) the current stresses of the patient's interpersonal life and the ease or difficulty in resolving them, and (5) the nature, timeliness and duration of the treatment.

TREATMENT OF PHOBIC NEUROSES

Psychotherapy of Phobic Neuroses

The main method of treating phobic neuroses is interview treatment, in which the patient seeks to resolve the emotional difficulties arising from past interpersonal conflicts and from current interpersonal stresses. The resolution of this emotional turmoil frees the patient of his phobia. Chapter 21 deals at length with the details of psychotherapy, but we shall give here a clinical illustration of the way in which psychotherapy is carried out in phobic neuroses.

The process of psychotherapy in a patient with a phobia is well demonstrated by the case of a 43-year-old, married businessman who consulted me for a severe claustrophobia of several months' duration. He could not enter elevators or small rooms of any kind, and he was very anxious when circumstances required that he ride in his automobile. He came for twice weekly interview sessions for 12 months.

The psychotherapy of this patient can be divided roughly into three broad periods: (1) the first two months of treatment dealt mainly with his inability to express assertive and hostile feelings in a wide variety of current interpersonal situations; (2) in the next three months of psychotherapy he discussed the emotional problems in his marriage and in other intimate relationships in his life; (3) in the last seven months he dealt with emotionally traumatic experiences in his childhood and adolescence.

In the first two months of treatment the patient discussed his inability to express any assertive or angry feelings. His passivity led him to be exploited and dominated by people in his family relationships, in his business activities and in his social life. Behind his inability to be assertive or angry lay a profound fear that even minor assertiveness would lead to rejection by people and to social isolation. He felt a desperate need to be well liked by everyone, and he felt that suppression of all assertive feelings was necessary to achieve this end. He felt very uncomfortable if anyone became irritated or angry at him, and he went to great lengths to avoid even the mildest kind of friction with people around him.

We discussed how his passivity led to much simmering anger being stored up within him. We explored how his unassertiveness caused people to exploit him and produced even more suppressed fury within him. We examined at length the unreality of his fears that everyone would reject him if he was assertive, and that actually he would be treated with more respect and consideration if he was reasonably assertive. He began to work on these problems in his daily life. He was able to become more aggressive and to cease bottling up all his angry feelings. People gradually stopped exploiting him and dominating him, and they treated him with more consideration and respect. We explored how some of his pent-up feelings contributed to the emotional turbulence that caused his phobia. As he made progress in this area, the severity of his phobia diminished to a certain extent.

During the next three months or so of treatment, the patient discussed problems in his marriage and in other intimate interpersonal areas of his life. He had profound yearnings for emotional closeness with his wife, but he had never achieved a truly comfortable relationship with her. His passivity and dread of arousing even minor friction in his marriage had prevented him from talking with his wife about any problems that had ever arisen between them. Their marriage gradually had drifted into a stale, distant relationship with little warmth and infrequent sexual activity; he retreated into his business affairs while his wife was busy with social activities and club work. They spent little time together, and their only area of interpersonal warmth was their mutual interest in their three daughters. This man, whose mother had died when he was nine, had a profound yearning for emotional closeness with a woman, and the absence of this closeness in his marriage stirred much anguish in him. He felt a confused mixture of yearning, resentment and disappointment in his marriage, but covered it over with a veneer of placid passivity.

As we discussed these difficulties, he was able to begin to talk out these problems with his wife. His new-found assertiveness helped him open up these areas with her. Fortunately, she was a sound person emotionally, and when she grasped how their marriage had drifted into stagnancy and how painful this was to her husband, she became much warmer and more affectionate. Over a period of several months their marriage gradually improved, and the patient and his wife found a warmth and companionship which they had not had previously.

The patient also was much upset by problems in his relationship with his three daughters who ranged in age from 5 through 10. He had never been able to be firm with them in any way, and they exploited his vacillating passivity; they had little affection for him, and in vain he sought their love by endless indulgence. In the end, he could be neither affectionate nor firm with them, and the emotional distance between him and his daughters upset him much. As we examined these problems he gradually developed the capacity to be firmer with his daughters, and he also developed a feeling of comfortable affection toward them, which they in return began to show toward him. These interpersonal improvements, accompanied by improvements in his marriage, resolved many of the patient's unmet needs for affection and his dependent yearnings which formerly had generated much anxiety in him.

In the last seven months of his psychotherapy the patient explored childhood emotional traumas which contributed markedly to his phobia. At first he could remember little that had happened prior to his mother's death when he was nine, and the only recollection he had of his mother was a memory of her lying ill one afternoon in bed. However, as he began to talk about his childhood he slowly uncovered an extensive set of painful repressed childhood experiences.

The patient was the last of three children, and he was born six years after his next oldest sibling. His mother was physically ill for several months after his brith, and when he was four years old his mother had a psychotic illness for which she was psychiatrically hospitalized for six months. On one occasion the patient was taken to see her in the psychiatric hospital, and he came away very upset and frightened. His mother recovered from her psychosis, but her physical health remained poor. When the patient was nine, his mother died at home in an acute crisis of a chronic pulmonary disease, which probably was tuberculosis.

Throughout these first nine years of his life, the patient's mother constantly attributed her physical and mental illnesses to the strain of giving birth to the patient and the work of caring for him. She was chronically hostile toward him, and often blamed him for all her suffering. Thus, her death precipitated immense guilt and anxiety in him, and these feelings persisted until early adolescence. During early adolescence, however, repression erased from his awareness all memories of the first nine years of his life, except for a few scenes which he could not connect with each other. His mother's illnesses, her hostility toward him, and his profound feelings of guilt and terror about what he felt had been his role in causing her suffering, were all lost to his conscious recollection. However, unresolved conflicts and emotional turbulence within him later erupted and contributed to his severe phobia in adulthood.

As he worked out the details of these childhood experiences, two further points became clear. Firstly, his phobia had begun when he was 43, the age at which his mother died. Basically, he had a strong unconscious fear that in some dreadful way he was to be punished for the illnesses he allegedly caused his mother by dying at the same age at which she had died. Secondly, a further aspect of his phobia became evident in studying a frightening dream which he had had many times. In this dream he saw himself lying in a closed coffin while a funeral service was in progress. Careful examination of the dream revealed that many of the details of the funeral were identical to the details of his mother's funeral, which he had attended and which had frightened him badly. Many psychiatrists would postulate that the patient's dread of being enclosed in small spaces, producing his claustrophobia, was a symbolic substitute for a more basic fear of dying and being enclosed in a coffin, in retribution for his guilty feelings that he had been responsible for his mother's illnesses, death and burial. After working through this material, the patient's phobia was resolved and treatment was terminated. Seven years later he returned to see me for four sessions because of transient mild anxiety he had at the time of his father's death; this anxiousness subsided quickly. During this seven-year interval he had not had a recurrence of his phobia and had not had any other neurotic problems.

This case illustrates two features of the interpersonal approach to the treatment of phobias and other neurotic disorders. Firstly, to use a simile we have employed before, the exploration of a neurotic disorder may be likened to progressively peeling back the layers of an onion. In therapy the patient first explores the current interpersonal problems on the day-to-day surface of his life. He then proceeds to examine deeper issues in his current and past interpersonal relationships, and then gradually proceeds into older, more deeply buried areas of his childhood experiences. The exploration of all these layers contributes to the resolution of the patient's neurosis.

Secondly, the causes of a neurosis are multiple; there are many contributing factors, some of which are large and others of which are minor. These multiple causes are to be found in the patient's past and present life situations, which must be explored in a joint enterprise with the therapist. (Much more material on the technics of psychotherapy is given in Chapter 21, and the special methods used in treating children and adolescents are discussed in Chapter 24.)

Other Aspects of the Treatment of Phobias

Suggestions to the family physician, internist and pediatrician in dealing with phobias. The treatment of phobias of severe or moderate degree lies in the province of the psychiatrist, but the family physician or internist sometimes can manage minor, transient phobias in the patient whose basic personality structure is reasonably sound and whose interpersonal stresses are of minor degree. Similarly, the pediatrician often can manage some of the minor phobias which are so common in children.

In dealing with a minor, transient phobia, the family physician first of all should reassure the patient about his phobic symptom. The phobic patient often fears that he will "go to pieces" in public if he encounters the phobic object and that other people will notice his fearfulness and will be alarmed by his reactions or will be contemptuous of him. Such things are extremely rare in patients with phobias, and the physician can reassure the patient on these points. The doctor's strong reassurances often give the patient the initial strength which starts him moving toward overcoming his phobia. Often the patient with a minor or moderate phobia must confront his phobic object or situation in carrying out his normal day-to-day activities. The physician may point out that by facing his phobia and by going through the experience successfully, a patient often feels a good deal of reassurance. The patient can tell himself that he faced his phobia and did not "go to pieces" in the process, and this gives him increased confidence in the doctor's support and reassurances.

In managing a minor phobia, the family physician should explain the emotional nature of the problem to the patient. He should explain that a phobia is caused by current and past interpersonal stresses and pent-up feelings. He should point out that perhaps the patient can inventory current interpersonal problems in his life and solve some obvious day-to-day emotional stresses. The family doctor, or internist, and the patient can discuss to some extent any obvious tensions in the patient's life, especially those which have begun recently. At times the physician can suggest a few steps for the patient to consider in resolving minor interpersonal difficulties. The family physician should not attempt detailed, prolonged interview work, but by a limited amount of flexible, common sense counseling he often can aid patients to resolve minor phobias of recent origin.

Token amounts of medication sometimes can help a patient in overcoming a minor transient phobia. A mild antianxiety medication taken before encountering his phobic object or situation often aids the patient to go through the experience comfortably. Frequently, the suggestive role of the mild sedative or minor tranquilizer is as important as its pharmacologic effect; the medication carries tangible remembrance of the physician's reassurances and gives the patient added self-confidence in facing his phobia successfully and comfortably. I feel that the physician should explain this to the patient: "The value of this medication is as much psychological as pharmacological; it will take the edge off your anxiousness by 20 per cent, and that will help you overcome the rest."

Some psychiatrists balk at the idea of family physicians and internists handling some of the minor or moderate phobias of recent origin, but these problems are so common, and so many patients refuse psychiatric consultation for them, that I feel the nonpsychiatric physician can render a service to many patients by helping them in these ways.

In a similar manner, the pediatrician sometimes can manage the minor phobias that are so common in children. When the parent-child relationship is basically sound and the child's phobia is mild, the pediatrician sometimes can aid in resolving it. By strong reassurances, by explaining the emotional nature of the phobia to the parents and the child, by discussing with the parents and the child any obvious interpersonal stresses in the child's life and examining ways of removing them, the child's phobia sometimes can be resolved. However, when the child's phobia is severe, or when it has been present for many months or longer, or when the parents are unable to alter emotionally unhealthy ways of dealing with the child, the child and his parents should be referred for child guidance psychiatric help.

By using similar technics, the pediatrician also can help to resolve mild school phobias of recent origin in prepuberal children. A basic principle is that the child must continue to attend school, regardless of his discomfort and even if his mother must stay with him during the first hour to two of the school day. When a prepuberal child with a school phobia is allowed to stay out of school, the phobia becomes much more difficult to treat. Moderate to severe school phobias, and all school phobias in patients over the age of 10, require the attention of a psychiatrist or child guidance clinic services.

Behavior therapy of phobias. In Chapter 3 we outlined the principles of *behavior theory* and its clinical application in *behavior therapy;* we also gave a brief sketch of its application to the treatment of phobias, probably its most promising area of clinical usefulness.

In brief, behavior theory views a phobia as a conditioned reaction (or, in oversimplified terms, a conditioned reflex) of anxiety to a particular object or situation. Through a series of experiences, or a single highly traumatic experience, in which much anxiety is associated with a specific type of object, the patient develops an invariable reaction of panic when he comes in contact with the object. In examples given by one writer on behavior therapy, a patient developed a phobia of dogs by being viciously attacked and dragged by the hair by a large dog when she was 5, and another patient developed a phobia of water and heights at the age of 38 after falling from a high dock into water between the dock and a large, lurching ship.

Although many variations of behavior therapy are used in treating phobias, almost all of them employ some form of desensitization, or deconditioning. By slow degrees, the patient's conditioned reaction (or conditioned reflex) of anxiety to his phobic object or situation is diminished by increasing exposure to it while the therapist works to substitute relaxation and anxiety-free responses for his panic reactions. A "hierarchy" of desensitization steps is used; often there are 20 to 35 steps in this process, and each step occupies, as a rule, one or more sessions. Thoughts and daydreams about the phobic object, as well as physical approximation to it, are used.

For example, a patient with a phobia of automobiles begins by thinking of an automobile and, in a daydream manner, visualizes himself as walking by it; while he does this he practices muscular and emotional relaxation technics in ways suggested by the therapist, to substitute anxiety-free relaxation for his reaction of anxiety. In further steps in his hierarchy of desensitization, the patient visualizes himself getting into an automobile, driving it, refueling it at a filling station, and washing it. If he is a child, he may play with toy automobiles and draw pictures of them. Then, always using relaxation technics, he looks at actual automobiles, goes near them, gets into one, starts the motor and lets it idle by the curb, drives it, and so forth. Each step occurs on separate days, or weeks.

Some behavior therapists combine deconditioning technics, or other behavior therapy methods, with the kinds of interpersonal psychotherapy illustrated in the cases given earlier in this chapter.

Most psychiatrists feel that the behavior therapy view of the etiology of phobias is oversimplified, or even erroneous, but they recognize that behavior therapy is nevertheless effective in eliminating many phobias. Moreover, there is increasing evidence that most patients who lose their phobias by behavior therapy do not develop other phobias or different neurotic symptoms in their places. Many psychiatrists who are skeptical about the claims of behavior therapists in other psychiatric conditions such as obsessive neuroses, homosexuality, and others, have come to accept behavior therapy as a useful treatment for phobias. It is most likely to work in patients who have only one phobia (as opposed to several) and who have relatively healthy current life situations. In fact, it is quite possible that for some such patients behavior therapy is less time consuming, less expensive, and more effective than other types of therapy.

Detailed studies of treatment of unselected phobic patients by various forms of therapy, and their prior and subsequent evaluation by neutral observers, are yet to be done, and are immensely difficult to do, but it appears that behavior therapy has a valid, perhaps important, place in the treatment of phobias. In our opinion, phobic patients who have unhealthy current interpersonal life situations and have had traumatic, long-term experiences in past life circumstances, should have exploratory, interpersonal psychotherapy in addition to any behavior therapy they have.

BIBLIOGRAPHY

Agras, W. S., Chapin, H. N., and Oliveau, D. C.: The natural history of phobias. Arch. Gen. Psychiatry, 26:315, 1972.

Freud, S.: Analysis of a phobia in a five-year-old boy. In Collected Papers. vol. 3. London, Hogarth Press, 1953.

Gehl, R. H.: Indecision and claustrophobia. Int. J. Psychoanal., 54:47, 1973.

Glick, B. S.: Conditioning therapy with phobic patients: success and failure. Am. J. Psychother., 24:92, 1970.

Kaplan, D. M.: On shyness. Int. J. Psychoanal., 53:439, 1972.

Kazuhiko, A.: Phobias and nervous symptoms in childhood and maturity. Brit. J. Psychiatry, 120:275, 1972.

Lassers, E., Nordan, R., and Bladholm, S.: Steps in the return to school of children with school phobias. Am. J. Psychiatry, 130:265, 1973.

Lautch, H.: Dental phobia. Brit. J. Psychiatry, 119:151, 1971.

Lazarus, A. A. (ed.): Clinical Behavior Therapy. New York, Brunner Mazel, 1971.

MacKenzie, K. R.: The eclectic approach to the treatment of phobias. Am. J. Psychiatry, 130:1103, 1973.

Marks, I. M.: The classification of phobic disorders. Brit. J. Psychiatry, 116:377, 1970.

Radin, S. S.: Job phobia: school phobia revisited. Compr. Psychiatry, 13:251, 1972.

Solyom, S., Shugar, R., Bryntwich, S., and Solyom C.: Treatment of fear of flying. Am. J. Psychiatry, 130:423, 1973.

8

Obsessive and Compulsive Neuroses

An obsession is a persistent, anxious thought the patient is unable to put out of his consciousness. For example, the patient may have a peristent fear of death running through his mind, or he may have the consistant thought that he has a particular disease such as heart disease or cancer.

A compulsion is a strong urge to perform a physical act to relieve tension. For example, some compulsive patients urgently feel that they must count every step in all flights of stairs they ascend, or that they must wash their hands repeatedly because of their fear of germs or dirt.

Obsessions and compulsions sometimes occur in the same patient, and hence they usually are considered together in psychiatric writing. Obsessions may be present in a patient without compulsions, however; this is particularly true of obsessive fears of death, disease and violence. On the other hand, the patient with compulsions usually has obsessive ideas, producing the classical picture of an obsessive compulsive neurosis. Both obsessions alone and obsessive compulsive disorders are commonly seen in psychiatric practice.

CLINICAL CHARACTERISTICS OF OBSESSIVE AND COMPULSIVE NEUROSES

Obsessive Neuroses

We can get a better insight into the nature of obsessions by considering the minor kinds of obsessive ideas that occur at times in most people. A rhythmic jingle or melody sometimes becomes a persistent, annoying preoccupation, and the person wishes he could get rid of it. A television slogan or an advertising phrase may run repetitively through an individual's mind in a somewhat irritating manner. Mark Twain once wrote an amusing short story about a man who developed a distressing obsessive thought stimulated by a notice in a tram to remind the driver to punch the tickets of the passengers. The jingle ran: "Punch, brothers! punch with care! Punch in the presence of the passenjare!" These normal obsessions help us better to understand the obsessive thoughts of the obsessional patient. The obsessive thoughts of the obsessive patient, however, carry much anxiety or even panic with them. Also, the obsessive patient usually has multiple obsessive ideas.

Common obsessive thoughts that bring a patient to psychiatric attention are obsessions of germs, dirt, diseases, death, illnesses of close relatives, obscene words, lewd sexual practices, and possible violent assaults of the patient on other people. Other obsessive thoughts take the form of abstract ideas often involving philosophical or religious subjects.

Obsessive fears of diseases are common, and they vary from mild worries to severe preoccupations that are almost constantly present. Among the more common obsessively feared diseases are cardiovascular disease (especially "heart attack" and "stroke") and psychiatric illness (usually expressed by the patient as "nervous breakdown," "mental disease," or "losing control and doing something terrible"). In general, the public considers cardiovascular disease and psychiatric illness to be often abrupt in onset and catastrophic in nature, and capable of striking anyone without prior warning; these factors probably influence the frequency of obsessions of cardiovascular and psychiatric illness. The public often envisions a psychiatric illness as some kind of "loss of control" in which the person wildly runs amok; the patient envisions himself as constantly on the verge of such behavior, and often he has lurid daydreams of unrestrainable sexual and hostile assaults which he fears he may carry out while in such a state. Obsessive fears of cancer, venereal disease and "germs" are common.

Obsessive ideas of violent or immoral acts are frequently encountered in psychiatric practice. The patient may fear that he will commit violence to himself or others. For example, coupled obsessions of infanticide and insanity in young mothers form a frequent clinical syndrome. They fear that they may at any moment murder their children, and they feel that such a dreadful thought circulating repetitively in their minds indicates incipient insanity. Patients of all age groups and both sexes may have similar obsessive fears of violence to others. Obsessive fears of harming oneself constitute another common group of obsessive ideas. The patient may fear obsessively that at some unpredictable moment he will hurl himself from a high window, or crash his speeding automobile into an oncoming vehicle, or impulsively swallow a large amount of sedatives or poisonous substances. Some obsessional patients fear constantly that they will commit lewd sexual acts in public, or carry out sexual assaults, or suddenly shout obscene words in social settings. Fears of other immoral acts, such as abruptly stealing things from a store or impulsively committing armed robbery, are less common.

It should be emphasized that the obsessive patient has no *urge* to carry out his obsessive thoughts or to experience their consequences. Rather, he has a profound *dread* that these things will come to pass and mobilizes every possible resource to prevent their occurrence. For example, he has no urge to commit violent or scandalous acts in public, but rather he has a nagging dread that he may do it against his will; similarly, he has no desire to experience heart disease, but rather he has a continual, obsessive fear of having a heart attack.

Another group of obsessive ideas is composed of repetitive word formulations and ruminative speculations concerning abstract philosophical or religions subjects. Repetitive sentences or expressions run through the minds of some obsessive patients; sometimes these sentences concern obscene sexual topics or blasphemous religious notions. At other times the obsessive ideas involve religious quandries or philosophical absurdities. For example, I recall a patient who endlessly speculated on whether the Archangel Gabriel had a beard and whether or not he was bald. Another patient was constantly obsessed with speculations about what the world would be like without gravity and about the nature of darkness.

Some patients have repetitive doubts causing them to check and recheck their actions. I recall an obsessive patient who always checked and rechecked to make sure all the water faucets and the gas outlets were turned off before he left home. After going out the door he usually reentered and checked these points again, and sometimes did this two or three times before driving away from his house. After arriving at his destination he would still ruminate obsessively that he had forgotten to turn off some gas or water outlet, and he would call home or return there again to make sure everything was all right. Some patients have obsessive indecisiveness; they shift constantly from one point of view to another, and back again, and cannot reach decisions about even minor activities. Some patients are almost socially incapacitated by such obsessive doubting and indecisiveness.

Some obsessive patients ruminate about past actions. I recall a patient who for many years was obsessed with wondering if she forget to close the door of a toilet she used in a restaurant on a tourist trip to Florida. Another patient ruminated obsessively about whether or not 12 years before he had burned a letter he had started to write about an illicit love affair he had had; he spent several hours each day debating back and forth in his mind whether he had remembered to burn it. Another patient was obsessed for years with whether or not she had washed a key in her mother's house before using it to unlock a closet, and whether she might in this way have caught a disease from her mother.

The anxiety of the obsessive patient often is increased by the superstitious awe he has of his own thoughts. He frequently dreads that in some magical way his thoughts have power to make their contents come true. For example the patient with an obsessive fear that a particular member of his family will die often fears that in some magical way his thought will bring about the death of that person. Such feelings about the magical powers of obsessive thoughts are especially strong in obsessive children, but they also occur in many adult obsessional patients.

Patients with mild obsessions may accept them as "worries" and consider themselves merely to be very "worrisome" people. However, patients with severe obsessions frequently are profoundly disturbed by them. They often are in continual discomfort and feel that such unjustified but persistent thoughts must be signs of imminent "insanity." Often they fear to talk about their obsessions to physicians or others for fear they will be dismissed as hopelessly insane.

Compulsive Neuroses

A compulsion is a strong urge to perform a physical act to relieve tension. The performance of the act relieves the person of anxiety he felt prior to the act. Typical compulsions are repetitive washings of the hands, repetitive movements of the arms and hands, touching various objects specific numbers of times, and many other similar acts. We can grasp better the feelings of the compulsive person if we consider the minor compulsions of many normal people. For example, many people feel a strong urge to knock on wood after they speak about the recent absence of misfortune in their lives. They may treat the matter as a joke, but they feel more comfortable if they carry out this small compulsive act. Other persons do not engage in certain activities unless they first touch a particular good luck charm or carry out some special act. If they do not carry out these acts they feel anxious. The compulsive patient differs in that he feels overwhelming anxiety if he does not perform his compulsive acts. Moreover, his compulsive acts are numerous throughout the day, and some compulsive patients are ridden by compulsive urges in virtually every area of their lives.

Compulsive problems may vary from mild annoyances to incapacitating systems of acts that are present all day long. I recall a 52-year-old woman who had a severe compulsive neurosis of eight months' duration. She washed her hands and arms for two to three hours each morning to clean herself of "germs and dirt," and she then washed each item in her bathroom with an antiseptic. She then went through an elaborate two-hour ritual in dressing, which was designed to avoid contamination with dirt and germs, and this was followed by more washing of her arms and hands, which were chronically red and rough from excessive washing. Similar rituals occupied her entire day, and frequently she was awake until the small hours of the morning cleaning her bathroom and bedroom.

Compulsions frequently take the form of repetitive acts that must be carried out a specific number of times. I recall a 46-year-old woman who had a compulsive need to say, "Thank you, doctor; you're a fine doctor" three times at the end of every office interview. She then shook hands three times with my receptionist and thanked her three times before leaving the office. After that she shook hands three times with each of the five elevator operators in the office building in which my office was located, and similarly shook hands with the elevator dispatcher. After leaving the building she often was overcome by doubts that she had carried out all these actions and she returned later to shake hands with the receptionist and the elevator attendants three times more. Her entire day was occupied by such routines both at home and whenever she went outside her house.

Bedtime rituals are common in compulsive patients. I recall a 27-year-old man who had to close the cabinet door in his bathroom in such a way that the last thing he saw in the cabinet was the letter "C" on the label of his toothpaste tube. He then arranged his shoes and bedroom slippers in such a way that their toes were lined up on a particular crack in the bedroom floor. He then got in and out of bed two times, rolled over and back in bed two times and then felt relaxed enough to sleep. In sexual intercourse he penetrated and withdrew three times before proceding with the sex act.

Some compulsive patients feel a necessity to count each step of every stairs they climb and must descend the stairs and recount the steps if they lose count. Some compulsive patients have rituals they must follow in passing through a door or in entering and leaving a house. The distinguished 18th Century English literary figure Samuel Johnson had a severe compulsive neurosis from which he suffered most of his adult life. Boswell's *Life of Johnson* contains classical descriptions of Johnson's compulsions. For example, Boswell records that Johnson had

> . . . an anxious care to go out or in at a door or passage by a certain number of steps from a certain point, or at least so as that either his right or left foot (I am not sure which) should constantly make the first actual movement when he came to the door or passage . . . I have, upon innumerable occasions, observed him suddenly stop, and then seem to count his steps with a deep earnestness; and when he had neglected or gone wrong in this sort of magical movement, I have seen him go back again, put himself in a proper posture to begin the ceremony, and having gone through it, break from his abstraction, walk briskly on, and join his companion.

Boswell also describes Johnson's other counting rituals, his compulsive gestures and mannerisms, and his compulsive mutterings of slogans and word formulas. Boswell's descriptions are given with an acumen that rivals the most accurate clinical descriptions.

Obsessive fears usually lie behind compulsions, forming the classical obsessive compulsive disorder. For example, the patient with compulsive hand washing and cleaning rituals usually has obsesive dreads of diseases which he fears he will get from the "germs" and dirt of unclean objects. The person with counting compulsions and elaborate rituals of repetitive actions usually fears that severe illness, death or some other calamity will overtake him if he does not carry out these compulsions to ward off such misfortunes. The patient with bedtime rituals usually fears that unless he goes through his routines he will not be able to go to sleep, and that chronic insomnia will cause physical or mental deterioration leading to severe illness. However, when a patient has had compulsions for many months or years, he may carry them out without conscious awareness of the obsessive fears that originally accompanied them; on initial clinical examination, it may appear that the patient's compulsions are not associated with obsessive ideas. However, when the early stages of the compulsive disorder can be recollected, or when the patient carefully searches his feelings and thoughts in relation to his compulsions, the original obsessive thoughts that accompanied the compulsions usually can be elicited. In compulsive disorders of a few weeks' or a few months' duration, the obsessive ideas usually are clearly linked to the compulsions.

A further feature of the patient with a compulsive neurosis is his return to a kind of primitive, magical thinking characteristic of early childhood. Though he has difficulty explaining it or putting it into words, he feels that his compulsive actions and routines have a type of magical power to avert calamities and to rid him of guilty and anxious feelings. He attaches much significance to the power of words, and they acquire for him the magical ability to ward off misfortunes. The compulsive patient often has sayings or word slogans that he repeats many times during the day in his chronic battle against impending disasters. I recall a patient who muttered under his breath dozens of times each day, "May it not be so" whenever he spoke of anything undesirable or heard anyone refer to misfortune or illness. Boswell in his *Life of Johnson* records that Johnson in his severe compulsive neurosis muttered to himself dozens of times each day, "Lead us not into temptation." Psychiatric theory holds that in his neurosis the compulsive patient returns to early childhood forms of thinking in which symbolic actions and words have magical powers to influence events and to rid the person of guilty and anxious feelings. However, the compulsive patient's anxiety and guilt are so great that the respite he gains by his compulsive acts is only momentary, and his compulsions must be repeated many times.

Obsessive and compulsive neuroses most commonly appear between middle adolescence and the early 40's, but they also occur in children, and they may appear for the first time in persons between the middle 40's and 60. It is rare for obsessive and compulsive neuroses to appear for the first time in patients over the age of 60.

INTERPERSONAL CAUSES OF OBSESSIVE AND COMPULSIVE NEUROSES

Interpersonal Causes of Obsessive Neuroses

Harry Stack Sullivan had a special interest in patients with obsessive neuroses, and his contributions to understanding them are of particular value. As he pointed out, the obsessive person is manipulating words and sentences in special ways to encapsulate and control anxiety. Instead of becoming aware of painful past and present interpersonal experiences, he is binding his anguish into words, which become symbols of those experiences. However, since the turbulence within him constantly threatens to break into his awareness, he must repeat the words and sentences endlessly, or think about them unceasingly. This obviously is a sick and only partially successful solution to the patient's problems, and it is achieved at the cost of the continual distress of the obsessive word formulas themselves. However, this distress is less than that which the patient would feel if he were to come to grips with the full brunt of his inner turmoil.

Thus, the person who is struggling with hostile feelings and urges which he cannot consciously face may find these angry feelings rising to the surface in the form of word formulas and repetitive thoughts concerning violence and death, either to himself or others. Guilt over masturbation or unacceptable sexual acts may become encapsulated in obsessive preoccupations with words representing filth, such as "dirt" and "germs." A patient with guilty feelings over unresolved conflicts with a parent or a sibling who died suddenly of heart disease may ruminate endlessly about "heart attack" and "death."

Words by their very nature lend themselves to the type of substitutive process that occurs in an obsessive neurosis, since words are merely symbols of other things. Thus, c-a-t is not a cat; it is a three-letter word, or a monosyllabic sound, which is a symbol for a furry domestic animal. However, once we agree that the word "cat" is a spoken and written symbol for the furry domestic animal, we can manipulate this symbol easily. We can talk about cats in both real and unreal ways; for example, we can talk about the real cat on the rug in the family room, or we can talk about the unreal, magical Chesshire cat in *Alice In Wonderland* which could disappear at will and leave only its smiling teeth visible.

Basically, the patient with an obsessive neurosis is doing the same thing with words; he has simply gone one step further. He has invested certain words, word-thoughts and repetitive word-phrases with the capacity to encapsulate anxiety. Looking at it from a slightly different point of view, he is using certain words and thoughts (thoughts, for the obsessive person, are merely set sequences of words) as symbols in which he binds and camouflages painful past and present interpersonal experiences which he cannot face consciously.

In addition, as noted above, the obsessional patient has given to words the magical qualities that words have for small children. During the first several years of life a child fails at first to recognize that the word-symbol and the real object are not the same thing, or that they are not closely linked. He feels that the word c-a-t and the furry domestic animal are the same thing, or nearly so. He also feels that by uttering the word and thinking about it he can manipulate the furry animal in much the same way that he could if he picked it up and carried it about. Thus, he invests words and the word-sequences of sentences with attributes we consider magical. The obsessional patient has either retained this feeling about words, or has returned to it, in his efforts to control anxiety by encapsulating painful interpersonal experiences in words and the word-sequences of sentences.

This process has various consequences for the patient with an obsessive neurosis. His emotional life becomes shifted away from people and close interpersonal relationships; he lives in a formal, cold, mechanical world in which words and word formulas, rather than interpersonal relationships, predominate.

Sullivan felt that in almost all instances the patient with an obsessive neurosis had during childhood and early adolescence a prolonged, brutal, cruel relationship with a close person, often a parent. However, the person who treated the patient with cruelty hid behind a mask of apparent affection and consideration for him. The child dimly perceived, but was baffled by, this relationship which traumatized him but was disguised as helpful to him. For example, the parent brutally rejected the child emotionally but told him that he was teaching him to be self-reliant and independent. Thus, the parent was, in a sense, teaching the child to use words as symbols for encapsulating and camouflaging painful experiences; this is, of course, what the patient later does in his obsessive neurosis.

The obsessive compulsive patient, Sullivan felt, has never had the experience of intimate, comfortable success in an interpersonal relationship, and, as a poor, second-best way of life, has fled into a world of words, word-sequences and slogans. He has substituted word formulas for interpersonal closeness. This process, having been stamped on him in childhood, persists into adulthood. Underneath this, however, the obsessive patient has low self-esteem and lives in constant dread of being revealed as the degenerate, worthless person he fears he is. He is, through his obsessive symptoms, unceasingly trying to ward off feelings of shame and guilt and to remove threats of anxiety from significant, close people. This basic process explains many aspects of obsessive neuroses; for example, obsessive doubting (did I turn off all the gas jets and water faucets, or didn't I?) keeps the patient so mentally and physically busy that he can avoid the challenges and opportunities of interpersonal life, which he finds threatening and anxiety-provoking.

The ways in which these processes and their causative interpersonal traumas can produce an obsessive neurosis are demonstrated in the case of a 33-year-old man whom I saw for obsessive fears of heart disease and death. He had severe obsessive ruminations that he would die suddenly of a heart attack, and these fears plagued him most of the time. He carefully arranged his daily activities to avoid "strain" of any kind. He never climbed even small flights of stairs, he did not engage in any kind of strenuous physical exertion, and he walked at a studiously slow pace. Repeated examinations by several cardiologists indicated that he did not have heart disease, but these reassurances did not affect his obsessive fears.

The patient's father was a demanding, hostile man and his relationship with the patient was always tense. The patient's mother was a withdrawn person who gave the patient little affection, and throughout his formative years the patient did not have a close, reassuring interpersonal relationship with anyone. The conflicts between the patient and his father became more intense in the patient's late adolescence when the patient became openly rebellious to his father. At times the patient had death wishes toward his father and he speculated that everyone in the family would be happier if the father were dead. When the patient was 19, and his conflict with his father was still open and bitter, the father died suddenly of a coronary thrombosis without previous evidence of heart disease. The patient was very upset and felt immensely guilty about his father's death, and at that time went through a mild depression for about one year, but he recovered without psychiatric help.

The patient was a tense, hard working man who in early adulthood became quite successful in business. However, he was unable to form close interpersonal relationships, and held people off by a glib talkativeness which disguised the feelings of anxiousness that any opportunity for interpersonal intimacy aroused in him. He also had underlying feelings of inadequacy which spurred him constantly to prove to himself and others by social and economic achievement that he was not the inferior, degenerate person that his childhood experiences led him to fear he was.

Despite his personality difficulties the patient had no further psychiatric disturbances until he was 33. At that time he began to have marked conflicts with his business partner, a man in his early 60's. These conflicts centered around details of the financial transactions by which the patient gradually was buying a controlling interest in the partnership. In the context of his conflict with his business partner, who in many ways was a father figure substitute to the patient, the patient abruptly developed the severe obsession that he suddenly would have a heart attack and die. He first came to see me eight months later, after the repeated reassurances from cardiologists failed to help him.

In twice weekly interview sessions over a 10-month period, we analyzed how he basically was afraid that he would die as his father died, and that his obsessive fear of his own death was a substitute for lingering, unconscious guilt feelings over the death of his father. We spent much time working through his anger, guilt and terror in his relationship with his father, and how his yearnings for closeness had been rebuffed by his mother. We traced how these old conflicts had been rekindled by his current conflicts with his business partner, who was a father figure to him. We analyzed how these conflicts had led to his obsessive fears of death by heart disease. We also traced how his relationships with both parents during his formative years had led him to remain aloof from close involvement with people, and had caused him to substitute verbal glibness for warm, meaningful communication. His fears of personal inadequacy and his attempts to quell them by socioeconomic success were explored. He recovered from his obsessive disorder. Six years later he returned because of a mild recurrence of his obsession which occurred four months after his partner's death in an automobile accident. However, this recurrence was brief and his obsession disappeared after six interview sessions. I met him socially three years after that and he indicated he was doing well.

The interpersonal causes of obsessive neuroses are well illustrated in the syndrome of simultaneous obsessions of infanticide and insanity, a common type of obsessive neurosis in young mothers. These patients, usually between the ages of 20 and 40, have severe obsessive fears that they will murder their children, and they feel that the occurrence of such thoughts must mean they are on the verge of insanity. Many of these young mothers are passive persons who keep all their anger pent up within themselves. They feel guilty if they become angry or assertive in any way. This pattern of passivity, and the feelings of worthlessness and inadequacy that accompany it, usually arose in the patient's early relationship with one or both parents who made her feel guilty and inferior whenever she was assertive in any manner. As a mother, this patient is usually too passive to be able to be firm and decisive with her children, and her relationship with them deteriorates into a chronic, frustrating tug of war. The patient's impotent anger in her attempts to deal with her children is added to the simmering mass of repressed anger of many years' duration. The patient is flooded with terror as she feels (in ways she cannot clearly express or become aware of) that her repressed fury may break its bonds and erupt in chaotically hostile behavior. She fears it may emerge in the most horrid type of hostile expressiveness, the murder of her children. Her inner turmoil becomes encapsulated, and finds limited expression, in her painful obsessive thoughts, which are substitutes for feelings of hostility in past and current interpersonal relationships. As a rule, this type of patient does well in interview therapy, which helps her gain insight into the origins of the obsessions and also enables her to develop the capacity for comfortable, reasonable expression of her assertive feelings.

Many other kinds of past and present interpersonal traumas can contribute to the production of obsessive neuroses. The life experiences of each patient must be searched to find the particular constellations of interpersonally damaging experiences which have led to his neurosis.

Interpersonal Causes of Compulsive Neuroses

Compulsions are caused by the emotional turmoil of past and current interpersonal stresses which flood the patient with severe anxiety and guilt; his compulsive actions and rituals are attempts to subdue this anxiety and guilt by repetitive physical actions. The interpersonal causes and emotional processes in compulsive neuroses are quite similar to those of obsessive neuroses. The difference between obsessions and compulsions is that in obsessions the patient's turmoil finds unhealthy release in repetitive ideas, whereas in compulsions it is expressed in a strong need to perform repetitive physical acts. In obsessions the patient encapsulates his emotional distress in words and word-sequences, which have awesome, symbolic significances for him; the compulsive patient does the same thing with physical actions in his efforts to control anxiety and guilt.

The guilt and anxiety that underlie a compulsive neurosis usually arise from both childhood and adult experiences. For example, guilt over masturbation in an adolescent or young adult may reawaken emotional conflicts from childhood and produce a compulsive neurosis. I recall a 22-year-old patient whose compulsive symptoms were precipitated by her marked guilt feelings after masturbation. She feared that in masturbating she had slightly soiled her pajamas and she washed them repeatedly. She then feared she had soiled her hands in the process of washing the pajamas and began to wash her hands compulsively several times each day. Her cleansing compulsions spread to various articles in her bathroom, and over a several-week period she developed a severe compulsive neurosis with many cleansing rituals, which occupied three or four hours each day. After several months she no longer was aware of the original connection of her cleansing routines with guilt over masturbation; she mechanically carried on her cleansing compulsions in an endless, anxious quest to free herself from contamination and guilt.

However, guilt over masturbation was only an immediate precipitant that reawakened old conflicts from this patient's childhood. Because of her parents' personality problems and their absorption in their marital difficulties, she never had a truly secure relationship with anyone throughout her formative years; she became a bookish, hard working girl who fled into reading and her studies to avoid the pain of her childhood home. She was subjected to much sexual trauma in childhood; many times she heard her parents late at night arguing bitterly and crudely over sexual intercourse. During childhood and puberty the patient many times heard her parents having sexual intercourse and she became sexually excited while listening to them. She felt very anxious and guilty about her sexual excitement at these times. The patient's mother was a disturbed woman who warned the patient from the age of five years onward that the father was an immoral man and that the patient should report immediately to the mother if the father ever made sexual advances to her. Because of all this sexual trauma in childhood and puberty, the patient's feelings toward men and sexuality in her adolescence and young adulthood were a chaotic mixture of terror, fascination, hostility and sensuous arousal. Sexuality produced much guilt and anxiety in her, and in this context her masturbatory activities precipitated her compulsive neurosis.

In other instances, hostile impulses, and guilt and anxiety related to them, lie at the root of a compuslive neurosis. I recall a 27-year-old married man with a compulsive disorder of four years' duration. He carefully counted his steps most of the time, had rituals in dressing and undressing, had bedtime rituals, and he muttered repetitive sentences at specific intervals many times during the day. The patient had been reared by a harsh, domineering father who criticized him endlessly and by a passive, whining mother who chronically complained to the patient about her mistreatment by the father. The patient was reared in the drizzle of his mother's tears and the blast of his father's anger. Throughout childhood and adolescence the patient was a quiet, timid boy who suppressed all angry feelings behind a cowed façade. However, in middle adolescence his suppressed rage broke into a defiant rebellion which took the form of delinquent acts, including robbery, which kept his father in agony for several years. The rebellion of the patient persisted until he was about 21, when he gradually retired back into the passive, conforming behavior that had characterized his childhood, and again he began to repress his hostility. His father once more dominated him with harsh criticism. At the age of 23 the patient abruptly developed a severe compulsive neurosis. His dammed up fury and resentment, which formerly had found release in adolescent rebellion and delinquency, now found expression in his compulsions.

Psychiatric theory suggests that there is usually a symbolic relationship between the compulsive symptom and the emotional forces finding unhealthy expression in it. Thus, the patient with a repetitive compulsion to wash his hands is struggling with feelings of moral dirtiness, unworthiness and guilt. The person who feels that he aggressively must stamp on each crack in the sidewalk as he walks along is expressing pent-up hostile impulses with which he cannot come to grips consciously. Compulsions to touch and handle parts of one's own body or the bodies of others are felt to be the expressions of sexual impulses that have been repressed and are finding devious release in these symptoms. The patient who must count his steps carefully or organize all his activities in meticulous, stylized routines has deep fears that he will lose control of his actions, and he must keep rigid count and control of his every step and movement to prevent his behavior from deteriorating into disorganized chaos. The patient, of course, knows little of his basic conflicts and feelings; he only feels an urgency to carry out the physical acts through which his unconscious conflicts are finding a partial, distorted expression.

Psychiatrists who adhere to the Freudian-psychoanalytic point of view believe that the roots of many compulsive neuroses begin in the toilet training period during the second and third years of life. They feel that a hostile struggle occurred between the mother and the child during toilet training, and that bowel functioning, cleanliness and meticulous order become anxious preoccupations in the child. They feel that much of the anxiety and guilt of the compulsive patient first arise in his hostile tug of war with his mother at this time, and that compulsive symptoms that deal with dirt, cleanliness and counting things are derived from aspects of traumatic toilet training. In my opinion, harsh, hostile toilet training periods sometimes play a part in the etiology of some compulsive neuroses; however, in such instances the hostile mother-child struggle over toilet training is merely one part of a generally harsh relationship between the mother (and often the father too) and the child.

Patients with compulsive neuroses often have characteristic personality features. They tend to be meticulous, conscientious and tenacious. Their relationships with others usually are mechanical and cold. They understand duty and responsibility as interpersonal bonds much better than they comprehend warmth and affection. They often are frugal collectors and accumulators of things, and they have strong needs for orderliness and cleanliness. Mildly compulsive persons sometimes are good organizers and prodigious workers, though they seldom have warm bonds with those around them.

Compulsive persons tend to have these kinds of personality difficulties because words, word-formulas and specific kinds of physical behavior have taken the places of relationships with people in their emotional life. The compulsive person's verbal operations are not truly communicative; the form is present, but not the emotional content. The compulsive person says "I love you" because the situation requires these words, not because he feels anything intense toward the person to whom he says them. He seems to communicate, but does not; as Sullivan says, he "miscommunicates, misinforms and misdirects." Constant, meticulous industriousness enables the obsessive compulsive individual to keep busy with words and things, and to avoid closeness with people. Compulsive persons sometimes have a glib facility with words, unaccompanied by the feelings usually associated with them, and this quality may make them successful in some business and professional fields. The glib, efficient salesman who never becomes truly friendly with either his customers or his colleagues, the persuasive executive whom none of his associates really knows well, and the charming professional person who moves from client to client without ever forming a sound relationship with any of them—are examples of the mildly compulsive person whose personality defects have been harnessed in socioeconomic ways. All these persons can function only in superficial relationships; relationships which become intense soon become stressful, and the person flees from them back to work or isolation.

The above comments refer mainly to persons with mild compulsive personality structures. Individuals with moderate or severe compulsive personality problems often become so embroiled with the minute details of their activities that they have much trouble in getting large tasks done; they become mired in swamps of small, uncoordinated fragments of uncompleted tasks and projects. (More material on the characteristics of the compulsive personality pattern that often exists in a patient with an obsessive compulsive neurosis is given in Chapter 12 on personality disorders.)

CLINICAL COURSE OF OBSESSIVE AND COMPULSIVE NEUROSES

Course of Obsessive Neuroses

Minor or moderate obsessions not accompanied by compulsions often spontaneously disappear in time, especially if they occur during a period of obvious interpersonal stress in the patient's life. However, when an obsessive neurosis of moderate severity undergoes spontaneous remission, the patient is prone to develop other obsessive ideas if he later experiences marked emotional tension. However, the patient with an obsession of minor or moderate degree usually resolves his neurosis more quickly if he receives psychotherapy and thus solves some of the emotional problems that caused his obsessive disorder. When the patient's obsessive neurosis is severe, the chance of spontaneous disappearance of his symptoms is much less likely. Some obsessive neuroses, even when not accompanied by compulsive symptoms, often last for years or decades, though they usually fluctuate much in intensity; their response to interview treatment often is disappointing, especially when they were present for many months or years before treatment started.

The obsessive neuroses of children, regardless of their severity, almost invariably disappear in time; they rarely extend beyond puberty. However, if the child's emotional problems and interpersonal stresses remain unresolved, he is prone to develop new obsessive symptoms or other neurotic difficulties in adolescence or adult life. Hence, children with obsessive neuroses should have psychiatric child guidance treatment, if possible.

Course of Compulsive Neuroses

The prognosis of a patient with a compulsive neurosis, or with a combination of obsessive and compulsive features to form the classical obsessive compulsive picture, is much more guarded than when the patient has obsessions alone. Compulsive neuroses often persist for years or decades. They sometimes begin in adolescence or early adulthood and last during the patient's entire life. However, they undergo wide fluctuations in degree, varying much from month to month and from year to year. However, in clinical practice one sees some exceptions to this general tendency. I have seen severe, incapacitating compulsive neuroses erupt for the first time in early adulthood or in middle age, last for several months and then disappear entirely. In other compulsive patients most of the compulsive symptoms resolve spontaneously in time, but a small residual of the symptoms persists for months or years afterwards. Prompt psychotherapy improves the chance of a favorable result.

The results of psychotherapy of acute compulsive neuroses that have been present from a few weeks to a few months are good in some cases, and the patient may be largely or entirely relieved of his neurosis. However, a psychiatrist usually sees compulsive neuroses after they have been present for many months or several years, and the prognosis of such entrenched compulsive neuroses is poor even with prolonged psychotherapy. Nevertheless, such patients may benefit to a certain extent from psychotherapy, but their symptoms rarely undergo more than a 50 per cent improvement.

Depressions and periods of marked anxiety are common in patients with chronic obsessive compulsive neuroses. These depressive and anxious periods often respond well to psychotherapy, sometimes with accompanying antidepressant or antianxiety medications, even when the basic obsessive compulsive symptoms are little changed by the treatment. In many instances, the chronic obsessive compulsive patient comes periodically for a few weeks or a few months of psychiatric treatment when depressive or anxious problems arise or when his chronic obsessive compulsive problems become temporarily more severe than usual. He benefits from such help, but does not persist in treatment when his exacerbation subsides.

The vast majority of obsessive compulsive patients never become psychotic, although many of them chronically fear they are on the verge of "violent insanity." In general, these patients get significant relief from repeated, strong reassurances that their likelihood of psychotic development is very small. Some psychiatrists believe that obsessive compulsive patients have an increased chance of becoming schizophrenic, but I do not believe this is so. In my experience, the chance of an obsessive compulsive patient becoming schizophrenic is no greater than that of a person in the general population. Obsessive compulsive patients have a higher chance of developing moderate depressions, but these depressive episodes usually respond well to psychotherapy, often supplemented by antidepressant medication.

It should be pointed out, however, that a schizophrenic or a depressive patient occasionally has a brief flurry of obsessive or compulsive symptoms as he proceeds into his schizophrenic or depressive psychosis. For example, I recall a 55-year-old man who over a period of 30 years had five depressive psychoses. Each psychosis began with a two- or three-week period of obsessive worry over his bowel movements. Other patients develop obsessive fears of cancer, venereal disease or bizarre body infirmities as they proceed into depressive or schizophrenic illnesses. However, the vast majority of schizophrenic and depressive patients do not have compulsive or obsessive symptoms preceding their psychotic illnesses or at any time during them. (This point in the differential diagnosis of depressive and schizophrenic disorders is discussed further in Chapter 14 on schizophrenia and Chapter 15 on severe depressions.)

Compulsive neuroses in children may last from a few months to several years, but they usually disappear in time. However, if the underlying emotional turmoil of the child is unresolved, he may develop new compulsive symptoms or other neurotic disorders in adolescence or adulthood; hence, the child with a compulsive neurosis should have psychiatric help whenever possible.

TREATMENT OF OBSESSIVE AND COMPULSIVE NEUROSES

Obsessive Neuroses

Obsessive neuroses unaccompanied by compulsive symptoms often respond well to psychotherapy. The interview treatment seeks to explore and resolve the emotional stresses arising from the patient's unhealthy past and current interpersonal relationships that have led to the obsessive neurosis. (The principles and technics of such interview treatment are discussed in Chapter 21. Illustrative examples of the general conduct of psychotherapy in neurotic disorders are given in Chapters 7 and 9.)

Suggestions for the family physician and internist in dealing with obsessive patients. The family physician or internist often can help resolve the minor obsessional fears of a patient who basically has a sound personality structure but who is under transient interpersonal stress. This is particularly true of obsessive fears of illnesses such as heart disease, stroke, cancer and others. Minor obsessive fears of this sort are commonly seen in medical practice, and firm reassurance and explanation by the family physician frequently helps to resolve them. Physicians often underestimate the value of early, firm reassurance in such instances. Sometimes the family physician or internist also can discuss a few recent interpersonal stresses in the patient's life and point out their relevance to the patient's obsessive fear. For example, minor obsessive fears of heart disease sometimes are precipitated by the sudden death by cardiac illness of one of the patient's relatives or work associates.

The family physician occasionally can help patients with other minor obsessive fears besides those of disease, but all patients with moderate or severe obsessive problems should be referred for psychiatric interview help whenever possible. Mild antianxiety medication is sometimes useful in patients with obsessive disorders of recent origin if they have much accompanying overt anxiety, but the patient should understand that past and current interpersonal stresses have caused his difficulty and that resolution of them is the main avenue of therapy.

Compulsive Neuroses

Compulsive neuroses that have been present more than a few months are very difficult to treat and even prolonged, skillful psychotherapy may give only limited relief. Medications are of little value unless the patient has marked anxiety or depression accompanying his compulsive neurosis; in such instances, antianxiety or antidepressant medication may be useful for the anxiety or depression, but they do not affect the main compulsive disorder.

The compulsive patient does poorly in psychotherapy for various reasons. He tends to approach psychotherapy in a cold, impersonal, mechanical way, with the attitude of a man who is discussing the mechanics of an electric gadget rather than the emotional difficulties of his own life. He is prone to talk with careful, meticulous glibness about his life, but he does not really become emotionally involved in examining his past and current life situations. He can discuss facts, but not feelings, and he maintains a frigid, obstinate reserve in his interpersonal relationship with the psychiatrist. The compulsive patient often develops an arid, impersonal, intellectual insight into his problems, but this does not help him much because he is not able to deal with his feelings and emotions.

Because he has never had a truly close, reassuring relationship with a significant person, and hence has substituted a vast array of word formulas and physical busyness for feelings and interpersonal intimacy, the severe obsessive compulsive patient often has a hard shell that is difficult to penetrate. Attempts to pierce this shell, whether in psychotherapy or in his daily life circumstances, tend to flood him with panic, and he resists all efforts to do so. Also, his glibness and adroitness with words often make therapy a smooth but emotionally empty process. He is so accustomed to using words as tools to ward off anxiety and guilt that he has much trouble employing them in emotionally meaningful communication in psychotherapy.

I have seen severe obsessive compulsive patients who had up to six years of Freudian psychoanalysis and other forms of psychotherapy without apparent benefit, and I have read of patients who had up to 12 years of psychotherapy without improvement. After extensive psychotherapy, many of these patients can talk with almost professional skill about the causes of their compulsive neuroses, but since they have divorced words so completely from feelings this insight does them little good. If a therapist adopts a too aggressive role in attempting to pierce the compulsive patient's defenses and make him confront the emotional turbulence which is camouflaged by his cold verbal fluency, the patient often becomes strongly anxious or depressed; in many cases he abruptly terminates treatment.

Hence, many psychiatrists question the wisdom and justifiability of continuing psychotherapy with a compulsive patient whose resistances to emotional involvement in it are marked. Each compulsive patient may be given a trial of treatment if he is motivated for it, but it is doubtful if long-continued treatment with minimal results is worthwhile and advisable. However, as pointed out earlier, the compulsive patient in psychotherapy often gets relief for periods of depressiveness or marked anxiety that may from time to time assail him, and he may get partial relief for some of his more distressing obsessive compulsive symptoms. The patient often discontinues treatment, or the therapist may terminate it, after these limited but useful goals are reached, and he may return periodically for further short episodes of interview help when he is depressed or particularly anxious, or is undergoing an exacerbation of his compulsive symptoms. (The material of Chapter 21 and the illustrative cases in Chapters 7 and 9 demonstrate the general psychotherapeutic approach in neuroses.)

BIBLIOGRAPHY

Adams, P. L.: Obsessive Children. New York, Brunner Mazel, 1973.

Barnett, J.: Therapeutic intervention in the dysfunctional thought processes of the obsessional. Am. J. Psychother., *26*:338, 1972.

Beach, H. R.: Ritualistic activity in obsessional patients. J. Psychosom. Res., *15*:417, 1971.

Binswanger, H.: Theoretical aspects of compulsive illnesses. Contemp. Psychoanal., *9*:83, 1972.

Goodwin, D. W., Guze, S. B., and Robins, E.: Follow-up studies in obsessional neurosis. Arch. Gen. Psychiatry, *20*:182, 1967.

Lesse, S.: Anxiety—its relationship to the development and amelioration of obsessive-com-

pulsive disorders. Am. J. Psychother., *26*:330, 1972.
Mills, H. L., Agras, W. S., Barlow, D. H., and Mills, J. R.: Compulsive rituals treated by response prevention. Arch. Gen. Psychiatry, *28*:524, 1973.
Schimel, J. L.: The power theme in the obsessional. Contemp. Psychoanal., *9*:1, 1972.
Sullivan, H. S.: Obsessionalism. *In* Clinical Studies in Psychiatry. New York, W. W. Norton, 1956.
Walker, V. J.: Explanation in obsessional neuroses. Brit. J. Psychiatry, *123*:675, 1973.

9

Hysterical Neuroses: Conversion and Dissociative Types

Two types of disorders are included under the general term *hysteria*. They are (1) *the conversion type of hysterical neurosis* and (2) *the dissociative type of hysterical neurosis*. In order to shorten these diagnostic phrases into more easily used terms we shall throughout this chapter refer to them as *conversion hysteria* and *dissociative hysteria*, or *conversion neurosis* and *dissociative neurosis*.

Conversion hysteria includes various kinds of emotionally caused disorders of movement, sensation and special sensory perception. These disorders are called conversion neuroses since it is felt that in them emotional forces have been *converted* into specific types of physical symptoms. Common types of conversion symptoms include hysterical paralyses, anesthesias and visual difficulties.

The dissociative neuroses are clinically related to the conversion neuroses and are characterized by disturbances of awareness and memory. They include such disorders as hysterical amnesias and stupors.

CLINICAL CHARACTERISTICS OF CONVERSION HYSTERIA

Conversion hysteria may produce many kinds of symptoms, which characteristically occur in the muscular, sensory and special sensory systems. The family physician and the internist, as well as the psychiatrist, often encounter small conversion symptoms such as minor conversion pains and muscular weaknesses. The major conversion symptoms such as extensive paralyses and anesthesias occur less frequently, but are occasionally seen in various fields of medical practice.

Conversion symptoms occur in the muscular groups under voluntary control and in those sensory systems whose interpretation is under conscious surveillance. For example, hysterical paralysis or rigidity can occur in the leg, a part of the body under conscious control. However, conversion symptoms cannot occur in intestinal musculature, because it is not subject to the patient's conscious control. Conversion anesthesia can occur in the arm or conversion blindness in the eye, because both of these sensations are subject to conscious interpretation. However, types of sensation such as autonomic or kinesthetic sensation, which are not subject to precise conscious interpretation, are relatively free of conversion symptoms. For example, a patient may have a hysterical pain in an area of the abdominal wall, but he cannot have hysterical pain in his small intestines.

The patient who develops a hysterical symptom, although his disorder is caused by unconscious emotional forces over which he has little control, is influenced by his conscious knowledge of the body in determining his particular type of symptom. Thus, a conversion paralysis of the hand involves those muscles and movements that the patient considers the functioning elements of his hand. Such a paralysis of the hand does not involve combinations of muscular weakness that would occur in a neurologically caused paralysis of the hand. Similarly, a conversion anesthesia of the hand usually stops abruptly at the wrist, covering what the patient considers to be his hand, rather than covering areas that would be involved in an anesthesia caused by nerve injury. This feature of conversion hysteria, coupled with the fact that it is more common in poorly informed or emotionally immature persons, often gives the hysterical symptom a striking quality which leads the casual observer to suspect malingering. Such an injustice should not be done to the hysterical patient. Conversion disorders occur in both sexes. In my experience, the old concept that they are more common in women is probably not justified. Conversion hysterical symptoms occur most commonly between middle adolescence and the middle forties, though they also occur in patients older than that and are occasionally seen in children.

Conversion neuroses should be clearly distinguished from psychosomatic (psychophysiologic) illnesses. In a conversion neurosis the patient has a physical dysfunction caused by emotional factors, but he does not have an organic lesion. For example, a patient with a hysterical paralysis of the leg does not have an organic lesion in his leg; he has an emotionally caused inability to move his leg. On the other hand, the patient with a psychosomatic illness has true organic pathology produced by emotional forces. For example, a duodenal ulcer is an organic lesion produced by emotional turmoil. Common psychosomatic illnesses are peptic ulcers, emotionally caused colitis states, some cases of urticaria, some cases of asthma, and others. (The psychosomatic illnesses are covered in Chapter 11.)

Conversion Symptoms in Muscles

Conversion paralyses may involve one arm or one leg, both arms or both legs, both limbs on one side of the body or all four limbs. The paralyses may be flaccid or rigid, and they may be complete or partial in any particular area. The paralysis follows what the patient considers to be an anatomical unit; for example, the paralysis of an arm or leg follows the skin distribution of the layman's concept of an arm or leg and not the distribution of neurological and muscular components of a limb. The gait of the patient with hysterical paralysis is bizarre and often varies from one hour to the next. He characteristically leans on the wall, and when he loses his balance and falls he rarely bruises himself and often falls into the receptive arms of a hospital attendant or a relative.

The differentiation of a hysterical paralysis from a neurologically caused paralysis usually offers few problems. The deep tendon reflexes are not lost in flaccid paralysis, and they often are dramatically exaggerated in rigid paralysis. Clonus is not present, and the Babinski and other neurological signs are normal. Hospitalized patients can be observed to move normally in their sleep, or they can be stimulated to move normally after profound drowsiness is induced by the intravenous injection of amobarbital (Amytal) and mild painful stimuli are applied to the arm or leg. Some patients can move a group of affected muscles in one type of movement, but not in another. For example, in getting on and off a bedpan the patient often uses muscles otherwise inactivated by the hysterical paralysis. Hysterically paralyzed muscles do not atrophy and the patients do not get bedsores.

Conversion seizures consist of bizarre sequences of movements and contortions bearing little resemblance to the tonic and clonic movements of grand mal convulsions. Conversion seizures may last from a minute or so to an hour or two. A hysterical seizure often consists of rigidity of the entire body, with clenched fists and tightly closed or blankly staring eyes. The patient may remain conscious during the seizure, or he may have amnesia for what occurred during it. During a hysterical seizure the patient does not bite his tongue, urinate or defecate, as may happen in organic seizures. Fainting episodes, often called "black-out spells" by the patient, are a common form of hysterical seizure. The patient collapses limply to the ground or onto a chair and remains unresponsive for from a few seconds to a couple of hours, while the vital signs and all aspects of the physical examination are normal. Aimless thrashing of the arms and fluttering of the eyelids are common in such fainting spells. Hysterical seizures characteristically occur only when other people are present. I recall a 17-year-old girl whose many fainting spells occurred only when her solicitous, handsome, 20-year-old boy friend was present.

Hysterical tremors consist of fine or gross shakings of the arms, legs or head, which on careful scrutiny bear little resemblance to the tremors of basal ganglia disease or other types of neurological illness. They vary immensely in amplitude from time to time; on some occasions the hysterical tremor may be scarcely noticeable, and at other times it is very prominent. They often are absent when the patient is alone or feels he is not being observed, and they are marked when he is being medically examined. I recall a patient whose hysterical tremor was scarcely noticeable while she was alone in my waiting room. The tremor was marked when I examined her and it was much more prominent when she appeared in Workmen's Compensation Court at the time of her compensation hearing. The opposition lawyers thought she was malingering, but her tremor continued for two years after her compensation was settled.

Minor conversion symptoms of muscles are common. They include weaknesses and limitations of movement of small muscle groups. The familiar writer's cramp is generally considered to be a minor conversion symptom, since the muscles that cannot comfortably be used to write can be used for other types of activities. Hysterical aphonia is common. The patient with hysterical aphonia may be mute or he may talk only in whispers and complain of a "weak voice." Visualization of the laryngeal cords in conversion aphonia reveals them to be normal in configuration and movement.

Conversion Sensory Symptoms

Conversion sensory symptoms include anesthesias, paresthesias and hysterical pain. Major hysterical anesthesias as a rule are easily diagnosed, since they follow skin surface concepts of body divisions rather than neurological patterns of sensation. For example, a hysterical anesthesia of the hand usually stops abruptly at the wrist, forming a glovelike pattern of sensory loss; it does not follow a pattern of neurological innervation. A hysterical hemianesthesia stops abruptly at the midline and covers the head, body and both limbs on the affected side.

Hysterical pain, conversion paresthesias and vague sensory discomforts described by patients as "numbness" are often seen clinically. These difficulties often are vague in location, and may shift in position from one day to the next. However, they may have precise locations, such as the commonly encountered burning or "numb" areas on the top of the head or the continuous severe pains in the coccygeal region. Hysterical paresthesias are described as feelings of "pins and needles" in the affected area. Paresthesias often present difficult diagnostic problems, since they may also be produced by neurological and vascular dysfunctions, which sometimes follow erratic patterns of distribution.

Conversion hysterical pain may be sharp, burning, aching or dull, and it tends to be continuous. Pain described as being of uniform intensity without cessation or fluctuation over periods of weeks or months is highly suspect of being hysterical. Virtually all organically caused pain is fluctuating and usually has at least brief periods of remission. The patient with hysterical pain often describes it as being excruciating and continual, but he does not appear to be in distress. The patient often states that the pain is present night and day, but his relatives say that he sleeps well. Conversion pain often is uninfluenced by narcotics and analgesics. However, frequent exceptions to these general rules occur, and hysterical pain sometimes fluctuates and may diminish temporarily in response to medication.

Hysterical pain is at times one of the most difficult diagnostic problems in clinical medicine. Hysterical pain syndromes in the lower abdominal region, the low back, the rectum and the pelvic area are particularly treacherous. Much diagnostic skill and caution often are required to avoid unnecessary surgical operations or prolonged treatment for nonexistent physical diseases.

Conversion Symptoms of Special Sensory Perception

Conversion problems of sight and hearing are encountered occasionally in clinical practice. Visual difficulties are by far the more common of the two, but hysterical deafness is seen at times. Hysterical deafness may occur at any time from childhood to old age. The diagnosis of hysterical deafness requires the use of special audiologic equipment by an experienced otolaryngologist.

Conversion visual disturbances may take the forms of blindness, constricted visual fields, cloudy vision, "spots in front of my eyes" and distortions of objects into larger or smaller dimensions than their actual sizes. A common hysterical visual symptom is constriction of the visual fields peripherally into "gun-barrel vision," or "tunnel vision." Monocular diplopia, in which the patient sees double images out of one eye with the other eye closed, usually is hysterical, but not invariably so. Binocular diplopia usually is not hysterical. In hysterical blindness the patient often describes his blindness as a "white blur" though at other times he may describe his vision as black or darkly clouded. Hysterical blindness may be monocular or binocular. Hysterical hallucinations may occur in suggestible, immature persons, or in individuals who do not have significant basic personality problems but are under great stress; such hallucinations tend to be gratifying and reassuring (as when they deal with religious themes) rather than frightening. Visual disturbances, like many hysterical symptoms, often appear suddenly in full-blown form and may disappear and reappear with equal abruptness.

Some General Clinical Features of Conversion Hysteria

A common characteristic of the patient with a conversion disorder is his apparent lack of concern about his dysfunction. His distress over his symptoms is much less than in patients with similar dysfunctions caused by organic diseases. For example, the patient with hysterical blindness often is remarkably unconcerned about a catastrophic incapacitation such as sudden, total blindness, and the patient with a conversion hemiplegia takes his trouble with unusual calmness. I recall a 24-year-old married woman with a complete hysterical paralysis of both legs of four days' duration; she was girlishly jovial and stated that she was sure she would be well enough in 10 days to leave the hospital and attend her cousin's wedding; she did. The hysterical patient's lack of concern about his symptoms is called his "bland indifference," or, in the older literature, his "belle indifférence." However, "bland indifference" sometimes is not present, especially in patients with multiple minor hysterical symptoms, and the patient may express much concern and agitation about them.

Hysterical symptoms sometimes are superimposed on organic diseases. For example, hysterical pain may be superimposed on orthopedic problems of the low back or on disorders of the pelvic and perineal regions. Such hysterical overlays occur in patients who are emotionally predisposed to develop hysterical symptoms and who have organic disorders that become the nuclei to which hysterical symptoms become attached. Such patients may present very difficult diagnostic and treatment problems, and their care requires the utmost clinical acumen.

A hysterical symptom sometimes is difficult to remove because it enables the patient to sink into a semi-invalid or invalid role in which he avoids interpersonal stresses. Thus, a passive, shy woman unconsciously may find that hysterical pain in the abdomen or low back enables her to become a housebound, chronic semi-invalid, and she thus avoids venturing into social situations in which she is uncomfortable. A worker who is injured on the job may develop a persistent hysterical overlay on top of his original injury; this overlay prevents him from going back to a job that he detests, and it may enable him to collect financial compensation during his period of invalidism. These complications, which are common in hysterical disorders, are called "secondary gains," because, although they are not caused by the basic interpersonal problems of the patient, they secondarily give his symptoms an added emotional premium. In some hysterical disorders the "secondary gain" becomes a bigger problem than the original emotional difficulty or physical injury that produced the dysfunction, and treatment of the patient becomes immensely more difficult. This is particularly true in hysterical disorders that become the basis of financial compensation or litigation, as may occur in industrial injuries and automobile accidents. We shall give special attention to these problems later in this chapter.

Hysterical disorders are more common in poorly educated persons of low socioeconomic status than in well-educated persons of high socioeconomic status. For example, in the British Army in the First World War hysterical disorders were much more common in enlisted men than in officers. On the other hand, anxiety neuroses were much more common in officers, who were better educated and came from higher socioeconomic groups. Naive, unsophisticated concepts of body functioning seem to predispose a patient to a hysterical disorder when he is under stress, whereas the well-educated person is prone to develop other types of neurotic illnesses. Also, hysterical neuroses tend to be more common in immature persons whose emotional development and interpersonal capacities are stunted at childish levels. Although women with hysterical disorders are sometimes coy and childishly flirtatious, they often are emotionally uncomfortable with sexuality and are sexually nonorgasmic (frigid).

CLINICAL CHARACTERISTICS OF DISSOCIATIVE HYSTERIA

Dissociative disorders are clinically related to conversion disorders; they are called dissociative disorders because they are characterized by a splitting apart, or dissociation, of the patient's activities from his conscious awareness of them.

In dissociative neuroses there are disturbances of awareness and memory. The dissociative neuroses include hysterical amnesias, hysterical depersonalization, dissociative personality states, fugues, hysterical stupors and hysterical twilight states, or deliriums. The dissociative disorders are much less commonly seen in clinical practice than the conversion disorders.

The patient with hysterical *amnesia* may be seen during the period of amnesia or after it is over. If he is seen during his amnesic state he may have a complete loss of memory about who he is and his entire previous life up to the time he is being examined; however, sometimes his memory loss covers only the preceding few hours or few days. When the amnesic patient is seen after the amnesic episode has ended, his memory is accurate except for a specific block of past time which may involve a period of days, or weeks, or months. Most frequently the patient's amnesic period covers several days to two or three weeks of his recent past life; people who saw the patient during this period may not have noticed abnormalities in his behavior, or they may have found him unable to identify himself and unable to remember his past life. A hysterical amnesic episode characteristically begins and ends abruptly, and often there are obvious emotional stresses in the patient's life just preceding the amnesic episode. The patient usually accepts his memory loss placidly and does not seem much upset by it. He does not have the troubled perplexity of the patient with organic memory loss who searches anxiously for clues that will help him recover his memory.

Depersonalization states may be produced by dissociative processes. In them the patient feels that in some strange way both he and his environment have changed, but he does not feel that he is someone else. (Depersonalization has been discussed in Chapter 3, and the controversial diagnosis of depersonalization neurosis is covered in Chapter 10.)

Multiple personality states, which are sometimes called *dissociated personalities,* constitute an interesting but extremely rare type of dissociative disorder. The patient with a multiple personality disorder has two separate personality states. His primary personality is his day-to-day personality, and his second personality is a different one into which he slips from time to time and in which his behavior is much different from his usual state. While in one personality state, he usually has complete amnesia for the other. Multiple personality states apparently were more common in the latter part of the 19th Century and the early part of the 20th Century, and the American psychiatrist Morton Prince was known for his study of this condition. However, multiple personality states are seen so rarely in modern clinical practice that it is difficult to find valid, firsthand accounts of them. In over a quarter century of psychiatric work I have never seen a case of this disorder, nor have I ever been present when such a case was discussed.

A *fugue* is a dissociative disorder in which the patient travels a long distance with complete amnesia for his actions during his journey. During his journey the patient may appear normal to the casual observer, but usually he is unaware of his true identity and past life. The patient with a fugue usually is seen after he has arrived in a city quite distant from the one he started in and after he has regained his memory except for the block of time during which he made his journey. Often a major emotional stress preceded the fugue, and the fugue literally may seem to be an unconscious flight from a painful interpersonal crisis in the patient's life.

Dissociative processes may produce disturbances in which the patient has clouding of consciousness and hallucinatory experiences. The patient with a hysterical *stupor* has clouding of consciousness. In the group of disorders variously termed hysterical *twilight states, dream states* or *deliriums* the patient has clouding of consciousness and also has hallucinatory experiences.

In a hysterical *stupor* the patient has marked clouding of consciousness. He is withdrawn from contact with people and may sit or lie quietly without apparent awareness of events in his environment. Sometimes the patient is drowsy or in an apparent deep sleep. The patient in a hysterical stupor may have occasional fluttering of the eyelids or bizarre movements and posturings of the limbs and body from time to time. Such stupors may last from a few minutes to several weeks or more, and they characteristically begin and end abruptly.

In the dissociative states variously termed *twilight states, dream states* or *hysterical deliriums,* the patient has clouding of consciousness and hallucinatory experiences. In this type of dissociative disorder, the patient may appear to live through again previous emotionally charged events in his life, or he may act out elaborate experiences he unconsciously desires. He may talk extravagantly to the hallucinated persons whom he sees and hears in his delirium and he may carry out physical actions. Hysterical dream states are rarely seen in modern clinical practice.

The *Ganser syndrome* is a special form of dissociative disorder which occurs in persons to whom mental illness offers a means of escaping responsibility for their acts. For example, it may occur in prisoners awaiting trial. The patient's behavior is irrational in extravagant ways which nevertheless have some relationship to the stimuli and events around him. His responses to questions are nonsensical and inaccurate, but they nevertheless indicate that the patient has some grasp of the nature of the question. For example, if the patient is asked the name of the current president of the United States, he may reply, "George Washington," and if he is asked the sum of 4 plus 4, he may reply "1,004." The patient may carry out grotesque acts, such as attempting to eat by putting his spoon in his ear or insisting to the examiner that his mother is under the bed. I recall a 30-year-old assistant bank cashier who was apprehended for embezzlement of a large sum of money from his bank. He developed a Ganser syndrome in which he was constantly engaged in pruning the roses and trimming the bushes in his jail cell while awaiting trial, and he spent much time showing his rose garden to each visitor who came to see him. The nature of the Ganser syndrome has been the subject of much dispute, since the patient derives obvious advantages from appearing mentally irresponsible at the time of onset of his disturbance. However, most psychiatrists consider the Ganser syndrome to be a special type of dissociative hysteria and do not consider it a malingered disorder. The person who develops a Ganser syndrome usually has a previous history of personality problems and emotional instability.

Dissociative disorders sometimes must be carefully distinguished from other types of psychiatric problems. Hysterical stupors, twilight states, depersonalization states and other dissociative conditions must be differentiated from early schizophrenic illnesses which on superficial observation might appear similar. Also, toxic, infectious, degenerative and acute traumatic brain disorders may produce amnesia and disturbed behavior which may at times be mistaken for dissociative conditions.

Some psychiatrists have advocated the use of interviews after intravenous amobarbital (Amytal) or thiopental (Pentothal) injection to distinguish dissociative syndromes from organic brain disorders. For example, one can sometimes recover in a barbiturate interview the lost memories of a patient with a hysterical amnesia, whereas one cannot do so if the amnesia is due to organic brain disease. In my opinion, however, this procedure is unreliable, for the patient with a hysterical amnesia may not give factually valid information under a barbiturate, and the patient with an organic brain disorder may tell confabulated stories which are difficult to distinguish from actual events. Moreover, if one mistakenly conducts a barbiturate interview with a borderline schizophrenic, the patient sometimes may be precipitated into a florid psychotic state. Hence, dissociative hysterical syndromes should be distinguished from early schizophrenic disorders and from acute organic brain syndromes on the basis of comprehensive study of the patient's emotional and neurological state and careful survey of his life history and personality structure.

INTERPERSONAL CAUSES OF CONVERSION AND DISSOCIATIVE HYSTERIA

Interpersonal Causes of Conversion Hysteria

In conversion hysteria the patient's past and current interpersonal stresses produce profound emotional turmoil which is converted into physical symptoms. The patient's emotional turbulence becomes encapsulated in the conversion symptom, and he does not feel the painful anxiety he would otherwise experience. Also, the patient does not have to face any of the past and current interpersonal conflicts that produce his anxiety. At the cost of developing a physical symptom, the patient unconsciously finds an unhealthy resolution for his anxiety and he avoids coming to grips with his interpersonal problems.

The particular hysterical symptom the patient develops sometimes has a clear symbolic relationship to the emotional problems causing it. In a sense, the patient with a hysterical muscular paralysis unconsciously is saying through his symptom, "I will not perform actions which are expected or required of me." The patient with hysterical blindness unconsciously is saying in a symbolic way, "I will not see or recognize my problems," and the patient with a hysterical anesthesia unconsciously is saying, "I will not feel my emotional distress nor be sensitive to it."

For example, I recall a 31-year-old man who had been transferred in his place of employment from an active job on the production line to a desk job of routine paper work which he detested. Shortly after this job change he developed a hysterical paralysis of his right hand and forearm. This paralysis made writing impossible and incapacitated him from doing paper work. The symptom was an unconscious rebellion against the change of jobs, and through his symptom he was, in a sense, symbolically saying, "I will not do the things demanded of me." Throughout his childhood, this patient had fought a hostile, tenacious battle with his harsh, domineering father. In his adult life the patient became very upset emotionally whenever he felt he was being subjected to arbitrary, callous acts by male superiors, whom he unconsciously interpreted as father substitutes. Thus, the job transfer, about which he had not been consulted, reactivated extensive childhood conflicts and resulted in his hysterical symptoms. The patient was transferred back to his former type of work on the production line, but the paralysis of the hand persisted for eight months more, during which I saw him in once weekly psychotherapy to help him resolve the turbulence of the past and current interpersonal stresses that had caused his conversion disorder.

The hysterical symptom brings two gains to the patient. In the *primary gain* of the hysterical symptom, the patient is protected from the painful anxiety he would otherwise feel if his emotional turmoil were not encapsulated in his symptom. By the *secondary gain,* the patient avoids interpersonal stress or achieves some form of gratification. For example, I recall a 28-year-old patient with a hysterical hemiplegia. Much emotional trauma in her childhood and adolescence contributed heavily to the production of her hemiplegia. However, it gave the patient a significant secondary gain, because it made her a housebound semi-invalid and enabled her to avoid many uncomfortable interpersonal relationships with her parents and siblings who lived in a city 200 miles distant. The entrenched secondary gain from her hemiplegia made her treatment difficult and prolonged, because recovery resulted in renewed contacts with her difficult relatives. The hysterical patient is not consciously aware of either the primary or secondary gains of his symptom. He merely knows that he has a dysfunction and that because of it his activities are to a certain extent curtailed.

In a hysterical fainting spell, the patient unconsciously shuts out awareness of emotional stress and avoids interpersonal action in a difficult situation. In some instances the fainting spell occurs in clear relationship to an upsetting interpersonal event; the spell abruptly removes the patient from a painful emotional situation and relieves him of the need for action about it. Many psychiatrists feel that hysterical seizures are symbolic expressions of hostile or sexual feelings that receive distorted expression in the bizarre posturings and movements characterizing conversion seizures.

Much of the material (outlined in Chapter 6) on the various interpersonal causes of anxiety is relevant to many cases of conversion neuroses, because in many instances a conversion disorder is a means of controlling and masking anxiety by the production of a particular kind of physical symptom. However, in some cases a conversion dysfunction arises out of certain characteristic personality patterns in which anxiety does not play a key role. (These personality patterns are outlined in a later section of this chapter titled "Further Interpersonal Concepts Concerning Hysteria," since they apply to dissociative disorders as well as conversion ones.)

Interpersonal Causes of Dissociative Hysteria

The patient with a dissociative disorder has a splitting off, or dissociation, of his actions from his conscious awareness of them; he may lose his conscious awareness of current actions he is carrying out, as in a fugue or hysterical stupor, or he may lose his conscious awareness of past actions, as in a hysterical amnesia. The dissociative disorder usually occurs when the emotional turbulence from the patient's past and current interpersonal stresses threaten to flood him with marked anxiety. In unconsciously protecting himself against this wave of profound anxiety, the patient loses his conscious awareness of past or current events in his life, and a dissociative dysfunction occurs.

In a fugue, the patient splits off conscious awareness of current emotional distress and literally flees from painful interpersonal stresses. In a hysterical amnesia, the patient protects himself from the pain of past events by splitting off his memory for a block of past events and loses his recollection of them. In hysterical depersonalization, the patient escapes from his emotional turbulence by developing the feeling that in some strange way his personality has changed and that he is different than he formerly was. In a hysterical stupor the patient is removed from his anxiety by the development of clouding of consciousness.

In a hysterical delirium, or twilight state, the patient loses awareness of his emotional difficulties by developing a profound clouding of consciousness, during which fragments of his past experiences and unconscious desires break through into expression, though they often are manifested in distorted ways. Thus, the patient may relive emotionally charged experiences with florid visual and auditory hallucinations. Such episodes may last from several minutes to several days or more, and they often have a dramatic, boisterous quality.

Further Interpersonal Concepts Regarding Hysteria

Harry Stack Sullivan's studies of hysteria are concentrated on one large group of hysterical patients—those who have the classic hysterical pattern of immature, naive, melodramatic personality features; these features form the picture often described as typical of hysterical patients. However, many other psychiatrists, including myself, feel that this pattern fits only about half the patients who develop hysterical disorders; the other half have other kinds of personality difficulties, and the causes of their hysterical symptoms lie in other types of emotional problems.

Sullivan felt that the hysterical patient basically was a self-absorbed, self-centered person whose emotional functioning, concepts and daydream life had been stunted and had remained at a childhood level. The hysterical patient is so self-centered that other people have no real meaning for him as persons; they are merely dim figures who suit, or do not suit, his impulses and convenience. He manipulates these persons by his hysterical symptoms, much as a child manipulates his toys as he plays out his games and fantasies with them.

The hysterical patient, Sullivan felt, was usually reared by very self-absorbed parents who never formed vibrant, intense relationships with the child. They neither rejected him, nor were hostile toward him, nor loved him, nor manipulated him. They treated him as a toy or an ornament in the home rather than a growing personality. On each contact with the child they soon grew bored and left him alone. The developing child was both neglected and indulged; he was blithely allowed to do what he wanted, and he grew into a self-centered individual who had no real grasp of what interpersonal relationships were all about. Also, there were no other people available during his formative years to establish close relationships with him and correct his personality warps.

As a result, the hysterical patient never developed emotionally beyond the level of middle or late childhood, and he has retained a facile, childlike ability to view people, reality and his own body functions in melodramatic, wish-fulfilling, daydream-like ways. He also has retained the emotionally labile qualities a child reveals in his play; he can shift abruptly from one extravagant mood to another. The hysteric is not hostile and he does not have low self-esteem; other people simply don't matter to him, except as an audience. Sullivan felt that these formulations held good for a large percentage of patients with both conversion hysteria and dissociative hysteria.

The hysterical patient's capacity for mature interaction with people in adult life is severely limited; he is incapable of sound, fully involved sexual relationships. Although she may put on a dramatic show of passion during intercourse, a hysterical woman is usually non-orgasmic (frigid). In marriage these patients are gay and playful when things go well and when they are indulged by their marital partners. However, when things go badly they tend to have melodramatic upsets, either of pouting anger or showy grief, from which they can recover abruptly if circumstances change or if their attention is diverted by pleasant events. When they encounter interpersonal impasses or become trapped in painful situations, they flee into conversion hysterical or dissociative hysterical symptoms to escape their interpersonal dilemmas.

This type of hysterical patient plays at life as if it were an entertaining game, and not a serious business. He agrees to anything on the spur of the moment and later finds irrelevant, often silly, excuses for not doing what he committed himself to do. He is a pleasant playmate, an irresponsible employee, and an unreliable marital partner. He treats his children as pretty dolls with which to play occasionally, or he ignores them altogether. His speech is strewn with colorful clichés, often thrown out as justification for his self-centered, impulsive acts.

Under stress the patient flees into a hysterical amnesia, or fugue, or twilight state to escape a problem in his marriage, or in child rearing, or in his economic life, or in his social relationships. In other instances he frees himself of responsibility by developing a physical incapacity, such as a conversion paralysis, or conversion pain, or conversion seizures. As would be expected in a person whose emotional growth was stunted at a childhood level, his symptoms conform to childhood concepts of body structure and functioning, and the connection between interpersonal problems and the abrupt onset and cessation of symptoms may be obvious to many people around him.

This type of hysterical patient is exemplified by a 19-year-old patient of mine. Her father was an egotistical, successful businessman who was rarely at home, and her mother was a vain, socially aspiring woman who paid little attention to her. They treated her as a china doll in whom neither had sustained interest, and she was indulged by maids and impecunious relatives who curried her favor and flattered her parents about her. She became a coy, self-centered, irresponsible, impulsive, gaily chattering girl. At 19 she married a man who was economically and socially inferior to her and treated him with amused raillery while she went through a series of brief, light affairs with other men. When her husband came home and discovered her in bed with another man she promptly developed paralysis of both legs, called an ambulance, and entered a luxurious apartment at the hospital. She spent three weeks receiving her friends and relatives there and recovered completely two days before she was due to leave on a vacation abroad.

As Sullivan points out, hysterical patients who fit this category are often very difficult to treat. They usually recover from their symptoms, but treatment has little impact on them. They cannot enter into a sincere, serious collaborative effort with the therapist; they treat therapy as an amusing game, though on the surface they may seem to comply with it, often in an exaggeratedly enthusiastic way. They often relate their childhood daydreams and speculations as if they were actual life events, and the therapist is led on an interesting but unrealistic trip. It takes considerable work and ingenuity for the therapist to find out what really went on, and is going on, in the patient's life, and when the therapist begins to discover the central realities of the patient's life he must go cautiously or the patient will find some minor excuse for stopping treatment. As Sullivan notes, one of the difficulties of Freudian psychoanalysis is that Freud spent the first 20 years of his psychotherapeutic practice working mainly with this type of hysterical patient, and most of his fundamental theories are based on this work. Moreover, Freud insisted that various personality features and developmental phenomena of these patients held true for all persons, both normal and abnormal. Although Freud in time realized that many of the things his hysteric patients told him were daydreams and not actual life events, he nevertheless accepted many other things they revealed as factual. Freud also assumed that all symptomatic recoveries of his hysterical patients were the results of his treatment; he never came to grips (at least in anything he wrote) with the fact that the vast majority of hysterical patients of this type recover from their symptoms regardless of what kind of treatment they receive, or even if they receive no treatment at all. It was not until many years later that psychotherapists began to be aware that they must be very cautious in evaluating whether a patient got well because of treatment or merely during it.

CLINICAL COURSE OF CONVERSION AND DISSOCIATIVE HYSTERIA

Conversion and dissociative disorders are uncommon in children under the age of 12. When conversion and dissociative difficulties occur in prepuberal children the prognosis for recovery from the symptom is excellent. Usually, the symptom persists only a few days or weeks and then disappears, even without any specific treatment. However, the child should have the advantage of child guidance evaluation when it is available. The child is still living in the interpersonal environment in which his basic personality structure is being formed, and psychotherapeutic work with him and counseling with his parents may prevent personality problems that would predispose him to further psychiatric difficulties both in childhood and later life.

The course and prognosis of a conversion or dissociative disorder that begins in adolescence or adult life depends on (1) the underlying personality structure of the patient, (2) the ongoing stresses of his interpersonal environment, (3) the nature of the secondary gains obtained from his symptoms and (4) the promptness and extent of the treatment which he receives. Moreover, some kinds of hysterical symptoms are more prone to persist than others.

The patient's basic personality structure is the most important factor in determining the course of a conversion or dissociative disorder. When the patient's hysterical disorder has been precipitated by severe current trauma (as in wartime battle or a civil disaster such as a flood) and his basic personality structure is reasonably sound, he has a good prognosis for recovery from his dysfunction and for remaining well after his current stresses have diminished. However, when a patient's basic personality structure is characterized by marked emotional immaturity and poor capacities for interpersonal relationships, and his disorder was precipitated by relatively minor current stress, a conversion disability may persist without interruption for years or decades, or a dissociative disorder such as hysterical amnesia may recur repeatedly at intervals of from several days to several months over a similarly long period of time. However, even in these latter cases the overall statistical probability for recovery, even with minimal treatment is good; only a small minority of patients have long-lasting disabilities.

The ongoing stresses in the patient's life

also affect the prognosis of a hysterical dysfunction. The patient with a healthy interpersonal life has a much better outlook than one whose day-to-day interpersonal conflicts drive him more fixedly into his symptoms. The nature of the patient's secondary gain from his symptoms is equally important. When the patient has a small secondary gain from his symptom the prognosis is much better than when the secondary gain is large and has become an ingrained feature of his life.

Prompt psychiatric management improves the prognosis of a conversion or dissociative neurosis. The longer a conversion disorder or a repetitive pattern of dissociative episodes persists, the more difficult it is to remove the disorder. This is particularly true when enough time has elapsed to allow the patient's secondary gain from his disorder to become an entrenched feature of his interpersonal adjustment. For example, the man who during many months or years gradually has sunk into the role of a chronic semi-invalid, dependent on the economic aid and personal services of others, usually is a poor candidate for successful treatment. Often it is impossible to convince such a patient that he has an emotional problem and needs psychiatric help. He tenaciously clings to the belief that his disorder is due to some kind of physical disease and rejects the idea of psychiatric care.

Certain types of hysterical problems have better prognoses than others. The patient with a single conversion symptom of recent origin, such as a paralysis of his hand or aphonia, has a much better outlook than the patient who has multiple conversion symptoms of insidious onset over a long period of time. Conversion pain is notoriously persistent; patients with multiple conversion pains, especially over the abdominal wall, in the pelvic region, over the perineum, or in the face, present very difficult treatment problems and they often reject psychiatric help. A dissociative dysfunction such as an amnesic episode or a fugue occurring when the patient is under stress has a better prognosis than dissociative stupors and deliriums often occurring repeatedly at intervals over long periods of time. A Ganser syndrome has a good prognosis, though it may go on for several weeks or several months. However, the patient with a Ganser syndrome usually has personality problems which lead in time to other kinds of social and interpersonal difficulties, and he usually rejects any kind of systematic psychiatric care.

TREATMENT OF CONVERSION AND DISSOCIATIVE HYSTERIA

Treatment of Conversion Hysteria

We shall consider treatment of conversion neuroses in two parts. First, we shall discuss interview treatment of conversion neuroses, which aims at helping the patient resolve the emotional problems causing his conversion disorder. Second, we shall discuss treatment measures directed toward the immediate removal of the conversion symptom itself.

When possible, removal of the conversion symptom by suggestive or other treatment often is desirable even while the interview treatment to resolve the patient's emotional turmoil is still in its early stages. As discussed earlier in this chapter, if conversion symptoms persist many weeks or months they have a marked tendency to acquire strong secondary gains, which make interview treatment difficult. Hence, early removal of the symptom gives the patient some immediate relief and also facilitates the task of psychotherapy.

Psychotherapy of Conversion Neuroses

The interview treatment of a conversion disorder should begin soon after the symptoms appear. Delay allows the symptoms to become ingrained and in some cases permits secondary gains to become a formidable problem. Above all, the patient should not pursue a long odyssey of many months or years of medical diagnostic procedures and organic treatments before the hysterical nature of his complaints is recognized and made clear to him. After such an odyssey the patient often becomes convinced that his symtoms are due to physical disease, and he cannot be persuaded that his problems have emotional causes and require a psychiatric approach.

(The basic principles and technics of psychotherapy are discussed in Chapter 21, and the application of psychotherapy to neurotic disorders has been illustrated in Chapter 7.) These principles and cases outline the general psychotherapeutic approach used in conversion neuroses. However, the patient with a conversion neurosis sometimes presents special problems. The psychiatrist often must work through an initial phase in which the hysterical patient engages in a childish fencing with him or a coy evasiveness of the work in hand. Moreover, hysterical patients are prone to develop erotically tinged dependent feelings toward a therapist of the opposite sex, which present special problems in therapy. Also, the patient may develop recurrences or exacerbations of his conversion symptoms during those stages of psychotherapy in which he is discussing emotionally painful past or current life situations. These problems in interview treatment require skillful management by the psychotherapist.

The process of psychotherapy in a patient with a conversion disorder is illustrated by the case of a 25-year-old married woman who at the time of psychiatric consultation had been a patient in the medical section of a hospital for six weeks for paralysis of both legs and severe pain in the lower back. She had had an extensive medical and neurological workup which had not revealed organic pathology. Various medical and physiotherapeutic treatments had been used in the hope that they would help the paralysis of her legs and low back pain by their suggestive power; they did not lessen her symptoms.

The interview treatment of this patient may be divided into three broad periods: (1) The first four weeks of treatment dealt with current interpersonal pressures in her life. It also included direct interpretations of the ways in which her symptoms were removing her from emotional stresses in her home; in addition, strong suggestions and urgings were used to diminish her symptoms so that she could leave the hospital and function at least partially as a mother and a wife. (2) In the next 14 months of psychotherapy, she worked to become more comfortable and adequate in handling many unhealthy interpersonal relationships in her current life situation. (3) In the final 12 months of therapy she explored the emotionally traumatic experiences of her childhood and adolescence which had produced her personality problems and had laid the basis for her conversion disorder.

During the first four weeks of treatment the patient was seen two or three times each week in the hospital for interview sessions. In the first interview, she blandly denied any interpersonal difficulties in her life, but in succeeding interviews she began to discuss the unhappiness and stresses in her marriage. At the age of 20 she had married a man four years older than herself, mainly to get away from an emotionally painful home situation. The man she married was an aggressive, persistent person who pressured her into marriage although she was not fond of him. After marrying him she discovered her husband to be a domineering, self-centered man who exploited her passivity and controlled her by angry tirades whenever she disagreed with him. In the seven years of their troubled marriage they had one child, who was by now a 2-year-old boy.

During the four-week period of psychotherapy in the hospital the patient discussed many facets of her marriage. She became aware that her inability to be assertive with her husband and her relatives made her unable to leave the marriage, and that she felt hopelessly trapped in it. She disliked sexual intercourse with her husband, though it occurred several times each week and she dared not refuse him. We discussed how her hysterical paralysis and back pain removed her from distasteful interpersonal and sexual relationships with her husband, and we discussed frankly how these unhealthy advantages she gained from her symptoms threatened to make her symptoms entrenched and difficult to remove. I gave her much strong encouragement to try to walk and to leave the hospital, and I held out the hope that in subsequent interview treatment we could resolve some of the personality problems preventing her from dealing adequately with various dilemmas in her life. The patient improved much and at the end of four weeks was able to return home where, although not fully recovered from her physical symptoms, she was able to resume many of her household responsibilities and could take care of her child. At this point I suggested to her husband that he seek psychotherapeutic help for his personality problems, but he refused.

In the second stage of her psychotherapy, in which she was seen two times each week in outpatient interview sessions, she worked on a wide range of current interpersonal problems. She discussed the profound feelings of inadequacy and worthlessness she had had since childhood, and she explored her marked passivity in all her relationships with people. She felt that everyone around her was more capable than she was and that they had better judgement than she had. Her husband dominated her in all household decisions and her stepmother and her cousins dominated her in all decisions in rearing her child. Emotionally she felt like a pygmy in a crowd of giants, and her relatives treated her as an inadequate person whom they patronized, criticized and exploited for their personal convenience.

We examined the unhealthiness of these relationships and the lack of realistic justification both for her views of herself and for the ways in which her relatives treated her. She began slowly to gain self-confidence and she became more assertive. She gradually became able to resist domination and exploitation by her husband and her relatives, and slowly she readjusted her interpersonal relationships with them on more mature levels; as she became firmer and more assertive with them, they ceased to treat her as an incapable child and began to accept her as a responsible adult. Her husband begrudgingly became somewhat less demanding and critical, but the marriage was still unhappy. The process of becoming more assertive precipitated repeated interpersonal stresses in her life in which her husband, her stepmother and other relatives lashed her with angry harangues, and during these stressful periods she had several brief recurrences of leg weakness and back pain which confined her to bed for one to four days but did not require hospitalization.

At the end of 14 months of work on these problems she was able to be reasonably assertive with comfort, and she had a much more self-confident and realistic view of herself. Her work in fully consolidating these interpersonal goals went on for many months longer, but she could carry out this personality development without devoting more of her interview time to discussing it. From this point on, she had no further physical symptoms.

In the process of resolving these current interpersonal stresses in her life the patient was relieved of much anxiety and emotional turbulence which had contributed much to the production of her conversion symptoms. She was relieved of feelings of profound inadequacy, and she no longer needed to repress the resentment which domination by her husband and her relatives formerly had produced in her. Before psychotherapy she had stored up all her feelings of anger and assertiveness and was fearful of the consequences of expressing them in any way. However, these pent-up feelings, most of which she did not consciously recognize, chronically threatened to erupt into conscious expression, and this threat flooded her with anxiousness. This anxiety and the emotional tumult that lay behind it constituted a significant part of the emotional forces which were *converted* into her physical symptoms. However, these forces involved only the current interpersonal causes of her disorder. The complete resolution of her conversion neurosis required an exploration of the unhealthy relationships in her childhood and adolescence, which had laid the deeper bases for her conversion disorder; this work occupied the final 12 months of her psychotherapy.

The patient was an only child and her mother died of carcinoma when the patient was nine months old. Her father was depressed and emotionally withdrawn for two years following the mother's death. The patient was raised by her maternal grandmother who felt unjustly burdened by the care of rearing the patient, and she openly rejected the patient emotionally. The grandmother also attributed the death of the patient's mother to the fact that she was pregnant with the patient at the time her carcinoma was discovered, and surgical treatment of the carcinoma had been delayed for three months until after the birth. It was not clear in psychotherapy whether or not this was actually so, but the grandmother made the patient feel it was so and left her with the devastating, guilty conviction that she had been the cause of her mother's death. The patient's mother had been a talented musician, the grandmother's favorite child and the center of family attention. Throughout her childhood and adolescence the grandmother and other relatives compared the patient unfavorably with her mother, and the patient was criticized bitterly for each shortcoming and was exhorted to be the talented, charming person her mother had been. As the years of her childhood rolled over her, she slowly became convinced that she was an inadequate, incapable, unlovable person.

Her grandmother, moreover, could tolerate no assertiveness or expression of anger from her, and made her feel guilty and worthless if she ever expressed any assertive feelings. Thus, she gradually was molded into a passive, timid girl with strong feelings of inadequacy, worthlessness and guilt. Periodically her grandmother took her to visit her mother's grave, and often the patient felt the urge to kick the headstone and to stamp angrily upon the ground under which lay the woman with whom she was unfavorably compared daily and of whose death she had been made to feel guilty.

Throughout the first 10 years of her life her father took little interest in her. She felt that his rejection and lack of interest in her confirmed her grandmother's contentions that she was an inadequate, unlovable person. When she was 10 her father remarried and she went to live with her stepmother and her father, who still paid little attention to her. Her stepmother had two children by a previous marriage, and found her an unwelcome intruder; she treated the patient with irritability and neglect. Thus, the patient's feelings of unworthiness and isolation were reinforced during a lonely adolescence. Beneath her passive, somewhat depressed façade lay large amounts of unconscious, smoldering anger, which periodically threatened to emerge into conscious expression and precipitated occasional anxiety attacks during her adolescence. When the patient was 20 her stepmother pushed her toward marriage with her future husband, and because of her passivity and her longing to leave home she entered into a marriage which she soon found an unhappy trap from which she could see no possibility of release.

In psychotherapy the patient for the first time gained a clear awareness of how her feelings of inadequacy and guiltiness had arisen and how her passivity had been produced. She became aware of her repressed anger against her grandmother, her stepmother and her father, and she realized that she resented her deceased mother who had been held up to her as an example of all she could not be. Many psychiatrists would say that the patient's paralysis of the legs was related to her angry, guilt-laden impulses to kick her mother's headstone and to stamp angrily upon her grave when her grandmother took her to visit the grave periodically throughout the patient's childhood.

At the end of treatment the patient was a much more self-confident, assertive person and she was free of the burden of repressed feelings of anger, guilt and unworthiness that had so painfully weighed upon her. Her marriage was still unhappy and her husband refused to participate either in marriage counseling or psychotherapy for himself. The patient began to attend teachers college to gain the education that would enable her to be self-supporting if she should later decide to dissolve the marriage. I did not see her again after she ended treatment, but eight years later I saw an aunt of hers in consultation. The aunt spontaneously mentioned that the patient had remained well, had separated from her husband, and was teaching grade school.

Other Aspects of Managing Conversion Disorders

A psychiatrist often wishes to remove a conversion symptom as soon as possible to allow a man to return to work or to enable a housewife to resume her responsibilities. The prompt removal of a conversion symptom reduces the chances of entrenched secondary gains, which make interview treatment very difficult. The three methods sometimes used for prompt removal of conversion symptoms are (1) persuasive, suggestive measures, (2) hypnosis, and (3) strong suggestions after the intravenous injection of a barbiturate. The use of any of these methods for removal of conversion symptoms should be followed by psychotherapy to resolve the emotional causes of the disorder.

For reasons I shall outline in later paragraphs, I prefer strong persuasive and suggestive technics for removing hysterical symptoms, and I am hesitant about the use of hypnosis and barbiturate interviews. Before using persuasive and suggestive measures the physician should first explain clearly to the patient that his symptoms are due to emotional factors. He may use the phrases "emotional tension," "emotional turmoil" and "stresses between you and people in your past and present life situations" in explaining what he means by emotional factors. He should indicate further that the complete solution of the conversion disorder lies in resolving the emotional problems that caused it, but that prompt removal of the symptom and rehabilitation of the patient to usual work or household responsibilities should be accomplished as quickly as possible.

In his use of persuasive and suggestive measures, the physician may exhort the patient to "rehabilitate himself." He may urge the paralyzed patient to begin to walk with the assistance of others, and he may urge patients with other types of conversion dysfunctions to take up their daily activities to the best of their abilities. The physician may advise the patient repeatedly and strongly, "You will get over this problem more quickly by being active rather than inactive." The psychiatrist may hold out the hope of complete resolution of the conversion disorder in psychotherapy after the patient has made sufficient improvement to become at least partially active socially and vocationally. The success of such persuasive exhortation and suggestions depends in large measure on the personality of the psychiatrist, his enthusiasm and his rapport with the patient. In a large number of instances these measures diminish the severity of conversion symptoms of recent origin. These suggestive technics, of course, do not affect the underlying emotional problems of the patient, but hysterical symptoms of recent origin are (unlike other types of neurotic symptoms) very sensitive to strong suggestion and, as an initial goal, their removal by suggestive technics is a useful procedure in the total treatment plan of the patient.

In addition, the physician may use other suggestive procedures. Self-suggestive technics for progressive relaxation of groups of tense muscles or graduated exercises for groups of weak muscles may be outlined. In occasional instances mild physiotherapy such as massage may be prescribed, but the physician repeatedly must emphasize that there is no organic disorder of the affected area and that the physiotherapy is merely to exercise or relax parts of the body not functioning well because of emotional distress. Such suggestive measures may help to reduce the severity of hysterical symptoms and thus diminish the possible occurrence of entrenched secondary gains. Long-term psychotherapy of the patient's underlying emotional problems then becomes a practical possibility.

Some psychiatrists, as the initial step in the patient's comprehensive management, use hypnosis to remove hysterical symptoms. Hypnosis has occasional usefulness for this purpose if employed by an experienced psychiatrist who previously has made a careful psychiatric examination. However, I am cautious about the use of hypnosis. The psychiatrist who employs it must have special training in its use, and even in experienced hands the results of hypnosis are not outstanding. Moreover, hypnosis is time-consuming, and many patients cannot be hypnotized even with hours of work by the hypnotist. In addition, hypnosis has certain dangers. It involves a special relationship between the physician and his patient, in which the physician plays a controlling, dominant role, and the patient adopts a submissive, pliable role. This is sometimes the source of erotic feelings of marked intensity by a patient toward a therapist of the opposite sex. Sometimes hypnosis may subtly corrupt the feelings of the hypnotist who finds himself exercising unusual powers over the consciousness of his patients. Occasionally, in patients whose personality integration is unstable, psychotic episodes or serious neurotic crises are precipitated by hypnosis. In my opinion, far better results are obtained with much less danger by using the suggestive technics outlined in previous paragraphs.

Some psychiatrists use the intravenous injection of a barbiturate, usually amobarbital (Amytal) or thiopental (Pentothal), to induce a state of slight drowsiness during which strong suggestions are employed to remove conversion symptoms. (The technic for beginning a barbiturate interview is outlined in Chapter 5.) The same limitations and problems which apply to hypnosis are, in general, applicable to barbiturate interviews. Induction of the state of altered consciousness is more rapid and more easily obtained than in hypnosis, but the degree of suggestibility of the patient is less. The same complications that may occur in hypnosis may occur in barbiturate interviews, but they are somewhat less common. In general, barbiturate interviews are more useful in hysterical disorders of recent origin precipitated by severe environmental stress, as in war or in civil disasters.

Suggestive technics should not be used alone. They should only be employed in the initial stage of a treatment plan that includes psychotherapy to resolve the patient's underlying emotional problems.

Recommendations for the family physician or internist in dealing with patients with conversion disorders. The family physician or the internist often is the first physician whom the patient with a conversion disorder consults, and his management of the patient in this initial medical contact frequently has an important bearing on the course of the patient's disorder. He should make the correct diagnosis promptly and should tell the patient the nature of his trouble, since hysterical symptoms have a strong tendency to become entrenched if they are mistaken for physical dysfunctions and are so treated medically.

The family physician or internist should examine the patient carefully, and if he feels the problem is a conversion disorder, he should discuss this possibility tactfully. He should proceed promptly to make whatever diagnostic tests are necessary to rule out possible organic disease. At the outset, the physician should say, "Mrs. Franklin, I am not completely sure from the physical examination what your trouble is. However, such symptoms often are due to emotional stress. We will run the necessary tests to rule out any physical disease, but I feel it is probable that we will find that your symptoms are due to emotional factors." If the doctor is convinced from the beginning that the patient has a conversion disorder, he should tell the patient so. The physician should never use the word "hysterical" in talking to patients or their relatives, for it alienates patients and leads relatives to assume that the patient is a silly, immature person who could "snap out of it if he really wanted to." The doctor should explain the trouble to the patient and his family as a physical dysfunction brought on by tension and emotional stresses, recent or past.

Despite decades of medical education to the contrary, psychiatrists still see all too many patients who for months or years have received physical treatments for hysterical disorders. A hysterical symptom should never be treated as an organic disease under the supposition that the medication or other procedures may remove the symptom by suggestion. Such treatment tends to prolong the symptom. After a patient has received prolonged organic treatment for a hysterical symptom, it is very difficult to persuade him that his trouble is due to emotional factors. The opportune time for psychiatric orientation and treatment has been lost, and the prognosis for recovery is poorer. Indeed, the prognosis of many hysterical symptoms is relatively good for spontaneous recovery without treatment in time, and can be made poor by complex, extensive physical treatment. Therapy by medications, injections and similar procedures sometimes alleviates a hysterical symptom or temporarily removes it, but the symptom, or others like it, may soon reappear. The patient returns for more organic treatment as before. The road to hysterical invalidism is easily entered by such a gate. Once started on this path, the patient can be turned back only with great difficulty; multiple hysterical symptoms draw a chain of endless medical treatments after them in a chronic course.

Treatment of Dissociative Hysteria

Dissociative neuroses are statistically much less common than conversion nueroses. Moreover, the patient with a dissociative disorder frequently is not well motivated for psychiatric treatment. Because of the episodic nature of dissociative conditions such as amnesias and fugues, the patient often is seen only after his dissociative episode has ended, and he then feels he has no need for treatment.

The patient with a hysterical stupor, or twilight state, or depersonalization state, or Ganser syndrome, more frequently is seen during his dissociative period, but after recovery from it he often is unmotivated to work on the emotional problems that caused his difficulty. The difference between conversion disorders and dissociative disorders in motivation for treatment lies in the nature of the symptoms; the patient with a conversion disorder usually has a persistent physical dysfunction which limits his activities and necessitates treatment, whereas the patient with a dissociative condition has a single episode or repetitive brief episodes of difficulty at widely spaced intervals, and he usually functions socially and vocationally in at least minimally adequate ways between his episodes.

When the patient is seen during a period of amnesic confusion, or in a stupor or a twilight state, he should be psychiatrically hospitalized. The patient almost invariably recovers from his dissociative episode in from a day or two to one or two weeks. If possible, after recovery from his dissociative episode the patient should be started in psychotherapy in the hospital, and it should be continued on an outpatient basis after he leaves the hospital.

CLINICAL PROBLEMS RELATED TO CONVERSION HYSTERIA

Compensation Problems

Psychiatric problems may play a major role in the disabilities that follow industrial accidents, automobile accidents and other types of injuries for which the patient becomes a candidate for financial compensation. The financial compensation may be given in weekly or monthly payments, as when the patient is disabled at work and receives compensation during his period of incapacitation, or it may be the subject of negotiation or litigation for a lump sum to cover medical expenses and personal suffering, as in automobile accidents and some types of vocational injuries.

The psychiatric problems that may be involved in these injuries fall in two groups: (1) problems in which the disorder following the injury is entirely of emotional origin, and (2) problems in which the patient has a significant physical injury on top of which a large emotional overlay is superimposed.

A large percentage of psychiatric problems in compensation cases are conversion disorders; anxiety neuroses rank second in the list of psychiatric conditions which may be precipitated by the emotional stress of physical accidents. However, phobic, depressive, obsessive or dissociative features may be added to conversion disorders or anxiety neuroses precipitated by injuries that become the basis of financial compensation. It should be emphasized that we are here discussing only those post-injury psychiatric problems that are due to emotional factors, and in which there is no impairment of brain tissue. (Organic brain injuries due to head trauma are covered in Chapter 18.)

These problems are sometimes labeled "compensation neuroses" or "accident neuroses." In addition, the term "traumatic neurosis" occasionally is applied to compensation problems, but this term also is used by different psychiatrists to cover a wide variety of conditions, in some of which financial compensation is not a factor. All these terms have been abandoned in the official medical nomenclature. They lack clinical precision and lead to cloudy thinking about the patient. It is much better to diagnose the specific psychiatric disorder of the patient and to state, for example, that he has a conversion disorder or an anxiety neurosis precipitated by the emotional stress of an industrial accident or other type of injury or environmental strain.

Virtually any kind of conversion symptom may occur in a compensation problem. However, the most common conversion symptoms are muscular weaknesses, paralyses, pain and tremors. Conversion anesthesias, paresthesias and visual problems are less frequently seen. Common accompanying symptoms are anxiousness, mild depressiveness, irritability, headaches, insomnia and fatigue. Often the patient is vindictive and resentful toward his employer and the employer's medical and legal representatives. (The symptoms of head injuries that become the subject of compensation have special features, discussed in Chapter 18.)

Certain personality characteristics and interpersonal problems predispose a patient to develop a psychiatric disorder which is precipitated by an industrial accident or by some type of compensable injury. For example, compensation problems are more likely to occur in dependent, emotionally insecure persons who unconsciously lean on physical disability as a way of securing economic support while withdrawing from the competitive stresses of modern industrial and commercial life. When the employee has resentment toward his employer and feels that he has been exploited and unjustly treated in his job, he is more prone to develop psychiatric symptoms after a vocational accident. Interpersonal conflicts in the job situation and unpleasant working conditions are sometimes important factors. Persons with paranoid personality features who feel that superiors at work are hostile to them and wish to defraud them of their rights are prone to develop compensation problems.

The development of compensation problems may be abrupt, gradual or delayed. For example, a conversion paralysis of the hand may occur immediately after an industrial accident, or it may develop over a period of two or three weeks following the injury. In many instances it develops after a symptom-free interval of several days or more following the accident; when this occurs, the symptom-free period is sometimes called the "incubation period" of the compensable difficulty. (As will be discussed in Chapter 18, head injuries constitute an increasingly common kind of compensable injury because of the high incidence of automobile accidents.)

A few basic principles are important in the comprehensive medical and psychiatric management of a patient who has a conversion disorder that becomes the focus of financial compensation. The patient should not be subjected to oversolicitous medical treatment nor to repeated medical examinations that are not explained to him. At an early point in his care he should have the advantage of consultation with a specialist whom he may choose with the help of his family physician, so that he will not feel that his only medical opinion is that of "the company doctor" who he fears may represent only "the company's" interests. He should be seen by a psychiatrist of his own choice, and perhaps by a specialist (such as an orthopedist or a neurologist) in the type of body dysfunction he believes he has. The patient then is more likely to accept the medical opinion that there are large emotional factors in his symptoms and that they must be taken into account in planning his rehabilitation. There should not be long delays before proper medical and psychiatric management is begun, and all physicians who examine the patient should be as reassuring and encouraging as the clinical facts will allow.

A prime rule is that the sooner litigation and a financial settlement can be made with fairness both to the patient and his employer, or the employer's insurance carrier, the better the prognosis of a compensation problem. Prolonged legal negotiations and delays in settlement tend to cause the patient's symptoms to become ingrained. The patient should never be accused of malingering, for such accusations do him an injustice and also tend to make his symptoms more severe and entrenched.

Psychotherapy of a patient with a compensable conversion disorder is difficult, and many psychiatrists feel that psychotherapy is usually not successful with a patient with a compensable disorder until after his litigation and compensation are settled. A major difficulty in treating a patient with a compensation problem is the economic secondary gain his symptoms acquire, which often is a greater problem in therapy than the primary interpersonal causes of his disorder. If the patient can become aware of the secondary gains of his symptoms and can resolve them, psychotherapy occasionally may be carried out to explore the patient's personality problems contributing to his disorder.

A major question that usually must be explored in psychotherapy is: What does the dysfunction mean to the patient in terms of his interpersonal life? Does the dysfunction allow the patient to withdraw from interpersonal stresses in his work situation? Does the injury permit a shy, insecure person with strong feelings of inadequacy to retire into a dependent, socially withdrawn role in life? Is this disorder, in part, a way in which the patient expresses resentment toward his employers or fear of returning to his job? The disorder usually has several meanings for the patient, and it offers him a way of seeking an unhealthy release from various personality problems and interpersonal tensions.

The psychiatrist and other physicians often are asked by attorneys and company officials what *caused* the disability of the patient with a compensable conversion disorder. Since a conversion disorder with compensation features is the product both of the patient's underlying personality problems and of the accident he experienced, a precise, fair answer to this question often is difficult. However, in most instances the physician can point out that, although the patient was predisposed by his personality problems and interpersonal stresses to develop a conversion disorder, this condition was *precipitated* by his industrial or automobile accident, and that his conversion disorder probably would not have occurred if the accident had not taken place. This conclusion must be based, of course, on a careful survey of the patient's physical, interpersonal and vocational effectiveness before and after the accident. In making such a survey the physician should interview carefully the patient and at least one of his relatives and he should review in detail all available records of the patient's medical history and vocational adjustment before and after the injury. The patient should be tested by a clinical psychologist, and the physician should write for reports from any physicians, clinics or other psychiatric facilities where the patient has been seen previously. After such a survey the physician can give his carefully weighed opinion with fairness to all parties concerned.

Malingering

The question of malingering by a patient occasionally is raised by work or school authorities, relatives, medical examination boards or others. They want to know whether or not a patient is pretending to have symptoms he really does not feel. This question may be brought up about patients with many kinds of neurotic and psychotic conditions, but it more often is raised about patients with hysterical disorders than patients with any other single group of psychiatric problems.

The subject of malingering is a difficult one. Many psychiatrists believe that the person who malingers usually has marked personality problems. An old psychiatric axiom states that persons who malinger psychiatric illness usually become psychiatrically ill in later years. Moreover, the person who malingers physical symptoms has a marked tendency to develop such symptoms, or similar ones, in later years. I recall two persons who malingered depression; one of them later committed suicide and the other one later had a marked depressive illness. I know of one instance in which a person malingered low back pain, and later developed low back pain on a conversion hysterical basis. I recall two instances in which persons malingered chest pain to escape unpleasant obligations, and in later years they had much obsessive fear of heart disease and chest pain on a conversion disorder basis.

Experiences such as these lead many psychiatrists to have a cautious view of malingering; they feel that most malingerers are indeed sick, though they may not have the particular disorder that they think they are malingering. The responsibility for making a decision about a patient who is accused of malingering an organic illness should be shared by two or three physicians, at least one of whom is a specialist in the particular kind of physical disorder under question; in addition, the patient should always have a thorough psychiatric examination. When the patient is accused of malingering a psychiatric disorder he should always be examined by a clinical psychologist, and the responsibility for the final decision should rest in the hands of two or three psychiatrists who have interviewed him carefully.

BIBLIOGRAPHY

Behrman, J., and Levy, R.: Neurophysiological studies in patients with hysterical disturbances of vision. J. Psychosom. Res., *14*:187, 1970.

Dickes, R. A.: Brief therapy of conversion reactions. Am J. Psychiatry, *131*:584, 1974.

Gelfman, M.: Dynamics of the correlations between hysteria and depression. Am. J. Psychother., *25*:83, 1971.

Ingraham, M. R., and Moriarity, D. M.: A contribution to the understanding of the Ganser syndrome. Compr. Psychiatry, *8*:35, 1967.

Kirshner, L. A., and Kaplan, N.: Conversion as a manifestation of crisis in the life situation. Compr. Psychiatry, *11*:260, 1970.

Levy, R., and Mushin, J.: The somatosensory evoked response in patients with hysterical anesthesia. J. Psychosom. Res., *17*:81, 1973.

Looff, D. H.: Psychophysiologic and conversion reactions in children. J. Am. Acad. Child Psychiatry, *9*:318, 1970.

Ludwig, A. M.: Hysteria: a neurobiological theory. Arch. Gen. Psychiatry, 27:771, 1972.

Meares, R., and Hovrath, T.: 'Acute' and 'chronic' hysteria. Brit. J. Psychiatry, 121:653, 1972.

Rice, D. G., and Greenfield, N. S.: Psychophysiological correlates of la belle indifférence. Arch. Gen. Psychiatry, 20:239, 1969.

Rock, N. L.: Conversion reactions in childhood: a clinical study on childhood neuroses. J. Am. Acad. Child Psychiatry, 10:65, 1971.

Sullivan, H. S.: Clinical Studies in Psychiatry. Chapter on Hysteria, p. 203. New York, W. W. Norton. 1956.

10

Other Neurotic Syndromes

The neurotic disorders, and their terminology, which we have discussed in Chapters 6 through 9, are accepted and employed by most American psychiatrists. Though some psychiatrists modify these terms somewhat (such as calling an anxiety neurosis an anxiety reaction or an anxiety psychoneurosis), these concepts may be considered firmly established in American psychiatry.

The current standard psychiatric system of diagnoses contains four further neuroses which are the subject of considerable debate. Only one of them (depressive neurosis) was in the official nomenclature prior to its revision in 1968; the other three (neurasthenic neurosis, depersonalization neurosis, and hypochondriacal neurosis) were introduced in the 1968 revised nomenclature to make American psychiatric diagnoses consistent with the international diagnostic system advocated by the World Health Organization. This international classification reflects many concepts prevailing in continental European and Soviet psychiatry, which have not found ready acceptance in the United States.

The state of these four diagnoses in current American usage may be roughly summarized as follows: (1) *Depressive neurosis* is a widely accepted and used term and concept. However, many psychiatrists feel it is somewhat artificial and prefer to classify depressions as *mild* and *severe*, rather than *neurotic* and *psychotic*. (2) *Neurasthenic neurosis* (also called neurasthenia in the official nomenclature) is employed by a minority of American psychiatrists. (3) The concept and term, *depersonalization neurosis*, is rarely used in American psychiatry. (4) *Hypochondriacal neurosis* is used by a small but significant minority of American psychiatrists; many psychiatrists object strongly to this term.

In this chapter we shall define and describe each of these neurotic diagnoses, but the amount of space devoted to each one will be proportionate to how commonly it is employed in day-to-day clinical practice.

DEPRESSIVE NEUROSIS

In traditional psychiatric terminology the depressive disorders are divided into neurotic depressions and psychotic depressions, and this distinction is maintained in the current standard nomenclature. Many psychiatrists, including myself, feel that this distinction is artificial, that depressions occur in a continuous spectrum that runs from minor to overwhelming, and that it would be clinically more valid and practical to label depressions as *mild* or *severe* and to consider them as a single type of disorder.

However, since many psychiatrists, and the official nomenclature, draw a distinction between neurotic depressions and psychotic depressions, we shall discuss the clinical characteristics attributed to neurotic depressions and their causes, courses and treatment. [The severe depressions (psychotic depressions) are discussed in Chapter 15, and the criteria often employed to distinguish neurotic depressions from psychotic ones also are listed there.]

The terms *reactive depression, depressive reaction, psychoneurotic depression,* and *situational depression* are all occasionally employed as synonyms of depressive neurosis.

Clinical Features of Depressive Neuroses

The basic feature of a neurotic depression is a pervasive feeling of emotional depressiveness. The patient may describe it as a feeling of sadness, or "low spirits," or "the blues." Sometimes he cannot express clearly how he feels until the examiner inquires, "Do you mean you're depressed, down in the dumps or melancholy?" His depressiveness usually is a persistent though fluctuating feeling that has been present from a few weeks to several months or more. Sometimes the patient can connect the onset of his depression with an upsetting event in his interpersonal life, and in other instances he cannot specify the factors that precipitated his depressiveness. Typical neurotic depressions may occur at any age from adolescence through old age. Depression in prepuberal children has special characteristics, and the term depressive neurosis ordinarily is applied only to adolescents and adults.

The patient finds that his usual activities have lost much of their appeal and meaning for him. He drags about his tasks without his customary sparkle and alertness. Friends and relatives may mention it. At times he may cover up his discomfort and only the most observant of his friends notice the change in him. Everything seems dull, flat, stale and saltless to him, and he looks at the world through gray-colored glasses. His appetite is not as good as usual, though he has had little loss of weight. His interest in sexuality is diminished; he usually is not impotent, but he is less interested. A depressed woman often is nonorgasmic (frigid). Frequently, there is a diurnal pattern in the patient's symptoms. He feels worse in the morning and somewhat better in the afternoon and evening. The patient often complains of fatigue and he may sleep somewhat poorly. He may also complain of vague physical malaise, constipation, headaches and poorly defined gastrointestinal discomforts. The patient continues to carry out customary vocational or household duties, but is somewhat less effective than usual. He may feel like crying at times and occasionally he breaks down in tears, though he cannot say what he is crying about.

The patient characteristically feels worthless, inadequate and guilty. In Harry Stack Sullivan's words, he feels an "all embracing negative self-appraisal." He feels he has not accomplished what he should in life; he magnifies his failures and overlooks his successes. He underestimates his talents and exaggerates his shortcomings and weaknesses. He ruminates over minor moral misdemeanors in his past and feels unduly guilty about them. In the patient with a depressive neurosis these feelings do not reach delusional proportions, but they color his views of himself and the world around him. The past seems discouraging, the present seems stale and the future seems unpromising.

Some psychiatrists describe a particular type of neurotically depressed patient who is demanding, tearful and bitterly critical of the people around him. This type of patient often fluctuates markedly in mood from one day to the next, and he attributes his depressiveness to what he feels are neglect and mistreatment he has experienced from members of his family and other emotionally close persons in his life. Though he has underlying feelings of worthlessness and guilt, he covers them with a façade of bitter castigation of the people around him and blames them for his emotional upset and all his difficulties. Such patients often are self-centered, immature persons who find themselves unable to cope with the complexities of mature adult life. They decompensate into floundering depressiveness and tearful agitation as they fail to adjust to interepersonal problems and crises in adult life.

The patient with a depressive neurosis often has other neurotic symptoms in addition to the basic depressive process. Chronic anxiety is common; he may be restless and tense much of the time. He may have obsessive worries about his physical health, his financial state, his family relationships and his work. Occasionally, the patient has mild phobias, especially of crowds and public places. Minor conversion symptoms such as abdominal pain and muscular weaknesses may occur in a patient with a neurotic depression. Sometimes a patient begins to misuse alcohol during a depression, and the underlying depressiveness may be obscured by his increasing problem with alcohol. In a similar manner, a few patients with neurotic depressions misuse sedatives and tranquilizers, and a few use marijuana and hallucinogens during their depressions.

Upon careful inquiry, the onset of a depressive neurosis can often be traced to an emotionally important precipitating event. Sometimes the patient is aware that his depression began in association with a specific interpersonal stress, and in other instances he is unaware of the association until it is pointed out to him. The precipitating event usually involves a loss of some kind to the patient or the imminent threat of a loss. The loss may involve people in the patient's life, or his possessions, or his prestige. For example, he may lose a member of his family by death or he may suffer a deprivation of the person's companionship and help by an incapacitating illness of the person. Often the loss occurs when the patient receives a decisive emotional rejection by a person on whom he is interpersonally dependent. Such a loss may occur when the patient loses his marital partner in a divorce or when a divorce seems imminent because of a marital crisis. A neurotic depression may follow the breakup of a love affair. Loss of possessions due to economic reverses, job dismissal, or failure in business may precipitate a neurotic depression. Sometimes the precipitating stress is loss of prestige in the eyes of the patient's family, friends or work associates; such a loss may involve school failure, job demotion, professional failure or the inability to live up to the expectations of family and friends.

Suicidal thoughts are less common in neurotic depressions than in psychotic depressions. Thoughts of suicide may occur at times in a patient in a neurotic depression, but, as a rule, he does not dwell on them and shrinks from such an act. Nevertheless, there are no entirely dependable rules in evaluating suicidal risk, and persons who are diagnosed as having neurotic depressions at times make serious suicidal attempts, some of which are fatal. Hence, although patients with neurotic depressions have a smaller risk of committing suicide than patients with psychotic depressions, the traditional psychiatric distinction between neurotic and psychotic depressions does not entirely differentiate between patients who do not present suicidal risk and those who do. (The problem of evaluating suicidal risk and preventing suicide is covered at length in Chapter 15.)

Interpersonal Causes of Depressive Neuroses

Psychiatric theory holds that in a neurotic depression the person unconsciously protects himself from feeling marked anxiety mobilized by the current interpersonal stress in his life. As Sullivan puts it, there is "a movement away from the experience of anxiety because depression is a more tolerable state than anxiety itself." The precipitating event, whether it is emotional rejection by a close person, or the loss of possessions or prestige by economic failure, arouses profound anxiety in the patient, which is masked by the development of a neurotic depression; there are, of course, in the patient's personality structure predisposing factors that were produced by unhealthy past interpersonal relationships.

The interpersonal causes of a neurotic depression can be approached by study of what the precipitating event means to the patient and how it reactivates old stresses in his life. For example, in some instances the patient with a neurotic depression experienced much hostility, criticism and emotional rejection in his childhood and adolescence, and these emotional traumas left him with profound doubts about his ability to be loved and esteemed. He felt worthless and he believed that he could expect no more in the world than he experienced at home. He often felt that the depreciation and criticism he received at home were justified by the inadequacies of his personality and his lack of attractiveness. However, these experiences were not so severe that they impaired persistently the patient's capacity for a reasonably sound emotional adjustment most of the time. He had enough healthy influences in his interpersonal relationships during his formative years to crowd his emotional trauma into the background. However, when in adult life he suffers loss of an emotionally close person, or loss of possessions or of personal prestige, these events reactivate old emotional conflicts that have long lain dormant, and a neurotic depression results.

The ways in which a current interpersonal

stress can reactivate old interpersonal traumas and lead to a neurotic depression are illustrated by the case of a 34-year-old woman whose depression had been present for several months when I first saw her. The patient was the second of two children. Her mother was a demanding, immature woman who had not wanted a second child and found the patient an annoyance from the beginning. Her mother chronically criticized her throughout her childhood; she depreciated her and made her feel guilty. In an immature way, the patient's mother competed with her for the attention of her father, a scholarly man who participated little in rearing her, leaving such care to the mother. In the context of these unhealthy interpersonal relationships the patient developed profound doubts about her worth as a person; she felt unloved and unlovable.

However, from middle childhood through adolescence she spent a great deal of time with an aunt and uncle who gave her much affection and esteem; these emotionally healthy relationships tended to diminish the effects of the emotional trauma at home. During her adolescence the patient had other healthy relationships which helped her develop a more self-confident view of herself. She had outstanding artistic talent and she did well scholastically and socially in high school and college. Her artistic and intellectual abilities gave her increased self-esteem and opened new areas of interpersonal activity.

At the age of 25 she married an advertising executive five years older than herself, and during the next six years she had two children. Shortly after the birth of her second child her husband began to drink heavily and to have extramarital affairs. He lost interest in his home and rejected the patient emotionally. When she was 34 her husband separated from her and filed for divorce, indicating his intentions to marry another woman after the divorce was obtained.

Until her marriage began to deteriorate, the patient's emotional adjustment in adult life had been good. She functioned well as a mother and a wife and she kept up her artistic activities, which were both emotionally and financially rewarding. However, the deterioration of her marriage and her husband's rejection stirred up the long dormant fears she had had in childhood that she was inadequate and unlovable. She felt her husband's rejection and the failure of her marriage were final confirmation that her early fears of worthlessness were actually justified. She felt that her rejection by both her husband and her parents indicated that anyone who got to know her well would in time discover her basic worthlessness and would turn from her in disgust and revulsion. Thus, the loss of her husband reactivated emotional traumas of her childhood and precipitated a neurotic depression.

This patient was seen in weekly psychotherapy for 18 months. As we explored the interpersonal events, both in her adult life and in her childhood, which had caused her depression, she gradually recovered from it during a six-month period. The rest of the time in which she was seen in psychotherapy was devoted to supportive counseling as she went through her divorce and faced the tasks of making a new home for her children and herself.

The patient with a neurotic depression often has much repressed anger about the emotional rejections he has received both during childhood and in his adult life. Some psychiatrists speculate that this repressed hostility is turned inward on the person himself because he at no time was able to give it adequate outward expression in the traumatic interpersonal relationships that caused it. When hostility is directed inward toward the person himself, he feels worthless and depreciated. The extreme result of inward directed hostility is to contemplate self-destruction by suicide. (However, the process of directing hostility inward operates more powerfully in the psychotic depressions we shall discuss in Chapter 15 than in the neurotic ones we are discussing here.)

When the repressed hostility of the depressed patient threatens to rise to the surface, it floods him with guilty feelings and anxiousness which become prominent symptoms of his neurotic depression. The patient's inability to express his resentment and anger arises in large part from his desperate need to try continually to seek the affection, approval and esteem of the people around him. In seeking their esteem and affection, any hostile feelings he may have toward them are repressed.

The self-esteem of a person who develops

a neurotic depression is in most cases acutely dependent on the continued affection and support of the persons to whom he is emotionally close; he needs continual reassurance of their love and esteem. His undue sensitivity to the presence or absence of reassuring love originally was developed during early parent-child relationships in which he did not have secure parental love (and got such love from no one else) and was desperately anxious for it. The abrupt withdrawal of the love or esteem of close persons in the patient's adult life floods him with the same lost, anxious, depressed, worthless feeling he had during the painful years of inadequate parental love and esteem in childhood. This basic emotional process may also occur in patients with psychotic depressions, but it is much more severe in them than in persons who develop neurotic depressions.

In a small number of cases a neurotic depression occurs after the death of a person who was emotionally close to the patient; in such cases the patient usually had strong, mixed feelings toward the deceased person. The patient's feelings toward the deceased person were a mixture of affectionate yearning and marked hostility. Both types of feelings are strongly activated by the death, and the patient is flooded with guilt over the hostile feelings he has within him toward the deceased individual. The patient may not be articulately aware of the nature of this turmoil within him; he may be aware only of the guilty feelings and the depressiveness which overwhelm him. This basic process may occur in psychotic depressions as well as neurotic depressions, but in psychotic depressions it is much more severe and malignant.

Clinical Course of Depressive Neuroses

An untreated neurotic depression usually lasts from several months to a year and a half, and then resolves spontaneously. However, some neurotic depressions may last two or three years. Most neurotic depressions have fluctuations during their courses, and they terminate by the gradual improvement of the patient over a course of several weeks or months. The patient usually continues his work or household duties during the course of the depression, but his efficiency is impaired. Psychiatric treatment considerably shortens the duration of neurotic depressions in the majority of instances.

The duration and course of a neurotic depression are affected by (1) the nature of the precipitating event and the severity of its emotional impact on the patient, (2) whether by chance or by intentional search the patient finds other persons or new socioeconomic gratifications to take the place of the person whose esteem and affection he lost or to replace his lost socioeconomic supports, (3) whether or not he suffers new emotional assaults by fresh rejections or losses, (4) the strengths and resources of his basic personality structure, which are largely determined by the nature of the healthy or unhealthy interpersonal relationships the patient experienced during childhood and adolescence, and (5) the timeliness and nature of psychiatric treatment.

When a patient with a neurotic depression suffers repeated emotional rejections or socioeconomic reverses over a period of several years he may undergo a series of neurotic depressions that stretch out over a period of several years or more. Such a patient may present a clinical picture of chronic depressiveness, but careful study of his personality structure and life history usually reveals the occurrence of multiple assaults upon his self-esteem and emotional security.

The good prognosis of the vast majority of neurotic depressions is clouded in occasional cases by the possibility of suicide. Suicide is much less common in patients with the clinical picture of neurotic depression than in patients with psychotic depressions. However, we do not have completely reliable criteria for predicting suicidal risk, and the distinction between neurotic and psychotic depressions (or, as many psychiatrists would prefer, between mild and severe depressions), though it helps in evaluating the possibility of suicidal risk, does not settle the question entirely. (Suicide and the criteria which help in determining its risk are discussed at length in Chapter 15; the management of suicidal patients is also discussed there.)

Treatment of Depressive Neuroses

The two methods of treating depressive

neuroses are (1) psychotherapy and (2) antidepressant medications. Many psychiatrists combine the two treatments; the patient in psychotherapy is also started on an antidepressant medication.

Many psychiatrists feel that exploration of the neurotically depressed patient's emotional problems and interpersonal stresses should continue even when an antidepressant medication clears his depressive symptoms in about 60 days, as it does in about 50 per cent of cases; however, in many instances the patient loses interest in psychotherapy once his symptoms have been removed, and such a patient may remain well for many years or indefinitely.

Psychotherapy of Depressive Neuroses. In psychotherapy, the patient with a neurotic depression should explore the interpersonal crisis that precipitated his depression, and he should analyze gradually the unhealthy interpersonal relationships in his childhood and adolescence whose emotional turmoil has been reactivated by the recent critical events in his life situation.

The therapist often must play a fairly active role in the interview treatment of the depressed patient, because the pessimism and lack of energy of the patient hinder him in free, spontaneous talk about his problems. Moreover, some depressed patients consider themselves unworthy of treatment and feel that the therapist should spend his time with persons who are more worthwhile than themselves. Many depressed patients find it difficult to talk about the emotionally painful events in their lives, and their guilt feelings are temporarily increased by discussing their hostile feelings toward rejecting people in current and past life situations. Some depressed patients fear that when the therapist understands them well he will be revolted by their inadequacies and, by terminating therapy he will reject them in the same manner that others have rejected them in past and current relationships. Because of these problems, and other difficulties, the psychotherapist usually must ask questions, offer comments and make interpretations in a more active way than in the psychotherapy of other types of neuroses if treatment is to be sustained and carried to a successful conclusion.

The patient must explore the repressed hostility he felt in past and current life situations, and he must come to grips with the guilt his hostility mobilizes in him. He must analyze the ways in which emotional rejection and depreciation during his early years left him unduly vulnerable to the emotional impact of rejection and loss of personal prestige in adult life. Often the patient also must explore his mixed feelings of affectionate yearning and hostile resentment toward the people who have rejected him and injured him emotionally. Coming to grips with these aspects of his life often mobilizes anxiety and guilt within him, and he needs the active explanations and interpretations of the therapist to make the process of psychotherapy sufficiently comfortable to ensure that he carries it to a successful termination.

(The general principles and technics of interview treatment are covered at length in Chapter 21, and detailed cases illustrating the general application of psychotherapy in the neuroses have been given in Chapters 7 and 9.)

Antidepressant Medications in Depressive Neuroses. Antidepressant medications are useful in selected patients with neurotic depressions. It is now generally agreed that, of the two available groups of antidepressant drugs, the tricyclic compounds are more effective and have a much lower incidence of serious side effects; the tricyclic compounds include imipramine (Tofranil), amitriptyline (Elavil), desipramine (Norpramin, Pertofrane), nortriptyline (Aventyl) and others.

The second group of antidepressant medications are the monoamine oxidase inhibitors, which include isocarboxazid (Marplan), nialamide (Niamid), phenelzine (Nardil) and others; a typical viewpoint of these medications is that of the American Medical Association's Council on Drugs which, in its publication *AMA Drug Evaluations*, recommends that, because of their lesser efficacy and potentially more serious adverse effects, the monoamine oxidase inhibitors should be used only in patients with a history of response to these drugs in previous depressions and patients who have not responded to tricyclic antidepressants. (The pharmacology, dosages, and possible complications of these medications are covered in Chapter 22.)

We shall discuss here the clinical criteria for

selecting the particular patients with neurotic depressions who are good candidates to benefit from their use. However, since serious adverse reactions to tricyclic antidepressants are immensely rare, many psychiatrists employ them routinely in neurotic depressions, after explaining to the patient that the drug may not be successful and that therapy will then consist mainly of psychotherapy, which can begin concomitantly with the employment of the antidepressant.

The mode of action of antidepressant medications is not known, although various biochemical theories have been advanced. However, clinical experience has shown that when the following clinical features are present in a neurotic depression there is increased chance that the patient will respond favorably:

1. The depression has a fairly clear-cut time of onset, before which the patient had functioned well emotionally for a period of several years or more.

2. The patient has marked feelings of worthlessness and guiltiness, and these feelings are present most of the time, though they may fluctuate somewhat in intensity.

3. There is a fairly consistent diurnal pattern in the patient's symptoms; he feels worse in the mornings and somewhat better in the afternoons and evenings.

4. The life history of the patient prior to the onset of his depression reveals little evidence of significant psychiatric disturbance, with the possible exception of one or two other clear-cut episodes of depression from which he completely recovered in time; he does not have a long history of various kinds of neurotic problems such as phobias, obsessions and conversion symptoms.

5. The patient has a weight loss of more than five pounds. Weight loss in a depressed patient is often a useful indicator of the degree of loss of appetite and loss of interest in life activities in general.

The patient whose clinical picture includes all five of these features has a good chance of responding favorably to antidepressant medication. When one or more of these characteristics are not present in the patient's clinical picture he has a much smaller chance of responding favorably to antidepressant medication.

When any of the following features are present in the patient's clinical picture, he is *unlikely* to respond favorably to antidepressant medication:

1. The patient has marked fluctuations in his depression; he may feel relatively well one day and very depressed the next day.

2. The patient has a long history of various kinds of neurotic symptoms, such as anxiety states and phobias, and it may be difficult to pinpoint any particular time as the time of onset of his current emotional upset.

3. The patient does not feel guilty or worthless; he feels that he has been mistreated and exploited by other people and he glibly blames them for his depressiveness and agitation.

When the patient's clinical picture includes one or more of these features, his chance of a favorable response to antidepressant medication is much reduced.

In my experience, when patients with neurotic depressions are carefully selected and meet all the criteria listed above, about 50 per cent of them will have a favorable response to antidepressant medication (the percentage of favorable responses in the *severe* depressions discussed in Chapter 15 is significantly higher). The dosage of the antidepressant medication must be large enough to be effective and the medication must be continued long enough for a thorough trial. (These details are discussed in Chapter 22.) As noted above, whenever possible, antidepressant medication should be accompanied by psychotherapy to explore the interpersonal roots of the patient's disorder.

Further Aspects of Managing Depressive Neuroses. As a rule, the patient with a neurotic depression should be urged to continue working at his usual job or routine. Rest at home and vacations usually do not help him. They often hinder his progress, because he feels even more guilty and worthless because he is not doing his usual job and handling his regular responsibilities.

The patient should not make any major life decisions during a depressive period. For example, he should not change jobs or make major financial decisions. The pessimism of a depressed patient and his low opinion of himself do not allow him to exercise his best possible judgement.

Some psychiatrists occasionally recommend a brief period of psychiatric hospitalization for a patient with a neurotic depression. The period of hospitalization may be used to facilitate daily contacts at the beginning of psychotherapy, or it may remove the patient temporarily from painful stresses at home until he is better able to handle them. Occasionally, psychiatric hospitalization is recommended when the patient seems to present suicidal risk. However, the vast majority of patients with neurotic depressions do not need psychiatric hospitalization and are best treated entirely on an outpatient basis. Electroshock therapy is not advisable in patients with neurotic depressions; it should be considered only in well selected patients with the more severe depressions (discussed in Chapter 15).

NEURASTHENIC NEUROSIS

The term *neurasthenic neurosis* is included in the current standard psychiatric nomenclature, which was issued in 1968; the word *neurasthenia* is given as a synonym of neurasthenic neurosis. For many years prior to 1968 neurasthenic neurosis was not included in the official American system of psychiatric diagnoses, and its reintroduction in 1968 was mainly to make American psychiatric diagnoses consonant with the diagnostic system promulgated by the World Health Organization; the World Health Organization's nomenclature markedly reflects the influence of continental European and Soviet psychiatric concepts.

As defined in the official system of nomenclature, a neurasthenic neurosis is characterized chiefly by a profound state of fatigue, or exhaustion. This fatigue state often is accompanied by anxiousness, mild depressiveness, insomnia and vague physical complaints. The terms *asthenia* and *psychasthenia* have occasionally been employed either as synonyms of neurasthenia or to designate closely similar states.

Few American psychiatrists feel that neurasthenic neurosis is a valid clinical concept, and the diagnosis is rarely used. Harry Stack Sullivan, for example, dismissed "so-called neurasthenia" as an ill-advised, poorly defined synonym for a mild depressive condition in which fatigue was a prominent symptom.

Fatigue is common in many kinds of emotional disorders, and to raise it to the level of a diagnostic category is no more valid than to use "fever" or "abdominal pain" as diagnoses. Most psychiatrists in the English-speaking countries therefore feel that the patient's basic emotional disorder should be diagnosed, and fatigue should be recognized as merely one of various symptoms of it.

The psychiatric disorders in which fatigue may be a major symptom include: (1) depressive disorders (both depressive neuroses and depressive psychoses), in which fatigue is characteristically a prominent symptom; (2) conversion neuroses, in which fatigue and weakness may be conversion symptoms, often intermingled with other conversion impairments; (3) anxiety neuroses, in which fatigue is produced by constant muscular tension due to anxiety; (4) early schizophrenic disorders, in which social withdrawal and early catatonic features may be inaccurately labeled fatigue; (5) phobic neuroses, in which the fatigue is secondary to the anxiety and tension of the patient and in which it also may be used to justify social inactivity in patients who fear social situations; and (6) other emotional disorders, such as some prostrating psychosomatic illnesses, in which fatigue is a prominent symptom. In each of these instances the physician must recognize that fatigue, which at times may be the patient's presenting complaint, is merely a symptom of some underlying process which must be identified accurately to allow correct treatment.

DEPERSONALIZATION NEUROSIS

The term *depersonalization neurosis* (of which *depersonalization syndrome* is an officially specified synonym) was introduced for the first time into the American standard psychiatric nomenclature in 1968 as part of the effort to make it similar to the diagnostic system advocated by the World Health Organization. This diagnosis, however, is very rarely employed in the English-speaking countries.

As discussed in Chapter 3, depersonalization, *as a symptom*, is an affective state in which a person has a persistent, eerie feeling that he and his environment have undergone a strange, unreal change. The individual feels estranged from himself, his body and his surroundings, though usually he cannot describe this estrangement clearly. Depersonalization may occur as a minor, often brief, feeling in early schizophrenic disorders, depressions, dissociative neuroses and some other psychiatric conditions. It may occur in some normal persons who are under unusual stress or in unfamiliar settings.

In over a quarter century of psychiatric work I have never seen a patient who fitted the diagnostic category of depersonalization neurosis, nor have I ever heard another psychiatrist refer to one of his patients as having this condition. A careful inventory of the published works of Harry Stack Sullivan reveals no reference to depersonalization, as either a symptom or a neurosis. Moreover, I could find only one reference to depersonalization in all of Freud's writings; he considered it as a transitory symptom, not a neurosis, in a letter written in 1936, which is included in his collected papers.

HYPOCHONDRIACAL NEUROSIS

Psychiatrists differ much in opinion about the concept of hypochondriacal neurosis and the use of this term. Only a minority of American psychiatrists use this expression in their day-to-day work with patients, and many psychiatrists object strongly to it. However, the number of psychiatrists who accept the concept of hypochondriacal neurosis is sufficiently large to justify detailed consideration of it.

We shall divide our discussion of hypochondriacal neurosis into two parts: (1) the concept of hypochondriacal neurosis, and (2) objections to the concept of hypochondriacal neurosis.

The Concept of Hypochondriacal Neurosis

The patient with a hypochondriacal neurosis is markedly preoccupied with his body functions and often feels that he has various kinds of diseases and physical dysfunctions. He discusses his symptoms, body sensations, medical treatments and diagnoses at length; these subjects occupy a large part of his conversation, and often it is difficult to divert him onto other topics. He may medicate himself with many kinds of nonprescriptive drugs and compounds, and he frequently consults physicians and nonmedical therapists of various kinds. Some hypochondriacs are gloomily worried much of the time, whereas others chat glibly and pleasantly about their many complaints. Their symptoms may cover the entire range of organ systems, but headaches, fatigue, insomnia, vague upper gastrointestinal complaints, constipation, low backache, chest pain, indistinct discomforts in the genital and perineal regions, low abdominal pain, pelvic pain, anxiousness and mild depressiveness are common. The diseases which the hypochondriacal patient most often fears are cancer, heart disease, venereal disease, obscure metabolic and hormonal imbalances, and vague neurological degenerations.

The course of hypochondriacal neuroses, as described in the psychiatric literature, tends to be chronic. However, this may be because the hypochondriacs who consult psychiatrists do so only after years of consultations and treatment by nonpsychiatric physicians. By the time they see psychiatrists their neuroses are ingrained. Persons who develop mild or moderate hypochondriacal neuroses perhaps recover in time, as their situational stresses lessen, and they may never arrive in psychiatric clinics and offices. For perhaps similar reasons, the psychiatric literature reflects a pessimistic view of the treatment of these patients; few of them are willing to embark on a systematic trial of psychotherapy, and those who do are often unable to talk on any level other than that of their symptoms and trivial life experiences. Many hypochondriacal patients are frankly skeptical that their problems are emotional, and reject a psychiatric approach.

It is frequently stated in the psychiatric literature that hypochondriacal patients have a much greater probability of developing schizophrenic psychoses and paranoid states than persons in the general population. I do not feel this is so. However, patients who are gradually slipping into schizophrenia, especially paranoid schizophrenia, may go through a several-week or several-month phase of intense body preoccupation and obsessive fear of disease. Often their fears of disease slowly become bizarre; for example, preoccupations with vague upper gastrointestinal complaints may in time become delusional beliefs that their internal organs "have all rotted away and there is nothing left inside" or that physicians and relatives are conspiring in malicious ways to hide their true physical states from them. In my opinion, the schizophrenic who passes through a hypochondriacal phase and the person with an ingrained hypochondriacal neurosis have quite separate types of disorders.

Freud wrote little about hypochondriasis; he himself suffered from multiple physical complaints during much of his adult life, and some of his biographers have speculated that he may have had a mild hypochondriacal tendency. Later psychoanalysts have advanced the suggestion that in a hypochondriacal neurosis the patient has bound up his libidinal (including sexual) urges and conflicts in various body organs and regions, and has become overly concerned with them. His anxiety has become invested in an all-consuming preoccupation with parts of his body and fears of diseases about them, thus deflecting anxiety from its original emotional sources. Other Freudian-psychoanalytic writers have speculated that the hypochondriacal patient has regressed to, or is fixed at, the infantile emotional level in which the person's concern focuses entirely on his own body, and the outside world is still nebulous and indistinct to him.

Harry Stack Sullivan, in his lectures and writings, dealt extensively with hypochondriasis. He felt that the basic process in a hypochondriacal neurosis was a shift of emotional interest from disturbing interpersonal relationships, both past and present, to an intense preoccupation with body functions and diseases. This may occur in a person with a prevailing negative, pessimistic view of himself and low self-esteem. Such personality problems tend to be produced by a persistent climate of censure, depreciation and disapproval throughout an individual's formative years, leaving him with feelings of social inferiority and worthlessness. These feelings often border on despair, especially as the future hypochondriacal person suffers one interpersonal failure after another during late childhood and adolescence. He becomes convinced (though he rarely is articulately aware of it) that he is not capable of being fully human, and he ceases to make both friendly and hostile contacts with people. As a result, his capacity to evaluate accurately his relationships with people, and to correct his maladjustments with them, deteriorates.

As the result of these personality impairments, Sullivan felt, the hypochondriacal person restructures all his interpersonal relationships on the level of continual discussions of his body sensations, symptoms, possible diseases, treatments and medical consultations. This becomes the façade he presents in all relationships with people; it is his only way of dealing with them. He is not looking for sympathy; on the contrary, his preoccupation with symptoms and constant discussion of them are barriers to intimacy and true rapport with people, since he found close relationships with people pervasively painful during his childhood and early adolescence. Nevertheless, he still wants to relate to people on some level, and he uses talk about his physical condition as a safe, neutral way to maintain such contact without becoming intimate and truly involved with them.

By his hypochondriasis the patient also blunts anxiety, turning it away from past and present interpersonal traumas and channeling it into body overconcern. All other aspects of his life recede in importance, as body functioning and feared diseases occupy his attention.

During the first decade, or more, of his psychiatric career, Sullivan devoted himself almost exclusively to the study of schizophrenia, and it remained one of his major professional interests throughout his life. Perhaps due to this, Sullivan felt that there was a rather fluid continuum between hypochondriasis and paranoid schizophrenia. He felt that, when under marked interpersonal stress or when undergoing strong internal turmoil, the hypochondriac has a tendency to shift his feelings of blame, guiltiness and worthlessness from himself to others; by the process of feeling "not I, but they," he finds release from mounting anxiety and guilt, and shifts his concern to others who he feels are persecuting him. As indicated above, many other psychiatrists, including myself, feel this is not so; schizophrenics may pass through hypochondriacal phases, but ingrained hypochondriacs rarely pass through schizophrenic phases.

Objections to the Concept of Hypochondriacal Neurosis

Many American psychiatrists, including myself, object strongly to both the concept and the term of hypochondriacal neurosis, and view its reintroduction into the standard nomenclature in 1968 as an unfortunate concession to the opinions of continental European and Soviet psychiatrists, who insisted that it be included in the World Health Organization's system of diagnoses.

Many psychiatrists feel that there is no clear-cut diagnostic category of hypochondriacal neurosis, and that this is merely a catch-all term for patients with other kinds of psychiatric disorders who have, as one of their major clinical features, marked preoccupation with body functioning and diseases. The psychiatric disorders in which body overconcern may be a significant feature are: (1) anxiety neuroses in which patients fear that the physical concomitants of anxiety (palpitation, muscle tension headaches, upper gastrointestinal complaints, and many others) are signs of physical illness; (2) obsessive neuroses in which the patient's major obsessions are fears of illness (this, and chronic anxiety neuroses, probably are the most common causes of the so-called hypochondriacal neuroses); (3) multiple conversion hysterical symptoms in patients who also have obsessive fears of diseases based on their conversion symptoms (this occurs particularly in conversion pain syndromes and other conversion sensory disturbances); (4) bizarre body concerns in early schizophrenics; (5) preoccupation over body dysfunctions in some depressed patients; and (6) preoccupation about body sensations and dysfunctions in persons with some kinds of personality disorders, especially schizoid personality disorders.

Most American psychiatrists feel that the term hypochondriasis should not be used since it has no specific psychopathological or clinical meaning. Moreover, in some circles the word hypochondriasis carries the connotation that the patient is an immature, aggravating person who could "snap out of it" if he really wanted to. The word hypochondriasis (or hypochondriacal neurosis) leads to inaccurate, foggy thinking. It disguises from both the doctor and the patient the true difficulty from which the patient is suffering, and it prevents the formulation of adequate treatment plans. Good medical treatment requires that the physician penetrate beyond the patient's concern about his body and preoccupation about illness and deal with the specific emotional disorder lying beneath this façade.

A further objection to this term in the standard nomenclature is that its use on hospital charts and clinic records, and its subsequent transposition to insurance reports and vocational records, can gravely damage the patient's vocational, economic and social interests. Insurance companies are loath to write policies on people who carry this label, and employers and their workmen's compensation insurers are leary of employing such people. To many laymen, and to all too many nonpsychiatric persons in the health professions, the term "hypochondriasis," or "hypochondriacal neurosis," indicates that the patient's condition is either hopeless or of his own invention. Such ideas are so ingrained in popular usage, and it is so widely believed that "hypochondriacs" are unreliable people or troublemakers, that it would require decades of public education to alter such prejudices. In general lay usage the term hypochondriac is often used as an epithet of ridicule, insult or scorn.

BIBLIOGRAPHY

Alarcon, R., and Covi, L.: Hysterical personality and depression. Compr. Psychiatry, *14*:121, 1973.

Covi, L., et al.: Drugs and group psychotherapy in neurotic depression. Am. J. Psychiatry, *131*: 186, 1974.

Friedman, A. S.: Hostility factors and clinical improvement in depressed patients. Arch. Gen. Psychiatry, *23*:524, 1970.

Hamilton, J. W.: Masked depression: progressive somatization as a response to object loss. Psychiat. Quart., *44*:583, 1970.

Jacobsen, E.: Depression: Comparative Studies of Normal, Neurotic, and Psychotic Conditions. New York, International Universities Press, 1972.

Ladee, G. A.: Hypochondriacal Syndromes. New York, Elsevier Publishing Co., 1966.

Lesse, S.: Hypochondriasis and psychosomatic disorders masking depression. Am. J. Psychother., *21*:607, 1967.

Lorand, S.: Adolescent depressions. Int. J. Psychoanal., *48*:53, 1967.

Myers, D. H., and Grant, G.: A study of depersonalization in students. Brit. J. Psychiatry, *121*:59, 1972.

Poznanski, E., and Zrull, J. P.: Childhood depressions. Arch. Gen. Psychiatry, *23*:8, 1970.

Sullivan, H. S.: Studies in Clinical Psychiatry. Chapter on hypochondria, p. 77. New York, W. W. Norton, 1956.

Tucker, G. T., Harrow, M., and Quinlan, D.: Depersonalization, dysphoria, and thought disturbance. Am. J. Psychiatry, *130*:702, 1973.

Wineberg, E. N., and Straker, N.: An episode of acute, self-limiting depersonalization following a first session of hypnosis. Am. J. Psychiatry, *130*:98, 1973.

Wolpe, J.: Neurotic depression: experimental analog, clinical syndromes, and treatment. Am. J. Psychother., *25*:362, 1971.

Uhlenhuth, E. H., and Paykel, E. S.: Symptom intensity and life events. Arch. Gen. Psychiatry, *28*:473, 1973.

Section Two

Psychosomatic Illness

Psychiatry and general medicine meet intimately in the study and treatment of psychosomatic illness. These disorders require comprehensive understanding of patients from both the organic and the interpersonal points of view. The following chapter presents the basic principles of psychosomatic medicine. It deals with the close interaction of physical and interpersonal functioning in each patient, and it presents a discussion of the various illnesses in which emotional factors play important etiologic roles.

11

The Common Psychosomatic Illnesses

The patient with a psychosomatic illness has a physical disease partially or entirely caused by emotional factors. The particular dysfunction in a psychosomatic illness may be physiologic, as in the irritable colon syndrome (mucous colitis), or it may lead to an anatomic lesion, as in peptic ulcer.

However, some psychiatrists employ the concept of psychosomatic medicine in a broader way. The course of a physical illness may be influenced by the emotional state and the morale of the patient even when emotional factors do not play a role in causing it. For example, the course of a patient with tuberculosis is often influenced by his emotional state. A depressed tuberculous patient with little desire to get well and little interest in following his medical regimen often does more poorly than an optimistic patient with a strong desire to recover. Thus, emotional factors may be important in affecting the course and outcome of an illness even when they did not play a role in causing it.

Psychosomatic medicine in its broadest sense stresses the intimate interaction of interpersonal and physical functioning in health and disease. It involves the study of the whole person. It insists that each disease must be seen as a disorder occurring in a particular person, with all his emotional forces and interpersonal relationships. It proposes that one cannot study a disease and ignore the person who has it.

In the official standard nomenclature of diseases the psychosomatic illnesses are classified as "psychophysiologic" disorders. For example, a duodenal ulcer is classified under psychophysiologic gastrointestinal disorders, and a hyperventilation syndrome is listed under the psychophysiologic respiratory disorders. However, the word "psychosomatic" is more widely used by physicians in talking about patients. The terms "psychosomatic" and "psychophysiologic" are synonymous.

In this chapter we shall consider some of the diseases in which emotional forces play important etiologic roles. We shall limit ourselves to those conditions generally accepted as psychosomatic and pay little attention to those in which the role of emotional factors is controversial or minor.

THE MULTIPLE LEVELS OF DISORDER IN PSYCHOSOMATIC ILLNESS

A psychosomatic illness may be visualized as a disease caused by disturbances on multiple levels of physical and interpersonal functioning. For example, the peptic ulcer of the patient in Figure 11-1 may be viewed diagrammatically as occurring on seven levels of dysfunction.

1. The duodenal ulcer of the patient in Figure 11-1 may be viewed as the result of prolonged hypervascularity, hyperacidity and hypermotility of the upper gastrointestinal tract, which in time lead to fragmentation of the duodenal mucosa and formation of the ulcer.

2. The autonomic nervous system and other physiologic pathways convey to the upper gastrointestinal tract the stimuli causing hypervascularity, hyperacidity and hypermotility. They thus participate in the etiology of the ulcer.

3. The hypothalamus, the autonomic nervous centers near the floor of the third ventricles, and other lower brain areas participate in the production and transmission of the excitatory impulses that flow to the upper

184 *The Common Psychosomatic Illnesses*

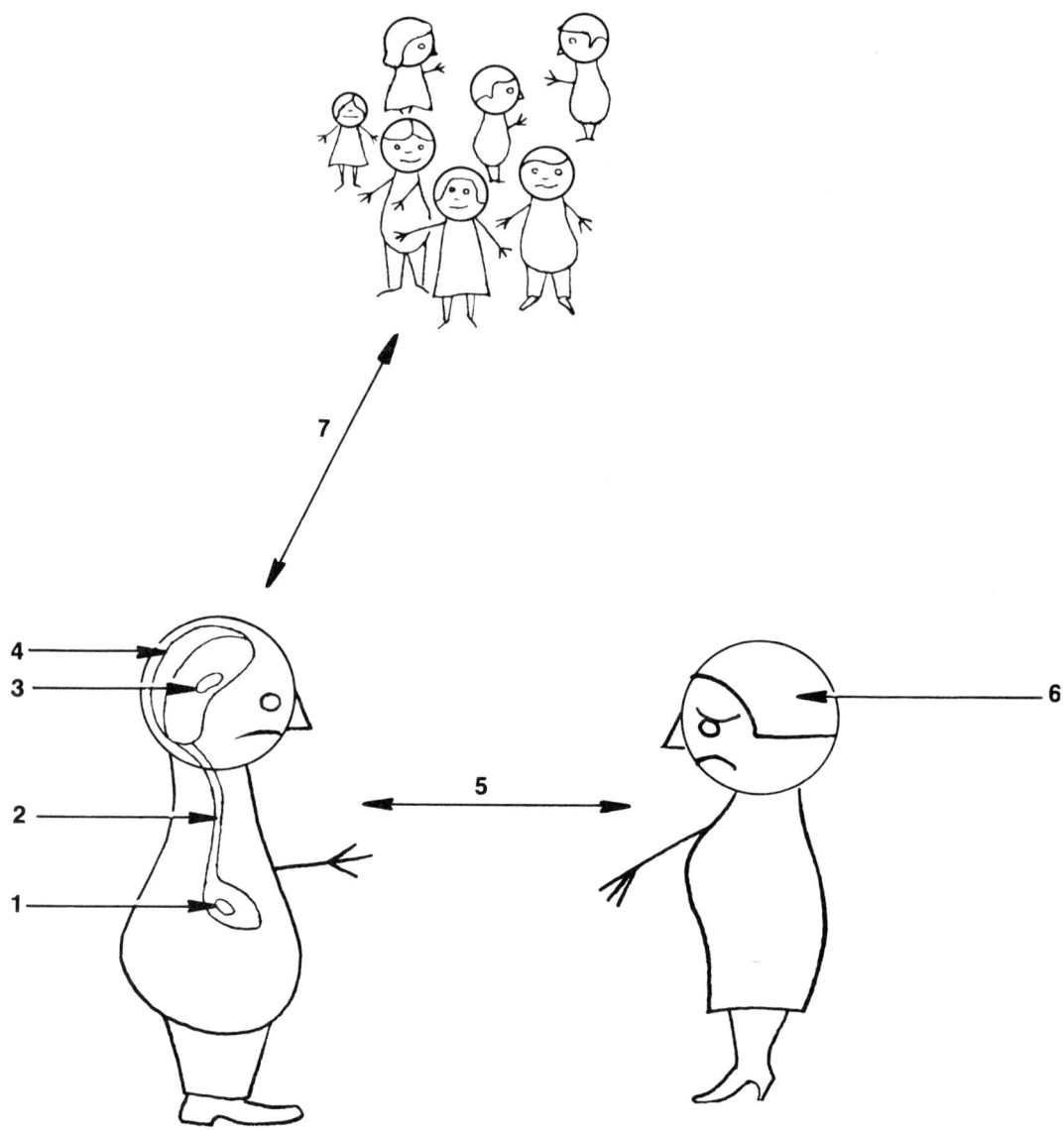

Fig. 11-1

gastrointestinal tract and cause its distorted functioning.

4. The patient's emotional life on its highest conscious and symbolic level is a function of the cerebral cortex. The memories and associations of the patient are stored here, and his interpersonal experiences and feelings are correlated and interpreted. Tensions of his past and present life may be transmitted from the cerebral cortex to lower brain centers, including the hypothalamus, and down the chain to the level of the gastrointestinal tract.

5. Major stresses in the patient's life may arise in a traumatic relationship with his emotionally upset wife. These interpersonal stresses keep the patient in continual emotional turmoil and constitute a further level of etiology in his psychosomatic disorder.

6. The disturbing behavior of his wife may in turn be due to personality problems in her.

These personality problems, arising out of her past and present interpersonal traumas, therefore constitute an additional level of etiology in the patient's psychosomatic illness.

7. The duodenal ulcer of the patient may also be influenced by social and economic forces in the community in which he lives. For example, if he is danger of losing his job or being demoted because of a business recession, or if he is distressed about the rising amount of street violence and illicit drug usage in his neighborhood, his ulcer may become worse. This is sometimes referred to as the psychosocial level of a psychosomatic illness.

Despite the fact that this type of schematization condenses many intricate details into a simple diagram, it is a useful way to make the psychosomatic approach to disease graphic and clear. In reality, patients are complex wholes, and any subdivision of their functioning introduces arbitrary and oversimplified concepts. The division of functions outlined in Figure 11-1 is a convenience to help us simplify data and think clearly about patients. Moreover, this type of drawing can be used by the physician in explaining to a patient what a psychosomatic illness is, and how interpersonal and organic factors interweave to produce a physical disease. To attempt to explain or understand a psychosomatic illness without such simplification is to risk becoming lost in vague generalities that lack clarity and emphasis. The practice of medicine requires that we flexibly bend our concepts and methods to meet the daily needs of patients.

Just as the concept of multiple levels of etiology has important connotations on the nature of psychosomatic illness, it has much to say about the types of treatment that should be given. If an illness is determined on multiple levels of functioning, it is best to treat it on these multiple levels. Thus, treatment of the local lesion should also be accompanied by attention to at least one or two levels of emotional and interpersonal difficulty. We shall cover the management of psychosomatic illness in the last section of this chapter.

We shall now proceed to discuss the various psychosomatic illnesses. We shall limit our attention to illnesses in which important psychosomatic correlations are generally accepted and well established; we shall not discuss those illnesses in which psychosomatic factors are controversial.

VARIOUS PSYCHOSOMATIC ILLNESSES

PSYCHOSOMATIC GASTROINTESTINAL DISORDERS

The gastrointestinal tract is subject to continual fluctuations in vascularity, motility and secretion. The autonomic innervation of the gastrointestinal tract is intricate and rich, and through autonomic pathways and other physiological channels, emotional states can cause rapid changes in gastrointestinal functioning. Hence, psychosomatic symptoms are common in all sections of the gastrointestinal tract. If one includes such complaints as "heartburn," "bloating" and vague dyspepsias, it is probable that 70 per cent of all gastrointestinal problems have psychosomatic factors.

Peptic Ulcer

Various kinds of emotional turmoil and interpersonal stress produce hypervascularity, hypersecretion and hypermotility of the upper gastrointestinal tract. When hypervascularity, hypersecretion and hypermotility are prolonged and severe, they lead to fragility and eventual fragmentation of its mucous membrane. Once the mucous membrane is broken, the continued hyperactivity of the upper gastrointestinal tract rapidly leads to ulcer formation, and the same hyperactivity that caused the ulcer tends to prevent its healing.

Many psychiatric studies have been made of patients with peptic ulcers. These studies indicate that persons with peptic ulcers often have profound, unmet yearnings for affection, and they have strong needs to be emotionally dependent on other people. However, these needs often are hidden behind a façade of bustling self-sufficiency and an anxious drive to succeed in vocational and social activities. The energetic drive of the patient with a peptic ulcer serves both to cover his deeper feelings of insecurity and to gain the recognition and esteem of people around him. Ulcer formation tends to occur when his needs for affection and for close relationships with important people in his life are not met; this may occur when the patient has stresses in his interpersonal relationships or when he suffers, or fears he will suffer, vocational or social setbacks that may lower him in the esteem and affection of other people.

In his anxiousness to be well liked, the patient with a peptic ulcer often stifles his hostile feelings and gives them little expression. When, on occasion, he gives limited expression to his hostile feelings as he pushes ahead in his drive for achievement, he is upset by them. His pent-up hostility smolders within him and gains partial, unhealthy expression through his hyperactive upper gastrointestinal tract.

However, some patients with peptic ulcers are socially retiring and unassertive in their interpersonal relationships. They are dependent, passive people who suppress all hostile and aggressive feelings, and they lack the façade of energetic accomplishment that characterizes many patients with peptic ulcers. These patients are prone to develop ulcers when they are emotionally exploited by others because of their passivity, or when they feel threatened with the loss of the affection of the people who are emotionally close to them.

Various psychiatric studies indicate that in many instances the patient who develops a peptic ulcer did not have warm, affectionate acceptance by his parents during his childhood. He emerged from childhood with profound unmet needs for love, and he has deep yearnings to be dependent on people who will give him the esteem and affection he did not have during his formative years. Both literally and figuratively, he is chronically hungry for affection. Some psychiatrists feel that in some instances the original emotional trauma of the patient with a peptic ulcer begins during the first year of life when the major mother-child contacts are centered around feeding the child; the child does not receive affection and emotional warmth at this time, and the same coldness is also carried into the later years of his upbringing. Hence, upper gastorintestinal functioning and the presence or absence of affection become emotionally linked. The hyperactive state of a hungry stomach becomes joined to feelings of unmet interpersonal needs for affection. When in adult life the patient's needs for affection are not met, he responds again with hyperactivity of the upper gastrointestinal tract; prolonged hypervascularity, hypersecretion and hypermotility lead in time to ulcer formation.

In the comprehensive medical management of a peptic ulcer, attention should be given to any current interpersonal stresses in the patient's life and to any personality problems causing him chronic discomfort in his relationships with people. When the ulcer is of recent origin and the patient has many personality strengths but has been under much recent tension, the family physician or internist may expand his medical regimen by including at least a brief inquiry into these areas. When the patient's emotional problems are ingrained and are deeply rooted in severe emotional trauma in his early life, such work should be undertaken only by a psychiatrist.

Ulcerlike Disorders

Emotional problems may produce a variety of symptoms caused by disturbed vascularity, secretion and motility of the stomach and duodenum. Many of these symptoms fall into the category of the ulcerlike syndromes which, however, are not associated with actual ulcer formation. Patients describe these difficulties as "heartburn," "bloating," "gas," "acid stomach," and other vague dyspepsias. In states of anxiety, insecurity and suppressed hostility, the upper gastrointestinal tract tends to be hypervascular, hypersecretive and hypermotile, leading to ulcerlike symptoms. In depression, the stomach and the duodenum are hypovascular, hyposecretive and hypomotile, leading to anorexia and vague dyspeptic symptoms.

Ulcerative Colitis

Emotional turmoil may produce hypervascularity, hypersecretion and hypermotility of the lower gastrointestinal tract. Prolonged lower gastrointestinal hyperactivity may lead in time to fragility and fragmentation of the colonic mucosa, and ulceration occurs. Subsequent infection in the ulcerated tissue and scarring complete the ominous picture of chronic ulcerative colitis. Many physicians who have carried out comprehensive studies of ulcerative colitis feel that emotional problems play a significant part in causing this illness, but many investigators feel that other factors, as yet undiscovered, must also play roles in its etiology. It should also be pointed out that many internists and gastroenterologists feel that there is little conclusive evidence that ulcerative colitis is a psychosomatic disease.

Many psychiatric studies have been made of patients with ulcerative colitis. In many instances, the patient with ulcerative colitis has much repressed rage and hostility which stem from traumatic interpersonal relationships both in his childhood years and in his current interpersonal relationships. His repressed hostility first arose in his relationships with harsh, demanding parents who left him with deep wells of bitter resentment. However, both in his early years and in his adult life he hides his feelings behind a façade of brittle self-control.

Psychiatrists often describe the patient with ulcerative colitis as a person whose hostility seeps out in bitter sarcasm and in subtly hostile actions in his dealings with people. Beneath this outer crust, however, the patient has marked needs for affection and a yearning to be dependent on a giving, protecting mother-like figure. Exacerbations of his ulcerative colitis often occur shortly after stressful events that threaten his emotional security or mobilize much rage within him. When his hostile feelings rise strongly to the surface, the patient may feel guilty and worthless; hence, the patient with ulcerative colitis tends to have periodic episodes of mild to moderate depressiveness. It has long been observed that if a patient with ulcerative colitis becomes severely depressed over a prolonged period of time, his ulcerative colitis undergoes a remission.

These emotional factors have a marked effect on the physiology of the colon. The repressed rage, the aching dependency needs and the chronic seepage of repressed hostility into his interpersonal relationships produce long-lasting hypervascularity, hypersecretion and hypermotility of the colon. The same hyperactivity that contributed to the etiology of the ulcerative colitis hinders the healing of the lesions once they are produced.

The results of psychotherapy in ulcerative colitis are difficult to evaluate. Since the disease is characterized by periodic remissions and exacerbations in a long, fluctuating course, it is difficult to ascertain if improvement that occurred during psychotherapy was due to the interview treatment or merely coincident with it. Moreover, the patients must be followed for many years or even decades to determine if psychotherapy influenced the eventual course and outcome of the disease. Many psychiatrists agree that psychotherapy often gives short-term improvement in these patients, but they disagree about the long-term results. In my opinion, the physician who is caring for a patient with ulcerative colitis should inquire into the patient's interpersonal life and should evaluate any personality characteristics causing him chronic emotional discomfort. When the patient is motivated to try a psychiatric approach, he should have the benefit of a trial of psychotherapy by a psychiatrist. Often the psychiatrist must be liberal with his interpretations, and he must give the patient many reassurances to assuage the anxiety and guilt that arise as the patient discusses his repressed anger and his bitterness about the interpersonal traumas of his life.

Ulcerative colitis is often a grim disease. Bowel perforation, peritonitis, hemorrhage, electrolyte disturbances, severe emaciation and other complications give it a varying but significant mortality rate throughout its various clinical stages. In patients who have had the disease for 10 years or more the incidence of secondary carcinoma of the bowel runs as high as 20 per cent in some series. Hence, psychiatric care must be carried out only in conjunction with careful medical care, and in some instances surgical intervention is necessary.

Irritable Colon Syndrome

The syndrome long known as mucous colitis or spastic colon is now called "irritable colon syndrome" or "adaptive colitis" by many writers on this subject. The disorder consists of fluctuating, varied symptoms of diarrhea, colonic cramping, delayed colonic evacuation, secretion of mucus in the stools, diffuse abdominal discomfort and poor appetite. An irritable colon syndrome may last for a week or so, or it may be present for many years. It may occur intermittently, with long remissions, or it may be a persistent difficulty.

A large percentage of cases of irritable colon are caused by emotional factors. In other instances similar clinical pictures may be due to food incompatibilities, improper dietary habits or residual colonic irritability after long-continued, low grade bacterial or protozoan infections of the lower gastrointestinal tract.

Irritable colon may be caused by various kinds of emotional distress. In many instances brief episodes of irritable colon occur in people who are reasonably well adjusted emotionally but are undergoing temporary situational stresses. For example, difficult job situations, marital problems and economic pressures may precipitate brief periods of irritable colon. The emotional stress produces fluctuating hypermotility or spasm of the colonic musculature. Brief episodes of colonic hyperactivity produce the periods of diarrhea.

Irritable colon may be a physical concomitant of a chronic anxiety neurosis. (Any of the personality problems and interpersonal stresses outlined in Chapter 6 in our discussion of chronic anxiety neuroses may cause irritable colon.) Thus, it may occur in association with a wide variety of different kinds of interpersonal stresses and personality structures. It may occur in an aggressive, self-confident businessman who is under much tension from business problems, and it may occur in a passive, retiring housewife who has difficulties in rearing her children and dealing with troublesome neighbors. A brief period of irritable colon may occur in a student who is approaching important examinations for which he fears he may not be well prepared. Irritable colon, in both its brief and chronic forms, is a common disorder encountered in medical practice. Investigation of traumatic aspects of the patient's interpersonal life and correlation of exacerbations of irritable colon with stressful events often constitute an important aspect of the patient's treatment.

Nausea and Vomiting

Nausea and vomiting often are caused by emotional stress. Much emotionally caused nausea and vomiting are so clearly associated with life stresses that the patient sees the connection and does not seek medical attention. In other instances, the relationship is not clear, and the patient comes to the physician with acute or chronic nausea and vomiting as his chief complaints.

Nausea and vomiting sometimes are associated with acute anxiety neuroses. (All the causes of acute anxiety states that are discussed in Chapter 6 may contribute to psychogenic nausea and vomiting.) Sometimes the patient presents nausea and vomiting as his only symptoms, and careful interviewing is required to uncover the acute anxiety states that lie behind his gastrointestinal symptoms. Chronic, intermittent nausea, which may occur daily or several times each week, is a common symptom in chronic anxiety neuroses.

Nausea and vomiting are prone to occur in some people when they are threatened with the loss or alienation of an emotionally close person. I recall a burly lieutenant in the Marines who vomited and retched for 24 hours after his wife asked him for a divorce. Psychogenic nausea and vomiting often occur in children with school phobias (which are discussed in Chapter 7). These children may have nausea and vomiting on each school morning for several months or more. Emotionally caused nausea sometimes occurs in patients with phobias of crowds and public places; the marked anxiousness of the phobia causes nausea whenever the patient prepares to go into a crowd or public place, and in time the nausea acquires the secondary gain of excusing the patient from participating in social situations in which he is uncomfortable. I have seen entrenched psychogenic nausea of several decades' duration in phobic patients of this type.

The syndrome of nausea and vomiting that occurs when a person travels in an automobile, bus, airplane, boat or other vehicle is termed *motion sickness*. Much motion sickness is caused by unusual stimulation of the vestibular apparatus of the inner ear when the person is in motion. However, in some instances motion sickness is partially or entirely caused by emotional factors. Fear of traveling in automobiles, airplanes or other vehicles may be causes behind the nausea or vomiting, and careful evaluation of the patient sometimes is needed to uncover this. In some patients the fear of traveling in a particular kind of vehicle, most often airplanes or automobiles, is so severe and invariable that it constitutes a true phobia, of which the nausea and vomiting are superficial physical symptoms.

Infantile Colic

Infantile colic often is due to anxiousness and rage in a baby who feels the anxiety, coldness or irritability of his mother as she goes through her daily tasks of caring for him. Though half of all cases of infantile colic are due to dietary incompatibilities and food allergies, the other half are caused by emotional factors.

During a bout of colic the infant cries, thrashes about, flexes his legs and fusses for from several minutes to two or three hours. This distress sometimes appears to be associated with abdominal discomfort, but at other times such a relationship is speculative. Colic is more common in firstborn children, and it occurs mainly in the first three months of life. With each succeeding child, the incidence of colic becomes less. The probable reason for this difference of incidence is that the mother is more tense and ill at ease with her first child as she learns how to care for a baby, but with later children she is more relaxed.

The psychiatric studies of babies with colic and their mothers indicate that babies can inarticulately perceive the anxiousness or the emotional coldness with which they are handled. Colic in many instances is a diffuse reaction of anxiousness and rage in a baby who senses the tenseness and irritability of his mother. Frequently the physician's most important measure in managing infantile colic is reassurance to the mother. The doctor should explain to the mother the necessity of relaxing as she takes care of the baby. The mother should talk to the baby in a gentle, pleasant way as she cares for him. Changes in the baby's diet sometimes help, but they should be accompanied by relaxed, self-confident, affectionate handling of the child.

Anorexia

Loss of appetite is a common symptom of emotional stress. A depressed person characteristically has a poor appetite, and anxiety or fear may take away the desire for food. The relationship of anorexia to emotional distress often is clear both to the patient and to those around him.

Anorexia nervosa is a syndrome that may occur from puberty through young adulthood, and it occurs mainly in girls and young women. The patient eats very little and may vomit food that is forced upon her. Over a period of from several weeks to several months she suffers a profound weight loss and becomes emaciated. Despite her emaciation the patient remains a bright-eyed, active girl who shows no signs of lassitude. Amenorrhea and a low basal metabolic rate may accompany the emaciation, but the patient shows no other signs of physical dysfunction. In some instances, the patient was plump and may have experimented with dieting during the several-month period before the onset of the anorexia nervosa.

The patient with anorexia nervosa may be a shy, passive person or she may be stubbornly resistant and assertive. She often has experienced subtle rejection and emotional neglect from her parents; this sometimes occurs in the context of open favoritism shown to other children in the family. Often there is much subtle, hostile tension in the parent-child relationships, and the patient expresses her hostility unconsciously in a defiant refusal to eat. The patient's progressive weight loss soon acquires a large secondary gain by moving her into the center of her parents' anxious attention and concern that she should eat. Some psychiatrists feel that an added cause of anorexia nervosa lies in the discomfort of the adolescent girl or young, single adult woman over sexuality; the anorexia, by its physical emaciation and amenorrhea, serves as a physical denial of sexual urges about which the patient has conflictual, uncomfortable feelings.

I recall a 12-year-old girl with anorexia nervosa who lost 32 pounds in a three-month period. Prior to the onset of her anorexia she was a pleasant, passive girl who rarely showed anger or assertiveness. Her father was an ambitious, successful attorney who was active in political affairs and paid little attention to his daughter, and her mother's time was filled with club activities and social affairs. Both parents gave much more attention to the patient's eight-year-old brother whom they openly favored. Beneath her pleasant, passive façade the patient felt much resentment toward her parents and her brother.

A few months prior to the onset of her anorexia nervosa the patient lost six pounds by intentional dieting because she felt she was slightly overweight. A few months later her anorexia started gradually and in a few weeks her food intake dropped to less than 1000 calories each day. She rapidly became the center of her parents' anxious concern; without success, they pleaded, threatened, bribed and coaxed her to eat. Coincident with the onset of anorexia her behavior toward her parents changed. She became sullen, hostile and stubbornly resistant to whatever they wanted. When they tried to kiss her she angrily turned her head away, and she stared sullenly at the floor when her parents tried to talk to her. She was, moreover, depressed to the point where her teachers, scout leaders and relatives commented on it. She spent little time with her family. She often paced to and fro in her room for an hour or two at a time, but she always paced in such a way that her parents could see or hear her.

The patient required psychiatric hospitalization, careful nursing supervision of her eating, and intensive psychotherapy to resolve the acute phase of her anorexia nervosa. Prolonged child guidance clinic help for the patient and her parents followed her discharge from the hospital. In this instance, anorexia nervosa clearly was part of a diffuse, hostile rebellion against negligent, rejecting parents. In most patients with anorexia nervosa the hostile rebellion lies hidden behind the patient's anorexia and is expressed only through it; the patient's interpersonal behavior remains unchanged.

In addition to psychiatric help, the patient with anorexia nervosa often needs hospitalization, which may be on a psychiatric or a medical floor. The patient's food intake must be increased by firm, careful nursing care. In rare instances, tube feeding must be employed to avoid the intercurrent infections and physical debility that severe emaciation may lead to, but tube feeding should be used only if firm, careful nursing care does not lead to improved nutrition. Separation from her family is often a useful aspect of hospital care, and hospitalization also allows psychotherapy to begin on an intensive basis.

Constipation

Constipation is a common complaint that patients present to doctors. Many patients devoutly believe in the myth of the imperative necessity of the daily bowel movement at a "regular" time. If this anxiously awaited event does not occur, they fear that they will suffer from irritability, headaches, "dizziness," "sluggishness," fatigue, dyspepsia, emotional lability and other vaguely defined but much dreaded symptoms. These beliefs are strongly encouraged by the laxative manufacturers who flood the various advertising media with advertisements that vary from the repulsive to the ridiculous.

The medical research on this subject indicates that, if ignored and left alone, the healthy colon often is very irregular, with perhaps several days between bowel movements in some patients. If a patient develops symptoms from delayed evacuation they are caused in the vast majority of instances by his worry about it rather than by any physiological processes. Constipation is usually a supra-orbital disease rather than an infra-umbilical one, except in aged, debilitated or immobilized patients, or in patients taking certain medications which harden stools or delay evacuation.

When patients spend much time each morning straining on the toilet to squeeze out the morning quota of feces, they may after many years of such exertion develop hemorrhoids. Thus, in a sense, hemorrhoids are sometimes psychosomatic, since they can be the result of incorrect ideas about bowel evacuation.

The cure is education, not colonic evacuation. Bowel movements are available to the inspection, the evaluation and the speculation of the individual, and he often pays much attention to them in interpreting the state of his health. Moreover, ideas about bowel functioning may be passed from one generation to another in some families without their validity being questioned. In educating a patient about his incorrect ideas on bowel functioning, the physician may render a service to the patient's family as well as to the patient himself.

Psychosomatic Skin Disorders

Some investigators have described psychosomatic factors in a large number of skin disorders. However, we shall restrict our attention to the skin disorders often considered as having psychosomatic aspects.

Urticaria

Urticaria may be caused by ingested, inhaled or injected substances, and it may also be caused by emotional factors. In some patients the relationship of urticaria to emotional stress is clear to the patient and to people around him. I recall a bookkeeper who had urticaria around the first and fifteenth of each month, the times at which she was under marked stress in her work. In occasional instances, urticaria occurs when the patient comes in contact with a particular person or contemplates encountering him. However, the relationship of urticaria to stress usually is less obvious. Emotionally caused urticaria occurs mainly on exposed surfaces such as the face, neck and arms, but it may be generalized over the entire body. In a sense, blushing is a type of diffuse skin reaction related to urticaria which occurs in many people under obvious emotional stress.

The differential diagnosis between allergic and emotionally caused urticaria often may be made by correlating the patient's episodes of urticaria with situational stresses in his life. Because urticaria is an episodic skin disorder that often appears rapidly and disappears in from a few hours to a week or so, the correlation of emotional stress with the onset of symptoms is more easily determined than in any other skin disease. When the physician directs the patient's attention to the possibility of psychosomatic factors in his urticaria, the patient sometimes can begin to note correlations between emotional stress and episodes of urticaria. In other instances, the patient can establish such correlations only by examining his interpersonal relationships in detailed interview work with the physician. Skin testing, of course, is useful in discovering allergens in some cases, and in some patients both emotional stress and allergens are etiologic factors.

Some psychiatrists have reported that patients with psychosomatic urticaria usually are insecure, passive people who have strong needs to be dependent on others. They tend to have their episodes of urticaria when they are in stressful situations or when their relationships with people on whom they are dependent are threatened by rejection or hostility.

The comprehensive medical management of a patient with urticaria often should include exploration of the possible relationship of emotional factors to his episodes of urticaria. When both allergic and emotional factors are present, antiallergic medications and desensitization procedures can be used in addition to counseling on interpersonal stresses in the patient's life.

Atopic Dermatitis

Atopic dermatitis is now the preferred name for the disorder long called eczema. At times atopic dermatitis is also called disseminated neurodermatitis, but from a psychiatric point of view any use of the term neurodermatitis is confusing.

Constitutional, allergic and emotional factors may play etiologic roles in chronic atopic dermatitis, and the individual importance of these factors varies much from patient to patient. When constitutional, allergic and emotional factors play variable roles in an illness, it is difficult to decide the relative importance of each factor in a particular patient. Moreover, demonstration of interpersonal problems in a patient with atopic dermatitis does not prove that his interpersonal difficulties play a causative role in his skin disease; interpersonal problems are common, and interpersonal problems and atopic dermatitis may merely coexist in the same patient and not be etiologically connected. In my opinion, proof of the role of emotional stress in the etiology of a case of atopic dermatitis demands that exacerbations of the atopic dermatitis are correlated with periods of emotional turmoil, and that improvements in the atopic dermatitis are associated with diminution or resolution of interpersonal stress.

Atopic dermatitis is common in childhood, and the chronic aggravation of severe skin lesions may cause emotional tension in the child. Moreover, the prolonged difficulties of caring for a child with severe atopic dermatitis for many years may cause the mother to have feelings of irritability and rejection toward her burdensome child. Hence, it is often difficult to decide whether the mother's rejection and irritability preceded the atopic dermatitis or came after it. A vicious circle of atopic dermatitis in the child and irritability in the mother may occur, and it may be difficult to decide whether the atopic dermatitis or the maternal hostility came first. Psychiatrists who have studied children with atopic dermatitis describe them as insecure, anxious, aggressive and irritable.

In my opinion, emotional factors play a role in the etiology and course of about 25 per cent of patients with chronic atopic dermatitis. In adults, exacerbations of atopic dermatitis occasionally are clearly related to emotional stress, and a patient who has been free of atopic dermatitis for many months or years may have a flareup when he undergoes marked interpersonal stress. In children with chronic atopic dermatitis the emotional factors often are enmeshed in a vicious circle between the child and his parents. The child lives with an unpredictable, aggravating skin disease and at times he may be irritable and demanding. His parents are burdened with the difficulties of his care, and they may have much impatience and irritability in their handling of him. The parents may feel guilty about their hostile feelings toward the child and they may become oversolicitous and indulgent, or they may become chronically annoyed and callous. The basis for these developments in the parent-child relationship possibly existed in early unhealthy attitudes of the parents toward the child, but the occurrence of the atopic dermatitis precipitated interpersonal trouble, which otherwise might not have occurred or would have evolved in less difficult ways.

Flexible counseling or interview therapy sometimes is useful in the comprehensive management of atopic dermatitis both in children and adults. Some psychiatrists have reported favorable results with children with atopic dermatitis and their parents in interview treatment, but relapses of the dermatitis may occur when the child faces later stressful situations. Because atopic dermatitis may be characterized by remissions and relapses, it may be difficult to decide whether improvement occurred because of psychotherapy or merely during it.

Acne

Emotional factors probably do not play a role in the etiology of acne. However, acne may have a significant influence on the interpersonal adjustment of an adolescent or young adult who has it. Adolescence is a time when the individual often has many doubts about his personal attractiveness, his talents and his social skills, and severe acne of the face may accentuate feelings of shyness, personal inadequacy and social ineptitude. In a similar way, severe acne may have an unfortunate effect on the interpersonal adjustment of a young adult.

The comprehensive treatment of acne in an adolescent should include some counseling to ensure that social withdrawal and feelings of social inferiority do not occur. Such counseling should include the teenager's parents as well as the adolescent himself. Counseling sometimes should be included in management of a young adult with acne. I have seen a few cases in which the emotional effects of severe acne were so devastating to the person that psychotherapy with a psychiatrist was necessary and useful.

Other Skin Disorders

Emotional factors play a significant role in some cases of *pruritis*. This is particulary so in pruritis of the perineal region, the genitals and the rectal area; conflicts over sexual urges and guilt over masturbation often lie behind pruritis in these areas. Psychogenic pruritis of the rectal and perineal areas is somewhat common in homosexuals and in persons who have strong unconscious homosexual urges. However, psychosomatic pruritis may occur in other areas of the body or it may be generalized over the entire body. Pruritis may lead to much scratching which in turn may produce rough, raw, erythematous lesions which can become secondarily infected. Some psychiatrists feel that psychosomatic generalized body pruritis may be caused by either sexual conflicts or by repressed hostility and guilt which are expressed in this self-punishing way. The differential diagnosis of organically and emotionally caused pruritus often is difficult and requires careful, comprehensive study of the patient.

The term *neurodermatitis* is used in a variety of ways. It is employed to designate a particular skin syndrome in which chronic scratching causes excoriated and lichenified areas on the back of the neck, the wrists, the ankles and other areas. Many dermatologists feel that in this form of dermatitis the pruritus that leads to the scratching has a large emotional factor, though the original stimulus may have been an insect bite or some minor irritant. However, the term neurodermatitis is employed by some dermatologists to designate other types of skin disorders, and, unfortunately, it is sometimes used to designate all skin diseases in which emotional factors play a part. The terms "psychosomatic" and "psychophysiologic" should be employed to describe skin lesions with emotional determinants. From the psychosomatic point of view, the term "neurodermatitis" has little usefulness in any connotation.

Excessive perspiration, or hyperhidrosis, is often due to anxiety and it may be episodic or chronic. Though it does not cause skin disease, it can be distressing to patients. *Warts,* or verrucae, are caused by a virus, but there is an extensive medical literature presenting evidence that warts often can be removed by strong suggestion (painting them with inert substances or exposing them briefly to a heat lamp) or hypnosis; such data raises the question of psychosomatic factors in warts. *Factitial dermatitis* consists of self-inflicted skin lesions, which the patient presents as a skin disease. He conceals his role in producing them and denies it when questioned. Many psychiatrists feel that factitious dermatitis is a means by which patients with much guilt find relief in self-punishing acts. In other instances, factitial dermatitis may have both exhibitionistic and masochistic features.

Psychosomatic Cardiovascular Diseases

Tachycardia

Paroxysmal or prolonged tachycardia often is a physical manifestation of acute or chronic anxiety neuroses. The patient describes his increased heart rate as his "pounding heart" or "racing pulse," and he often fears that his tachycardia is a sign of heart disease or an imminent "heart attack." The patient's fear of heart disease adds much tension to the original anxiety that caused the tachycardia, and in some instances the tachycardia sets off a chain of fearful speculations which terminate in panic.

The patient with emotionally caused tachycardia and concurrent obsessive fear of heart disease often develops fatigue, "dizziness," shortness of breath, chest pain and fear of any kind of physical effort. This syndrome, especially when it becomes chronic, sometimes has been labeled "neurocirculatory asthenia," "cardiac neurosis" and "effort syndrome." The use of such terms is misleading, since it fastens attention on the concept of cardiac illness and overlooks the fact that the patient actually is suffering from an acute or chronic anxiety neurosis with secondary obsessive fear of heart disease. The causes and management of these syndromes is that of acute and chronic anxiety neuroses and obsessive neuroses.

Hypertension

The systolic blood pressure of most people is somewhat elevated when they are excited, angry or anxious. Tense people who are examined in hospital emergency rooms often are found to have systolic elevations of blood pressure which subside after an hour or two of rest. Many clinicians believe that in some patients essential hypertension may be the result of sustained emotional tension caused by various kinds of personality problems. In many instances the patient with essential hypertension is a passive, unassertive person who keeps his anger pent up within himself. He is on an endless treadmill to please other people at the expense of suppression of his feelings. The hypertensive patient also is described as a systematic, overly neat individual who feels uncomfortable if his affairs are not in meticulous order.

The emotional problems of the patient cause prolonged elevations of systolic blood pressure, and the elevated blood pressure may in time lead to secondary renal and cardiovascular changes which, in turn, increase the hypertension and make it persistent. The management of a patient with early essential hypertension should include inventory of his interpersonal life and counseling to diminish stress and correct personality difficulties whenever possible. Even when irreversible renal and cardiovascular problems are present in late hypertension, the interpersonal life of the patient may be evaluated to help resolve stresses which raise his blood pressure to even higher levels.

Extrasystoles

The frequency of extrasystoles may be influenced by emotional factors. People who have extrasystoles often tend to have them when they are anxious or upset. Extrasystoles often worry the patient much and precipitate much fear of heart disease. The patient with benign extrasystoles often needs strong, repeated reassurance from his physician, and the doctor may point out that when the patient is under stress his extrasystoles may be more frequent.

Coronary Artery Disease

It has long been clinically observed that emotional stress may precipitate attacks of angina pectoris and at times may precede myocardial infarction. The oft-quoted words of the 18th Century Scottish clinician John Hunter, who had angina, that "my life is in the hands of any rascal who can worry me" were proved accurate by his death from myocardinal infarction shortly after a heated argument. Anxiety, panic, anger and agitation may increase the hear rate, raise heart blood flow requirements, and cause angina, and perhaps infarction, in a person who has coronary artery insufficiency.

However, there is much controversy about whether emotional factors in themselves can produce coronary artery disease. Recent psychosomatic research has tended to take a much broader view of patients with coronary artery disease, and to consider their comprehensive life styles. In these studies the person who is predisposed to develop coronary artery disease is described as one who works hard, plays little, eats a diet high in lipids, and smokes a lot. All these factors are seen as products of his personality structure, his aims and his general approach to life; the same factors which cause him to work hard also lead him to smoke much, overeat and engage in strenuous, rather than relaxed, recreational activities. The hard-working, chain-smoking, tense businessman who drinks and eats too much while entertaining customers and business colleagues is the caricature of the coronary artery disease candidate.

The current trend in psychosomatic research is to look beyond the personality features of the patient and to examine how his personality structure affects his dietary habits, his use of tobacco and other harmful substances, his work pattern, his recreational activities and his socioeconomic aspirations. This broad approach to psychosomatic illness has been applied most systematically to the study of heart disease, but it probably will set the pattern for future psychosomatic investigations.

Similarly, congestive heart failure, which, of course, is often related to other disease processes than coronary artery illnesses, can be influenced by the life style and personality of the patient. The prudent, self-disciplined person with heart disease is much less likely to enter into decompensation than the impulsive, imprudent individual who disregards his medical regimen and the less active life pattern his physicians have recommended.

In addition, it is obvious that the poorly understood personality factors which, despite public knowledge that smoking is dangerous, cause some people to smoke heavily and others to abstain, have a decided influence on the incidence and course of coronary artery disease, as well as other diseases such as lung cancer and emphysema. In a sense, all these diseases are psychosomatic since they are heavily related to the emotional factors which lead people to observe or disregard the well known perils of smoking.

Migraine

Interpersonal stress and personality problems may play important roles in migraine headaches. The term "migraine" sometimes is incorrectly applied to muscle tension headaches of the temporal and frontal regions (discussed later in this chapter). Nausea may accompany severe muscle tension headaches, but visual scotomata rarely occur. Muscle tension headaches usually are bilateral as opposed to classical migraine, which is unilateral. The differential diagnosis of muscle tension headaches and migraine headaches may require careful, prolonged study of the patient. The term "migrainous" is confusing and some muscle tension headaches are given this label. Muscle tension headaches and migraine headaches should be carefully distinguished from each other, since the vascular constricting drugs used in migraine are not helpful in muscle tension headaches, and the measures used for the latter have limited usefulness in true migraine.

Emotional stress, operating through the autonomic nervous system, can produce constriction or dilation of arteries. The initial constriction and subsequent dilation of the arteries of the upper face and scalp which lead to a migraine headache are affected by the patient's emotional state. The psychiatrists who have studied patients with migraine describe them as perfectionistic, hard-driving persons who unduly inhibit anger and have strong needs to win the affection and esteem of others by achievement. The vascular instability that produces the migraine headache is felt to be a physiological expression of the patient's suppressed rage. Vascular changes in the face and scalp are common in angry people. Many persons become pale or flushed, due to constriction or dilation of facial and scalp blood vessels, when they are angry. The patient with migraine has a more subtle, prolonged vascular reaction to the pent-up rage he feels, and the constriction and subsequent dilation of his facial and scalp arteries cause his headaches. Though other factors probably are active in migraine besides emotional forces, the comprehensive evaluation of a patient with migraine should include inventory of the patient's personality structure and interpersonal life.

Psychosomatic Respiratory Tract Disorders

Bronchial Asthma

Bronchial asthma is mainly caused by inspired or ingested allergens, but emotional forces play an important role in many cases. Both factors are present in many cases of asthma, and the relative proportions of these two etiologic forces vary much from one patient to another. The incidence of each type of factor in asthma is not known, but an old psychiatric axiom states that one third of bronchial asthma is caused by allergens, one third is due to emotional forces, and a final third is due to combinations of these two etiologic forces. Asthma caused by allergens and asthma caused by emotional factors are clinically similar, and the eosinophile count may be raised in each type.

Psychiatric studies of patients with emotionally caused asthma indicate that they have profound, unmet needs for affection. The child with emotionally caused asthma often has experienced coldness and subtle rejection in his relationships with his parents, and he has deep, painful yearnings for affection and esteem. A depressive thread runs through the child's personality structure, and some psychiatrists feel that the asthmatic attacks are substitutes for stifled urges to sob and cry for affection from the parents.

However, after the asthma begins, it draws to the child the anxious concern of his parents. The disease thus acquires the unfortunate secondary gain of obtaining through physical sickness the parental care and attention the child unconsciously yearns for. This secondary gain often makes the asthma more severe and more difficult to treat, because the disease becomes ingrained as the major avenue through which the child receives parental attention. This type of secondary gain may become the dominant cause of the asthma, and it may occur both in emotionally caused asthma and in asthma originally caused by allergens. The emotional determinants in asthma in adults are similar, but they are related to the emotional trauma both of childhood experiences and of adult interpersonal stresses. The adult with emotionally caused asthma transfers his dependency needs to people in his current environment.

The influence of interpersonal stress on asthma sometimes is obvious. I recall a 26-year-old single woman who had asthma only when she went to visit her parents in a distant city. Whether she went by private car, bus or airplane, she developed asthma a day or so before she started on the trip and it left her only when she returned. She did not have asthma during trips to other cities. At times the influence of interpersonal conflicts on asthma is easily demonstrated. Asthmatic patients who are interviewed before groups of medical students in psychiatric demonstration clinics sometimes cease to have asthmatic breathing, or it diminishes much in severity, within 5 to 10 minutes after the interview begins, and they recommence their asthma when they return to the waiting room or while they wait for the elevator to take them back to their hospital floors. The comprehensive medical care of many children and adults with asthma often should involve evaluation of the patient's interpersonal life and appropriate interview help.

Hyperventilation Syndrome

Hyperventilation was mentioned briefly in Chapter 6 in our discussion of anxiety neuroses, since hyperventilation is a common physical symptom of acute and chronic anxiety states. The patient in an episode of hyperventilation breathes in rapid, gasping respirations which may be shallow or deep. His anxiety often is severe, and in many instances he fears he is having a heart attack or some other physical illness from which he may die suddenly. If severe hyperventilation continues more than one or two minutes, the patient begins to get symptoms from the respiratory alkalosis caused by his overbreathing. He may be giddy and weak, and he develops tingling in the toes, fingers and perioral region. Hyperventilation attacks usually last from a few minutes to half an hour or so, but I have seen them persist, with fluctuations, for several days in hospitalized patients with severe anxiety states. Hyperventilation attacks may occur daily, or several times each week, or at long intervals, and they vary from minor discomforts to incapacitating episodes.

The hyperventilation syndrome is usually a clinical form of acute or chronic anxiety state in which overbreathing becomes the dominant physical manifestation of the patient's anxiety. The patient usually first consults his family physician or internist about hyperventilation, and the physician should make the correct diagnosis promptly and should explain it to the patient. Extensive laboratory and hospital investigations for possible cardiac or pulmonary disease are unwise. They tend to fix in the patient's mind the idea that he has a serious cardiac or pulmonary disease which has not yet been elucidated. Prompt diagnosis and firm reassurance from the physician often diminish the severity and frequency of his hyperventilation episodes. (The causes, treatment and prognosis of most cases of hyperventilation syndrome are those outlined in Chapter 6 on anxiety neuroses, and that material is relevant to the interpersonal causes and psychiatric management of hyperventilation.)

Sighing respirations consists of occasional deep inspirations during which the patient feels that he is not getting enough air and is anxious about it. Sighing respirations may be accompanied by feelings of tightness in the chest and throat. Sighing respirations constitute a mild variation of hyperventilation. Reassurances and explanations to the patient often are useful.

Psychosomatic Musculoskeletal Disorders

Muscle Tension Syndromes

Emotionally caused muscle tension syndromes are common, and they tend to occur in groups of muscles which in the course of evolution had important uses in lower mammals but have less importance in man. Some of these muscles persist in man though they have no useful functions, and others are more extensive than they need to be for the purposes of modern man. Hence, muscle tension symptoms are common in the muscle groups of the posterior neck and occipital region, the lower back, and in some other neck and shoulder girdle muscles. Though these muscles were necessary in arboreal animals, they are overdeveloped for man in an upright posture pursuing his customary urban activities. Muscle tension symptoms are also common in the thin muscle layer of the skull and cranial base, which have lost any real use for man; muscle tension symptoms here cause various types of headaches. Emotionally determined muscle tension syndromes are much less common in useful groups of muscles, such as the muscles of the legs, arms and hands. However, no muscle group is entirely free of muscle tension symptoms, for they occasionally occur in the anterior chest wall, the hamstrings and other parts of the body.

The pain of acute or chronic muscle tension may be dull or sharp, continuous or throbbing, mild or severe. Patients sometimes describe it as burning or as a weight pressing down on the involved area. Muscle spasms may produce acute, severe pain, but often the muscle tension is less marked and the symptoms are milder. Muscle tension symptoms may last only a few minutes or they may produce chronic discomforts that affect the patient intermittently for years.

Emotionally caused muscle tension symptoms of the low back and the anterior chest wall are common clinical problems. In many cases of backache in the lumbar region the patient has no objective findings except local soreness, and roentgenologic studies do not reveal abnormalities. Psychosomatic factors should often be considered in the differential diagnosis of lumbar backache. Even when orthopedic pathology exists in this area, the psychosomatic overlay may be a large part of the problem. Moreover, pain in the mid-dorsal region of the back, especially in the rhomboid muscles, often is due to emotionally caused muscle tension. In a similar manner, the pectoralis musculature of the anterior thorax is sometimes the site of psychogenic muscle pain. This sometimes creates problems in the diagnosis of angina pectoris.

Spasmodic Torticollis

Spasmodic torticollis consists of continuous or intermittent spasms of the neck muscles resulting in rotation of the chin and head sharply to one side. Torticollis is produced mainly by spasmodic contractions of the sternocleidomastoid muscle on one side, but the trapezius and other muscles of the same side are involved to a lesser extent. The chin and head are turned toward the side opposite to that of the spastic muscles; for example, contraction of the right sternocleidomastoid turns the chin and head sharply toward the left shoulder. The head usually remains rotated constantly, with chronic, minor jerking movements. The neck muscles relax and the patient does not have torticollis when he is asleep.

Some cases of spasmodic torticollis are due to diseases of the cerebral vertebrae or the basal ganglia, but others are caused by emotional factors. Early psychotherapy has been reported to help some patients with emotionally caused spasmodic torticollis, but in many instances the patient does not come for psychotherapeutic help until he has pursued a long course of orthopedic treatments, during which time his symptoms have become entrenched. If the patient is not seen soon after the onset of his disorder, the chances for successful psychotherapy are much diminished. I recall a 37-year-old woman with a two-year history of severe spasmodic torticollis. She was a passive, shy person who was dominated by her husband. Frequently, he forced her to engage in fellatio despite her protests that she found it repulsive. Her torticollis began one night when she turned her head persistently to one side and refused fellatio, but her husband bullied her into it despite her protests. Her torticollis began that night and her head remained rotated to the same side to which she had turned it in her attempts to avoid fellatio. The torticollis persisted unchanged during two years of orthopedic treatments which included neck braces, neck traction and procaine injections of the cervical plexus. At the end of two years she came for psychiatric consultation, and in 14 months of psychotherapy her symptoms were relieved a good deal, but her torticollis was not removed entirely.

Muscle Tension Headache

Muscle tension headaches of the posterior neck are common; probably from 25 to 40 per cent of all persons suffer from muscle tension headaches of the occipital and posterior nuchal regions at some time during their lives, and some people frequently have them. The pain of such headaches may be mild or severe, sharp or dull, brief or prolonged. They sometimes produce painful spots on the occipital prominences where the neck muscles insert over the entire posterior cranium or the pain may descend into the shoulders and upper back. Millions of aspirin tablets and other analgesic compounds are bought by the public each year to alleviate muscle tension headaches. Some types of nonmedical practitioners thrive on these problems and apply their crude physiotherapies and manipulations to these regions.

Muscle tension headaches are common in the thin muscular layer present in the scalp extending over the entire cranium. This muscular layer forms a thin skullcap covering the head and it inserts into bone in a bandlike circle which passes around the forehead, the temples, the mastoid areas and the occiput. These muscles have no useful function in man, and they are the site of various types of headaches. Emotionally caused tension in this muscle layer often causes discomfort along the line where the muscle layer inserts at the base of the skull. It may produce headaches, which the patient describes as feeling like a tight band circling the head and drawn painfully around the forehead. Dull or throbbing headaches in the temporal regions also may be produced by tension in this muscle layer. It may also cause burning spots or pressure sensations on top of the head. Various kinds of facial pain are due to emotionally caused tension of facial muscles. Periorbital headaches often arise from similar tensions in the muscles of the periorbital region.

The majority of headaches are due to emotionally caused muscle tension in the muscles over the posterior neck, the cranium and the face. The importance of dental decay, eyestrain, sinus infection, nasal congestion and vague facial neuralgias in causing headaches often is overestimated. The role of intracranial pathology and vague systemic dysfunctions in the production of headaches has been overemphasized. Though the physician should be alert to the many various organic processes that may produce headaches, he should remember that the vast majority of them are psychosomatic. Chronic anxiety states are the most common cause of psychosomatic headaches, but any psychiatric disorder accompanied by anxiety may also produce them.

Rheumatoid Arthritis

Among the possible causes that have been suggested for rheumatoid arthritis are infections, hypersensitivities, vascular disorders, endocrine abnormalities and metabolic disturbances. None of these etiologies is generally accepted, however. Many clinicians feel that emotional factors may play at least a partial role in the production of rheumatoid arthritis.

It has long been observed that the onset of rheumatoid arthritis, or exacerbations of it, may be associated with periods of emotional stress. Psychiatrists who have studied this disorder report that the patient with rheumatoid arthritis inhibits the expression of both his affectionate and hostile feelings. He is inclined to be physically active and intellectually busy. He has a strong need to be of service to others, and he busies himself in many activities which make him useful to the people around him. However, behind his strivings for usefulness to others are hidden marked dependency needs; he attempts to bind himself to other people by making himself indispensible to them, since he cannot express affection in more direct ways. The suppressed hostile feelings of the patient are partially discharged in impulses toward excessive physical exertion, and he has an anxious need to try to control people in his environment by making them indebted to him. The patient with rheumatoid arthritis often was reared in an interpersonal environment in which his needs for affection were not met and in which there was much competitiveness between the patient and his siblings or between the patient and his parents.

The onset of rheumatoid arthritis, or exacerbations of it, may coincide with an event in which the patient's needs to be emotionally close to people are rudely shaken. Such stress may occur when the patient is rejected by an important person in his life, or when the patient loses a close person by death. Though feelings of anger may be produced by rejection, or grief may be caused by the death of a close person, the patient gives neither of these feelings open expression.

Some psychiatrists have reported favorable results with psychotherapy of patients with rheumatoid arthritis. These psychiatrists advocate a supportive, encouraging, reassuring role by the therapist. However, rheumatoid arthritis is characterized by remissions and exacerbations, and there are as yet no carefully controlled studies to prove that psychotherapy alters the long-range course of this illness.

Psychosomatic Endocrine Disorders

Hyperthyroidism

Since the earliest clinical descriptions of hyperthyroidism physicians have commented on the precipitation of this disorder by emotional stress. Psychiatric investigators have found that the hyperthyroid patient often is an insecure, anxious person with strong, unmet needs for emotional dependence on others. The patient clings to the people on whom he is emotionally dependent and is anxious to please them, though he may have much repressed, unconscious hostility in deeper personality layers. The patient's early relationships with his parents left him with strong, unmet yearnings for affection. He is very sensitive to how people feel about him and reacts with anxiousness and mild depressiveness when people are hostile or reject him.

Clinical hyperthyroidism may be precipitated when the patient experiences emotional rejection or faces separation from an important person in his life. The precipitating interpersonal stress may arise in the patient's relationship with his marital partner, his parents, his children or other close persons. The comprehensive management of the patient with hyperthyroidism should include evaluation of his emotional life as well as appropriate general medical treatment. Psychiatrists who have worked in thyroid clinics have reported that the results of combined psychotherapy and medical treatment are better and longer lasting than the results of organic medical management alone.

Diabetes

Though emotional stress may result in a brief elevation of blood sugar, and though much has been written on the possibility that emotional factors may play a role in causing diabetes, the evidence for a psychosomatic etiology of diabetes is unconvincing.

However, the patient's personality structure and his interpersonal life often have a marked effect on the course and treatment of this disease. Diabetes has the unique feature that deviations from the prescribed medication or dietary regimen may result in serious medical trouble within a few hours. The depressed, discouraged diabetic who gives up the struggle to maintain the proper dietary and medication schedule may soon be in diabetic coma or insulin shock. The adolescent diabetic who uses noncompliance with his medical regimen to rebel against his parents may be in grave medical trouble within a matter of hours. Hence, the successful management of a diabetic patient sometimes requires careful attention to his interpersonal relationships and his emotional state. This is particularly true of the patient who repeatedly has episodes of insulin shock or diabetic coma despite careful medical management.

A good physician-patient relationship often is important in treating diabetes. The patient needs a counselor who understands his interpersonal background and can help him make a successful adjustment to his illness. In many cases of diabetes the successful management of the illness requires a thorough knowledge of the person.

Psychosomatic Central Nervous System Disorders

Seizures

Epileptic seizures are produced by neurophysiologic disturbances in the brain, which may be caused by inborn disorders of the electrochemical discharges of the brain, as shown in electroencephalographic dysrhythmias, or by inflammatory, traumatic, neoplastic or degenerative brain lesions that disrupt its normal physiology. It has long been observed, however, that emotional stress may increase the frequency of organically caused seizures. It is doubtful that emotional stress alone can produce epileptic seizures; a strong dysrhythmic predisposition must first exist in the brain. However, in the person with an electrochemical dysrhythmia or other predisposing brain pathology, emotional stress may play a crucial role in determining the frequency of seizures. It may in some patients be the crucial factor that determines whether seizures are an infrequent occurrence or an incapacitating disability.

The ideas and emotional experiences of a person have their highest, most articulate neurophysiologic organization in the cerebral cortex. The less refined, cruder emotions are represented in the lower brain centers. Both these regions of the brain are involved in the periodic electrochemical discharges that spread a wave of disturbance through cerebral tissue and precipitate a clinical seizure. When the turmoil of emotional stress in the cortex and lower brain centers is added to an underlying neurochemical predisposition, the total excitation may exceed the seizure threshold, and a convulsion occurs. Thus, the interpersonal life of the patient may become an important facet of his epilepsy.

In some instances, successful management of an epileptic patient requires evaluation of his interpersonal environment and resolution of stressful relationships in his life. This is particularly true of epileptic patients whose seizures are refractory to pharmacologic management. I recall a 9-year-old boy who had one or two seizures each day despite adequate doses of diphenylhydantoin and phenobarbital. Evaluation of his family relationships revealed that he was subjected to constant hostility and depreciation by his stepfather, who viewed him as an annoying leftover from his wife's first marriage. Except for occasional irritable criticism, his mother paid little attention to him. The parents refused to participate in counseling to work on these problems, but they agreed to allow the boy to live with an aunt who took a warm interest in him. When he left his parents' home and went to live with his aunt, his seizures immediately dropped from one or two each day to one seizure every six to eight weeks, despite the fact that his medication was unchanged.

The comprehensive management of the epileptic patient should include attention to his social and economic adjustment. The fear an epileptic patient has of having a seizure in public may cause social seclusiveness and vocational incapacitation. Supportive counseling often must be combined with the use of vocational counseling and rehabilitation services. I have seen adult epileptic patients who were socially withdrawn and could not work because of ingrained fearful attitudes toward their seizures despite the fact that improved regimens of medication had reduced the incidence of their seizures to once every six months or so.

The majority of cases of idiopathic epilepsy begin during childhood, and successful management of the epileptic child demands careful attention to the child's interpersonal development as well as a good regimen of medication. The fear of having seizures in public may cause the epileptic child to become socially withdrawn, and the sedative effects of large doses of some anticonvulsant medications may add to his withdrawal and isolation. The combination of slight drowsiness and social withdrawal occasionally gives the epileptic child a false appearance of mental retardation. If, because of his apathy and social withdrawal, the child does not function at his best possible level on I. Q. testing, the test result may be much lower than his true intelligence merits. These children should not be misdiagnosed as being mentally retarded or as having diffuse organic brain damage, when the main problems are social withdrawal because of fear of having seizures in public and apathy due to anticonvulsant medication.

In treating children with epileptic seizures, the physician should advise the parents and the child to take appropriate measures to avoid interpersonal withdrawal by the child. I urge parents to encourage their child to do everything that other children do except those activities involving "wheels, water and heights." For example, the child should not ride a bicycle, swim or climb trees. However, the physician and the parents should encourage him to engage in all other social, athletic and scholastic activities in which children participate. Only a small victory is gained if the child's seizures are well controlled by medication but he is interpersonally crippled by the emotional impact of having a convulsive disorder.

Psychosomatic Genitourinary Disorders

Menstrual irregularities sometimes are caused by emotional stress. It is common medical knowledge that a woman sometimes may skip from one to several menstrual periods after an upsetting emotional experience. In other instances, emotional trauma may precipitate a menstrual period a week or two before it is due. Prolonged menstrual bleeding occasionally is caused by emotional tension. These menstrual irregularities may occur in a woman who is basically well adjusted but who undergoes an emotional shock, such as a marital crisis or severe illness in a close person. Menstrual irregularities also may occur in women with various kinds of psychiatric disorders during exacerbations of their problems.

Pseudocyesis is a syndrome in which the patient stops menstruating, has apparent distention of the abdomen, has breast changes and is convinced that she is pregnant, though in fact she is not. Pseudocyesis occurs in women with various kinds of personality problems who have either strong wishes for pregnancy or strong fears of it. Though some psychiatrists consider pseudocyesis a type of hysterical conversion disorder, the abdominal distention, breast changes and cessation of menses are psychosomatic effects of the patient's emotional state. I recall a patient in a prominent university medical school hospital whose pseudocyesis was so realistic that the true diagnosis was not made until she entered the hospital in apparent labor. Her appearance of pregnancy was so convincing that one physician had even noted on her chart that he thought he could hear the fetal heart beat. The patient with pseudocyesis requires careful psychiatric evaluation and psychotherapy for the underlying personality difficulties that led to the pseudocyesis.

Dysmenorrhea may be related to conflictual feelings about sexuality and childbearing, and it sometimes in linked to a deep dislike of the female role in life. Dysmenorrhea is somewhat more common in women who as girls were unprepared for the menarche and whose first menstruation was a fearful, guilt-ridden, puzzling experience.

Premenstrual tension occurs in a large number of women; for several days prior to the onset of menstruation they are somewhat anxious, irritable or depressed. Mild premenstrual tension occurs in so many women who are reasonably well adjusted emotionally that it must be considered within the normal limits of emotional and physiological functioning. However, severe premenstrual emotional instability may be a sign of underlying personality problems which undergo exacerbations in the premenstrual period. Premenstrual tension also is associated with physiological changes such as fluid retention, sodium storage and increased steroid hormone activity.

Premenstrual tension probably is caused by a combination of physiological and emotional factors, and the importance of these two types of factors probably varies much from patient to patient. Premenstrual tension may be related to conflictual feelings the patient has about sexuality, pregnancy and her role as a woman. A strong fear of pregnancy, a strong desire for pregnancy or strong mixed feelings about pregnancy may accentuate premenstrual tension. The comprehensive medical management of severe premenstual tension often should include personality evaluation of the patient and exploration of the emotional problems that may play a role in her difficulty.

Urinary tract dysfunctions. Dysuria and *frequency* may be caused by anxiety and guilt over masturbation or other sexual activities. These symptoms are common during adolescence and young adulthood when the individual is struggling to achieve a comfortable adjustment with sexuality. Homosexuals are prone to develop dysuria, urinary frequency and vaguely defined urinary tract symptoms caused by their conflictual feelings about their sexual activities. In some instances, urinary frequency is a symptom of acute or chronic anxiety. Some students have urinary frequency while tensely preparing for important examinations.

Urinary retention in women often is due to emotional problems. When a woman has persistent urinary retention and urological examination does not reveal obvious pathology, her retention is usually due to emotional difficulties. I have seen women with emotionally caused urinary retention that necessitated daily catheterization for periods ranging up to eight weeks in duration, and from whom as much as 1200 cc. of urine was obtained in a single catheterization. These women often are immature, passive individuals with long-standing conflicts over sexuality. The urinary retention may be precipitated by marital stress, and often the urinary retention acquires the secondary gain of relieving the patient from participation in sexual intercourse, which she finds distasteful. The patient frequently has marital conflicts that she is unable to deal with on an articulate level. Some psychiatrists classify emotionally caused urinary retention in women as a hysterical conversion disorder since the muscles involved in micturition are to a large extent under voluntary control.

[Enuresis is covered in Chapter 25, and problems of sexual adjustment such as impotence, premature ejaculation, orgasmic dysfunction (frigidity) and dyspareunia are discussed in the same chapter.]

Psychosomatic Disorders of Organs of Special Sense

Glaucoma. It is doubtful that emotional problems can cause glaucoma. However, in the patient with established glaucoma emotional stress of either acute or chronic nature can further increase intraocular tension and accentuate the severity of the process. Because of their rich autonomic innervation, the iris and its neighboring structures are very sensitive to anxiety and changes in mood. Glaucomatous exacerbations often are clearly related to episodes of anger, fear or agitation in the patient. The comprehensive medical management of some glaucomatous patients demands attention to the patient's interpersonal life and requires lessening of emotional stress when possible.

Rhinitis. In many instances the emotional state of the patient has a marked effect on the vascularity and secretions of the nasal mucosa. Acute and chronic nasal problems may be caused or much influenced by the patient's interpersonal life. Both chronic hypertrophic rhinitis and atrophic rhinitis may be related to psychosomatic forces. In some patients, allergic, physically traumatic and emotional factors combine to produce chronic rhinitis.

Obesity

Overeating is the major cause of obesity, which rarely is caused by endocrine disorders and other physical dysfunctions; even if some people are somewhat predisposed to become obese because of the ways in which they metabolize and store food, they do not become fat unless they eat excessively. Obesity may be related to family eating customs, individual eating habits, social customs and emotional problems. Since various types of physical illness are more common in obese persons, obesity is a significant health problem.

Emotional factors often play a role in the etiology of obesity that begins in those periods of life in which obesity is least acceptable socially. Hence, marked obesity that begins in late childhood, adolescence or young adulthood is more likely to have strong emotional determinants than obesity that begins in middle age, when it is more accepted socially. Psychiatric studies of obesity reveal that the obese patient sometimes is reared by a hovering, overprotective mother who unconsciously uses excessive feeding of the child and the resultant obesity as a means of binding the child close to home. The mother's clinging to the child may arise from her need to dominate him or from her emotional insecurity, which leads her to tie him close to her as a comforting companion. In some instances the obese child initially was rejected and unwanted by the mother, and by overprotecting and overfeeding the child the mother attempts to hide from herself her guilty feelings about her underlying hostility toward him. These events during the child's formative years may establish in him trends toward overeating and obesity which become ingrained and lay the basis for obesity in adolescence and adult life.

Obese persons sometimes use overeating as a way of assuaging feelings of anxiety and insecurity. The patient finds that the physical gratification and self-attention of excessive eating lessens anxiousness, and overeating becomes a frequent recourse when he is emotionally upset. Feelings of inferiority, loneliness and mild depressiveness are occasionally diminished by overeating. Some persons use excessive eating before bedtime as a way of relaxing and combating insomnia; the pattern of overeating at night is sometimes a major contributant to obesity.

Obesity may be a way in which some individuals escape from interpersonal tensions. For example, marked obesity in adolescence or young adulthood may be the means by which the patient unconsciously flees from the discomfort he feels about dating persons of the opposite sex. Obesity, especially in adolescent girls and young women, creates marked problems in social acceptance by persons of their own age group. Obesity offers them a rationalization which hides from themselves and others their marked anxiety about close relationships with the opposite sex. Obesity also may offer a rationalization for social failures that actually stem from personality problems too painful for the patient to recognize consciously.

Sudden increases in weight sometimes follow major emotional stresses, such as a death in the family, vocational failure or marital unhappiness. The patient retreats into the self-centered gratification of overeating as a way of easing his emotional pain. In some instances, over a long span of time periodic gains and losses of weight may be correlated with the presence or absence of interpersonal stresses in the patient's life.

The treatment of obesity sometimes should include evaluation of the patient's interpersonal life. The therapist should explore the emotional significance of obesity to the patient, in terms of both past and current interpersonal experiences. Resolution of old emotional conflicts and current interpersonal difficulties may be an important contributant to successful weight loss and the persistent maintenance of the patient's weight at a lower level. It must be remembered that after he loses weight, the obese patient must adjust his daily food intake to a permanently lower level than when he was obese, for he no longer needs the extra food that formerly went into the daily metabolism of his lost obese bulk.

OTHER PSYCHOSOMATIC DISORDERS

In this survey of the organ systems of the body we have covered only the more common and well established psychosomatic illnesses. The list of disorders that have been studied from the psychosomatic point of view is long. Much more is yet to be learned about the intimate correlations of interpersonal relationships, emotional forces and the functioning of the body in health and disease. Comprehensive medical practice does not allow the study of disease with disregard of the interpersonal life of the patient. They constitute a single process.

THE COMPREHENSIVE MANAGEMENT OF PSYCHOSOMATIC ILLNESS

In discussing the comprehensive management of psychosomatic illness, we shall cover each of the seven levels of dysfunction in the psychosomatic process listed in the first part of this chapter and diagrammed in Figure 11–1. The seven levels are: (1) the disease process in the involved organ or organ system, (2) the autonomic nervous and other physiologic pathways through which emotional stresses are transmitted from the higher levels of organization in the brain to the particular organ system, (3) the lower brain areas in which emotional and autonomic nervous system forces interrelate, (4) the cerebral cortex, where the feelings and ideas of the person have their highest level of neurophysiologic organization, (5) the interpersonal relationships of the patient with the emotionally important people in his life, (6) the personality structures of those persons who cause emotional turmoil in the patient and (7) social and economic stresses in the community in which the person lives, which have an adverse emotional impact on him.

The best treatment of a psychosomatic illness involves therapeutic measures on multiple levels of functioning. The number of levels involved in a treatment plan varies, of course, with the type of psychosomatic illness and the nature of the patient's emotional problems.

Treatment on the Level of the Local Lesion

The first step in the comprehensive medical management of a psychosomatic illness usually is treatment of the local lesion. The patient with peptic ulcer, urticaria or convulsive seizures should receive the appropriate medications that will help the local disease process. Some psychosomatic illnesses require vigilant medical attention, and major crises such as perforation of a peptic ulcer or carcinomatous change in ulcerative colitis demand surgical intervention.

The patient should understand, however, the role of medications and other direct treatments of the local lesion in the total management of a psychosomatic illness. He should understand that the problem is much broader than a dysfunction in a single organ of his body. He must understand that measures directed at the local lesion are treating merely the final result of a chain of causes that extends into his emotional and interpersonal life. The role of medication should be explained in this light. In explaining the role of medication, the physician at times may roughly sketch the diagram of Figure 11-1, and he can use it to explain how medication works on the level of the local lesion.

Treatment on the Level of the Autonomic Nervous System and Other Physiologic Pathways

The autonomic nervous system is an important avenue through which many organs receive the impulses by which emotional stress is transmuted into physical disease. However, in addition to the sympathetic and parasympathetic channels, vascular, peripheral nervous, endocrine and other pathways also are involved. Treatment directed at interrupting the passage of these pathways may be used to diminish the severity of the psychosomatic process. Medications that block the action of sympathetic and parasympathetic impulses are useful in some diseases. Sympathomimetic or parasympathomimetic medications sometimes can help to reestablish an autonomic equilibrium unbalanced by emotional turmoil. Surgical procedures have been used occasionally to interrupt autonomic pathways in some disorders. Endocrine products such as steroid hormones are used in some allergic disorders and sexual hormones sometimes are employed to correct persistent psychogenic menstrual irregularities. When such medications are used the patient should understand that they merely are intervening at useful points in the long chain of interpersonal and physical processes producing the psychosomatic illness.

Treatment on the Level of Lower Brain Centers

Some medications used in psychosomatic illnesses act upon the physiology of the hypothalamus, the reticular system, the basal ganglia and other lower brain centers. This field is relatively new and its full possibilities await pharmacologic exploration. For example, prochlorpromazine (Compazine) is useful in treating nausea and vomiting, whether it is of emotional or organic origin. Isocarboxazid (Marplan) and some other monoamine oxidase inhibitors have been advocated as adjuncts in treating angina pectoris which is resistant to other medications. The phenothiazines (Thorazine, Stelazine, Mellaril and others), which appear to exercise much of their activity on lower brain centers, are sometimes used to assuage emotional turmoil in patients with psychosomatic illness. The development of these medications has stimulated much research, which in time may increase the number of therapeutic agents for alleviating emotional distress and psychosomatic disorders by action on lower brain centers. When such medications are used, the patient should understand their intermediate role in the sequence of emotional and physical dysfunctions causing his illness.

Treatment on the Level of the Cerebral Cortex

The emotional and interpersonal functioning of a person has its highest level of neurophysiologic integration in the cerebral cortex. The memories, ideas, feelings and fears of an individual are organized here in their highest articulate and symbolic form. When we speak of guilt, dependent needs, hostile thoughts and daydreams, we are talking mainly of functions of the cerebral cortex, because without a well-functioning cerebral cortex man is capable of only the crudest types of emotional and physical responses to his environment. Successful communication with other people requires complex activities of the cerebral cortex; hence, it is an important level in the chain of functions involved in a psychosomatic illness.

A remarkable property of a cerebral cortex is that it can influence the functioning of the cerebral cortices of other people. When a domineering wife berates her husband and makes him feel guilty, her cerebral cortex is exercising a marked effect on her husband's cerebral cortex, and a harshly critical husband can similarly affect his wife. When a physician talks to a patient about the patient's psychosomatic illness, the cerebral cortex of the physician is acting immediately on the cerebral cortex of the patient; new plans, new ideas and new feelings arise in the cortex of the patient. In a schematic sense, most interpersonal relationships involve the complex interactions of the cerebral cortices of various persons on one another.

The cerebral cortex of a patient may be influenced by talking with him or by giving him medications. Some sedatives, such as amobarbital and phenobarbital, act mainly on the cerebral cortex and occasionally are used to diminish the severe anxiety and agitation that may accompany exacerbations of peptic ulcer, irritable colon syndrome, and other psychosomatic diseases. However, the most useful treatment on the level of the cerebral cortex is talking with the patient. In the treatment of a psychosomatic disorder, the physician in many instances should survey the interpersonal life of the patient and assess his emotional and personality status. He may point out areas of stress, and he may help the patient evaluate the ways in which he handles his feelings of affection, aggressiveness and self-esteem. The doctor may be able to define correlations between the onset or exacerbations of a psychosomatic disease and emotional stresses in the patient's life. (The interview technics outlined in Chapters 4 and 21 may be used to orient the physician in this work.) In many instances, the internist or the family physician can include some counseling of this type in his comprehensive treatment plan for a patient with a psychosomatic illness. When the patient's problems are deeply rooted and the patient will accept psychiatric referral, psychotherapy with a psychiatrist may be advisable.

Treatment on the Level of Interpersonal Relationships

Disturbed interpersonal relationships between the patient and the people around him constitute a further level of dysfunction in a psychosomatic illness. Improvement of interpersonal relationships often aids in the treatment of a psychosomatic illness. When the patient recognizes his interpersonal problems and understands their relation to his psychosomatic disorder, he sometimes can take constructive action to ameliorate his difficulties. Improvement of marital situations or elimination of vocational tensions can sometimes be accomplished by a patient when he understands how such problems are related to his illness. Increased assertiveness by a patient may terminate the upsetting exploitation of him by relatives, friends and employers.

When the patient sees his psychosomatic illness as the product of disturbed interaction with people, his outlook becomes much broader. He no longer sees his problems merely as a search to find the appropriate medication. His orientation is changed, and his opportunity for ameliorative action is greater. Talking things out with aggravating relatives or a difficult work supervisor becomes more than a matter of interpersonal adjustment; it becomes a matter of physical health or illness. Sometimes a difficult marital partner can modify his behavior when he sees that something more is at stake than being dominant in all marital decisions. Some patients with psychosomatic illnesses are not deeply disturbed emotionally, and they are able to use a broader understanding of their illnesses in decreasing interpersonal stresses. In some instances, the family physician may carry out limited counseling about unhealthy relationships with people. However, the physician should consider referral to a psychiatrist or to an appropriate counseling service, such as a marriage counseling facility, when the patient's interpersonal problems are severe and his psychosomatic illness is uninfluenced by the physician's treatment plan.

In dealing with a psychosomatic illness in a child the physician often should talk with the parents to evaluate any stresses in the child's environment. The doctor may be able to do some useful counseling on ways to reduce tension in the child's life. When the parents have deeply ingrained unhealthy attitudes toward the child, referral to a child guidance facility may be advisable if the parents will accept it.

Treatment on the Level of Personality Problems of Persons in the Patient's Environment

Another level of etiology of a patient's psychosomatic illness may lie in the personality problems of important people in his environment. For example, the personality problems of a martial partner who is a chronic alcoholic or of a rebellious, delinquent adolescent son or daughter may be important in the etiology of a psychosomatic illness.

The internist or family physician cannot deal effectively with the personality problems of persons in the patient's environment. However, he may at times find it necessary to point out their possible connection with the patient's psychosomatic illness. He may recommend that the emotionally disturbed member of the patient's family seek psychiatric help for his personality problems. Sometimes, when the family member realizes that his personality problems are not only causing great disturbances in his own life but also are adversely affecting the health of the patient, he accepts the psychiatric help he previously has refused. In a similar manner, the parents of a child with a psychosomatic problem sometimes try to solve their emotional problems or improve an upset marriage when they realize that these emotional disturbances are affecting the health of their child.

Treatment on the Level of Psychosocial Factors

As a rule, the physician can do little about the impact of stressful social and economic forces on a patient, except to indicate their possible relevance to his psychosomatic illness. For example, the influence of living in a violence-filled, drug-ridden neighborhood, or employment in an ominously declining industry, or being trapped in a struggle to maintain a standard of affluent living which is clearly beyond his means, may sometimes be pointed out as socioeconomic factors which are adversely affecting a patient's emotional and physical health.

However, these things lie in a middle ground between medicine and sociology, and physicians differ much in opinion about whether they should comment on such aspects of patients' living circumstances and life styles. Nevertheless, some psychiatrists feel that there is something basically unhealthy about the way that many Americans live, that in many families the home has become a base of operations rather than a close emotional unit, that two marital partners who are highly absorbed in their respective jobs cannot also be effective marital partners and parents, and that all the expensive, needless gimcrackery of the affluent way of life is eroding family relationships and social comfort. The most that the family physician or internist can do is occasionally to ask: How much time, outside of meals and bedtime, do you spend with your martial partner each week? How much time do you spend talking, or doing anything else, with your children every week? Do you feel that the neighborhood you live in, the job you work at, and the standard of living you are struggling to maintain, are emotionally healthy or unhealthy? Do you think that all these things have any bearing on your peptic ulcer? In other words, do your living circumstances and life style constitute a final level of etiology in your psychosomatic illness?

BIBLIOGRAPHY

Brown, D. G., and Bettley, F. R.: Psychiatric treatment of eczema. Brit. Med. J., 2:729, 1971.

Bruch, H.: Eating Disorders: Obesity, Anorexia Nervosa and the Person Within. New York, Basic Books, 1973.

Budzynski, T. H., Stoyva, J. M., Adler, C. S., and Mullaney, D. J.: EMG biofeedback and tension headache. Semin. in Psychiatry, 5:397, 1973.

Cobb, S., and Rose, R. M.: Hypertension, peptic ulcer and diabetes in air traffic controllers. J. A. M. A., 224:489, 1973.

Heine, B.: Psychogenesis of hypertension. Proc. Roy. Soc. Med., 63:1267, 1970.

Kasl, S. V.: Blood pressure changes in men undergoing job loss. Psychosom. Med., 32:19, 1970.

Liebman, R., Minuchin, S., and Baker, L.: The use of structural family therapy in the treatment of intractible asthma. Am. J. Psychiatry, 131: 535, 1974.

Liljefors, I., and Rahe, R. H.; An identical twin study of psychosocial factors in coronary heart disease in Sweden. Psychosom. Med., 32, 1970.

Lind, E., and Theorell, T.: Sociological characteristics and myocardial infarctions. J. Psychosom. Res., 17:59, 1973.

Liss, J. L., Alpers, D., and Woodruff, R. A.: The irritable colon syndrome and psychiatric illness. Dis. Nerv. Syst., 34:151, 1973.

McKegney, F. P., Gordon, R. O., and Levine, S. M.: A psychosomatic comparison of patients with ulcerative colitis and Crohn's disease. Psychosom. Med., 32:153, 1970.

Sacks, O.: Migraine: The Evolution of a Common Disorder. Berkley, University of California Press, 1973.

Spilken, A. Z., and Jacobs, M. A.: Prediction of

illness behavior from measures of life crisis, manifest distress and maladaptive coping. Psychosom. Med. 33:251, 1971.

Stunkard, A.: New therapies for eating disorders. Arch. Gen. Psychiatry, 26:391, 1972.

Surman, O. S., Gottlieb, S. K., Hackett, T. P., and Silverberg, E. L.: Hypnosis in the treatment of warts. Arch. Gen. Psychiatry, 28:439, 1973.

Thiel, H. G., Parker, D., and Bruce, T. A.: Stress factors and the risk of myocardial infarction. J. Psychosom. Res., 17:43, 1973.

Voth, H. M., Holzman, P. S., Katz, J. B., and Wallerstein, R. S.: Thyroid "hot spots": their relationship to life stress. Psychosom. Med., 32:561, 1970.

Section Three

Personality Disorders

Unhealthy interpersonal relationships during the individual's formative years may cause persistent problems in his basic personality structure. These personality disorders limit the person's capacity for comfortable, successful social living. In the first of the two chapters of this section we shall consider the nature of the common personality disorders and we shall discuss their interpersonal causes and psychiatric treatment. In the second chapter of this section we shall discuss the personality problems that contribute to abuse of alcohol and drugs, and we shall examine some of the emotional and social results of alcoholism and drug abuse.

12

The Various Personality Disorders

The kinds of emotional problems we have discussed in previous chapters are characterized by clinical symptoms that distress the patient in some way. The patient finds his phobia, obsession or psychosomatic disorder painful, and he can see it objectively as a difficulty for which he wants help. In this chapter we shall deal with those disorders in which the unhealthy interpersonal relationships in the patient's life lead to persistent distortions or defects of personality structure sufficiently great to bring the patient into significant trouble in social living. In these disorders the emotional difficulties of the patient do not produce symptoms in the usual sense of the word, but cause difficulties in his relationships with people and in his personality structure.

The person who has a personality disorder may be aware to some extent that he has a problem. However, his personality problems often are so entrenched that he cannot see any problems in himself, but attributes his continual difficulties with people to what he feels are the defects of everyone around him. For example, the individual with a paranoid personality disorder usually cannot see that he has a problem; he believes that his suspiciousness about people is justified by their maliciousness and hostility toward him. The person with a pathologically aggressive personality disorder is unaware that he has a problem; he feels that his chronic hostility and aggressiveness are justified by the aggravating behavior and shortcomings of other people. Other persons, such as individuals with pathologically passive personality structures or homosexuals, may be able to see that they have personality problems, but find it difficult to change their behavior.

When we talk about an individual's personality, or personality structure, we (as pointed out in Chapter 1) are not speaking about a rigid, fixed, material thing. *Personality consists of the long-term characteristic ways in which an individual interacts with the people around him, and the ways in which he feels and thinks about himself and others.* The word "personality," or "personality structure," is merely a verbal convenience we use. We can never see, hear, touch, or otherwise directly evaluate a "personality." The only things we can directly observe are the things a person does when he is with us and other people, and how he talks about himself and them.

As Harry Stack Sullivan emphasized, the concept of personality has meaning *only in the context of interpersonal relationships.* A passive person seated alone in a room cannot express his passivity unless someone else, with whom he can be passive enters the room, and a paranoid person must have someone to be paranoid about. Moreover, we cannot discuss, let alone treat, an individual's passivity or his paranoid problems unless we first set up an interpersonal relationship with him.

The interpersonal approach to psychiatry emphasizes that we never deal with a highly speculative thing called the patient's "mind," in which his "personality," or "personality structure," resides, and we cannot proceed validly to divide such a "mind" or "personality" into component parts, such ego, id and others. When we talk about the "mind" and such components we are dealing with things that can never be proved or disproved, and must therefore forever remain subjects of speculation and doubt. Like the concepts of "Divine providence" and "evil," such propositions can be used to explain much that happens to men, but they can never be scientifically demonstrated because of the manner in which they are set up. However, when we base our concepts of "personality" on interpersonal relationships, which can be directly scrutinized, we are on far sounder ground.

The Concepts of Normality and Emotional Maturity

The range of personality disorders extends from minor problems that are borderline normal, to difficulties of such severity that the person is socially incapacitated. A continuous spectrum extends from the normal range of personality structure to severe personality problems. Often it is difficult, and at times arbitrary, to define the point where normality ends and mild personality disorders begin.

Every person has at least a few minor personality problems and occasional emotional difficulties. If "normal" is to mean that there are persons without emotional difficulties and personality problems, then there are no "normal" people. There are, simply, a large number of people of whom we say, not that they are "normal," but that they are "within normal limits." However, all these people have at least a few minor personality problems and occasional small emotional difficulties. "Normality" and "abnormality," then, are parts of a continuous spectrum that fades imperceptibly from one division into the next. The precise point at which "within normal limits" ends and "abnormality" begins may be hard to define in many instances, and it is influenced by cultural standards and the prevailing attitudes of the particular social group in which the person lives.

Moreover, there are no generally accepted standards for defining emotional maturity; however, there are some general concepts, and by examining some of them we can arrive at an idea of what emotional maturity is.

Emotional maturity has been defined as a comfortable capacity for a wide variety of interpersonal relationships with other people in adult life. The emotionally mature person can adjust reasonably well in marriage and he has good capacities to give affection to his marital partner and his children. When his interests require it, he can be firm with other people, but he does not exploit them with undue aggressiveness. He can adjust reasonably well in his work situation and can establish economic self-sufficiency. He can become angry with people occasionally, but he is not continually irritable and bitter. He can impose upon himself the limitations and restrictions that society requires for reasonably harmonious community living. The emotionally mature woman can find satisfaction as a wife and mother, or in a vocational career. She has affection for her family and reasonable capacities for getting along with other people. From time to time the emotionally mature person has difficulties with other people and occasionally he has brief, minor emotional upsets, but he has the personality resources to resolve these problems and to make reasonable decisions about the occasional dilemmas he faces in life.

Some psychiatrists define emotional maturity in terms of continually wider circles of interpersonal activity in the person's life. An infant's first circle of interpersonal life consists only of himself and his mother. In the latter part of the child's first year of life the circle begins to widen to include the father, the child's brothers and sisters and other relatives. This circle of interpersonal activity enlarges a great deal when the child starts to attend school and enters into other groups. During puberty and adolescence, his relationships with persons of the opposite sex take on new meaning and intensity, and his circle of interpersonal activity stretches into wider areas. When he reaches adulthood he enters into vocational areas of activity, takes on economic responsibilities and usually marries and establishes a new family of his own. Then, he watches his own children start the process again in their life journey toward maturity.

If the person gets stuck at any stage in the sequence of continually widening circles of interpersonal activity, his emotional maturity is impaired. For example, the person who never enlarges his circle of close interpersonal relationships beyond an attachment to his mother and father remains emotionally immature and restricted in his life adjustment. Though he may achieve prominence in vocational and economic activities, he is immature in his ability to adjust comfortably in a broad spectrum of interpersonal relationships. Some persons cannot extend their circles of interpersonal life to include comfortable relationships with persons of the opposite sex. Other people cannot give love and warm acceptance to their children. Hence, emotional maturity may be measured in terms of the individual's capacities to enter comfortably into continually widening circles of emotional and social adjustment.

A similar but somewhat different way to evaluate maturity is to use Harry Stack Sullivan's concept of *intimacy*. Intimacy is a state in which the welfare of another person is as important to an individual as his own welfare. A person first becomes capable of some degree of intimacy in late childhood, but its full development occurs in adolescence and early adulthood; its most common adult manifestations in our culture are in marital relationships and parent-child relationships. To the extent that a person's capacity for such intimacy is impaired, his maturity may be considered to be defective.

An inventory of the interpersonal capacities of an adult is yet another way of attempting to define maturity. Has he been successful in his educational and vocational pursuits? Does he assume economic responsibilities? Does adjust reasonably well with people in work situations, in the neighborhood, in social organizations and other areas? How well does he adjust as a marital partner and a parent? What kinds of personality traits and what types of emotional problems are revealed by careful examination by a clinical psychologist?

All these concepts should be employed in evaluating the personality structure of a person and in seeking to define his degree of emotional maturity. Personality can be assessed only by a comprehensive study of the past and current interpersonal relationships of the individual and by a thorough understanding of his emotional functioning.

THE COMMON PERSONALITY DISORDERS

We shall now consider systematically the common kinds of personality disorders. Although there are various systems for classifying personality disorders, we shall use, with some minor modifications, the classification and terminology employed in official standard medical nomenclature. All the personality disorders listed in the standard nomenclature will be covered, but the amount of space devoted to each disorder will depend on how commonly it is used by psychiatrists and other mental health professionals in talking and writing about patients.

Schizoid Personality

A schizoid person is withdrawn and shy, and he fears close interpersonal relationships. He cannot engage in warm, intimate activities with people and he may be unable to express self-assertive and hostile feelings. He struggles with feelings of inadequacy and inferiority, which he may attempt to assuage by extensive daydreaming of accomplishments and fame. Since he finds interpersonal relationships uncomfortable, often he retreats into a world of fantasy. He may spend much time in solitary intellectual pursuits, mechanical work or household duties. Beneath his outer façade of emotional flatness and interpersonal distance from people the schizoid person usually is very sensitive to how people feel about him. His "antennae" are sensitively tuned to note hostility or friendliness in people around him.

The emotional withdrawal of the schizoid person is produced by life experiences in childhood and early adolescence that leave him apprehensive about close relationships with people. The coldness and criticism of rejecting, hostile parents during the child's formative years cause him to expect similar treatment from the world at large; he expects no more from the world than he received at home. Such feelings and ideas may be so ingrained in his personality structure that he is not consciously aware of them, and he may offer various rationalizatons to himself and others to justify his social withdrawal. The schizoid personality pattern often is evident during childhood, but it becomes more obvious during adolescence and young adulthood when wider circles of interpersonal activity are expected and social withdrawal is more noticeable. The schizoid person hesitates a long time before becoming comfortable in a new interpersonal relationship. He needs strong assurances of acceptance before making a new friendship or entering a new group of people.

Some schizoid persons cover their shyness with a thin façade of talkativeness or an energetic, bustling manner, and they may be quite successful vocationally. However, they tend to seek circumstances in life where few interpersonal demands are made of them. Some schizoid persons are emotionally cold in their marriage relationships and with their children. However, others can establish warm bonds in a small family circle, but outside it they are shy and retiring.

The terms "schizoid" and "schizophrenic" must not be confused. Schizoid persons have firm contacts with reality; they merely find warm interpersonal relationships difficult. A schizophrenic has lost contact with reality and has entered a psychotic world of hallucinations, delusions and profound withdrawal from people. The prepsychotic personality of a schizophrenic often was characterized by marked schizoid features, but only a very small percentage of schizoid persons ever develop schizophrenic psychoses.

Schizoid persons vary much in their motivation for psychiatric treatment and their ability to benefit from it. Sometimes they find their interpersonal isolation painful and can use psychotherapy to resolve some of their deeply rooted fears of closeness with people. However, psychotherapy should not be conducted too aggressively with schizoid persons, for they may become very anxious if they come to grips too abruptly with the painful relationships in their early lives that led to their schizoid problems. In some instances, when psychotherapy is conducted aggressively or when the patient is subjected to abrupt penetration of his personality structure by such measures as hypnosis or barbiturate interviews, a schizophrenic episode may be precipitated. The psychotherapy of a schizoid person demands skillful sensitivity by the psychiatrist to the patient's limits for new insight at each stage of therapy. If the schizoid person's anxiety about probing his personality structure and life experiences is too severe, psychotherapy may be unwise.

Compulsive Personality

The person with a compulsive personality disorder (*obsessive compulsive personality,* and *anankastic personality* are synonyms of *compulsive personality*) is characterized by excessive orderliness, frugality and a cold, mechanical quality in his relationships with people. He cannot tolerate disorder, dirt and uncompleted tasks, and he carries out all his activities with systematic meticulousness. He may be capable of a great amount of work, but his work lacks flexibility and interpersonal warmth. He drives with unfeeling, rigid energy toward accomplishment, order and cleanliness. As a housewife, the compulsive person is an endless arranger and cleaner who cannot relax from her work to spend time with her family. As a businessman, the compulsive person is a tireless worker who is insensitive to the feelings of his fellow workers.

The person with a severe compulsive personality disorder may decompensate into depressiveness or marked anxiety when he is deprived of his usual routines and work schedule. He is restless and lost on weekends unless he can substitute a work schedule at home to take the place of his weekday work schedule. He is a classic candidate for the so-called weekend neurosis in which the person becomes anxious when deprived of the harness of his usual weekday activities. He often finds vacations difficult and he tends to feel guilty when he is not working. The compulsive person is overly conscientious and feels that he must justify each day by accomplished work and achievement. He may be scrupulously moralistic and observant of religious obligations. He rigidly pursues the letter of the law while unable to feel its spirit, and is hounded by guilty feelings when he feels he has not fulfilled his obligations. In some instances, the compulsive person becomes torn between conflicting impulses, and he wavers anxiously from one point of view to another in paralyzed indecisiveness.

There are various degrees of compulsiveness in people. A mild degree of compulsiveness can be an asset. Many of the world's most creative persons have channeled their compulsive tendencies into well organized, constructive effort. Indeed, a complete lack of compulsive features may leave the individual mired in disorganization and disorder. However, as one moves toward more severe degrees of compulsiveness this personality quality becomes less an asset and more a barrier to achievement and to warm relationships with people. Persons with severe compulsive personality disorders become so enmeshed in meticulous details that they cannot accomplish the larger, more important tasks. They become emotionally cold, aloof from interpersonal relationships and embroiled in the minutiae of life.

Compulsive personality disorders are produced by the same interpersonal causes (outlined in Chapter 8) which lead to obsessive-compulsive neuroses, but the interpersonal causes of compulsive personality disorders usually are less severe than those of compulsive neuroses. Indeed, there is a continuous spectrum of compulsive problems ranging from the mildest types of compulsive personality disorders to the most severe kinds of obsessive and compulsive neuroses. We need not repeat here the various kinds of interpersonal traumas (outlined in Chapter 8) leading to obsessive and compulsive patterns. The vast majority of persons with compulsive personality disorders never decompensate into frank obsessive or compulsive neuroses; however, a small percentage of them do so, especially when they are subjected to severe interpersonal pressures. Though the patient with an obsessive or compulsive neurosis often has a history of a long-lasting compulsive personality disorder prior to the onset of his neurosis, only a very small percentage of persons with compulsive personality disorders ever decompensate into frank obsessive or compulsive neuroses. Compulsive personality disorders are immensely more common than obsessive and compulsive neuroses.

The results of psychotherapy of persons with compulsive personality disorders are quite variable. Psychotherapy rarely results in complete resolution of a compulsive personality disorder, but often the patient can be helped to develop greater warmth in his relationships with people and more flexibility in his ways of managing his affairs. In many instances the person with a compulsive personality disorder does not seek psychotherapy until a series of upsetting interpersonal events precipitates much anxiety or an exacerbation of his compulsive problems. After such an exacerbation, psychotherapy usually can help the compulsive patient back to his former level of adjustment, and perhaps can help him to soften some of the brittle rigidity of his compulsive personality disorder. In many instances, the compulsive person is seen psychiatrically when problems in his marriage or in rearing his children cause him to seek marriage counseling or child guidance clinic help.

A major obstacle in psychotherapy of the person with a compulsive personality disorder is that he approaches psychotherapy with the same mechanical, meticulous coldness with which he approaches his other activities. Often he does not become emotionally involved in the process of resolving his interpersonal problems, but treats them with cold objectivity. Hence, he may develop a certain amount of glibness in talking about his personality difficulties, but he does not deal with his feelings and he does not resolve emotional issues. This frigid barrier to psychotherapy is most marked in persons with severe compulsive personality disorders, who may glibly engage in long periods of psychotherapy with little improvement. Persons with mild or moderate compulsive personality disorders often are able to deal with their emotions more deeply in psychotherapy and can make better progress in ameliorating problems.

Passive and Aggressive Personality Disorders

Persons who are unduly passive or excessively aggressive in their relationships with people are included in this group. We shall consider separately the personality problems of the overly passive person and those of the overly aggressive person.

Passive Personality. The person with a passive personality disorder is unable to express hostile feelings or to assert himself adequately in his relationships with people. Whereas most people can express a reasonable amount of their angry feelings in a socially acceptable manner, the passive person can express little or no anger. He fears that hostile and assertive actions will cause him to be disliked, isolated and alienated from people. He continually tries to please other people and goes to elaborate lengths to avoid friction with them. He feels devastated and crushed if others get angry at him. These patients are "allergic to anger"; they are uncomfortable both with their own anger and with the anger of other people toward them.

Passive patients sometimes can be capable, achieving people despite their personality problems. Their inability to be assertive with people often is a hindrance to achievement, but by patience and ingenuity they may partially compensate for this difficulty. Their easygoing passivity may cause them to be well liked, and people may praise them for being "able to get along with everybody." However, in many instances they are dominated by their work associates, marital partners and friends. Their inability to refuse the demands of other people puts them chronically in tense positions. These impositions and exploitations of others arouse still more resentment in them, which in turn is bottled up. Thus, a vicious circle is set up which often keeps the passive person chronically anxious. Persons with passive personality disorders are somewhat prone to develop phobias, anxiety states, some kinds of psychosomatic illnesses and other kinds of psychiatric difficulties because of their large amounts of pent-up hostile feelings.

Passive personality disorders are divided into two subtypes: (1) *passive-dependent type* and (2) *passive-aggressive type*. The person with a passive-dependent personality is emotionally dependent on other people. He leans on them to make decisions for him and to guide him in his activities. He is indecisive, timid and easily dominated by other people. The person with a passive-aggressive personality cannot be assertive or express angry feelings, but he resists the aggressiveness of others by foot-dragging obstructionism, evasiveness and procrastination. He may appear placid while he passively resists the wishes of others, or he may at times retreat into a whining sullenness or a silent withdrawal.

During his childhood and adolescence the passive person usually was dominated by his parents and other close persons who made him feel guilty and unloved whenever he was assertive or angry. Such parental suppressiveness caused the child to feel much anxiety and guilt each time angry feelings arose in him, and he soon began to repress those feelings. His parents' affection was purchased at the price of his docile obedience, and the child gradually developed the feeling that assertiveness led to emotional rejection and social isolation. He dreaded the torrent of guilt-slinging he got from his parents each time he asserted himself at home, and he developed the fear that the world would treat him similarly if he was assertive outside his home. In time the passive child or adolescent lost his ability to recognize his angry and assertive feelings or to be aware of them; although much hostility smoldered deeply within him, he protested that he never had angry feelings or assertive urges.

The patient with a passive personality disorder in many instances is well motivated for psychotherapy and can make much progress in it. He may be able to trace the origins of his fears of assertiveness to interpersonal trauma during his formative years, and he may begin to lose his dread of the consequences of expression of reasonable amounts of anger. Sometimes the patient can use the patient-therapist relationship in his first experiences in being assertive. I recall a 29-year-old woman whose first assertiveness occurred when one day she angrily expressed her indignation because, after exceeding the speed limit to get to my office on time for her appointment, she had to wait 25 minutes to see me because I was running behind in my schedule. She was able to express her irritation without anxiousness or guilt and without fears of rejection or retaliation by me. In time she learned to be comfortable with assertiveness in a wide spectrum of interpersonal activities. The passive person in many instances can overcome gradually the personality problems that make him unduly dependent on others and fearful of reasonable assertiveness. However, the patient with a passive-aggressive type of passive personality disorder often brings into his relationship with the therapist the same foot-dragging resistances that have become ingrained in many of his interpersonal activities, and their resolution may present difficult problems in psychotherapy.

Aggressive Personality. The person with an aggressive personality disorder is irascible and easily irritated; he has excessive assertiveness and marked expression of anger. Such persons often fly into rages when they meet the normal frustrations and stresses of life, and often they are domineering toward the people around them. When they have their way they often can be pleasant and well liked, but when their wishes are obstructed they become abruptly angry. If they are talented and well coordinated in their dealings with people, they may be driving and successful in vocational and social activities. If they are ineffective and lack ability, they may be bitter, chronically irritable persons in continual conflict with those around them. The person with an aggressive personality disorder can maintain sufficient self-control to avoid antisocial and delinquent actions. However, persons with severe aggressive personality disorders at times may border on the category labeled "antisocial personality disorder" (discussed in a later part of this chapter). Behind his aggressiveness the overly assertive person sometimes has dependency needs that he cannot consciously face. His aggressiveness in many instances is a blustering façade to disguise from himself and others his underlying anxieties and insecurities.

Over aggressive personality disorders may be produced by a variety of interpersonal backgrounds. Often the overly aggressive person received much hostility and little love during his childhood and adolescence. He emerged from his formative years as an angry rebel, diffusely hostile toward a world that he experienced as cold and punitive. In other instances, the aggressive person was overly indulged and few limitations were placed on his impulses and desires; he was reared without affection and without discipline, and as an adult he is aggressive and angry when people do not yield promptly to his wishes, as his parents and others in his childhood did. Sometimes the aggressive person was reared with brutality, and aggressive harshness in turn became his ingrained method of handling all interpersonal problems. The aggressive person may have formed an unhealthy identification with a chronically hostile mother or father, and he may imitate unconsciously the behavior of this dominant parent.

In general, the person with an aggressive personality disorder is an unpromising candidate for successful psychotherapy. The aggressive person often is irritable and impatient with the therapist whenever the therapist does not concur spontaneously with his opinions and feelings; this presents marked problems in therapy, and the patient often stops treatment after a few sessions. Moreover, the aggressive person often spends his time in therapy talking about the provocations he feels he receives from others, and he is unable to examine his own personality problems. However, a minority of aggressive persons benefit from psychotherapy, and any well-motivated aggressive patient may be encouraged to undergo a trial of interview treatment to seek improvement of his personality problems. In many instances, the aggressive patient is seen when his personality problems precipitate marriage difficulties or child-rearing problems, which bring him and his family to psychiatric counseling services. In such circumstances, the aggressive patient often can recognize the marital or child-rearing problems but cannot accept his own behavior as contributants to their causes. Psychotherapy of the aggressive patient rarely is successful when his relatives push him into it; successful treatment depends on some degree of spontaneous desire to change.

Cyclothymic Personality

An individual with a cyclothymic personality disorder (also at times termed an *affective personality disorder*) has periods of energetic exhilaration which alternate with periods of mild depressiveness. The mood changes of the cyclothymic person may shift once every several weeks, or once every few months, or once every few years. During his periods of exhilaration the cyclothymic person feels buoyant, energetic, self-confident and cheerful. He makes plans, carries out projects, and relates warmly to people; this is sometimes called his euphoric period. During his depressed periods he feels somewhat discouraged, fatigued, sad and inferior. He is less active, is somewhat seclusive socially, and ruminates on what he feels are his shortcomings and failures. However, in the vast majority of cyclothymic persons the exhilarated phases are never sufficiently marked to justify being termed manic disorders, and his depressive periods are relatively mild. Often the person's family and friends take for granted that he has his "high" periods and "low" periods and think little more about it.

As opposed to the schizoid person (with

whom he is often contrasted), the cyclothymic person usually feels comfortable in a wide range of interpersonal activities. He is gregarious and has good capacities for giving affection to others and for receiving it. He can express most of his feelings openly and comfortably. He prefers activities with people and shuns solitary pursuits. Whereas the schizoid person prefers work that removes him from intimate contact with people, the cyclothymic person prefers a job in which he is in continual interaction with many people.

Psychiatrists feel that the mood fluctuations of the cyclothymic person are caused by a deeply hidden depressive current running through his personality structure. His bouyant, exhilarated periods are defenses against the tendency of this depressive current to rise to the surface. In a sense, by ebullient, gregarious behavior the person unconsciously tries to deflect the depressive current out of his awareness. Hence, the exhilarated moods of the cyclothymic person sometimes have a somewhat overeager, forced quality, as if the person unconsciously were saying, "If I were not exhilarated, I would fall into sadness." However, the hypomanic defense against depressiveness does not entirely resolve his personality problem. From time to time his mild depressive current rises to the surface and a depressive period occurs.

The causes of the cyclothymic person's mood swings lie in subtle emotional trauma during his formative years that left him with lingering doubts about his adequacy, self-esteem and value as a person. Emotional rejection, depreciation and hostility from close people in his early years left the patient with a tendency to depressiveness which he covers with his exhilarated moods. He reaches out eagerly for contacts with people to reassure himself constantly that by their acceptance of him and affection for him he is shown to be an esteemed and loved person. He uses achievement as a further avenue to continuing support of his self-esteem. (These emotional problems basically are similar to those outlined in Chapters 10, 15 and 16 on depressive and manic disorders, but the problems of the cyclothymic person are much less severe.)

Most cyclothymic persons are not strongly motivated for psychotherapy since their mood swings usually do not reach sufficient proportions to cause them significant interpersonal difficulties. They can see no need for psychotherapy during their exhilarated periods, and the discomforts of their depressive phases usually are not painful enough to give them motivation for treatment. However, if a person with cyclothymic personality problems is motivated to engage in psychotherapy to resolve his underlying emotional problems, he sometimes benefits from it.

Patients with manic or depressive psychoses, or neurotic depressions, sometimes have histories of preexisting cyclothymic personality structures. However, only a very small percentage of persons with cyclothymic personality structures ever develop manic or depressive psychoses, or neurotic depressions.

Paranoid Personality

The person with a paranoid personality disorder suspects the people around him of having hostile, malicious feelings toward him. His paranoid feelings may be diffuse or circumscribed. He may suspect everyone of malicious intentions, or he may suspect only a few people or a particular group of persons. A mildly paranoid person may say little about his paranoid feelings, though he may sometimes mention them. Other paranoid persons talk openly about their suspicions and they may embarrass or upset their families and friends by doing so. Persons with paranoid personality disorders often suspect the intentions of relatives, work associates or neighbors. Suspicions of infidelity by their marital partners are common in paranoid persons.

Many persons with paranoid personality disorders are cold, aloof individuals who nurse grudges, ruminate over minor injuries from others and are sullen and retiring in manner. They have much simmering irritability which they hide behind a fragile façade of formal self-control, but their irritability breaks out in unpredictable bursts of anger and hostile suspiciousness. Their marriages often are difficult, and their children receive little warmth from them. Some paranoid people appear gregarious and socially outgoing on the surface, but underneath this veneer is much paranoid sensitivity and hostility, which occasionally seeps to the surface. The paranoid person usually cannot establish lasting friendships or close interpersonal relationships. Though his paranoid feelings may vary in intensity, the underlying personality structure of the person tends to remain persistently tinged with paranoid preoccupations. In occasional instances, the paranoid feelings may seem to disappear for long periods of time, but they are prone to return when the individual is under stress.

There is a wide spectrum of paranoid difficulties extending from mild suspiciousness about the intentions of other people to elaborate delusions of persecution. Minor degrees of paranoid sensitivity are common and may interfere relatively little in the person's interpersonal life. A paranoid personality disorder of moderate degree may be compatible with a successful vocational career, but it usually causes many problems in the person's intimate interpersonal relationships and hinders a comfortable adjustment in many social areas. In severe paranoid problems the person's thinking is dominated by paranoid suspicions, which are diffuse and often bizarre. At the more severe end of the spectrum of paranoid disorders, persons with marked paranoid disturbances no longer are classified as having paranoid personality disorders, but are classified as suffering from paranoia, or paranoid state or paranoid schizophrenia (discussed in later chapters), depending on the severity of the process and the bizarreness of the patient's persecutory delusions. In this chapter we are discussing only the mildest types of paranoid problems which are grouped under the category of paranoid personality disorder.

Paranoid ideas occur when an individual projects onto other persons various strong feelings of his own with which he cannot come to grips. For example, the man with suspicions of marital infidelity about his wife is projecting onto her impulses of marital infidelity he himself has, but which he cannot recognize or accept. He rids himself of these uncomfortable feelings by casting them out of himself onto his wife and suspecting her of his own unconscious, forbidden wishes. The person who suspects others of hostility to himself actually has much unconscious hostility toward others.

Harry Stack Sullivan viewed paranoid processes in a somewhat different way (which we shall also disucss in Chapter 17). He felt that a paranoid slant occurs when (1) an individual has deep feelings of inadequacy and (2) transfers blame to others. He cannot become articulately aware of either his feelings of inadequacy or the process in which he transfers blame to the people around him; he merely feels a deep distress and uneasy threat to his self-esteem and worth, which he resolves by saying, as it were, "The problem is not that I am inadequate and worthless, but rather that malicious persons are scheming to make me appear worthless and of no value." From this point, over a period of years, the person slowly evolves ideas of specific ways in which people are trying to malign him, exploit him and despise him. Thus, he maintains a feeling of self-respect and personal worth at the cost of developing paranoid ideas.

Moreover, Sullivan pointed out, the development of this paranoid outlook destroys the individual's capacity to engage in close, comfortable interpersonal relationships, the only way by which his paranoid warp could be corrected. Thus, a vicious circle is set up. The paranoid person withdraws from people and becomes aloof, and the more isolated he becomes the more easily he can misinterpret the intentions and feelings of others. Whether this process stops at the relatively mild level of a paranoid personality disorder or proceeds gradually into a bizarre paranoid schizophrenic process depends on how profound the persons' sense of inferiority is, how desperate his need is for reassuring delusions that others are to blame rather than himself, and how isolated from people he becomes.

The paranoid person's deep sense of personal inadequacy begins in early childhood and is reinforced by his interpersonal experiences during later childhood and adolescence. He experienced coldness, rejection, hostility and depreciation from his parents and other close people. Thus, he developed what Sullivan called the "malevolent transformation"; he came to view himself as ugly and unworthy, and the world as menacing and malicious toward him. Nowhere during his formative years did he find the warm, reassuring relationships which would have given him feelings that perhaps he was a reasonably worthwhile person and that the world was not entirely threatening and punitive toward him. By the time he reached middle adolescence he had developed so ingrained a suspiciousness of people that he no longer could form the close relationships that might have helped him.

Many psychiatrists feel that, in addition to these factors, the paranoid person has much repressed hostility about the way he was reared, and that he cannot deal with this hostility in any conscious, healthy way. In later years he therefore tends to project this hostility onto others. Instead of coming to grips with the bitterness and pent-up hostility within himself, he attributes it to everyone around him, and sees them as hostile and vengeful toward him.

Freudian-psychoanalytic theory suggests that paranoid ideas arise out of unconscious homosexual impulses. It is as if the person desperately seeks to escape his homosexual feelings by saying, "I do not love him, but rather I despise him, and my dislike of him is justified by his continual maliciousness toward me." This basic process can be elaborated in various ways to account for the diverse expressions of paranoid feelings. (This view of paranoid problems is further considered in Chapter 17 on other kinds of paranoid disorders.)

The person with a well-ingrained paranoid personality disorder usually is very resistant to all types of psychiatric treatment. A patient who has long had scarcely noticeable paranoid trends may have a flareup of paranoid ideas when he is under special stress, and such an exacerbation often subsides spontaneously. However, in psychiatric practice one more commonly sees patients with long patterns of paranoid suspiciousness which have periodic exacerbations. Persons with paranoid personality disorders in most instances are reluctant to enter psychotherapy and do poorly in it. Some psychiatrists are skeptical of the advisability of attempting psychotherapy with paranoid patients because they may become agitated and more suspicious if therapy is conducted too aggressively.

In some instances a person who has long adjusted at the level of a paranoid personality disorder may decompensate into one of the more severe types of paranoid illnesses (discussed in Chapters 14 and 17 under paranoid schizophrenia and the various paranoid psychotic states). Decompensation into a psychotic paranoid illness may occur so insidiously that it is difficult to state when the patient passed from the milder area of paranoid personality disorder into the more severe area of paranoid psychosis. In other instances, a life situational crisis or a series of upsetting interpersonal stresses may abruptly precipitate an exacerbation of a paranoid psychosis. Such paranoid psychotic illnesses may occur in middle aged and elderly persons who had mild paranoid personality disorders during their earlier adult years. In middle aged persons, such paranoid psychoses are precipitated by the problems of adjusting to the many emotional stresses of middle age (outlined in Chapter 25). In elderly persons paranoid psychoses may be precipitated both by the emotional difficulties of old age and by the problems of making new interpersonal adjustments while subtle senile deterioration of brain tissue is diminishing the individual's intellectual and emotional flexibility.

Inadequate Personality

The diagnosis "inadequate personality" was first introduced into the standard nomenclature in 1952, and, although some psychiatrists feel that the term is somewhat undesirable and that its characteristics are vague, it has proved useful for some kinds of personality problems which do not fit any other category, and it has been carried into the current nomenclature.

The person with an inadequate personality disorder has normal intelligence and he does not have physical defects. However, his interpersonal adjustment is characterized by irresponsibility, ineptness and poor judgement. He makes erratic adjustments in his scholastic, vocational and economic activities, and he usually drifts from one uncompleted venture to another. He does not persevere in his projects, for neither the rewards of success nor the discomforts of failure spur him to sustained, well-planned activities. He may be blandly good-natured and gregarious, or he may be ill at ease and awkward with people. He adapts poorly to new situations, and he has little ingenuity and few emotional resources in meeting the day-to-day problems of life.

The person with an inadequate personality disorder has problems in his emotional, economic and social adjustments. He is emotionally dependent on his parents, his marital partner or others, and relies on them to repair his failures and to take on the responsibilities he does not assume. His relationships with other people are always superficial, for he can neither give nor receive deep affection, though he leans on other people in an immature way. The inadequate man often is economically dependent on his family, though sometimes he makes a marginal adjustment in a routine, poorly paying job that demands little of him. The woman with an inadequate personality disorder flounders as a wife and a mother, and others fill in for her deficiencies in rearing her children. In many instances, the marriage of the inadequate person drifts chaotically until it terminates in divorce. This general pattern of interpersonal inadequacy becomes apparent by middle or late adolescence and usually persists throughout the person's adulthood.

Various kinds of unhealthy interpersonal relationships during the individual's formative years may contribute to the formation of an inadequate personality structure. In some instances, the inadequate person was reared by overprotective, hovering parents who did not allow him to develop independence, self-reliance and social adaptability. The parents' overprotective guidance of all his acts and decisions left the patient with the conviction that he was an inferior, inept person who could not make sound decisions or carry out projects effectively. Hence, he fears to attempt things and does not persevere when he encounters problems in any sphere of activity. In other instances, the person with an inadequate personality was emotionally neglected during his formative years and received little love or guidance. In some cases, the inadequate person's relationships with both his parents were so distant that he could not identify himself with either one of them, and he did not develop the ideals, standards and goals that would have given him strength and direction in his life activities. In still other cases the inadequate person was subjected daily to parental criticism and depreciation, and he lacked other close interpersonal relationships in which he could have developed a more optimistic, self-respectful, confident view of himself; he feels inferior and inept, and, when faced with a problem he either wallows in indecisiveness or makes an impulsive, unwise decision.

The person with an inadequate personality disorder rarely has the motivation or the persistence to engage meaningfully in psychotherapy. In those instances in which he is seen in psychiatric consultation, he usually is brought by his relatives who hope that psychotherapy can correct some of his personality problems. However, the patient usually gives only halfhearted cooperation and finds little to talk about in psychotherapy. Hence, treatment usually falters, and the results are poor. Occasionally, when threatened by a life crisis such as impending divorce or job failure, the patient can summon up sufficient motivation to benefit from short-term psychotherapy, but the therapist usually must play an active role to keep psychotherapy going and to make it meaningful.

Antisocial Personality Disorder

The person with an antisocial personality disorder is in chronic conflict with the people around him and with the moral standards of society. He has a defective sense of the rights and feelings of others, and he exploits them unfeelingly. He does not have the capacity to form sincere, affectionate interpersonal relationships; he uses people like objects that are either convenient or inconvenient to his desires of the moment. The antisocial person has a profound self-centeredness, which excludes perception of the sufferings, wishes and rights of others. He runs roughshod over other people and uses deceit, callousness and unscrupulousness to achieve his self-centered ends. He has little concept of the demands and rights of society; his own wishes, impulses and emotions crowd all other considerations to the wall. In the older systems of nomenclature, antisocial personality disorder was labeled "psychopathic personality," and the individual with this personality structure was called a "psychopath." "Sociopathic personality disorder" was a related but not exactly synonymous term in the older nomenclature.

The individual with an antisocial personality disorder has little guilt, anxiety or shame about his acts. His pathological lack of guilt and anxiety about his antisocial behavior leads some psychiatrists to say that he has "Swiss cheese morality," or a "Swiss cheese superego." He often is irresponsible in his economic life and in his duties as a marital partner and parent. He has little ability to bear frustration or to postpone satisfaction of his desires. He is unable to tolerate the routine, tedious tasks of life. The goals of the antisocial person are short-term, and he is unable to work patiently toward the achievement of long-term goals.

The person with an antisocial personality disorder does not learn from punishment or failure. He barges carelessly from impulse to impulse, seizing immediate gratifications at the cost of eventual disasters. When the consequences of his acts catch up with him he often tries to evade them with florid, persuasive lying, which may at first seem convincing, but which is found to be false when his statements are checked against the facts. Frequently, he is melodramatic and exhibitionistic in a crisis, with vehement protestations of innocence or accusations against other people.

Some persons with antisocial personalities are glib, pleasant and even charming on superficial acquaintance. They may tell elaborate, untrue tales about their accomplishments and family connections. Other antisocial persons are angry, belligerent rebels against society, its customs and its morals. Some antisocial persons descend into criminal paths and are repeatedly in legal trouble. A large number of petty swindlers, cheats, prostitutes and recidivist criminals fall in the category of antisocial personality disorder. The antisocial person learns little from previous apprehension in antisocial acts, and he flounders from one crisis to the next.

The interpersonal problems of the individual with an antisocial personality disorder often begin to be apparent during late childhood. He may even then be evasive, rebellious and deceptive in his relationships with his parents and schoolmates, and his tendency to avoid the consequences of his acts by elaborate lying may begin. His antisocial problems usually become more marked during adolescence as his interpersonal life becomes more complex and he is expected to assume more responsibility. In adolescence his scholastic and sexual irresponsibility may become prominent, and he may go into sullen, evasive rebellion against his parents, school authorities and other adults. He may engage in delinquent and illegal acts, and he has more than average probability of drug abuse.

In his adult years, the antisocial person often goes through a series of turbulent marriages and divorces. He pays little attention to the children of his marriages and leaves a trail of damaged people behind him. As he proceeds through his adult years, the social and legal consequences of his antisocial behavior often begin to close in on him, and his deceit and evasiveness no longer enable him to get out of the interpersonal dilemmas his behavior creates. Chronic alcoholism is common in antisocial persons in adult life, and narcotic addiction and chronic drug misuse occasionally occur.

An antisocial personality disorder may be mild, moderate or severe. Some persons with mild or moderate antisocial personality disorders may achieve economic success, but when they do so it is usually in vocational fields, such as some types of sales work, where sustained, close contact with people is not necessary. In a similar manner, persons with mild or moderate antisocial personality disorders may achieve social or professional prominence, but they do so by moving quickly in a wide social circle in which few people ever get to know them well. However, beneath the veneer of economic or social prominence, the antisocial person's family life and other close relationships are chaotic. The person with a severe antisocial personality disorder is chronically involved in severe interpersonal problems in all areas of his life, and often he is economically and socially incapacitated.

Various kinds of unhealthy interpersonal relationships during childhood and early adolescence may contribute to the formation of antisocial personality disorders. In many instances the child had painful relationships with both his parents and did not form a warm, healthy identification with either one of them. Often, both parents rejected the child emotionally, and treated him with cold indifference or irritability while they were preoccupied with their own pleasures and problems. No one else stepped in to fill the child's needs, and he grew out of his formative years without an interpersonal model on which to pattern his life. A person's sense of morality, social conformity and interpersonal harmony is largely developed out of healthy relationships during childhood and adolescence. When the person does not have at least a minimum amount of healthy interpersonal life in his formative years, he may emerge without the moral and social standards necessary for successful community living, and he develops an antisocial personality disorder. As outlined in Chapter 1, a person's moral standards (psychoanalytically included under the term *superego*) are developed as a child gradually patterns his behavior and his ideals on the models provided by parents with whom he has healthy, affectionate relationships. When the child's relationships with his parents are cold, distant and chaotic, he may have no models from which he can assimilate standards of moral and social conformity; also, he does not develop a capacity for the warm interpersonal give-and-take on which all intimate associations are based.

In other instances the person with an antisocial personality disorder was treated by his parents and other close persons with such marked hostility and neglect during childhood and adolescence that he emerged from his formative years an angry rebel against society and all its standards. His diffuse hostility overflows into all his interpersonal relationships and pushes aside other feelings and considerations. In some cases, the antisocial patient throughout his childhood witnessed, and was subjected to, the continual cruelty of a brutal parent, and the patient unconsciously identified himself with that parent and adopted his behavior characteristics and standards. In other instances, the child becomes a pawn in a hostile struggle between his parents, and one parent encourages the child's antisocial tendencies in order to use him as a vengeful tool against the other parent. Other kinds of interpersonal traumas also may contribute to the development of an antisocial personality disorder. The life history of each patient must be studied carefully to determine the particular kinds of emotional traumas that have led to his antisocial problems.

There is some resemblance between severe antisocial personality disorders and the personality changes that may occur in some patients who have had encephalitis or other types of diffuse, subtle damage of the cerebral cortex. For example, after encephalitis or a severe head injury that causes persistent brain damage, a person may become impulsive, irritable and insensitive to the feelings of others; he may fabricate untrue stories to evade the consequences of his misdemeanors and he may be explosively angry at times. Hence, some psychiatrists feel that in some cases antisocial personality disorders are caused by encephalitis or other diffuse cerebral cortical brain damage. They speculate that such damage occurred in encephalitic illnesses or other forms of brain damage that were not correctly diagnosed when they occurred in childhood, and in this way they explain the absence of a clear-cut history of brain damage in the patient's past life. In other instances, the personality disturbance is felt to be due to subtle brain damage that occurred before, during or shortly after birth. In most cases the evidence for such brain damage is speculative, and neurological studies are normal. Often the evidence rests on borderline electroencephalograms or doubtful findings in psychological testing. Most psychiatrists now feel that organic brain disease is the cause of antisocial personality disorders in less than one per cent of cases. The physician should insist on clear, compelling evidence of organic brain disease before accepting it as a cause of an antisocial personality disorder. Borderline or questionable evidence should be rejected, and the causes of the patient's antisocial behavior should be sought in his interpersonal environment during his childhood and early adolescent years.

Occasionally a psychiatrist is called upon to give an opinion about the psychiatric state and legal responsibility of a person with an antisocial personality disorder who is charged with a criminal act. (The difficult subject of the psychiatric criteria for responsibility for criminal acts is covered in Chapter 27 on the legal aspects of psychiatry.)

The vast majority of persons with antisocial personality disorders are not motivated to enter psychotherapy to work on their personality problems. When they do enter psychotherapy they usually do so because of pressure from relatives or legal authorities who press it on them as the alternative to punitive action, and the patient often sees therapy as a way to avoid punishment for illegal or socially reprehensible acts rather than an earnest effort to change his personality structure. Some psychiatrists feel that persons with antisocial personality disorders are untreatable.

The antisocial person does not have the stimulus of painful anxiety and guilt to spur his motivation for psychotherapy. Moreover, his inability to establish meaningful interpersonal relationships inhibits the use of the therapist-patient relationship as an avenue of therapy. The antisocial patient often carries into psychotherapy the same hostility, deceptiveness and evasiveness that characterize his other ventures, and psychotherapy fails in the same way that the antisocial person's other interpersonal activities fail. In many instances the antisocial person breaks off therapy after a few visits unless he is compelled by legal authorities or his family to continue it.

However, some psychiatrists report successful psychotherapy with selected patients who have antisocial personality disorders. As a rule, the patients who benefit from psychotherapy are in their adolescence or early adulthood, and they have at least a minimal amount of anxiety and guilt to motivate them in treatment. Their antisocial personality problems are mild or moderate in degree and they have a few healthy personality features that can be used in therapy. The patient with a severe antisocial personality disorder, especially if he is beyond his early adult years, rarely benefits from psychotherapy.

Dyssocial Behavior. A distinction is made between the individual with an antisocial personality disorder and the person who has *dyssocial behavior*. The dyssocial person is in chronic conflict with society because he was reared in an environment in which the usual standards of morality and social conformity were not followed. In many instances he was reared in a social splinter group in which illegal activity was common and accepted. Within his special group the person with dyssocial behavior may be capable of developing close, loyal interpersonal relationships, but he is in conflict with the broader social groups outside his own circle. He adheres to the standards of his own group and rejects the moral and cultural standards of society as a whole. Many professional gamblers, petty thieves and traffickers in illegal goods fall in the category of persons with dyssocial behavior. Help for individuals with dyssocial behavior must come from the social, legal and psychiatric groups that work in this field.

A condition which should be distinguished from both antisocial personality disorder and dyssocial behavior is *kleptomania*. This is a very rare disorder; in over a quarter century of active consultative and therapeutic psychiatric work, I have seen only one case of true kleptomania. The kleptomaniac gets a profound sensual thrill from the act of stealing; in some cases he may experience sexual orgasm during a theft. The one kleptomaniac I studied stole objects of many kinds, including two-foot square oil paintings, from stores over a 10-year period, but was never apprehended. This patient got a profound exhilaration from thefts; the objects stolen thereafter had no meaning and were either stored in the basement or given away. Except in this area, the patient had reasonably sound marital, vocational and social relationships. Although the medical literature contains some psychiatric case reports of kleptomania, the well studied cases are so few that its emotional origins and interpersonal roots cannot be confidently stated.

OTHER PERSONALITY DISORDERS

The standard system of psychiatric diagnoses contains three further personality disorders: *asthenic personality, explosive personality* and *hysterical personality*. These three diagnoses were first introduced into the official American nomenclature in 1968 to make it consonant with the diagnostic system advocated by the World Health Organization. The first two of these terms (asthenic personality and explosive personality) are little used by American psychiatrists and other mental health professional workers.

The third of these diagnoses (hysterical personality) is not widely used in hospital charts, clinic records, insurance forms and other records where diagnoses are officially given, since the word "hysterical" implies to many laymen and nonpsychiatric medical persons that the patient is a weak, annoying person who could "pull out of it if he (or more often, she) really wanted to." Also, the term "hysterical personality" tends to cause confusion with the hysterical conversion and dissociative neuroses, which are discussed in Chapter 9; the vest majority of patients who are labeled "hysterical personality" do not have hysterical conversion and dissociative symptoms. However, in day-to-day talk about patients, and occasionally in the psychiatric literature, psychiatrists and other mental health professional workers sometimes use the term and concept "hysterical personality"; if, in this context, its limitations are recognized the term has some usefulness.

The amount of space devoted here to these three diagnostic categories will be in proportion to the extents to which they are employed in American psychiatry.

Asthenic Personality. As described in the current standard nomenclature, the individual with an asthenic personality has little energy, poor initiative, easy fatiguability, little enthusiasm in any area of his life, and little tolerance for either unpleasant stress or pleasant excitement. Since the introduction of this term in 1968 so little has been written about it, and it has been so little employed in American psychiatry, that the causes, course and treatment of this condition cannot be confidently discussed. The standard nomenclature states that "asthenic personality" must be differentiated from "neurasthenic neurosis." (The infrequent usage and vague characteristics of "neurasthenic neurosis", which also is little employed in American psychiatry, are covered in Chapter 10.)

Explosive Personality. An individual with an explosive personality disorder has frequent outbursts of violent rage during which he verbally storms at the people around him. Occasionally, he is physically abusive to others during some of his outbursts. After an episode of fury he is repentant and chagrinned, and may ask forgiveness for his uncontrollable behavior. He is unable to control his actions during his tirades, and they may occur daily or once every few weeks. The patient remembers clearly what he does when he is furious. Between these episodes he usually adjusts well to people, and may be gregarious and well liked.

Presumably, the person with an explosive personality has much repressed hostility, perhaps mixed with guilt and anxiety, which he controls most of the time but which erupts in his "explosive" behavior when he is subjected to various kinds of stresses and tensions. However, so little has been written about this diagnostic category, and it is so rarely used in American psychiatry, that its psychodynamics, course and treatment cannot be definitely discussed.

In the standard nomenclature, the term "epileptoid personality disorder" is given as a synonym of explosive personality disorder. This is confusing to American mental health professional workers since these patients usually do not have epilepsy. This synonymous term is given to make this diagnostic category consonant with the continental European and Soviet psychiatric concept that there is some poorly understood connection between the explosive person's outbursts and the cerebral dysrhythmias on eleclectroencephalograms that are characteristic of epilepsy. Also, the term "epileptoid personality" harkens back in a poorly defined way to the old concept that epileptics have special personality characteristics; this concept was long ago abandoned in American psychiatry.

Hysterical Personality. The individual with a hysterical personality disorder (in the standard nomenclature, *histrionic personality disorder* is listed as a synonym for this condition) is immature, self-centered, vain and at times dramatic in his behavior. He also tends to be petulantly demanding and attention-seeking. In many cases he is coyly seductive with persons of the opposite sex and blatantly parades his sexuality in exhibitionistic ways. He is emotionally labile, shifting from gayness to sobbing despair or temper tantrumish fury, and back again, within a matter of minutes.

For unclear reasons, this diagnosis is more often applied to women than to men, though this may be a clinical artefact; this condition probably is equally common in both sexes. The woman with a hysterical personality disorder is a gay, chatty person who often behaves in a sexually provocative way toward men as a means of manipulating them, or perhaps because she knows no other way of relating to men. Beneath this veneer of sexy bravura, she usually is nonorgasmic (frigid), though she may put on a passionate show during intercourse. She is too immature and childish to become truly involved sexually and to have orgasms. When her wishes are granted and things go her way, she can be charming in a girlish manner, but when her desires are thwarted and she faces stress she flounders in an agitated manner, or becomes poutishly angry or panicky. Brief, melodramatic bouts of depressiveness, which begin and end abruptly when her wishes are granted or refused, are common.

The hysterical person may adjust fairly well socially during his adolescence and early 20's, since he has relatively little responsibility at this time and few demands are made of him. However, as he begins to assume obligations as a marital partner and a parent, for which he does not have the necessary maturity and emotional resources, he often decompensates. He looks about for someone on whom he can lean and for people who will assume the responsibilities for which he is ill equipped. When he does not find such social and emotional supports, he often decompensates into panic states, episodic depressiveness, chronic physical symptomatology of psychogenic origin, and alcoholism. Such interpersonal deterioration is common during his 30's and 40's.

The characteristics and life history of a person with a hysterical personality disorder are illustrated by a 36-year-old woman whom I treated for a period of several weeks. An only child, she was reared by self-centered, negligent parents who gave her whatever she wanted, left her to be reared by maids, and handed her money whenever she sought companionship from them. She grew into a vain, egocentric, superficially charming young woman whose social behavior was a caricature of the sexy siren. She dropped out of college in her second year and dabbled at a succession of jobs and careers during her 20's while her parents supported her financially. She married impulsively at 30 and a year later had a child; she was unable to cope with the duties of a mother and the role of a wife, and was sexually nonorgasmic, though she feigned melodramatic ecstasy during the sex act. Having never had a sound, mature interpersonal relationship during her childhood and early adolescence, she could not form mature bonds as an adult. She became panicky and had brief depressive periods, and saw four psychiatrists for short times during a 12-month span. She apparently did well in psychotherapy with each psychiatrist for a few weeks, but broke off therapy when the psychiatrist would not comply with her petulant demands that he enter into her home life and, in conferences with her husband and parents, quickly solve all her problems. During this time she made three suicidal gestures with small quantities of antianxiety tablets. On another occasion, psychiatric hospitalization was precipitated when she struck a pose in the living room with the point of a kitchen knife directed at her larynx and then called her husband into the room to tell him farewell. After the brief period during which she was under my care, she saw several other psychiatrists and went through three further marriages.

During his formative years the individual with a hysterical personality disorder receives neither affection nor realistic limitations on his behavior. Never having had a mature, intimate interpersonal relationship during childhood and adolescence, he remains self-centered, childish and demanding. For him, people are merely convenient or inconvenient objects which satisfy, or do not satisfy, his whims and needs. The hysterical person tends to act out childish daydreams of romantic love affairs and vocational achievements without clear perception of how unrealistic his aspirations and behavior are, and how his daydreams clash with the day-to-day reality of his life. In marriage he expects rose-tinted, unalloyed bliss without effort on his part, and in jobs he expects instant, spectacular success.

These patients are very difficult to treat psychiatrically. Never having had a meaningful interpersonal relationship, they have great difficulty setting up one with a therapist. They see the therapist as someone who will magically solve their problems, perhaps by haranguing their families, and who by his authority will manipulate their environments to suit their needs. Often this type of patient alternates between seductiveness and nasty sparring with the therapist, and he sometimes threatens suicide to corral the therapist into some course of action he wants. The patient's suicidal gestures are usually benign, but occasionally, either by accident or because of a moment of true despair, he makes a serious, or even fatal, suicidal attempt. Psychiatric hospitalization, though sometimes necessary, is treacherous for this kind of person; it offers him a way out of his life situational problems and puts a premium on being ill, and he may flee into psychiatric hospitalization each time he faces stresses at home, at work, or in social groups.

Occasionally the hysterical patient in his 30's or 40's develops multiple physical complaints, such as abdominal pains, headaches, thoracic pains, low backaches and many others, and retreats into the role of a semi-invalid whom others care for. He thus escapes the responsibilities and stresses of adulthood by chronic, vague, emotionally caused physical symptomatology. However, true conversion hysterical symptoms and dissociative hysterical problems (described in Chapter 9) occur in only a small percentage of patients with hysterical personality disorders.

PERSONALITY DISORDERS ASSOCIATED WITH SEXUAL DISTURBANCES

Some personality disorders result in the deviation of sexual urges into abnormal channels. The sexual deviations we shall discuss are (1) homosexuality, in which the individual prefers persons of his own sex as sexual objects (the controversial 1974 action of the American Psychiatric Association in removing the term homosexuality from the psychiatric nomenclature and substituting the ambiguously defined category "sexual orientation disturbance" is considered at the end of our discussion of homosexuality), (2) exhibitionism, in which the person achieves sexual gratification from exposing his genitals, (3) pedophilia, in which the person seeks children as sexual objects, (4) transvestitism (also written transvestism), in which the individual gets sexual stimulation by dressing in the clothing of persons of the opposite sex, (5) fetishism, in which the individual gets sexual gratification from a specific object belonging to a person of the opposite sex, such as a shoe or a lock of hair, (6) voyeurism, in which the individual achieves sexual gratification by watching other people during their sexual activity or by spying on them when they are naked, (7) sexual sadism, in which the person gains sexual gratification through brutality to others, (8) sexual masochism, in which the individual obtains sexual gratification by submitting himself to the cruelty of others, (9) sexual activity with animals, which is sometimes termed bestiality or classified as a form of sodomy and (10) the controversial category of transsexualism, in which the individual has a profound desire to be a member of the opposite sex, feels himself to be innately so, and seeks genital surgery and hormone therapy to achieve this objective. We shall also discuss the subject of incest.

Homosexuality

The sexual urges of a homosexual are directed toward persons of his own sex, and he has a deeply rooted discomfort about sexual intimacy with persons of the opposite sex. Homosexuality is the most common disorder of sexual behavior; although statistical speculations vary a good deal, most psychiatrists feel that about 3 per cent of adult persons of both sexes are homosexual. (The much contested action of the American Psychiatric Association in dropping the term homosexuality from the psychiatric nomenclature in 1974 and substituting the ill-defined category "sexual orientation disturbance" is discussed later in this section.)

A limited amount of homosexual experimentation in puberty and early adolescence, particularly among boys, is common, and it can be considered within normal limits if it is brief. For example, puberal and early adolescent boys sometimes engage in mutual masturbation as they struggle to adjust to their strong sexual impulses. Homosexual physical contacts are less common in adolescent girls than in adolescent boys, but they may sometimes develop brief infatuations with other girls or older women.

The initial homosexual yearnings of the person who in his adult years will be a homosexual usually begin during adolescence, though the adolescent may not at first be clearly aware of what he is experiencing. The first homosexual strivings of the puberal or adolescent child may come into his awareness in the daydreams he has during sexual excitement or masturbation. The adolescent boy discovers that he tends to identify himself with the woman's role rather than the man's role in his daydreams of sexual activity. He finds men more stimulating as sexual objects than women, and he is infatuated with boy friends rather than girl friends. The adolescent may accept these feelings easily, or he may be troubled and puzzled about them at first. During his adolescence he comes in contact with other homosexuals or he hears about homosexuality, and he becomes more articulately aware of his homosexual feelings. He may daydream of using his anus and mouth as receptive sexual orifices after he has read or heard more about homosexuality. A few teenage boys and girls are alarmed by their feelings, tell their parents and seek psychiatric help, but the vast majority of them carefully conceal their homosexuality from their parents, and their parents do not realize the sexual problems of their children.

The homosexually inclined boy or girl during his adolescence usually encounters other homosexuals and is introduced by them into the homosexual circles which exist in every large city. Many male homosexuals have effeminate manners and are attracted to the activities and vocations that usually interest women, and many female homosexuals dress and groom themselves in mannish ways. However, neither male nor female homosexuals can be positively identified by their grooming, their public behavior or their interests. Many mannish women and dainty men are not homosexuals, and many homosexuals have no apparent signs of their sexual deviation in their public behavior. The homosexual often dates persons of the opposite sex, but into such relationships he carries feelings of passionless comradeship rather than alert sexual interest. Many homosexuals can engage in sexual intercourse with persons of the opposite sex, but they are usually anxious about such heterosexual activity. Some homosexuals, however, have such profound dread of intimate sexual contact with persons of the opposite sex that they cannot engage in any kind of physical intimacy with them. Despite their discomforts in heterosexual activity, many homosexuals marry in their early or middle adult years, but their adjustments in marriage often are unstable. Many homosexuals continue their homsexual liaisons after they marry, and they often adjust poorly as marital partners and parents. Sometimes they manage to suppress, or at least to conceal from general notice, their homosexual activities after they marry, but often in later years they return to an active homosexual role and leave a chaotic marriage and disturbed children behind them.

Male homosexuals, though often pleasant and charming in their public behavior, are basically self-centered, and their capacities for relationships with people are defective in many areas. They have much deeply rooted hostility toward persons of both sexes, and their relationships with their homosexual paramours often fluctuate between fickle affection and marked hostility. Competition among homosexuals for the attention of each others' paramours creates a bitter chaos behind the façade of urbane sophistication. Male homosexuals are much more prone than the general population to depressions, anxiety states, psychosomatic disorders, schizophrenic disorders and other psychiatric problems. Homosexual men often develop psychogenic symptoms in their anal and perineal regions and consult physicians about them.

Female homosexuals, who sometimes are called lesbians, often make easier adjustments in their sexual deviations than male homosexuals. Long-lasting attachments may occur. It is socially acceptable for women to wear male clothing, such as trousers, and it is socially acceptable for single women to live together for long periods of time as a convenient economic arrangement. Hence, the suspicion of homosexuality is less frequently raised in women than in men, and female homosexuals may live in less conspicuous ways. Female homosexuals occasionally marry, but often they periodically lapse back into homosexual liaisons during their married years. Other psychiatric problems, such as anxiety states and depressions, are more common in homosexual women than in the general female population, but they are not as common as in male homosexuals.

The causes of homosexuality lie in unhealthy interpersonal relationships during childhood and early adolescence. The homosexual did not make a healthy identification with the parent of the same sex, but instead identified himself emotionally and sexually with the parent of the opposite sex. For example, the homosexual man during his childhood and early adolescence did not identify his emotional and sexual role with that of his father, but instead he identified himself with his mother. A boy may do this when his father is an ineffective, passive person who plays a weak role in the boy's emotional life and his mother is the dominant, important person in the family. In other instances, the father rejects the boy and abandons him emotionally to be reared by the mother; the only parent with whom the boy has a meaningful interpersonal relationship is the mother, and he unconsciously patterns his personality structure on the model she provides. When these kinds of interpersonal relationships persist throughout the boy's formative years, and no other close persons form sound associations with the boy which may correct his identifications, he does not have an admired, firm masculine model with which he may identify and on which he may pattern his emotional and sexual identification. He unconsciously retreats into an identification with his mother and adopts feminine orientations and attitudes. During adolescence and early adulthood his sexual urges become stronger and he seeks the male sexual partners whom a woman would seek. The homosexual girl identifies with her father, patterns her attitudes on masculine models and seeks out the female sexual partners toward whom a man would be attracted.

In addition, the person with a homosexual personality disorder dreads sexual intimacy with persons of the opposite sex; the homosexual woman has a strong revulsion from sexual intimacy with men, and the homosexual man is frightened of sexual intimacy with women. Hence, the homosexual is sexually drawn toward persons of his own sex and repelled from sexuality with persons of the opposite sex. This double force makes a homosexual personality disorder very difficult to change once it is established.

The homosexual emerges from the traumatic relationships of his formative years with profound resentment toward both parents, and toward the other close persons in his life who might have intervened to help him but did not, because all of them in his own way failed the patient emotionally. The homosexual carries this deeply rooted hostility into his later relationships with persons of both sexes, and his diffuse, basic hostility erupts unpredictably and erratically in his relationships with people. His relationships with his paramours and other homosexuals often fluctuate between coy seductiveness and bitter hostility. This underlying hostility makes the homosexual undependable and untrustworthy in his interpersonal dealings, and it often poisons long-term relationships with persons of both sexes. There are exceptions to these broad generalizations, but they hold true for most homosexuals.

Moreover, because neither of his parents, and no other close persons, satisfied his emotional needs, the homosexual unconsciously retreated into a marked self-centeredness and self-preoccupation. His self-centeredness adds a further obstacle to close, long-term relationships with people. He is preoccupied with his own feelings, his own needs and his own pleasures, and he has only superficial sensitivity or sympathy for the needs and feelings of others. His egocentricity, however, may be camouflaged by a thin veneer of charm and apparent interest in other people. Some psychiatrists feel that this profound self-centeredness is a basic factor in the homosexual's choice of sexual objects; he seeks sexual partners whose bodies are similar to his own. The homosexual often is fastidious in the care of his body and in grooming and dress. Some psychiatrists have suggested that, in addition to interpersonal causes, there may be constitutional factors, such as genetic or metabolic disorders, in homosexuals, but the evidence supporting such a point of view is unconvincing.

Harry Stack Sullivan pointed out that, in addition to individual emotional forces, there are cultural and social factors that often play a role in tipping a person toward homosexuality. He felt that in many cases homosexuality is a "developmental mistake" which is to a large extent determined by the fact that our culture makes homosexual outlets for lustful feelings easier than heterosexual ones during late childhood, puberty and early adolescence.

Society erects strong barriers against heterosexual experimentation by a boy or girl between the ages of 11 and 15, whereas homosexual experimentation is always easily found. The boy or girl, who at this time is somewhat confused in sexual orientation, may become fixed in a homosexual pattern, Sullivan felt, if his first long-term sensual experiences in sexuality are homosexual. The barriers to heterosexual expression, and the readiness with which homosexual contacts are found, vary much from one individual to another, and these variables play significant roles in determining the individual's eventual sexual orientation. Most psychiatrists feel that Sullivan's essentially sociological explanation of homosexuality cannot account fully for this disorder, though it adds a further dimension to our understanding of this type of personality problem.

Most homosexuals do not wish to engage in psychotherapy to try to change their sexual orientation, but they often seek psychiatric help for psychosomatic problems, depressions, anxiety states and other emotional problems. Most psychiatrists feel that the basic sexual orientation of a homosexual usually is not altered even by prolonged psychotherapy, though psychotherapy often helps the homosexual resolve other emotional problems and aids him to achieve a more comfortable social adjustment. However, some psychiatrists have reported encouraging results in changing the basic sexual orientation of well selected homosexual patients who were motivated to engage in psychotherapy over long periods of time.

Homosexuality is a major public health problem, since, at a conservative estimate, six million persons in the United States are homosexuals. Since the majority of homosexuals are not well motivated to change their sexual orientation and the results of treatment often are poor, prevention is more promising than treatment as a way of dealing with this widespread problem. Prevention lies in an interpersonally healthy family life in which the child during his formative years has a good opportunity to form a firm identification with the parent of the same sex. Programs of community psychiatry and public education perhaps offer a hopeful way to help parents provide emotionally healthy family environments that prevent the development of homosexual personality disorders.

In recent years some organizations whose aim is to create more public understanding and tolerance of homosexuals have proposed that homosexuality is not a psychiatric disorder, but merely a different life style chosen by the individual. Proponents of this viewpoint state that the homosexual is an emotionally healthy person who simply has elected to direct his sexual feelings toward persons of his own sex. This point of view is not consistent with the overwhelming body of psychiatric experience. As noted above, homosexuals have deeply rooted emotional problems with persons of both sexes, and they have many other interpersonal difficulties than merely their choice of sexual partners. Although psychiatrists deplore scornful or ridiculing attitudes toward homosexuals, and feel that laws against private homosexual acts (except with nonconsenting partners and with minors) should be abandoned, they feel that homosexuals have personality warps that make them vulnerable to many kinds of emotional and interpersonal misery.

It should be noted that in 1974, after a great deal of controversy, the Board of Trustees of the American Psychiatric Association voted to remove the term "homosexuality" from the standard nomenclature of psychiatric disorders and to substitute the term "sexual orientation disturbance" in its place. In its statement, the Board said that "homosexuality . . . by itself does not necessarily constitute a psychiatric disorder," but added that, this "is not to say that homosexuality is 'normal' or that it is as desirable as heterosexuality." Many psychiatrists find this statement confusing. Few psychiatrists would agree with the concept that a person whose main sexual orientation is toward persons of his own sex is an emotionally healthy individual. All leading psychiatrists of all theoretical viewpoints, including Freud and Sullivan, throughout the evolution of modern psychiatry have felt that a primary homosexual orientation constituted a psychiatric disorder. Moreover, virtually all current psychiatrists who have devoted themselves to

Exhibitionism

In exhibitionism, which occurs only in males, the person gets sexual stimulation from exposing his genitals to women. He does this in parks and other public places and then flees before he can be identified and arrested for indecent exposure. Exhibitionism is one of the most common sexual deviations. An exhibitionist rarely comes willingly for psychiatric help, but he frequently is compelled by police authorities, criminal courts and his relatives to seek psychiatric consultation. When he enters psychotherapy he usually does so on the demand of legal authorities who offer him a choice of treatment or prosecution, and he sees psychotherapy as a legal maneuver rather than an opportuntiy to change his personality structure. Only in occasional instances does the exhibitionistic patient have a sincere motivation for psychiatric help.

Psychiatrists who have studied exhibitionism report that the exhibitionist has deeply rooted fears of sexual inadequacy. Unconsciously he fears that his genitals are inadequate for satisfying a sexual partner, and he seeks to reassure himself repeatedly about his sexual prowess by exposing his genitals to women. Exposing the body is a preliminary step in normal sexual intercourse; however, the exhibitionist has such deep fears of his sexual ineffectiveness that he stops at this preliminary, partial stage of sexual intercourse and seeks his full sexual gratification in it.

In many instances the exhibitionist was reared by a domineering mother who gave him affection only so long as he submitted himself to her control. His father often was a weak, ineffective person who did not play a significant emotional role in the patient's upbringing. The patient emerged from childhood with a weak identification with the masculine role, with feelings of sexual inferiority, and with a need to prove his masculinity to women in immature, defiant ways. These personality problems lead to his exhibitionism, which begins in late adolescence or early adulthood and usually continues sporadically through most of his adult years.

Pedophilia

Pedophilia, in which the individual chooses children as his sexual objects, occurs only in men. The pedophiliac seduces girls, usually between the ages of 4 and 10, to engage in mutual masturbation or frank sexual intercourse, and he uses threats and bribes to prevent them from telling their parents. Such sexual seduction of young girls occurs much more frequently than the public realizes, and pedophilia is a fairly common type of sexual deviation. The pedophiliac may seek out children in his neighborhood, children whom he meets casually, or children who are relatives of his. I have seen pedophiliacs who seduced nieces, stepchildren, foster children and grandchildren. The pedophiliac often begins to practice his sexual deviation in middle or late adolescence, and he usually continues it episodically throughout his adult years into old age. In many instances, the pedophiliac becomes skillful in threatening or cajolling the children he seduces into silence about their sexual activities with him, and he may escape detection for many years or several decades.

Sexual seduction by an adult is a devastating experience for a small child. It leaves strong feelings of guilt and anxiety in her, and she feels a mixture of terror, anger and fascination toward her seducer. Such sexual exploitation often leaves the girl with chaotic feelings toward men and toward sexuality, and she is predisposed to develop anxiety states, phobias, obsessive disorders and other psychiatric problems in adolescence and adulthood. Parents should be aware of this common type of sexual trauma to young girls and should be vigilant in protecting them against it.

The pedophiliac, like the exhibitionist, has deeply rooted feelings of inadequacy about mature heterosexual activity, and as substitutes for adult women he seeks out children as his sexual objects. Children are less threatening sexual partners to him than adults. Moreover, a strain of marked emotional immaturity in the pedophiliac is an added factor that draws him toward children sexually. The causes of a pedophiliac personality disorder lie in unhealthy interpersonal relationships during the patient's formative years. The pedophiliac emerged from childhood and early adolescence with profound doubts about his sexual capacities and a gnawing discomfort about sexual activity with adult women.

A pedophiliac rarely comes voluntarily for psychiatric help. When he enters psychotherapy he usually is forced into it by indignant relatives or by legal authorities to whom complaints have been made about his sexual approaches to young girls. Hence, he rarely does well in psychotherapy and often stops it as soon as the pressures that forced him into it cease. However, an occasional pedophiliac is genuinely troubled about his problem, is motivated for therapy, and benefits from it.

Transvestitism

In transvestitism (which is also written transvestism) the individual gets sexual stimulation by dressing in clothing of persons of the opposite sex. Transvestitism is a much more common clinical complaint in boys than in girls. To a large extent, this is probably because it is socially acceptable for girls to dress in trousers, men's shirts and other articles of men's clothing. A girl who dresses mannishly goes largely unnoticed in public, whereas a boy who dresses in girls' clothing is readily noted and ridiculed. Although psychiatrists feel that transvestitism as a psychiatric problem is much more common in boys than in girls, this may be a clinical artefact rather than a true difference in the incidence of this type of sexual difficulty.

Moreover, since parents bring transvestitite boys and adolescents for psychiatric consultation, and adult transvestitites rarely seek psychiatric help, transvestitism is generally felt to be more common in boys and adolescents than in adults; this too may be a clinical artefact. However, valid knowledge about transvestitism as a sexual deviation is largely limited to boys in late childhood and adolescence. Transvestitism, as a special type of sexual deviation, should be clinically distinguished from homosexuality. In transvestitism the patient gets his major sexual stimulation from dressing in female clothing and in most instances he does not engage in physical homosexual activity with other persons. In homosexuality, though the patient occasionally may dress in female clothing, wearing female attire is only a small part of his sexual problem and it does not constitute the major source of his sexual stimulation; the homosexual's major sexual deviation consists in physical sexual urges and activities with persons of his own sex. The possible relationship of transvestitism and homosexuality is discussed in later paragraphs of this section.

The transvestitite boy or adolescent may put on female underwear, girdles, brassieres, dresses, stockings and shoes. As a rule, he does it in secret, though occasionally he may go out in public wearing articles of female clothing; in many cases the transvestitite wears female underwear beneath male clothing when in public. Though in some instances transvestitism begins in early childhood it more commonly starts in late childhood and adolescence. Though accurate information on the long-term course and prognosis of transvestitism is not available, some psychiatrists feel that transvestitism often stops in early adulthood, though the basic personality problems persist and may cause other types of emotional difficulties. The psychiatrists who have studied transvestitism feel that only a small percentage of transvestitite boys become homosexuals during adolescence and early adult life, and that most transvestitites appear to adopt a heterosexual pattern of behavior in their adult years.

The transvestitite patient has a confused sexual identification; he feels in some ways identified with women and in other ways identified with men. In the sexual excitement he feels when dressed in female clothing, the transvestitite adolescent boy sometimes fantasies himself in the male role and sometimes daydreams of himself in the female role. During masturbation he sometimes daydreams of himself as a man in sexual intercourse and at other times he visualizes himself as a woman. The interpersonal causes of transvestitism are similar to those of homosexuality, but they are much less severe. The transvestitite's mother usually played a much more important role in the patient's life than his father, and the patient felt closer to her emotionally than to his father and partially identified himself with her. The father, though less close to the patient than the mother, nevertheless played a sufficiently prominent role to provide a masculine model on which the patient could make a partial identification. However, the patient's identification was not strong enough with either parent to incline him completely to either a heterosexual or a homosexual role, and a confused identification resulted which produced his clinical transvestitism. In many cases there were other close persons, such as older siblings or grandparents, who played significant roles in the patient's personality formation and prevented the severer personality warping which might have led to a homosexual pattern. In addition, social forces in adolescence and early adulthood press the transvestitite toward conformance with the male role, and they probably constitute a major factor in the transvestitite's eventual adoption of the heterosexual role in early adult life. However, his underlying emotional difficulties may cause problems in his role as a husband and a father.

The transvestitite child or adolescent should be evaluated in a child guidance clinic or other appropriate psychiatric service for children and adolescents, and psychotherapy for the patient and counseling for his parents should be undertaken whenever they will accept such help. Though the symptom of transvestitism has a good chance of disappearing eventually, the child's underlying personality problems merit attention. Adult transvestitites rarely are motivated for psychotherapy, and valid information about the results of psychotherapy with them is not available.

Other Sexual Deviations

The sexual deviations we have discussed in the preceding pages—homosexuality, exhibitionism, pedophilia and transvestitism—are the most common types of sexual disorders. In the following paragraphs we shall consider briefly the less common sexual deviations. Though they have much interest from a psychiatric point of view, they are much less commonly encountered in clinical practice and, accordingly, we shall give them less detailed consideration.

Fetishism. In fetishism, a sexual deviation that occurs only in males, the individual gets his sexual gratification from caressing articles of female clothing such as underwear, or shoes or stockings; a lock or braid of female hair may be a fetish. The fetishist achieves sexual orgasm in fondling his fetishistic object and he may engage in normal sexual intercourse only on infrequent occasions. The fetishist has profound anxiety about genital sexual contact with women, and he seeks a symbolic substitute as his source of sexual stimulation and gratification. During his childhood and early adolescent years the fetishist's interpersonal experiences left him with a deeply rooted dread of intimacy with women. Though heterosexual in orientation, he cannot approach women sexually and therefore seeks symbolic substitutes for contact with them.

Voyeurism. Voyeurism is a sexual deviation in which the individual achieves sexual gratification by watching other people during their sexual activity or by spying on them when they are naked. Though it occurs in both sexes, voyeurism is much more common in men than in women. The voyeurist, like the fetishist, often has anxiety about sexual activity with women and seeks substitute sexual gratification by watching other people in sexual intercourse or by spying on women while they are undressed. He sometimes masturbates during these activities and he daydreams of himself in sexual intercourse with the woman he is watching. In some instances, the voyeurist also engages in normal heterosexual activity, but he finds it does not satisfy his sexual needs and he seeks further sexual gratification in his voyeurism. Some psychiatrists have speculated that the voyeurist during his early childhood witnessed his parents in sexual intercourse and that in his voyeuristic activities he is attempting repeatedly to master the emotional turmoil which that experience left in him. The term "scoptophilia" is sometimes employed as a synonym for voyeurism.

Sexual Sadism. In sexual sadism the individual achieves sexual satisfaction by physical brutality to his sexual partner. It occurs almost exclusively in men. Sexual sadism includes physical cruelty before or during the sex act, vicious sexual assault, mutilation of the sexual victim and rape. In some instances, the sexual sadist achieves orgasm during brutality to his victim without engaging in sexual intercourse with her. A variety of personality disorders may lie behind sexual sadism, but all of them are characterized by deeply rooted hostility toward persons of the opposite sex. Moreover, in many instances the sexual sadist has marked doubts about his sexual adequacy and masculinity, and he attempts to assuage these doubts by exaggerated aggressiveness in his sexual activities. During his formative years the sexual sadist underwent much emotional trauma which left him with his profound hostility toward women and doubts about his sexual capacities. Some sexual sadists have severe antisocial personality dosorders and a few are schizophrenics.

Sexual Masochism. In sexual masochism the individual achieves sexual gratification by submitting himself to cruelty from his sexual partner. This relatively rare sexual deviation occurs in both men and women. In occasional cases an individual alternates between sexual sadism and sexual masochism, and is termed a sado-masochist.

The psychiatrists who have studied sexual masochism report that the sexual masochist has profound feelings of guilt and unworthiness. He cannot relax and achieve sexual orgasm unless he first undergoes physical suffering which he feels absolves him of the guilty feelings which gnaw at him. He feels unworthy to enjoy sexual pleasure unless he first pays for it by physical suffering. The sexual masochist also has much repressed hostility about which he feels guilty and of which he feels he can be cleansed only by physical punishment. The formative years of the sexual masochist left him with profound guilt feelings, marked passivity and a strong need repeatedly to gain brief relief from his guilt feelings by physical humiliation. His sexual masochism usually is only one aspect of a need for suffering in various areas of his life.

Sexual Activity With Animals. Sometimes termed bestiality or classified as a form of sodomy, this sexual deviation is encountered occasionally in clinical practice. It may occur in adolescents or adults and is restricted to males; it is more common in persons who live on farms. I have seen patients who performed sex acts with sheep, cattle, dogs and other farm animals. Though some persons who have sexual activity with animals are mentally retarded, most of them are not. There is very little psychiatric literature on the incidence, personality structures or psychiatric treatment of persons who are detected in sexual activity with animals. Presumably, it occurs in individuals who have emotional problems that inhibit them in normal sexual pursuits and who therefore seek sexual activity of this kind.

Transsexualism. In recent years the term transsexualism has been employed to designate a highly controversial clinical concept and various medical procedures linked to it. The few physicians who accept this concept state that the transsexual, who is almost invariably male, has throughout his life regarded himself as female, despite the fact that he is in all physical and endocrinological ways a male. He furthermore strongly wishes to adopt the female role sexually and socially, and is anxious to undergo whatever surgery and endocrine therapy is necessary to enable him to make this change. A number of transsexual surgical changes, which have attracted much attention in the lay press, have been made in Europe and the United States. In such a procedure, the penis is amputated, the testicles are removed, and the scrotum is turned inward to form a mock vaginal pocket. Female breast development and other female secondary sexual characteristics are achieved by massive female hormone treatment. The patient thereafter adopts female clothing, a female name and all other features of a female life style.

The few surgeons and psychiatrists who advocate these procedures state that they are merely correcting anatomical and social anomalies in a person who is psychologically female but is prevented from assuming a female role by anatomical and endocrine hindrances. However, most psychiatrists feel that there is no such clinical entity as "transsexualism," and that so-called transsexuals are merely homosexual men who want to assume the female role and are willing to undergo disfiguring surgery and endocrine therapy to achieve that aim. Many of the homosexual men who have undergone such procedures are very dissatisfied and bitter about the results, and find that they are no happier in the female role than they were in the male one. There also are dubious ethical, legal and social problems in the performance of transsexual procedures. Many psychiatrists feel that it is ethically and clinically unjustified to engage in clumsy attempts to turn a patient's pathology into mock reality.

Incest. Incest is sexual activity between members of the same immediate family. Incest is uncommon, but it occurs more frequently than the public and many physicians realize. Sexual acts between fathers and daughters and between brothers and sisters constitute the most common incestuous relationships. Incest between mothers and sons is immensely rare. Incest occurs more frequently when there is no blood relationship between the participants, as between stepfathers and stepdaughters and between foster fathers and foster daughters. I recall three instances in my clinical practice in which incest occurred between mothers-in-law and sons-in-law. Though incest is reported to be more common among persons who are impoverished, culturally deprived or mentally retarded, it may occur in any level of society. In several instances I have encountered incest in well-educated, well-to-do families.

Incest is a very disturbing emotional experience for the child or adolescent who engages in it, and it creates strong emotional conflicts in him. The emotional trauma of incest predisposes the child to the later development of phobias, depressions, anxiety states and other psychiatric problems. Incest often leaves the child with chaotic feelings about sexuality and about persons of the opposite sex, and it predisposes the child to marital and sexual maladjustments in adult life. The adult who engages in incest usually has a marked personality disorder, though he may present an appearance of social conformity to the community. In many instances the incestuous adult has an antisocial personality disorder or a schizoid personality structure. Some incestuous adults are mentally retarded or have organic brain disease. The elderly incestuous adult often has early senile degenerative or arteriosclerotic brain disease that his family does not recognize as a serious problem until he makes incestuous overtures to his nieces or grandchildren. Some incestuous relationships occur while the adult is under the influence of alcohol. Women who have incest with their sons usually are schizophrenic or grossly mentally retarded.

Children who have been subjected to incest should have careful psychiatric evaluation, and in many instances should receive psychotherapy to resolve the emotional problems created by the incest. The incestuous adult should also be psychiatrically evaluated, but in most instances he will not engage in psychiatric treatment. Court officials and social welfare agencies should not hesitate in removing children from homes in which incest has occurred and seems likely to recur; the children should be placed in foster homes to prevent further emotional damage to them by the incestuous adults. Incestuous relationships of both heterosexual and homosexual nature between brothers and sisters are more common than is generally realized, and after the first few years of life siblings should not sleep in the same bed with each other.

BIBLIOGRAPHY

Adler, G., and Shapiro, L. N.: Some difficulties in the treatment of the aggressive acting-out patient. Am. J. Psychother., 27:548, 1973.

Artiss, K. L.: An administrative behavioral pattern of certain obsessional characters. Comtemp. Psychoanal., 6:93, 1970.

Borriello, J. F.: Patients with acting-out character disorders. Am. J. Psychother., 27:4, 1973.

Buckner, H. T.: The transvestite career path. Psychiatry, 33:381, 1970.

Bursten, B.: The manipulative personality. Arch. Gen. Psychiatry, 26:318, 1972.

Evans, W. N.: On the nature of obstinacy. Psychoanal. Rev., 60:419, 1973.

Giovacchini, P. L. Characterological problems: the need to be helped. Arch. Gen. Psychiatry, 22:245, 1970.

Gonen, J. Y.: Negative identity in homosexuals. Psychoanal. Rev., 58:345, 1971.

Kernberg, O. F.: Factors in the psychoanalytic treatment of narcissistic personalities. J. Am. Psychoanal. Ass., 18: 51, 1970.

Keutzer, C. S.: Kleptomania: a direct approach to treatment. Brit. J. Med. Psychol., 45:159, 1972.

Luisada, P. V., Peale, R., and Pitteard, E. A.: The hysterical personality in men. Am. J. Psychiatry, 131:518, 1974.

Maddocks, P. D.: A five year follow-up of untreated psychopaths. Brit. J. Psychiatry, *116*: 511, 1970.

Resnik, H. L. P., and Wolfgang, M. E. (eds.): Treatment of the Sex Offender, Boston, Little Brown, 1972.

Stoller, R. J.: Male transsexualism: uneasiness. Am. J. Psychiatry, *130*:536, 1973.

Stoller, R. J., et al.: Should homosexuality be in the APA nomenclature? Am. J. Psychiatry, *130*:1207, 1973.

Sullivan, H. S.: The Interpersonal Theory of Psychiatry. Chapter on introductory concepts, p. 3. New York, W. W. Norton, 1953.

————: The Fusion of Psychiatry and Social Science. Chapter on personal identity, p. 198. New York, W. W. Norton, 1964.

13

Personality Disorders Contributing to Alcoholism and Drug Abuse

In this chapter we shall discuss the personality disorders which lead to, and become complicated by, the misuse of various kinds of substances and drugs. The chapter is divided into three main sections: (1) *personality disorders associated with alcoholism,* in which we consider all aspects of alcoholic abuse except the organic brain syndromes which may be caused by alcoholism (they are covered in Chapter 18 on the common kinds of organic brain disorders), (2) *personality disorders associated with narcotic addiction,* in which we discuss addiction to heroin and other opiates, and (2) *personality disorders associated with other forms of drug abuse,* including sedatives and antianxiety medications, marijuana, amphetamines, hallucinogens, and cocaine.

PERSONALITY DISORDERS ASSOCIATED WITH ALCOHOLISM

Excessive use of alcohol occurs in persons with various kinds of personality disorders. The number of chronic alcoholics in the United States is estimated at more than five million, and more than 12,000 persons die each year from physical diseases produced by alcoholism. Two or three times that many persons die each year in automobile accidents and other accidents in which alcohol plays a causative role. The number of work hours lost in business, industry and the professions each year because of alcoholic abuse is staggering. In addition to its effects on the abusers of alcohol, alcoholism leads to much hardship and suffering among the families, work associates and friends of alcoholics. In addition, alcoholism in some cases leads to organic brain disorders, such as delirium tremens and alcoholic hallucinosis, (discussed in Chapter 18).

Alcoholism is said to be much more common in men than in women, but this belief may be based on a statistical artefact produced by cultural conditions. Alcoholic men commonly become intoxicated in public, whereas alcoholic women drink more at home and their alcoholic excesses draw less notice. An alcoholic man often has vocational and economic problems which soon attract attention to his alcoholism, whereas the alcoholic housewife may attract little attention in her solitary drinking at home. In my clinical practice I have seen almost as many alcoholic women as men, and I have seen almost as many alcoholic psychoses in women as men. However, the number of men admitted to public mental hospitals for alcoholism and alcoholic psychoses is much greater than the number of women admitted for alcoholic problems to the same institutions.

In former times alcoholism was said to be less common in some ethnic and religious groups, but with the progressive assimilation of these ethnic groups into the American culture such differences in the incidence of alcoholism are rapidly disappearing. It sometimes is stated that alcoholism is much more common among the economically deprived, poorly educated segment of society, but this belief also is subject to doubt. Prolonged alcoholism often leads to vocational instability and a consequent decline in the economic status of the alcoholic and his family. Hence, poverty often is the consequence of alcoholism rather than its cause. Moreover, the well-to-do alcoholic less often attracts the notice of social welfare agencies and public hospitals than the poor alcoholic; hence, statistics tend to focus more attention on the amount of alcoholism occurring among the poor and the underprivileged. Alcoholism is most common between the ages of 30 and 55, but the physician also encounters alcoholic problems in older adolescents, young adults and elderly persons. Better medical care in recent years has resulted in an increasing number of alcoholics living into their 60's and 70's while still drinking excessively.

There are various patterns of drinking among alcoholics. Some alcoholics drink mainly on weekends and others misuse alcohol sporadically for periods of several days or several weeks with variable intervals of abstinence between their episodes of alcoholic excess. Some alcoholics drink mainly in solitude, but others drink heavily both in public and alone. The severest alcoholics begin drinking in the morning and continue throughout the day until they collapse prostrate into bed in late afternoon or at night, but these persons form only a small percentage of alcoholics. If, as some students of alcoholism suggest, alcoholism is a physical addiction, it is among these severe, around-the-clock drinkers that such dependence can be shown, rather than in the vast majority of alcoholics who have regular abstinence periods of from a couple of days to several days. An alcoholic may drink any kind of alcoholic beverage, but whiskey, rum, gin and vodka are most commonly used. Alcoholics usually shun beverages with low alcoholic content such as beer, but wine drinking occurs in some alcoholics. Some alcoholics also misuse sedatives, such as barbiturates and antianxiety medications, and a few severe alcoholics become physically addicted to these drugs. An alcoholic is especially prone to misuse sedation when he cannot get alcohol, but some alcoholics use sedatives and alcohol concomitantly.

There is much dispute about the medical definition of alcoholic intoxication. However, many physicians who have studied alcoholism define alcoholic intoxication as the mental and physical state of a person who has 150 mg. or more of alcohol in 100 cc. of blood, or equivalent levels in his breath, saliva or urine. However, reactions to alcohol vary immensely from person to person. Some individuals become disorganized in their behavior if they imbibe a small quantity of alcohol, whereas others may continue to function fairly well after drinking much more. In clinical practice it is best to avoid difficult discussions with alcoholics and their families about what constitutes being "drunk." If a person's behavior deteriorates significantly after drinking, then he certainly is "behaving under the influence of alcohol." The extent of the deterioration of his behavior may be variable, but any degree of deterioration is undersirable. This is the crucial point, rather than whether the individual has passed some arbitrary line to qualify him for "drunkenness."

The physician sometimes is asked whether a particular patient should be considered an alcoholic. In some cases, as when the patient is drinking each day to the point of intoxication or when he has had a recent episode of delirium tremens, the answer is obvious. In most cases seen in daily practice, the answer is not so clear-cut. Some persons maintain that if they drink mainly in social company, or if they can on occasion abstain from alcohol for a week or more, they are not alcoholics. The physician should avoid such hairsplitting discussions, and in dealing with some patients it is wise to avoid the word alcoholic altogether. It often is better to say that the patient "has a problem with alcohol" rather than to argue with him about whether or not he is an alcoholic. If the patient drinks alcohol to excess, and if it is causing any significant problem in his social, economic, family or emotional adjustments, then the patient has a problem with alcohol and he should take appropriate steps to resolve it. If the physician surveys with the patient and his family the influence of the patient's drinking on his social, vocational, family and emotional adjustments, it is usually easy to declare whether or not the person has a problem with alcohol and how severe it is.

In the standard psychiatric nomenclature alcoholism is divided into three categories of increasing severity: (1) *Episodic excessive drinking,* in which the person becomes intoxicated between 4 and 12 times a year. (2) *Habitual excessive drinking,* in which a person becomes intoxicated more than 12 times a year or is recognizably under the influence of alcohol, "even though not intoxicated," more than once a week. (Many psychiatrists and other mental health professionals find these first two categories so broad and vague that they would include between 20 and 30 per cent of the adult population, and hence feel that the standard nomenclature's definitions and divisions of alcoholism are unworkable.) (3) *Alcohol addiction,* in which the person drinks every day, presumably to the point of intoxication, or when "heavy drinking" has occurred for three months. The instructions for use of the standard nomenclature state that such a person is physically dependent (that is, addicted) on alcohol and that he has withdrawal symptoms when he is deprived of it. However, as will be discussed later, there is much controversy about whether alcohol is a physically addicting substance in any sense analagous with opiates and sedatives, and whether withdrawal symptoms similar to those during withdrawal from narcotics and sedatives actually occur in the vast majority of alcoholics.

Physiological and Emotional Effects of Alcohol

Ethyl alcohol is absorbed quickly into the blood since it does not require digestion, and it accumulates in the body tissues because it is absorbed much more rapidly than it is metabolized. Its maximum blood level is maintained for about five hours after ingestion. Ethyl alcohol is uniformly distributed to the body tissues, but its accumulation and release in the brain and spinal fluid are slower than in other organs. The metabolism of alcohol occurs largely, but not exclusively, in the liver. It is first oxidized to acetaldehyde, and the acetaldehyde is then oxidized to acetic acid. In the final step, the acetic acid is oxidized to carbon dioxide and water. The clinical use of disulfiram in treating alcoholism (discussed later) is based on the ability of disulfiram to delay the metabolism of alcohol at the acetaldehyde stage.

With levels of 100 to 200 mg. of alcohol in each 100 cc. of blood, the patient is clinically intoxicated and shows exhilaration or other emotional reactions to the alcohol. With blood levels of 200 to 300 mg. the patient has marked physical incoordination and ataxia. Blood levels over 500 mg. may result in death. Persons who have drunk alcohol heavily over long periods of time are reported to be able to tolerate it with less marked central nervous system effects than occasional drinkers, but this may be a learned ability rather then a true physiological change.

Physicians differ in their opinions about whether a patient can become physically addicted to alcohol in the same way that a person can become physically addicted to narcotics due to their action on the central nervous system. Some physicians feel that a mild but definite central nervous system physical dependence on alcohol can develop in a person who drinks heavily and persistently over a long period of time. These physicians feel that abrupt abstinence from alcohol in such a patient may result in withdrawal symptoms such as weakness, tremors, agitation, craving for alcohol, nausea, tachycardia, fever and hallucinations. Other physicians feel that true physical dependence on alcohol does not occur, and that the patient's dependence is exclusively emotional. These physicians feel that the symptoms occasionally seen in heavy alcoholics who stop drinking are produced by the toxic effects of previously ingested alcohol and by malnutrition, which often accompanies chronic alcoholism. I incline toward this second point of view.

Some of the clinical studies often cited to support the thesis that a person can become physically dependent (addicted) on alcohol were carried out on long-term narcotic addicts who were serving prison sentences for narcotic offenses. Many psychiatrists (as will be pointed out later in this chapter), feel that long-term narcotic addicts are not emotionally and physiologically a reliable sample of patients for such studies; many investigators feel that after many years of narcotics usage these patients have special vulnerability to addiction to various kinds of drugs and substances. Moreover, not all the patients in these series had the reactions interpreted as withdrawal symptoms after a prolonged period of high alcohol intake and abrupt withdrawal. Also, other investigators have been unable to confirm these findings in other patient groups. If alcohol were an addicting substance, moreover, one would expect the administration of alcohol to cause the cessation or marked diminution of the presumed withdrawal symptoms, such as tremulousness and tachycardia, in delirium tremens and lesser states which are alleged to be withdrawal syndromes; administration of alcohol to these patients causes no significant changes in their clinical conditions. In clinical practice one sees many alcoholics who drink heavily each day for long periods of time and have no withdrawal symptoms when their families force hospitalization and abrupt abstinence on them. If alcohol is an addicting substance, it would appear to be so only in the severest alcoholics who have spent several weeks or much longer in continual inebriation and have undergone marked nutritional, as well as social and economic, deterioration during this time.

The question of whether alcohol is a truly addicting substance has significance in clinical practice. Through public education programs on alcoholism, many people have heard that alcoholism is an addiction, and one now frequently encounters alcoholics who resist treatment proposals on the grounds that they are "addicted" to alcohol and cannot do without it. Moreover, the concept that the alcoholic is "addicted" causes his family to hesitate in taking a firm stand on treatment in many instances, and, as they flounder in doubt, the patient goes on drinking. Of course, such patients might well find other grounds to resist treatment, but the concept of alcoholic addiction often adds a further hindrance to the already formidable ones in treating alcoholics.

Ethyl alcohol acts as a sedative on the central nervous system, and its first effect is to diminish the activity of the cerebral cortex. This decrease of cerebral cortical activity results in less inhibited behavior by the patient, and the nature of his uninhibited behavior depends to a large extent on his personality structure. Anxious, insecure persons may experience relief from their anxiety and become more relaxed and self-confident. Some persons become exhilarated, gregarious, talkative and jovial. Others become belligerent, arrogant and agitated, and some become morose and tearful. The person's judgement and intellectual alertness are impaired, though often he is unaware of this. As the blood level of alcohol increases, the motor areas of the cortex are affected and the patient's physical coordination deteriorates. With high blood levels of alcohol the midbrain and other lower brain centers are progressively affected. Ataxia, somnolence and coma result, and very high blood levels of alcohol cause malfunction of vasomotor, cardiac and respiratory centers in the medulla.

Emotional Causes of Alcoholism

A wide variety of personality problems may contribute to alcoholism. Alcohol is the most available legal sedative the public can buy and some people use it to allay the anxiety arising from many kinds of emotional problems. The person with a chronic anxiety neurosis, or diffuse phobias, or other neurotic problems in which anxiety is a prominent symptom may seek relief from his tension in the sedative effects of alcohol. These sedative qualities offer a seductive alternative to experiencing the pain of his anxiousness, and he gradually may use alcohol increasingly for relief. In time he may use alcohol not only to assuage his anxiousness, but also to blot out awareness of other emotional and interpersonal problems. Often the patient feels inadequate and ashamed about his misuse of alcohol, and he may seek to erase these additional painful feelings from his awareness by even greater abuse of alcohol. A vicious circle is set up in which the patient's alcoholism accentuates his emotional, interpersonal and vocational problems and leads to even greater alcoholic excesses. In some instances, the person first begins to drink to seek relief from strong guilt feelings, and the additional guilt he subsequently feels about his alcoholic excesses drives him into peristent misuse of alcohol.

Persons who struggle with feelings of inferiority and inadequacy may drink to gain the sensation of giddy self-confidence that some people feel when intoxicated. Thus, when under the influence of alcohol they may boast and fabricate stories of personal achievement. Remorse and even greater feelings of inadequacy when they recover from alcoholic bouts may lead to ever heavier drinking. Some drinkers can release other kinds of pent-up feelings while intoxicated; they may vent suppressed anger, social complaints, hidden fears and secret aspirations. Other persons become sexually aggressive or brazenly seductive after drinking, though heavy drinking often deprives a man of his penile erectile capacity.

Misuse of alcohol also may be a means of rebelling against domineering parents, of defying a nagging wife, or of refusing to conform with the standards of a social group that condemns the excessive use of alcohol. When serious problems exist in a teenager's relationship with his parents, a vicious circle may be set up in which the adolescent's misuse of alcohol increases his parents' hostility and criticism toward him, and the adolescent defies them even more strongly by yet heavier drinking. The same kind of vicious circle often is set up between an alcoholic and his wife: a passive man may use alcoholism to defy a harsh, domineering wife. A similar interpersonal pattern may exist between a callous, hostile husband and a passive wife who rebels through abuse of alcohol to defy others; such alcoholic misuse may be persistent or intermittent. Some patients go through periods of severe alcoholic excess for a week or 10 days once every six months or a year, and are abstinent between these episodes. Such patients usually are dependent, immature men who unconsciously feel that they periodically must show their independence by defying their families by an alcoholic spree.

Alcoholism may occur in persons who have difficulty in tolerating obstacles to their urges and needs. Hence, alcoholism is common in individuals with antisocial personality disorders when they find their impulses and desires persistently blocked by circumstances. Persons with antisocial personality disorders also may use alcoholism as a way of defying their families and the standards of a society that condemns alcoholic excess. Some psychiatrists feel that there is a strong thread of latent homosexuality in some male alcoholics. They feel that this finds sublimated expression in the cameraderie of men's drinking groups, especially when the group has a feeling of cohesive defiance against their families, which disapprove of their alcoholic bouts.

An occasional patient drinks heavily while going through a depressive illness, and his alcoholism may mask the underlying depression. Others drink excessively during a period of grieving after the death of a close relative or during the distress following an economic reversal, a vocational failure or other kinds of situational problems. In some instances, alcoholism accompanies psychological illnesses or organic brain disease; thus, a schizophrenic occasionally uses alcohol to assuage the agitation or panic that may be a feature of his schizophrenic process, and alcoholic excess also may accompany the personality deterioration that occurs in early, progressive organic brain disease, such as in slow-growing brain tumors or in senile or arteriosclerotic brain degeneration. As the personality structure of the patient deteriorates, he struggles to adjust to the stresses of life with less cerebral cortical capacity, and he feels anxiety, inadequacy and confusion, from which he may seek relief in the sedative effects of alcohol.

Clinical Course of Alcoholism

The clinical course and outcome of alcoholism are variable, and there are no reliable general statistics on the life courses of large numbers of unselected alcoholics. The psychiatrist who is engaged in individual private practice may be optimistic about treatment results, but the patients whom he treats usually are well motivated and have helpful families. On the other hand, the psychician who works in a large public hospital often sees patients who are further advanced in alcoholic social and emotional deterioration, and the statistical results of work with these patients are less encouraging. The statistical results of various treatment methods depend much on how patients are selected; selection may be intentionally determined by the psychiatrist, or it may depend on the nature of the treatment facility and its administrative and intake policies.

A sizable minority of alcoholics stop

drinking without medical aid after many years of alcoholism. For example, an alcoholic occasionally stops drinking because of religious persuasion or because of a major life crisis such as a threatened divorce or job dismissal. In some instances an alcoholic stops drinking after a severe illness due to alcohol, such as cirrhosis of the liver or delirum tremens, or after a serious automobile accident that occurred while he was inebriated. Though alcoholics who spontaneously stop drinking because of these reasons, or other similar factors, may do so in early or middle adulthood, some do not stop until they are in their 50's or 60's. Alcoholics who stop drinking for such reasons may continue to have difficulties with the underlying emotional problems that led to their alcoholism, but in some instances the interpersonal stresses in their lives and their underlying emotional problems have decreased and they make fairly good adjustments after they become abstinent. Diminution in interpersonal stress and emotional turmoil may be significant factors in the end of their alcoholism; the tensions that caused their alcoholism have receded sufficiently to allow them to recover from it.

Another group of alcoholics eventually stop drinking because of a therapeutic approach to their problem. This may come through a nonmedical approach, as in Alcoholics Anonymous, and in some therapeutic discussion groups organized under religious auspices. A significant number of alcoholics become abstinent through one of the medical approaches discussed in the following section of this chapter.

The remaining number of alcoholics, probably amounting to more than 50 per cent, continue to drink throughout their entire adult lives. With the improvements in medical care that have occurred during the past few decades, a small but significant percentage of alcoholics live into their 60's or even well into their 70's while continuing to drink heavily. I have found this especially to occur in female alcoholics and in business and professional people who periodically enter the internal medical divisions of hospitals for several weeks at a time for treatment of medical problems often related to their alcoholism. These patients usually do not suffer the dietary deficiencies that often accompany alcoholism. Frequently they are from well-to-do economic groups, and their affluence allows better medical care and a reasonable economic adjustment in spite of their alcoholism.

Another group of alcoholics develop serious physical diseases, often of the liver or the central nervous system, due to alcoholism, and they either die or become chronically incapacitated. In the United States at least 12,000 persons die each year of cirrhosis of the liver, delirium tremens and other diseases caused by alcoholism. A small percentage of alcoholics become permanently psychotic as the result of central nervous system damage. Many thousands more die because of diseases which alcoholism complicates, such as pneumonia, diabetes and cardiovascular disease, and many thousands of persons each year die or suffer grave injuries in automobile accidents and other kinds of accidents which occur while they are intoxicated.

A large group of alcoholics eventually undergo gradual socioeconomic, emotional and physical deterioration. This deterioration is primarily caused by the drastic effects of alcoholism as a way of life on the interpersonal and emotional adjustments of the patient. In some cases, this deterioration is secondarily influenced by minimal, subtle degeneration of cerebral cortical brain tissue due to the toxic effects of ethyl alcohol and the nutritional deficiencies that sometimes accompany chronic alcoholism. In some patients the interpersonal and neurological factors in alcoholic deterioration are so closely interwoven that they cannot be separated clinically; they comprise an indivisible, single clinical process. We are not discussing here the organic brain syndromes (discussed in Chapter 18) that may be caused by alcoholism; we are discussing the frequently encountered emotional and socioeconomic deterioration in long-term alcoholics that is primarily caused by the alcoholic way of life and may be influenced secondarily by minimal, diffuse cerebral cortical brain damage. In many patients with alcoholic deterioration, neither neurological nor electroencephalographic studies reveal abnormalities; these common instances emphasize the primary importance of emotional factors in producing this clinical picture.

The deteriorated alcoholic often is evasive

and unreliable. He makes endless promises which he does not keep, and he covers his shortcomings with lies and subterfuges. Often he lies profusely even when his falsehoods are sure to be discovered in a short time. In many instances he denies that he drinks excessively and he may deny that he drinks at all, despite obvious evidence to the contrary. He chronically engages in petty deceptions and he has a shallow craftiness in obtaining and hiding alcohol despite the vigilance of his relatives. He is irresponsible, blames others for his own shortcomings and accepts little or no blame himself for the ruinous circumstances of his life. He loses his ambition, his sense of decency and his personal integrity. All long-term goals and ethical standards are lost in his ever-recurring search to find oblivion in more drinking.

The deteriorated alcoholic is profoundly self-centered. He has no affection or real interest in his family or his former friends. His interest in sexuality declines; often the deteriorated male alcoholic is impotent and the deteriorated female alcoholic is indifferent to sexual intercourse. While drinking he may engage in a shallow camaraderie with his drinking associates, but this easily changes to belligerence or sullen withdrawal. Job instability, marital maladjustment often ending in divorce, economic destitution, and poor physical health often ensue.

All this deterioration may occur without clinical evidence of cerebral cortical brain damage, but in some instances the patient also develops signs of organic intellectual degeneration. He becomes forgetful, is partially disoriented some of the time, and his judgement and intellectual capacities undergo progressive impairment. Often he goes through one or more episodes of delirium tremens as these features develop, and in time he may shade gradually into one of the persistent alcoholic psychotic states (discussed in Chapter 18).

Treatment of Alcoholism

An important principle in the treatment of alcoholism is that the person who once has had a problem with alcohol cannot become a moderate, or social, drinker. He must abstain completely from alcohol. If he attempts to drink in moderation, he in time inevitably slips back into the misuse of alcohol. The physician must define complete abstinence as the only workable goal if the patient is to resolve his problem.

In covering the various approaches to alcoholism, we shall discuss (1) Alcoholics Anonymous, (2) psychotherapy, both individual and in groups, (3) conditioning therapy, (4) disulfiram (Antabuse) therapy, and (5) comprehensive social and vocational rehabilitation programs.

Alcoholics Anonymous. Alcoholics Anonymous consists of a nationwide system of small, separately organized groups of alcoholics who band together to help themselves and their fellow group members to achieve lasting abstinence from alcohol. Since it was founded in 1935 it has helped a large number of alcoholics to achieve long-lasting or permanent abstinence from alcohol. It is organized and run without psychiatric guidance, but its leaders intuitively have introduced some general principles of group psychotherapy into its operation.

Upon entrance into a group, the person declares openly to the group that he is an alcoholic and he pledges himself in earnest fellowship to seek abstinence for himself and to help the other group members when they are tempted to relapse. The group meetings have strong inspirational features and depend heavily on a feeling of cohesive fellowship. If a member of Alcoholics Anonymous is tempted to relapse at any time, he may call other members who will come to him at once to persuade him to remain abstinent. Thus, the group is bound together by ties of group loyalty, a common problem and a common goal.

In general, Alcoholics Anonymous offers its most effective help to the alcoholic who is well motivated to stop drinking and who is of better than average education, intelligence and social background. Alcoholics Anonymous helps only a minority of those who examine its approach, for many alcoholics go to only a few meetings and then stop. However, it has helped many alcoholics to achieve abstinence and a much better social adjustment. Alcoholics Anonymous also has group sessions for the marital partners of alcoholics where they can seek aid in understanding the problems of their alcoholic mates.

Psychotherapy. Most psychiatrists have

found that individual psychotherapy alone is rarely successful with an alcoholic unless a temporary obstacle to drinking has first been arranged. The most common obstacle employed is disulfiram therapy (discussed in succeeding paragraphs of this section). Once the patient has been placed on disulfiram and cannot drink because of the pharmacological properties of this drug, he often can settle down to work on the emotional problems and interpersonal stresses that led to his alcoholism. In some instances psychotherapy can be started in a psychiatric hospital where the patient has no access to alcohol, and the psychotherapy later continues on an outpatient basis after the patient has achieved enough psychotherapeutic progress to leave the hospital with a reasonable chance of remaining abstinent. As outlined in our earlier discussion of the emotional causes of alcoholism, its interpersonal roots are different from one patient to the next, and psychotherapy deals with particular emotional problems of each individual patient. It is unwise to prescribe antianxiety medication of any kind during the psychotherapeutic management of an alcoholic, for the person who has had a problem with alcohol is prone to take excessive amounts of sedatives, and in occasional instances may become physically addicted to them.

Without such obstacles to drinking as disulfiram therapy or a period of psychiatric hospitalization, psychotherapy flounders, for as the alcoholic discusses the painful emotional stresses of his life and deals with his day-to-day interpersonal difficulties he usually starts drinking again to assuage the anxiety he feels; he begins to skip treatment sessions and in time he discontinues treatment altogether. Psychotherapy alone is successful only in the patient whose problem with alcohol is mild and whose motivation for psychotherapy is strong. In such instances the patient usually has various emotional problems and interpersonal difficulties, and alcohol is only a small or moderate problem among several others; it is not the dominant, overwhelming feature of the clinical picture.

Group Psychotherapy. For many years group psychotherapy has been employed extensively with alcoholics. Some alcoholics can engage more effectively in group psychotherapy than in individual psychotherapy. In a group with other alcoholics they can discuss their problems with less anxiety than in individual sessions with a psychiatrist, and often they can accept the comments of other alcoholics more easily than the interpretations made in individual psychotherapy. In a group the alcoholic does not feel the moral censure he often feels in discussing his problem with a person who does not share his difficulty, and the group may achieve an atmosphere of fellowship that the alcoholic needs. Group psychotherapy is most useful for the passive, emotionally isolated alcoholic with strong feelings of insecurity and inadequacy. Such group psychotherapy may be conducted by a psychiatrist, or by a psychiatric social worker, or by a psychiatric nurse with advanced training in this field, or by a clinical psychologist, working in collaboration with a psychiatrist in a medical setting. (The therapist may use the principles of group psychotherapy outlined in Chapter 21.)

Conditioning Therapy. Various conditioning therapies have been employed in the treatment of alcoholism; they often are termed *aversive treatments* since they attempt to create a strong physical aversion to alcohol. The least sophisticated type of conditioning therapy, which has enjoyed periodic waves of use for more than 65 years, involves the production of nausea and vomiting by giving the patient an injection of an emetic drug shortly after he imbibes alcohol. This procedure is repeated daily in a hospitalized patient for several weeks until he develops a conditioned response of nausea and vomiting whenever he tastes or smells alcohol. This treatment obviously requires a well motivated patient who is willing to undergo the discomforts and hospitalization period involved. Group or individual psychotherapy should accompany the treatment.

Modern behavior therapists have experimented with more refined conditioning technics. Repulsive visual imagery (or daydreams) may be repeatedly associated with the idea of drinking or with smelling or tasting alcohol. As in all other treatments of alcoholism, the results of conditioning therapies are difficult to evaluate since they require well motivated, cooperative patients, and a certain percentage of such patients abandon drinking without special help. However, conditioning therapies probably help well selected patients who would otherwise waver at times about beginning to drink again.

Disulfiram (Antabuse) Therapy. Disulfiram (Antabuse) is an orally administered drug widely used in treating alcoholism. The person who is taking a daily maintenance dose of this drug has no effects from it unless he drinks alcohol. If he drinks alcohol he becomes ill quickly and is acutely uncomfortable. Disulfiram acts by inhibiting the metabolism of alcohol at the acetaldehyde stage, so that acetaldehyde accumulates in the patient and causes much physical discomfort.

I feel that when a patient is started on disulfiram he should, if feasible, be hospitalized for a brief period of time in the psychiatric division of a hospital. During the one-week period while disulfiram is being built up in the patient's body, he should be in a setting where he cannot get alcohol and where any side effects of the drug can be noted quickly and removed by immediate reduction of its dosage. There are various regimens of disulfiram dosage. I usually administer 0.5 gm. of disulfiram to the patient for seven consecutive days, and on the eighth day early in the morning I give him 30 cc. to 45 cc. of whiskey in a glass of water as a "test dose" to make sure he has an adequate level of disulfiram in his body. Within 10 to 15 minutes the patient begins to have flushing of the face, shortness of breath, headache, a feeling of tightness in his chest, tachycardia, aching in his limbs and body, and a profound feeling of malaise. Nausea and vomiting may occur. This "test dose" shows the patient convincingly the results of drinking alcohol while on disulfiram. During the test dose period, which usually lasts about two hours, the patient's blood pressure is checked every 10 minutes, since a moderate fall in blood pressure usually occurs. If the systolic blood pressure drops below 70 mm./Hg., the patient is given an intramuscular injection of a vasopressor drug, such as 5 mg. of metaraminol (Aramine). A fall of systolic blood pressure below 70 mm./Hg. is unusual, but the physician must be prepared for such an event with a vasopressor drug and, on very rare occasions, a set for the intravenous administration of plasma. After recovery from the test dose the patient is watched medically with blood pressure readings every 30 minutes for the rest of the day. The next day he may be discharged on a maintenance dose, which I usually set at 0.25 mg., but which in some instances may be 0.125 mg.

I always insist that the maintenance dose of disulfiram be given by a close relative at a regular time each day, because I have found that the probability of a patient's staying on the drug is much greater if the responsibility for administering it daily is given to someone else. The patient continues to take the drug from one to five years or more. If the patient stops taking disulfiram at any time, it still prevents drinking for about two weeks. If the patient drinks alcohol while taking disulfiram he should be rushed to a hospital at once for observation and possible treatment of cardiovascular collapse; he should carry a card in his wallet with instructions to this effect. In rare instances, fatal reactions to disulfiram have occurred when the patient ingested a large amount of alcohol quickly.

Disulfiram therapy should be given only by a physician who has experience in administering it. A certain number of patients develop a toxic psychosis due to disulfiram if the dosage is not skillfully adjusted during the buildup period. It passes within seven days when the medication is discontinued, and consists of a confusional state which resembles an organic brain disorder. There are few physical contraindications to disfulfiram; the most common is coronary artery insufficiency. The patient who is emaciated and malnourished should have a two-week inpatient period of physical recuperation before taking disulfiram. Some physicians use disulfiram on an outpatient basis when they feel the patient and his family are fairly reliable; the patient enters the hospital for one day when he has his test dose of alcohol.

Disulfiram therapy should be followed by individual or group psychotherapy if the patient will accept it. As pointed out above, disulfiram erects a chemical barrier to drinking which allows the patient to engage in psychotherapy and the anxiousness it may arouse. I have dealt with disulfiram therapy at some length because, in my hands, it is the most effective form of treatment of alcoholism; other investigators who have compared matched groups of patients who were treated with various technics have reached similar conclusions. Only a minority of patients to whom I propose disulfiram therapy accept it, but most of those who accept it stick with it and remain abstinent.

Social and Vocational Rehabilitation Programs. For the alcoholic working to rehabilitate himself there are various rehabilitation institutes, social welfare agencies and religious groups that sometimes can give him assistance. Vocational counseling, job training and placement, and personal encouragement are useful adjuncts in the comprehensive management of some alcoholics.

(*Treatment of the psychotic states* (*delirium tremems, Korsakoff's psychosis and others*) *which may be associated with alcoholism* is covered in Chapter 18 on the common organic brain disorders.)

PERSONALITY DISORDERS ASSOCIATED WITH NARCOTIC ADDICTION

The most common narcotic to which persons become addicted in the United States is heroin. Addiction also occurs occasionally to morphine, meperidine (Demerol), paregoric and hydromorphone (Dilaudid). Addiction to codeine is immensely rare, and many psychiatrists doubt that true physical addiction to codeine can occur.

Persons who become addicted to narcotics find that these drugs relieve them of emotional turmoil and also give them a sensuous feeling of well-being and physical comfort. These effects of narcotic drugs make them attractive to some persons with serious personality problems. The person who uses a narcotic first develops an *emotional dependence* on taking it periodically; he yearns for the relief of tension and the feeling of well-being it gives him, and he becomes emotionally dependent on taking it periodically. However, this emotional dependence soon gives way to a *physical dependence* on the drug as he continues to take it. He develops a physical *tolerance* to its effects, and finds that he must take increasingly larger doses to obtain the desired sensations. His central nervous system develops a physiological reliance on the drug, and if the patient goes more than 12 hours without it he begins to develop acute physical discomforts, which constitute the *withdrawal* syndrome, or *abstinence* syndrome. Individuals differ somewhat in the length of time required for physical addiction to occur, but in most instances a person becomes physically addicted if he takes significant amounts of a narcotic three or more times each 24 hours for three to four weeks; however, the emotional dependence of a drug user and his physical dependence are much more intertwined than neat separation of these two aspects of addiction implies.

There are various theories about how narcotic drugs function pharmacologically to produce physical addiction. The most widely accepted theory is based on the observation that the clinical features of the withdrawal syndrome are opposite in nature to the sedative features of the drug. As the addict uses the drug regularly over a prolonged period of time his central nervous system, and other body systems, gradually develop continual discharge mechanisms to counteract and cancel the effects of the drug. The body attempts to maintain its former homeostasis, or balance of forces, despite the presence of this new substance. Therefore, increasing amounts of the narcotic are needed to produce the relaxation the addict seeks. When the addict abruptly ceases to receive the drug, his central nervous system and other body systems continue to discharge the impulses with which they formerly counteracted the continual presence of the narcotic. However, in the absence of the narcotic these discharges produce central nervous system excitation and the various clinical features of the withdrawal syndrome. The features of the withdrawal syndrome tend to be the opposite of the effect of the narcotic; the person is panicky instead of sedated, his pupils are widely dilated instead of pinpoint constricted, and so forth. After a period of about 10 to 14 days without the narcotic the central nervous system reestablishes its normal equilibrium; other organs regain their steady-state, or homeostasis, and the withdrawal symptoms cease.

There is much controversy about the number of narcotic addicts in the United States, with the estimates running from 60,000 to 10 times that number. There probably are about 200,000 to 300,000 addicts and regular users.

A little over one per cent of all late adolescents and young adults experiment with narcotics a few times, but only a small fraction of them go on to become addicted. The rest desist because of the grim legal, social and economic consequences of addiction. In their desperate search to get the large daily sums of money they need to buy their narcotics, addicts account for a sizable percentage of the thefts, muggings, frauds and other crimes committed each year.

Clinical Characteristics of Narcotic Addiction

The person who becomes addicted to a narcotic usually first becomes acquainted with the effect of the drug through the suggestion of an acquaintance who is a regular user, or perhaps an addict. In many cases the person who introduces the novice to the drug hopes to gain money from the novice by selling the narcotic to him regularly after he becomes dependent on it. In this way the seller can obtain the money to buy his own daily supply of the drug from the criminal sources from which he gets it. Most persons who experiment with a few doses of a narcotic quickly abandon its use because of the ominous criminal and social consequences of taking it. However, a small but significant minority of persons with severe personality problems find that heroin assuages their emotional turmoil and gives them a feeling of sensuous well-being. They yearn for more heroin and soon are taking it two or three times each day. After three to four weeks they become physically addicted to it, though their increasing emotional dependence on it began somewhat earlier. A sizable number of persons who currently become addicted begin to experiment with herion during adolescence, whereas in former decades most addicts first used heroin in early adulthood.

Almost all heroin addicts in the United States administer their narcotics to themselves intravenously, or have other addicts perform the injections on them. The antecubital veins are most commonly used, and the addict usually has a telltale line of needle puncture marks on his arm and scars where infections have occurred after injections with poorly sterilized needles. An American addict probably takes between three and eight grains of heroin a day, but his daily intake may run higher than that when he can get the drug easily. However, accurate figures about daily narcotic intake are extremely speculative since addicts usually are not truthful in telling how much they take, and, moreover, their illegally obtained narcotics usually are adulterated with inert substances by the sellers so that the addicts actually do not know how much narcotic they are taking in each injection. In addition, the drug scene changes from month to month, and from one area of the country to another, depending on the ease or difficulty of heroin procurance, its price, the rigor of narcotic agents and other variables. It has been estimated that about 1 to 3 per cent of all long-term addicts die because of an overdose of heroin when they unknowingly get a much purer sample than they are accustomed to taking; however, these figures are difficult to verify. Some addicts also take antianxiety drugs or sedatives concurrently with their narcotics, and in time become addicted to both types of drugs.

The addict can get the narcotics to maintain his addiction only through criminal sources, and he soon sinks into an underworld of deception and illegal trafficking. He associates to a large extent with other addicts, and he is in continual danger of legal apprehension and imprisonment. Often he cannot hold a steady job because of his daily necessity for periodic self-administered intravenous narcotics and decreased job efficiency for several hours after each injection. Many narcotic addicts resort to thievery, fraud, prostitution and other illegal activities to get money to buy narcotics. The addict continually must increase his dosage to get the sensations he seeks from narcotics, and he is at the mercy of his criminal suppliers who frequently raise their prices and adulterate the narcotics with inert substances. The addict undergoes marked social, economic and interpersonal deterioration, and after a few years he usually has a record of several criminal arrests for illegal possession of narcotics and several brief, unsuccessful hospitalizations for narcotic addiction, which have been forced upon him. Since he neglects his health and nutrition, physical health problems are common in the addict. Suicide is common; the addict may commit suicide when he faces the agony of another withdrawal from narcotics because he can no longer get a supply of the drug.

It is very difficult for a narcotic addict to rise out of his emotional deterioration once he has sunk into it. He is deterred by his severe basic personality problems and his physical dependence on the drug. In addition, his interpersonal world is composed mainly of other addicts and he feels alienated from all other interpersonal circles. After he emerges from a period of enforced hospitalization for his addiction or from a prison term for possession of narcotics, in the vast majority of instances the addict seeks out his former addict associates and sinks rapidly back into addiction. Most psychiatrists who have worked with addicts agree that the prognosis for persistent rehabilitation of a narcotic addict is poor.

In recent years a few psychiatrists have spoken of narcotic addiction in many users as "a way of life," or "life style," and state that the addict takes such adulterated heroin that in many cases he is more accustomed to addiction as type of existence than truly dependent on the drug. They also state that a significant percentage of addicts drift away from narcotics by the age of 40. This may be true in selected, small samples of addicts, especially those seen in private psychiatric hospitals where patients undergo hospitalization for several months or more, but in my opinion it does not represent the general outlook and nature of narcotic addiction.

In rare instances, a person becomes accidentally addicted to narcotics because of injudicious medical administration of too much narcotics during a painful physical illness. This type of patient has a much better prognosis than the addict who becomes addicted through illicit channels of narcotic procurance.

I once worked for 15 months in a hospital that had a continual census of 300 narcotic addicts. The saddest cases of all were the physicians and nurses who had become addicted by the self-administration of narcotics easily available to them because of their professions. Every physician and nurse should be acutely aware of the dangers of self-administered narcotics under any circumstances.

The Emotional Causes of Narcotic Addiction

The emotional turmoil of various severe personality problems may contribute to narcotic addiction. The addict often has profound anxiety and marked feelings of insecurity and inadequacy. He finds relief from these painful feelings in the sedative effects and sensations of well-being that narcotics give him. Some addicts have, in addition, severe antisocial personality disorders, and the personality problems discussed in the section on antisocial personality disorders in the preceding chapter are present in them. This type of addict has a defective sense of guilt and social responsibility, and he tolerates frustration of his impulses and desires poorly. He is unable to engage in warm, meaningful interpersonal relationships, and he has a profound self-centeredness in which people are merely objects that serve his needs or frustrate them. He does not modify his behavior because of punishment or failure, and he has little perception of the feelings and rights of others and the demands of society. He proceeds from one impulse to another without consideration of the long-range results of his acts.

In his childhood the narcotic addict usually had traumatic relationships with both parents and with other close persons; in most cases he did not have a sound, affectionate relationship with any adult. He did not form a healthy identification with anyone, and often he emerges from childhood and early adolescence with profound hostilities which cause him to rebel wildly against his parents and against social conformity. His narcotic addiction and the criminal activities into which it leads him serve as a flagrant means of defying the standards and ethics of society. Narcotic addiction tends to be more common among individuals in socially deprived groups, for, in addition to disorganized family lives, they are damaged by the poverty, cultural neglect and racial discrimination in which they were reared and are still living. For them, narcotic addiction is a way of rebelling against both their families and the social system they hate. However, beneath their belligerent defiance many addicts have anxious cravings to be cared for in childlike ways. Many of them are very immature emotionally, and they live to a large extent in a world of unrealistic daydreams. They often describe their future plans with immature unreality, and their concepts of the world around them are so childlike as to be almost delusional at times.

The pharmacological experience of being addicted to heroin or any other narcotic aggravates the original personality problems of the patient. So many addicts, and the physicians who work with them, state that once an individual has been thoroughly addicted he is never the same person again, that there must be some truth is this cliché. After he becomes addicted he retreats even further into preoccupation with his own body and his own feelings. His emotional world becomes composed of himself and the drug, and other people and other things are pushed to a dim periphery of his emotional life. Hunger, pain, sex and all other body sensations recede as the physical dependence on the drug becomes dominant in his feelings and thinking. Interpersonally, the drug takes the place of people, and some addicts speak of their drug almost as if it were a personified being whom they endlessly seek for the sensuous placidity it gives them, and without whom life has little meaning or vitality.

In rare instances a person becomes addicted to narcotics while going through the suffering of a severe depressive illness; these patients have a better prognosis than most other addicts, and often can be cured of their addiction after the depressive illness terminates. A small number of narcotic addicts are schizophrenics, though many others could be classified as schizoid personalities. In rare instances narcotic addiction occurs during the progressive personality disorganization of early organic brain disease.

Treatment of Narcotic Addiction

We shall consider treatment of narcotic addiction under five headings: (1) withdrawal from narcotics, (2) psychotherapeutic and rehabilitative programs for narcotic addicts, (3) methadone maintenance programs, (4) group residential approaches to narcotic addiction and (5) medicolegal approaches to narcotic addiction.

Withdrawal from Narcotics. When a person who is physically addicted to heroin or any other narcotic is cut off from his supply of the drug he develops a characteristic withdrawal syndrome. After 12 hours of abstinence the patient begins to be increasingly restless and agitated. Yawning, perspiration, lacrimation, sneezing and nasal snuffling begin. After 24 hours the patient is very agitated and in acute distress with anorexia, severe generalized muscular pains and insomnia. His pupils are widely dilated, and he has gooseflesh and involuntary muscular twitchings. These symptoms continue at their peak for 48 hours to 72 hours, and then begin a gradual decline that lasts 10 days or so. However, the patient often complains of weakness, anxiousness, insomnia and minor muscular pains for several weeks to several months longer.

Withdrawal of an addict from narcotics must be carried out in a psychiatric hospital setting, since the physician must make every effort to prevent the patient from getting illicit narcotics during his withdrawal period and during his subsequent hospital rehabilitation. When an addicted person is withdrawn from narcotics in a hospital he usually is shifted to the synthetic narcotic methadone (Dolophine), and then he is withdrawn gradually over a 10-day period. There are various schemes of withdrawal dosages, but they all are complicated by the fact that many addicts intentionally exaggerate the amount of narcotic they have been taking so they can receive a high initial dose of the narcotic used in the withdrawal procedure. Also, many addicts can counterfeit withdrawal symptoms and thus can deceive the physician about whether he is giving the patient a reasonable dose of the withdrawal medication. In my experience in withdrawing narcotic addicts, a standard, average procedure is to stabilize the patient for two days on 40 mg. of methadone each day, given in four doses of 10 mg. each at six-hour intervals; the methadone is given orally in its liquid form.

After stabilization for two days on this dosage, the patient is withdrawn by gradually decreasing the drug over a 10-day period. The individual doses are decreased by regular decrements, so that after the first reduction the patient is getting 8 mg. four times each day at six-hour intervals, and so forth. However, even with gradual withdrawal the patient has a certain amount of withdrawal symptoms, which cannot be avoided. The patient's discomfort can be somewhat assuaged by the use of phenothiazines, such as chlorpromazine (Thorazine) during the withdrawal period. Phenothiazines are the only advisable sedatives to use with narcotic addicts, since physical addiction to phenothiazines cannot occur. The addict should not receive potentially addicting sedatives such as barbiturates, meprobamate (Miltown, Equanil), glutethimide (Doriden), chlordiazepoxide (Librium, Libritabs), diazepam (Valium) and others. However, if the addict also has been taking large amounts of illicit antianxiety drugs or sedatives before entering the hospital, he may also be physically addicted to them as well as to narcotics. In such an instance, the patient is also given an appropriate regimen for withdrawal from the barbiturate or other sedative while he is being withdrawn from the narcotic. The regimen for withdrawing patients from non-narcotic sedatives and antianxiety medications is given later in this chapter. Patients with myocardial disease or other severe physical illnesses should be withdrawn more slowly over a three- or four-week period.

Nalorphine (Nalline) and levallorphane (Lorfan) are narcotic antagonists which precipitate an abstinence syndrome in any person who has narcotics in his system. In my opinion their use in detecting narcotic addiction is dangerous, unnecessary and unreliable. If a person does not admit addiction, or reveal it by withdrawal symptoms or the telltale line of puncture sites and scars along his veins, it is medically dangerous and legally unwise for a physician to administer a narcotic antagonist against the patient's wishes and without his full understanding and written consent. The only permissible use of these drugs is in the resuscitation of addicts who are in dangerous comas after accidentally or suicidally taking a high dose of narcotics; even in such cases, however, narcotic antagonists can have perilous results if the patient also has taken barbiturates, antianxiety medications, and some other drugs.

Psychotherapy and Rehabilitative Programs for Narcotic Addicts. After withdrawal from narcotics the addict should remain in the psychiatric hospital for a minimum of four months of rehabilitation. In many instances the total period of hospital care should be six to eight months. Addicts who leave the hospital in less than four months have an extremely high rate of relapse back into narcotic addiction. The relapse rate is smaller in patients who remain in the hospital for four months or more following withdrawal. In addition to the direct therapeutic benefits of the hospital experience, it requires four to six months for the addict to lose his craving for the drug, and this time span also helps him to break his interpersonal bonds with the other addicts with whom he was associating.

Psychotherapy is perhaps practical with a few well selected addicts, but most psychiatrists with much experience in this field feel that it is so difficult to engage most narcotic addicts in meaningful individual psychotherapy that it is not a workable therapeutic measure. The addict's profound self-centeredness, his incapacity to form sound interpersonal relationships, his proclivity to rebel against any kind of social conformity or authority, and his intense dedication to his drug as almost a personfied, all-giving being, make psychotherapy with him very difficult. Group psychotherapy is perhaps a more useful approach to treating narcotic addicts in psychiatric hospitals. (The principles of group psychotherapy outlined in Chapter 21 may be employed.)

The major problem in psychotherapy of a narcotic addict is to reach across the interpersonal gap that separates him from the rest of society and to offer him an interpersonal relationship with the therapist that can be used to rehabilitate him. Even the well-motivated addict tests out the therapist with provocative rebellion and evasiveness many times before he feels any security in his relationship with him. The major part of psychotherapy with an addict can be carried out effectively only in a hospital setting, for during his provocative periods the addict will return defiantly to narcotics if he is being treated on an outpatient basis. However, the terminal phases of psychotherapy can be conducted on an outpatient schedule.

The addict usually needs vocational and social rehabilitation. Job placement and careful discharge planning often are advisable before he leaves the hospital. Counseling with his relatives should be carried out to try to arrange an interpersonal environment into which he may enter when he leaves the hospital, so that in his loneliness he will not seek out his old circle of addict acquaintances.

However, the vast majority of addicts will not stay in the hospital for several months of rehabilitative work unless they are forced by legal pressure to do so. Moreover, even with elaborate treatment plans most addicts relapse back into addiction after they leave the hospital. The poor prognosis of narcotic addiction causes a continual search for new ways to control this public health problem and to manage the addicted patient.

The withdrawal of the addict from narcotics and his subsequent rehabilitation should be in psychiatric hands. The family physician or internist should refer all addicted patients to private or public psychiatric facilities for care. Moreover, it is unwise to give the addict "just one shot to tide me over until I get to the hospital." When he receives narcotics from a physician under such circumstances, the addict usually defers hospitalization and returns with more pleas for narcotics. The family physician or internist may help the narcotic addict and his relatives to arrange hospitalization, but he should go no further in managing the patient's addiction.

The choice of hospital for an adolescent or young adult addict often poses a dilemma; my experiences with special federal, state and municipal hospital facilities for addicts has been discouraging. In such hospitals, or wards, the patient associates with long-term addicts, or addicts with little motivation to resolve their problem, and the constant talk is of the merits of various narcotics, sources of narcotics, and illegal ways to get money to buy drugs. The young addict often emerges no better, and perhaps worse, than when he entered. Whenever possible, therefore, an addict who has good motivation for rehabilitation should be hospitalized on a general psychiatric service where he will meet few, or no, other addicts. However, the difficulties of arranging such hospitalization frequently are formidable, since general psychiatric hospitals have had so many disappointing experiences with addicts that they tend to shun them. The addict should be committed whenever possible, since very few stay more than several days or a few weeks without legal means of holding them. Since most state laws do not permit committment on the basis of addiction alone, it is well to remember that a significant number of addicts commit suicide when they can no longer get their drugs and must come off them abruptly; the patient sometimes can be committed on this basis when state laws permit committment of a person "who is dangerous to himself or others" because of a psychiatric problem.

Methadone Maintenance Programs. In a methadone maintenance program the synthetic narcotic methadone (Dolophine) is given orally on an outpatient basis to proved addicts. This is sometimes called the Dole-Nyswander treatment after the physicians who developed it. The addict comes each day to the clinic where he receives between 50 and 100 mg., or more, of methadone in syrup, often mixed in fruit juice. The dose is adjusted to keep the addict comfortable but not to sedate him. Psychotherapy in individual or group form, rehabilitation services, and vocational counseling and job placement services are offered to the patient once he becomes stabilized on methadone and is a regular frequenter of the clinic. Most of these clinics operate in unimposing settings in inner city districts where there is a relatively high incidence of narcotic addiction. The urine of patients can be tested occasionally to determine if, in violation of treatment aims, they are still taking heroin.

Advocates of methadone maintenance programs feel that they free the addict from his dependence on his illicit heroin suppliers, decrease the amount of criminal activity by addicts who are desperate for money to buy drugs, and gradually lead many addicts into social and vocational rehabilitation. They cite increased employment rates, better social adjustments and less criminality by their patients as evidence of the usefulness of methadone maintenance regimens. Also, proponents of this approach state that methadone creates a "narcotic blockade" which prevents the addict from getting sensuous gratification if he injects heroin, but there is increasing doubt about how effective such blockading is.

In my opinion, methadone maintenance programs are useful for a sizable minority of addicts and also cause a discernible reduction in community crime rates. These programs are well worth the money and professional time put into them. However, a relatively small percentage of addicts become abstinent from narcotics because of methadone maintenance regimens. Moreover, long-term experience shows that some clinic frequenters continue to inject heroin occasionally, that many of them do not persist in clinic attendance for a long period, and that only a small fraction of them make good use of the available psychotherapeutic and rehabilitative facilities. Nevertheless, until better technics are evolved, a methadone maintenance clinic in every drug-ridden neighborhood would help many addicts and the potential victims of their criminal assaults. The related topic of licencing addicts and giving them their narcotics medically, as a social approach to this problem, is discussed later.

Group Residential Approaches to Narcotic Addiction. In some cities small numbers of addicts who are strongly motivated to abandon narcotics have banded together in small groups organized along lines similar to those of Alcoholics Anonymous, described earlier in this chapter. By mutual support and persuasion, they work to free themselves and their associates from drugs. They have adopted names such as Narcotics Anonymous and Synanon. Some of them live communally in large, old houses or in joined apartments. Such an approach probably is suitable only for a small percentage of addicts, and its degree of success is uncertain, but any sincere, reasonable effort to abandon addiction should be encouraged, and a physician may recommend such a group if one is available in his city. Local welfare offices, psychiatric hospitals, and family and children's service agencies know if such groups are available in any particular city and how reliable they are.

Medicolegal Approaches to Narcotic Addiction. As narcotic addiction has become a prominent public health problem in the United States and has contributed much to spiraling crime rates, some psychiatrists and other mental health professional workers have suggested a return to the system which existed in the United State before 1914. Until 1914 any addict could, with a physician's prescription, buy his drug in a pharmacy. This was the accepted system; for example, in Charles Dickens's novel *Bleak House*, Dr. Woodcourt, a minor hero, regularly prescribes narcotics for Captain Hawdon as a routine medical procedure. The Harrison Narcotic Act of 1914 (and all the subsequent federal, state and municipal legislation against narcotic usage) for the first time made possession and usage of narcotics by an addict illegal in the United States, and such legislation made narcotic trafficking a highly lucrative business, just as prohibition of alcohol in 1919 threw a major industry into criminal hands and created the affluent criminal underworld which still afflicts American society. Some psychiatrists have suggested that if narcotic addiction were made an exclusively medical problem, as it was before 1914, or if addicts were legally identified and given photo-bearing identification cards which permitted them to get their drugs from physicians or public clinics, the general problem would decrease greatly; this system is used in some European countries, and they have, apparently, far less addiction than the United States. It is becoming clear that punitive laws are not effective, and may even increase addiction by making it a profitable commercial enterprise for pushers and middlemen. At least, a return to treating addiction as a purely medical problem might be the lesser of two evils; I incline toward this point of view, but this highly controversial proposal can be argued both ways.

PERSONALITY DISORDERS ASSOCIATED WITH OTHER FORMS OF DRUG ABUSE

In this section we shall consider personality problems which contribute to, or are complicated by, abuse of (1) sedatives and antianxiety medications (minor tranquilizers), (2) amphetamines, (3) hallucinogens, (4) marijuana and (5) cocaine.

Sedatives and Antianxiety Medications

A person may become physically addicted to virtually all sedative-hypnotic drugs; addictable drugs include all barbiturates, chloral hydrate, ethinamate (Valmid), glutethimide (Doriden), methyprylon (Noludar), ethchlorvynol (Placidyl), methaqualone (Quaalude, Sopor, Parest, Somnafac), paraldehyde and others. Physical addiction also may occur to most antianxiety medications (minor tranquilizers); these drugs include chlordiazepoxide (Libritabs, Librium), meprobamate (Equanil, Miltown), oxazepam (Serax), diazepam (Valium) and many others. All these drugs, if taken two or more times each day in excessive doses over a period of several weeks or longer may cause physical dependence; if the addicted person stops the medication abruptly he undergoes a withdrawal syndrome, which may include a hallucinatory delirium and convulsions. The amount of drug that a person must take and the length of time he must continue on it, to produce addiction, vary much from one drug to the next.

We shall discuss in detail addiction to one set of these drugs, the barbituates, since more is known about them than the others. However, with the exception of the specific dosage figures given here, this discussion of barbiturates applies equally to all the other sedative-hypnotics and antianxiety medications enumerated above, and to many others not listed. The causes of addiction, the withdrawal syndromes and the treatment of physical dependence of these medications are more or less the same. Although the incidence of addiction to any one of them varies from one decade to the next, and from one region of the country to another, the general incidence of addiction to these various medications seems to be approaching that of the barbiturates.

A person who takes 800 mg. of a barbiturate in two or more divided doses each day for six weeks or more develops marked withdrawal symptoms upon stopping it, and lesser grades of physical dependence have been reported in patients ingesting from 300 to 700 mg. each day. Symptoms of withdrawal consist of anxiousness, weakness, insomnia, tremors and diffuse malaise, and in some instances the patient develops a psychosis with visual hallucinations, panic and marked agitation, similar to delirium tremens. Grand mal convulsions often occur in a patient going through a withdrawal syndrome from barbiturates. The basic physiological mechanism by which the addiction occurs is felt to be similar to that in narcotic addiction, described earlier in this chapter. The doses of sedative-hypnotics and antianxiety medications that must be taken for addiction to occur are usually three or more times the recommended daily total, taken around the clock in two or more divided doses; a typical meprobamate addict, for example, takes 1200 mg., or much more, three or four times during each 24 hours, making a daily total of 3600 mg. to 4800 mg., or more.

In many instances the person who becomes addicted to a barbiturate, or other sedative or antianxiety medication, has an underlying neurosis with much anxiety. He may have a chronic anxiety state, severe diffuse phobias, or an obsessive neurosis with much accompanying anxiousness. He takes ever increasing doses of a sedative or antianxiety medication to try to quell his uncontrollable anxiety levels until he in time becomes addicted. In other cases a depressed patient similarly misuses a medication to drown his feelings of guilt, agitation and melancholy. Adolescents and young adults may use sedative-hypnotics and antianxiety medications, often in combination with other drugs, to obtain the sensations of relaxed euphoria and giddy exhilaration they give. Intensive use occasionally leads to addiction; in some instances, addiction to these sedatives coexists with addiction to narcotics or alcoholism. A person with an antisocial personality disorder may, among his various motivations for drug abuse, misuse sedatives as a way of defying social customs which decry such usage of medications.

Addiction to sedatives and antianxiety medications usually is not associated with the severe socioeconomic and interpersonal deterioration that accompanies narcotic addiction, and the long-range prognosis of a person addicted to sedatives is distinctly better than that of a narcotic addict. However, addiction to sedatives is a serious medical problem and the patient usually has severe emotional problems which led to his misuse of the drug; relapses back to drug use, after withdrawal in a hospital, are common, but the probability of eventual long-term abstinence is much greater than in narcotic addiction.

The patient addicted to barbiturates, or any

other sedative-hypnotic or antianxiety medication, should be admitted to the psychiatric division of a hospital where he can be under careful medical supervision and can be prevented from getting additional self-administered sedatives. He is stabilized on whatever level of barbiturate, or other drug, he was taking and is gradually withdrawn over a three-week period. He should receive 100 mg. of diphenylhydantoin (Dilantin) twice each day to prevent convulsions during the withdrawal period. Following withdrawal the patient should begin psychotherapy in the hosptial for his underlying emotional problems, and he should continue the psychotherapy on an outpatient basis after he leaves the hospital. The patient who cannot engage in individual psychotherapy may be able to benefit from group psychotherapy, and rehabilitation work to reintegrate him into his college or vocational activities may be useful.

Amphetamines

Although some psychiatrists feel that a mild physical addiction to amphetamines can occur, with several-day mild withdrawal periods, most psychiatrists feel that physical addiction to this group of drugs does not occur. However, a patient may become emotionally dependent on them.

The most commonly abused amphetamines are amphetamine (Benzedrine), methamphetamine (Desoxyn, Drinalfa) and dextroamphetamine (Dexedrine). The drug usually is taken orally, but some abusers also inject it intravenously. These drugs give some patients feelings of pleasurable stimulation, excessive energy and giddy self-confidence. The patient who becomes emotionally dependent on them may take total daily doses of several hundred milligrams or much more. On large doses the patient becomes overactive, tremulous, agitated and distractible. He eats poorly, loses weight and often is thin and haggard. Abuse of amphetamines may produce toxic psychoses (which are described in Chapter 19 on organic brain disorders). Also, misuse of amphetamines occasionally precipitates an acute paranoid schizophrenic episode in a person with a schizoid personality structure. In poorly understood ways, heavy amphetamine usage occasionally causes sudden death; this is reflected in the youth culture sayings, "Speed can kill" and "Meth is death." In addition, amphetamine users, along with all other drug abusers, have a significantly higher incidence of injury and death in automobile accidents, household accidents, surfing mishaps, and other kinds of accidents when they are under the influence of drugs. There is also some evidence that amphetamine misuse can produce organic brain damage and necrotizing angitis, which is sometimes fatal.

The person who becomes emotionally dependent on amphetamines has marked underlying personality difficulties. In many instances he has strong feelings of emotional insecurity and inadequacy. In other instances he has antisocial personality problems and uses the drug as part of a rebellion against social conformity and authority. About 10 per cent or more of adolescents and young adults experiment with amphetamines a few times in seeking a thrill or in order to stay awake while studying for examinations. The persons who go on to misuse an amphetamine chronically find that the exhilaration it gives assuages their emotional turmoil and unhealthy personality needs.

The person who is emotionally dependent on large doses of amphetamines should be psychiatrically hospitalized. He should be withdrawn immediately from amphetamines and should be given moderate sedation. Although a barbiturate or chlordiazepoxide theoretically is the preferred sedative for this purpose, I prefer phenothiazines (Thorazine, Sparine and others) since it is impossible to become physically addicted to phenothiazines; thus, in using them one does not introduce the patient to another addictable drug, as one does when a barbiturate or one of the common antianxiety medications is used. A program of psychotherapy and social rehabilitation should follow withdrawal from the drug. The relapse rate back to the use of amphetamines after discharge from the hospital is fairly high, but the long-range prognosis is much better than that of narcotic addiction.

Hallucinogens

The most widely used of the drugs called hallucinogens is lysergic acid diethylamide, commonly termed LSD or "acid." This chemical was first used during the 1940's in psychiatric research to produce conditions that were felt to be schizophrenic-like psychotic states of several hours' duration. During the 1960's LSD became extensively used, mainly by late adolescents and young adults, for its exhilarating sensations, but as its dangers have become apparent its use has tended to decline since then.

The person who ingests LSD has marked changes in perception, feeling and thinking which he may describe as exalting, ecstatic, fascinating, terrifying or panicky. He often has brilliantly hued visual hallucinations, and he perceives objects in his environment in distorted, colorful, provocative ways. Some early enthusiasts of LSD proclaimed it to be "mind-expanding," but most psychiatrists now believe that it merely produces a brief, stimulating organic brain syndrome. The term "psychedelic" is sometimes applied to the experiences characteristic of LSD, but this word is also applied to similar visual and auditory sensations produced by the rapid, striking manipulation of light, sound and color in the environment without the use of drugs.

Many other chemicals and substances, loosely grouped under the term hallucinogens, may produce similar states. They include mescaline (obtained from the mescal cactus), psilocybin (extracted from a fungus), morning glory seeds, catnip preparations, nutmeg preparations, and many others. Similar states may be induced by inhaling the fumes of some aromatic glues, aerosol paint sprays, deodorant sprays and many other substances.

About 10 per cent of adolescents and young adults (the figures vary much from one social group to another and from one year to the next) experiment a few times with LSD, or other hallucinogens, but only a very small number become regular users. Individuals with much anxiety, subtle depressiveness, feelings of inferiority, feelings of meaninglessness, and other problems, may find the hallucinogenic experience very attractive and may become emotionally dependent on the use of a hallucinogen from once to several times a week. LSD also can be, in part, a tool of rebellion against parents, authorities and social groups who condemn it. Frequent users may undergo social, scholastic and vocational deterioration as their lives become increasingly centered on the drug and its attendant experiences. Although a person thus may become emotionally dependent on a hallucinogen, physical dependence cannot occur.

LSD is a dangerous drug; severe adverse reactions to it are fairly common. In a small percentage of users it precipitates psychotic states which are indistinguishable from schizophrenic illnesses, and these episodes may last from a few hours to several months or longer; in the jargon of the youth culture they are called "bad trips." Some psychiatrists feel that these are true schizophrenic disorders precipitated in persons with predisposing schizoid personality disorders, whereas others feel they are poorly understood toxic reactions to the drug. Their treatment is roughly the same as that for schizophrenia. Also, some LSD users have momentary or several-minute returns of hallucinations and visual distortions hours or days after the main LSD reaction has worn off; if these "flashbacks" occur while the person is driving a car, or swimming, or skiing, or working with complex heavy machinery, serious accidents can occur. There is fragmentary, controversial evidence that LSD may cause fetal abnormalities in pregnant women and chromosomal changes in both men and women, which may produce later fetal malformations. In addition, some psychiatrists feel that LSD usage predisposes a person to experiment with heroin, and perhaps later to become addicted to it; other psychiatrists feel that most such invididuals would have used heroin even if they had not first taken LSD.

There is not enough clinical evidence to indicate how dangerous other hallucinogenic substances, such as mescaline and psilocybin, are, but most psychiatrists feel that intensive use of high potency preparations of them involves many of the hazards of LSD. Persons who defend the use of these substances, or minimize their risks, often are unaware that most of them are generally taken briefly in very weak forms. Widespread, long-term use of these hallucinogens would probably result in the production of ever more potent preparations with higher incidences of serious adverse reactions.

A person who has a psychotic break, or a severe neurotic decompensation, because of LSD usage should be hospitalized and given large doses of an oral phenothiazine (Thorazine, Stelazine, Mellaril, or others). An uncooperative, panicky, assaultive patient may be given intramuscular injections of 50 mg. of chlorpromazine once every four hours. After recovering from his acute disturbance he should remain hospitalized for group or individual psychotherapy and subsequent social and vocational rehabilitation counseling. Any outpatient who is found to be using hallucinogens should be informed of their dangers and, if he will accept it, should have whatever psychotherapy or counseling he needs to stop taking them.

Marijuana

Marijuana is a substance obtained from plants of the genus Cannabis which grows wild in many parts of the United States; its distribution is worldwide. The flowering tops of the plant are dried and, in its most common form, made into cigarettes. In other forms, such as hashish, Cannabis products may be chewed, drunk or smoked. The person who uses marijuana gets feelings of sensuous euphoria, exhilaration and dreamy well-being from it. Hallucinations and distortions of the senses of time and space may occur. Claims that it increases sensitivity to music, appreciation of rhythm, and perceptual intensity have not been substantiated by objective clinical studies. The effects of marijuana last from one to six hours after smoking it. Physical addiction does not occur, but a person can become emotionally dependent on its alluring qualities. A person who uses marijuana rarely commits antisocial or criminal acts while under its influence, though he may indulge in imprudent sexual acts and behave in an irresponsible way (as when driving an automobile).

The euphoria, sensuous relaxation and exhilaration of marijuana may make it attractive to some persons who have strong feelings of inadequacy, insecurity, inferiority, anxiousness or depressiveness. A small number of marijuana regular users have antisocial personality disorders and flount it as a way of rebelling against parents and social authorities who disapprove of it. A quite small percentage of marijuana users sink into a life of irregular employment, scholastic irresponsibility and socioeconomic deterioration; however, many psychiatrists feel that most persons who do so would have followed a similar course without marijuana usage. The percentages of marijuana users vary a good deal from one social group to another. Between 25 and 40 per cent of late adolescents and young adults now experiment with marijuana at least a few times, but only about 10 to 15 per cent ever use it regularly over a significant period of time. The heavy use of marijuana tends to be more common among deprived socioeconomic groups in large cities.

The controversy about the harmfulness of marijuana continues. The American Medical Association, the American Psychiatric Association (which has more young members than old ones), and the National Institute of Mental Health state that its use is undesirable. Federal, state and municipal laws forbid its use, but these laws are now applied with erratic severity; conviction may draw a sentence that ranges from a reprimand to a several-year prison sentence. Most physicians feel that stringent punishment is unjust and ineffective, but few physicians favor legalization of marijuana. Legalization would involve the question of how it would be merchandised, distributed and advertised. Most important of all, legalization would probably result in the production of much stronger preparations. The essential ingredient of marijuana, tetrahydrocannabinal, can be extracted from it easily; simple kits for extracting it in the home are now illicitly available. The vast bulk of marijuana now used is very weak, but high potency preparations have an apparently greater tendency to produce emotional dependence and social deterioration.

Although some writers have spoken of "marijuana psychoses," there is little evidence that the incidence of psychoses and abruptly precipitated severe neuroses is any higher in marijuana users than in the general population. Whether this is true of persons who use tetrahydrocannabinal is not known. Some psychiatrists feel that marijuana users have a decidedly higher subsequent rate of heroin usage than nonusers of marijuana; other psychiatrists feel that heroin users would probably have experimented with heroin even if they had not first smoked marijuana. However, it is striking that alcoholics very rarely procede into heroin experimentation, whereas a significant small percentage of marijuana users do.

In my opinion, physicians, while not ranting on the subject, should point out the general medical attitude on marijuana to adolescents and young adults when the subject comes up in the course of medical practice. Marijuana users who have undergone marked scholastic, vocational, familial or socioeconomic deterioration should be referred for whatever group or individual psychotherapeutic help they will accept, and some can benefit from vocational and social rehabilitative services. In such cases, the physician should advise discontinuance of marijuana, though he can point out that it may be debated whether it is a cause or a symptom of the patient's interpersonal decline.

Cocaine

In the late 19th Century and early 20th Century cocaine, which is extracted from the leaves of Andean shrubs, was apparently a widely used intoxicant. From about 1915 to the late 1960's its use was rare in the United States, but since the late 1960's it has again become a commonly used drug, particularly among late adolescents and young adults. It is not physically addicting, but emotional dependence on it can occur. It gives feelings of sensuous exhilaration, pleasurable excitement and dreamy well-being. It may be chewed, sniffed or intravenously injected, and it often is taken in association with other drugs. Although statistics are unreliable in a rapidly changing drug scene, it appears that up to several per cent or more of young adults experiment at least a few times with cocaine, but only a small number go on to use it regularly.

The upsurge in cocaine usage is too recent to allow a general overview of just how dangerous cocaine is, but the old literature presents a very grim picture. Cocaine users were said to undergo the most severe interpersonal deterioration of all drug abusers; marked social and emotional deterioration was said to be common as the user progressively limited his life experiences to his drug and its sensations. A significant number of cocaine users develop toxic psychoses with florid hallucinations, paranoid delusions, assaultiveness and disorientation. Suicide, homicide and random destructiveness can occur during such psychotic bouts. Long-term users may develop the sensory hallucination that insects are crawling beneath their skin; this is called formication. Cocaine overdoses can cause fever, convulsions, delirium and death.

A person in an acutely agitated state due to cocaine should be hospitalized and sedated with barbiturates. Afterwards he should be engaged in group or individual psychotherapy if he will accept it, and rehabilitation services should be mobilized to help a cooperative patient. All physicians should point out the clear dangers of cocaine to any adolescent, young adult, or other person who is found to be using it. The long-term prognosis of cocaine usage is not known at present. It is possible that many persons use it for a short time and then, because of its obvious dangers, desist. In the late 19th Century such temporary cocaine users included such fictional and actual persons as Sherlock Holmes and Sigmund Freud. The percentage of cocaine users who descend into chronic social deterioration today is uncertain.

BIBLIOGRAPHY

Baekeland, F., et al.: Correlates of outcome in disulfiram treatment of alcoholism. J. Nerv. Ment. Dis., *153*:1, 1971.

Bowers, M. S.: Acute psychosis induced by psychotomimetic drugs. Arch. Gen. Psychiatry, *27*:437, 1972.

Clark, L. D., Hughes, R., and Nakashima, E. N.: Behavioral effects of marijuana. Arch. Gen. Psychiatry, *23*, 193, 1970.

Fisher, S., and Freedman, A. M. (eds.): Opiate Addiction: Origins and Treatment. New York, John Wiley & Sons, 1974.

Glass, G. S.: Psychedelic drugs, stress and the ego. J. Nerv. Ment. Dis., *56*:232, 1973.

Greene, M. H., and Dupont, R. L.: Heroin addiction trends. Am. J. Psychiatry, *131*:545, 1974.

Hendin, H.: Marijuana abuse among college students. J. Nerv. Ment. Dis., *56*:259, 1973.

Inaba, D. S., et al.: Methaqualone abuse. J. A. M. A., *224*:1505, 1973.

Isbell, H., et al.: An experimental study of the etiology of "rum-fits" and delirium tremens. Quart. J. Stud. Alchohol, *16*:1, 1955.

Khantzian, E. J., Mack, J. E., and Schatzberg, A. F.: Heroin use as an attempt to cope: clinical observations. Am. J. Psychiatry, *131*:160, 1974.

Kolansky, H., and Moore, W. T.: Effects of marijuana on adolescents and young adults. J. A. M. A., *216*:486, 1971.

Kupfer, D. J., Detre, T., Koral, J., and Fajans, P.: A comment on the "amotivational syndrome" in marjiuana smokers. Am. J. Psychiatry, *130*:1319, 1973.

McClelland, D. C., Davis, W. N., Kalin, R., and Wanner, E.: The Drinking Man. New York, Free Press, 1972.

Martin, W. R., et al.: Methadone—a reevaluation. Arch. Gen. Psychiatry, *28*:286, 1973.

Proskauer, S., and Rolland, R. S.: Youth who use drugs. J. Am. Acad. Child Psychiatry, *12*: 32, 1973.

Rathod, N. H., and Thomson, I. G.: Women alcoholics. A clinical study. Quart. J. Stud. Alcohol, *32*:45, 1971.

Smith, D. E., and Wesson, D. R.: Phenobarbital technique for treatment of barbiturate dependence. Arch. Gen. Psychiatry, *24*:56, 1971.

Snyder, S. S.: Uses of Marijuana. New York, Oxford University Press., 1971.

Taylor, R. L., Maurer, J. I., and Tinkelberg, J. R.: Management of "bad trips" in an evolving drug scene. J. A. M. A., *213*:422, 1970.

Section Four

Psychotic Disorders

There is no entirely satisfactory definition for the general term psychosis; it is traditionally used in medical nomenclature to designate those psychiatric states in which there is an extensive disintegration of personality structure and a marked loss of contact with reality. This loss of contact may be due to a profound withdrawal into an inner world of fantasy, with disintegration of thought processes, hallucinations and delusions, as in schizophrenia. Loss of contact with reality also may be due to a severe disturbance of mood which causes the patient to view the world unrealistically. Depressive psychoses fall in this group; the severely depressed patient sees the world and himself in such melancholy, depreciated ways that he ceases to have an emotionally realistic view of himself and the people around him. The psychotic patient usually suffers moderate to severe impairment in his social, vocational and close interpersonal activities, though in some instances he may for a time present a superficial façade of adequate behavior.

In this section we shall cover the psychoses which are accepted by most psychiatrists as mainly caused by severe interpersonal trauma; the psychoses caused by organic brain disease are discussed in Part IV. We shall here cover the interpersonally caused psychoses under the headings of (1) schizophrenia, (2) severe depressions, (3) manic psychoses and (4) other psychotic disorders, including the paranoid conditions.

14

Schizophrenia

Schizophrenia is the most common of the interpersonally caused psychoses. Schizophrenic patients comprise about 20 per cent of the first admissions to public psychiatric hospitals in the United States, and about 50 per cent of all the psychiatric beds in the United States are occupied by schizophrenics. About one per cent of the population between the ages of 15 and 45 will have a schizophrenic illness at some time during this span; the incidence before and after this period is much less. Though the majority of schizophrenics now recover and return to their former activities, schizophrenia still poses a major challenge for psychiatric treatment and research.

CLINICAL CHARACTERISTICS OF SCHIZOPHRENIA

The Basic Clinical Features of Schizophrenia

Withdrawal from Interpersonal Relationships. The fundamental process in schizophrenia is a profound withdrawal from interpersonal relationships and a retreat into an inner world of fantasy and self-absorption. The schizophrenic finds interpersonal life devastatingly painful, and unconsciously he flees from it into a private, inner life composed of his fantasies, sensations, preoccupations and turbulent emotional conflicts. He undergoes a loss of contact with reality, which may vary from mild to severe depending on the degree of his schizophrenic disintegration. The schizophrenic's withdrawal from reality is not a conscious, intentional process; it is a chaotic personality regression over which the patient has no conscious control and which he perceives only dimly through the emotional distortions produced by his illness.

The schizophrenic's withdrawal from interpersonal contacts and from reality may be manifested both in his emotional functioning and in his physical behavior. In his profound self-absorption the patient may become mute and motionless, and he may continue in this state for days, months or years. In other instances, the patient's withdrawal from reality is only partial, and he continues to interact with the people around him. However, the impairment of his contact with reality leads to inappropriate acts, delusions and hallucinations, which cause further disturbances in his interpersonal life. His withdrawal into an inner world and his loss of contact with reality may be so profound that it is immediately obvious to a casual observer or it may be hidden behind a brittle façade of seemingly adequate behavior.

Disturbances of Thought Association Processes. As he withdraws from people and reality, the schizophrenic regresses back to the primitive ways of thinking and feeling that occur in infancy and childhood. His thoughts no longer proceed in an orderly, logical way; his flow of thoughts is fragmented, and the disjointed fragments are attached to each other by emotionally charged associations rather than by logical sequences. Thoughts, symbols and words related by strong emotions jumble forth in a succession that has emotional significance to the patient, but that conveys no logical meaning to the casual observer. For example, the schizophrenic who sees a blue necktie may associate it with a blue necktie his father once wore, and he may feel that the person wearing it is an emissary of his father in disguise, or is trying to convey some message to him about his father by means of the necktie. The association of this particular blue necktie to his father and the patient's subsequent conclusions are not logical; they are produced by powerful emotional forces in the patient that sweep logical thinking aside and proceed to link one thought with another in a primitive, unhealthy way.

In his emotional withdrawal from reality the schizophrenic regresses back to thinking in terms of the kinds of symbolisms that are characteristic of infants and small children. Thus, he may feel that certain words, gestures or physical objects are symbols of supernatural powers or of particular persons. For example, he may feel that sunlight is a symbol of divine guidance radiating to him, or that certain colors or sounds represent malignant persons or organizations who are trying to harm him. I recall a schizophrenic patient who felt that electric light bulbs were symbolic representatives of a protecting power that was preventing people from harming him. The schizophrenic also may feel that things that look alike, or have similar sounding names, or are placed side by side, are identical to each other or are closely related. For example, I recall a schizophrenic patient who believed that because my last name was *Chapman* I was a member of the *chapter* of the fraternal organization to which he belonged, and that I had been sent to bring him secret messages.

At times the fragmentation of the schizophrenic's flow of thoughts results in sudden halts of speech called blocking; the patient abruptly stops talking and seems lost in inner puzzlement or preoccupation. At these times, conflicting fragmented thoughts crowd for his attention in jumbled confusion, and the patient ceases to speak. At other times a strong feeling or thought that has no relevance to his flow of speech erupts abruptly into his awareness and steals his attention away to a train of fantasies or silent preoccupations.

Disturbances of Emotional Responsiveness. As a consequence of his withdrawal from interpersonal relationships and his retreat into an inner fantasy world, the schizophrenic's emotional responses to events and people in his environment are altered. Often he shows no emotional responses to happenings around him. His face maintains a wooden impassivity and he does not manifest pleasure or sadness, or fear or rage about the events in his environment. He is said to have flatness of affect, or flatness of emotional response. His emotional interest has been transferred to his fantasies and inner preoccupation; he is unresponsive to things in the world around him because they now have less emotional impact on him.

In other instances, the schizophrenic's emotional responses to events around him are inappropriate. He laughs, smiles or grimaces without apparent provocation, or he may be frightened, agitated or morose without ostensible cause. These emotions are inappropriate to the realistic events in his environment, but they are appropriate to the strong feelings mobilized by his inner fantasy life and its attendant delusions and hallucinations.

Further Clinical Features of Schizophrenia

Disturbances of Physical Behavior. In about one third of cases of schizophrenia, the patient's loss of contact with reality leads to alterations in his physical behavior. As the result of his retreat into his inner fantasy world, he may sit motionless for long periods of time, not moving his body or altering his facial expression in any way. In some instances, the schizophrenic may hold his arms or legs in whatever position the examiner places them; this feature is called the waxy flexibility (or, in the older literature, cerea flexibilitas) of schizophrenia. At other times a schizophrenic patient may engage in repetitive physical gestures, stereotyped movements and elaborate mannerisms. These physical movements may continue for long periods of time, and they have symbolic significances for the patient that are not apparent to the casual observer. On some occasions an immobile schizophrenic may be resistant and negativistic to any action requested of him, and at other times, in response to the emotionally charged content of his inner fantasy life, he may become physically agitated, destructive or combative. In occasional instances, a schizophrenic has echopraxia, in which he imitates the actions of people around him, and in some instances he has echolalia, in which he parrots back whatever is said to him. The term *catatonic* is used to indicate the physical disturbances of schizophrenia.

Hallucinations. About 90 per cent of schizophrenics at some time during their illnesses have hallucinations. Most of the hallucinations are auditory, but in a small number of patients visual hallucinations occur. Hallucinations of smell, taste and touch are present in a few schizophrenics. The hallucinations are produced by the overpowering force of the inner fantasy life of the schizophrenic. The sensory perceptions of the world of reality lose their significance for him; crowding into their place come hallucinatory perceptions, which are produced by, and are in accord with, the content of his inner world of fantasy.

In his auditory hallucinations the schizophrenic hears voices speaking to him from outside his room, from the walls, from heating ducts, from electrical appliances, from television sets and radios, or from other sources. Often he describes the voices as being inside his head. The things the voices say to him are determined by the nature of his emotional turmoil. The voices may reaffirm what he dreads, or, in reassuring ways, they may tell him the opposite of what he fears. Thus, the patient who is struggling with feelings of inadequacy may hear voices that degrade and censure him, or he may hear voices of divine religious figures praising him and telling him that he has an important mission. The schizophrenic who is overwhelmed with guilt feelings may hear voices that curse him, condemn him or accuse him of immoral deeds. The patient who is suspicious and fearful of people may hear people talking about him in hostile ways in the next room or in the street. The patient usually has no doubt that the voices are valid sensory perceptions, but in some instances the patient occasionally wavers and is not sure whether or not the voices are "real."

The schizophrenic who has visual hallucinations may see people entering or leaving his room, often through the walls or windows. He may see divine figures who encourage him or malicious figures who threaten him. Occasionally a schizophrenic has olfactory hallucinations, which he may interpret as gas being pumped into his room by persecutors or as foul smells sent to annoy him. The schizophrenic may have hallucinations of taste in which he feels that he tastes "dope" or poison in his food. Tactile hallucinations may occur; a typical type of tactile hallucination is the feeling that someone is touching and manipulating the genitals, anus or perineal region.

Delusions. About 75 per cent of schizophrenics have delusions at some time during their illnesses. Persecutory and grandiose delusions are the most common. The patient with persecutory delusions feels that hostile persons are spying on him, plotting against him and trying to rob, harm or kill him. He may be convinced that the walls of his house are wired, that his telephone is tapped or that bizarre electronic devices are being used to spy on him. He may feel that things said or seen on television convey special malicious or favorable messages to him. He may believe that his persecutors are attempting to destroy his thoughts, or to control his mind or to dominate his actions. The patient may feel that his persecutors are prominent political figures, agents of foreign governments, criminals, members of his family, his work associates or others. In common usage, the word *paranoid* (as in paranoid delusions) is employed as a synonym of persecutory; the older, somewhat broader meaning of this term is outlined later in this chapter.

The patient with grandiose delusions feels that he is an exalted, important, powerful person. He may believe that he is an emissary of a divine figure or perhaps a divine personage himself. In other instances, a schizophrenic patient may feel that he is an important political or military figure or that he has supernatural powers that enable him to control the destinies of nations and the actions of large numbers of people.

Self-accusatory delusions may occur in schizophrenic illnesses. The patient may be convinced that he has killed people, committed robberies or carried out heinous sexual crimes and immoral sexual acts. He may feel that he is personally responsible for wars, the bombing of cities, fires and other public disasters.

Delusions of body distortions sometimes occur in schizophrenics. During the early stages of a schizophrenic illness the patient may feel that his body has changed in some strange way that he cannot define. Later in his illness the patient may feel that his body is deformed or that he has foul, loathsome diseases. He may feel that he has cancer or venereal disease or that parts of his body have rotted away. In some instances, the patient believes that he is dead, or that parts of his body are dead or are being destroyed in a bizarre way; such delusions, and delusions that all or part of his environment has been destroyed, are sometimes called *nihilistic* delusions.

The delusions of the schizophrenic patient are produced by the emotional tumult within him. After his withdrawal into an inner fantasy world, the real environment around him no longer puts firm limits on the form his ideas and feelings take; his feelings and thoughts push reality aside and become delusional. For example, the schizophrenic patient with strong feelings of inadequacy and inferiority has profound needs to feel important and significant; these needs, freed from the restrictions of contact with reality, may soar into grandiose delusions that he is an exalted, important, powerful, adored person. Psychiatric theory holds that delusions of persecution are produced when the patient projects his hostile feelings onto the outside world. He has pent-up hostilities that he cannot face, and he casts these hostile feelings out of himself onto other persons and groups of people; he perceives his own unacceptable feelings in others and then fears that they are hostile to him and are trying to harm him. (The subject of persecutory, or paranoid, delusions is discussed further in Chapter 17.)

Self-accusatory delusions occur when the schizophrenic is flooded with strong guilt feelings; unchained from realistic limitations, his guilt feelings assume the form of bizarre convictions that he has performed heinous acts and crimes. Schizophrenic delusions of body deformities arise from his dim, distorted awareness that in some strange way he has changed during his illness, and he arrives at the conviction that his body is diseased and deformed, or that he is dead.

Disturbances of Speech. The schizophrenic's withdrawal into an inner fantasy world and his disturbances of thought association processes may cause characteristic abnormalities in his speech. (Such speech abnormalities as the use of obscure symbolisms and blocking were mentioned in the early paragraphs of this chapter in discussing disturbances of thought processes in schizophrenia.) In addition, the schizophrenic may use words and phrases in ways that have private, unusual meanings that only he understands; for example, I recall a schizophrenic who talked much about the "big hats" and the "yellow balls" in referring to people who he felt were persecuting him. A schizophrenic may coin new words whose meanings are not clear to the casual observer; for example, I recall a patient who spoke of the "firlinks" and the "ranfelts" in talking about members of her family and her friends. These abnormalities of speech are noticeable in only a minority of acute schizophrenics whose illnesses are of recent origin. However, in schizophrenics who have been ill for a long time these abnormalities of expression may make the patient's speech a rambling sequence of disjointed phrases whose meaning is entirely obscure. Such incoherent schizophrenic speech is sometimes called verbigeration or a "word salad." Psychiatrists who work closely with schizophrenics may become skillful in unraveling the meanings hidden behind their obscure symbolisms, coined words, special phrases and fragmented sequences of ideas and feelings.

Other Clinical Features of Schizophrenia

As a patient proceeds into a schizophrenic disorder he may go through a phase in which he has neurotic symptoms lasting from several days to several weeks. When the onset of the schizophrenic process is very insidious this period of neurotic symptoms may last for several months or more. The patient may have acute or chronic anxiety symptoms, phobias, obsessions, compulsions, conversion symptoms, or dissociative features. These neurotic symptoms occur as the patient's emotional turbulence begins to increase and he becomes progressively disturbed. As he proceeds more deeply into his schizophrenic illness the neurotic symptoms recede and the picture of frank schizophrenia unfolds. About 10 per cent of schizophrenics go through a period of neurotic symptoms in the early phases of their schizophrenic illnesses. However, less than one per cent of all patients with neurotic symptoms ever develop schizophrenia.

Feelings of depersonalization may occur in

a patient as he begins to develop a schizophrenic illness. He has an eerie feeling that his personality has undergone a marked change. He cannot say what the change is and he does not feel that he is someone else, but he feels that in an unreal, strange way he is not the same person that he was. His feelings and actions seem alien and unreal to him. Feelings of depersonalization also may occur in some neurotic disorders and other psychiatric disturbances.

Manic or depressive features occasionally are present in a schizophrenic illness. The patient may have exhilarated, hyperactive, manic features added to a basic schizophrenic process, or he may have the depressed, self-depreciatory, guilt-ridden feelings that characterize a depressive psychosis. When manic or depressive features are prominent in a schizophrenic illness, the patient is said to have a schizoaffective disorder. (The schizoaffective type of schizophrenia is discussed in more detail later in this chapter.)

CLINICAL COURSE OF SCHIZOPHRENIA

In most instances schizophrenia first appears in late adolescence or early adulthood. The vast majority of cases of schizophrenia occur between the ages of 15 and 45, but occasionally schizophrenia may begin in childhood or middle age.

The onset of a schizophrenic illness may be insidious or abrupt. The onset often is so subtle and slow that the illness imperceptibly unfolds over a period of many months or years. The patient's withdrawal from interpersonal relationships and the appearance of other schizophrenic symptoms are so gradual that people around the patient may not be aware of his illness until it is far advanced. For many months they may notice only that the patient is quieter than previously or that he engages in eccentric acts or says something odd occasionally. Finally, his behavior startles their attention and they become aware that the patient has developed a serious psychiatric illness.

In other instances the onset of schizophrenia is abrupt, and during a period of a few days the patient develops a full-blown schizophrenic psychosis. His illness may begin with the sudden onset of a severe panic state, with marked agitation and terror. Florid persecutory delusions and auditory hallucinations may develop over a 48-hour perood, or the patient may withdraw into mute immobility. Schizophrenic disorders of sudden onset may be accompanied by belligerence, combativeness and destructiveness.

When a schizophrenic disorder is insidious in onset, the patient's relatives and friends usually cannot identify a precipitating cause, and many schizophrenic illnesses of abrupt onset are not preceded by any acute stress that the patient and his family can define. However, in other instances a schizophrenic illness begins after an obvious upsetting event. Interpersonal conflicts at home, at work or in other relationships with people sometimes disturb the patient immensely and trigger a schizophrenic disorder. The precipitating event, or series of events, unleashes a schizophrenic process to which the patient was predisposed by the emotional turmoil within him.

Prior to the introduction of modern treatment methods the prognosis of schizophrenia was dismal. The patient usually went through a series of partial remissions and relapses, and his general course was toward chronic psychotic incapacitation. He lived under the supervision of relatives or was institutionalized in psychiatric hospitals for long periods of time. However, a minority of schizophrenic patients recovered after one or two psychotic episodes and they remained well, and a few others had periodic psychotic illnesses throughout their lives with good remissions lasting several years or more between them. The original name of this disorder was dementia praecox (stressing its occurrence in young people and its tendency toward progressive deterioration), given to it by Kraepelin; the term schizophrenia was introduced in 1911 by Bleuler, and by the 1950's had displaced the older term in common usage and in the official nomenclatures.

The prognosis of schizophrenia has improved immensely in recent decades because of better methods of treatment. Statistics are difficult to evaluate, since psychiatrists working in different settings see different types of patients. The psychiatrist in private practice sees patients earlier in their illnesses and his patients usually have a high recovery rate. The patients who are admitted to public psychiatric hospitals often have not improved with previous treatment and have been sick longer periods of time; hence, recovery rates of patients in public psychiatric hospitals may not be as high as recovery rates in other settings. Nevertheless, a decided majority of schizophrenics who are today seen as new patients in public psychiatric hospitals recover, and many others improve markedly and are able to lead reasonably effective lives outside the hospital. In my practice, admittedly a somewhat selected group, more than 80 per cent of schizophrenic patients make a good recovery and, if they will remain for two years on outpatient maintenance doses of a phenothizine medication, maintain it; the number of my schizophrenic patients who must be counted as failures is less than 10 per cent. When I first began to work in psychiatry in the 1940's only about 25 per cent of private psychiatric patients made good recoveries, and even these patients often remained ill a year or two before recovering.

As a rule, the patient with a schizophrenic illness of abrupt onset has a much better prognosis than the patient whose illness began insidiously during a period of two or three years or more. The patient whose prepsychotic interpersonal adjustment was relatively good has a better prognosis than the patient who since childhood or adolescence has been seclusive and very tense. The prognosis is much better when the patient receives hospital treatment in the early weeks or first few months of his illness; a delay of many months or several years allows the psychotic process to become more entrenched. The prognoses of some clinical types of schizophrenia are better than others. (Some of these differences are mentioned in our discussion of the various clinical types of schizophrenia in the next section.)

The Clinical Types of Schizophrenia

In psychiatric nomenclature schizophrenia traditionally is divided into several different types. These types are defined in terms of the predominant symptoms of the patient. Thus, a patient whose illness is dominated by delusions and hallucinations is said to have the paranoid type of schizophrenia, and the mute, immobile schizophrenic is said to have the catatonic type of schizophrenia. Schizophrenic illnesses with other predominating symptoms are classified in other categories.

However, most schizophrenic patients go through periods when different kinds of symptoms predominate. For example, a patient who begins his illness with predominant delusional and hallucinatory features may later present mainly catatonic features. A patient whose schizophrenic illness begins with a strong depressive coloring, and is diagnosed as having the schizoaffective type of schizophrenia, later may lose his depressive features and may have mainly the delusional and hallucinatory symptoms of paranoid schizophrenia. Hence, most psychiatrists view the different types of schizophrenia merely as ways of describing the predominant symptoms of a patient. They feel that the various types of schizophrenia are merely aspects, or phases, of a single kind of illness, and that the main emphasis should be placed on studying the emotional turmoil of each individual patient and understanding the long-range interpersonal traumas that have caused his illness.

However, since these clinical types are an established feature of psychiatric nomenclature and thinking, they should be defined in our discussion of schizophrenia. Moreover, if their limitations are recognized, they have some clinical usefulness. For example, the prognoses of some clinical types are better than those of others. The patient with a catatonic schizophrenic disorder of abrupt onset and recent origin has a better chance of recovery than a patient with a hebephrenic schizophrenic disorder of insidious origin. The patient with simple schizophrenia has less chance of responding to treatment than a patient with a schizoaffective schizophrenic illness. In addition, the various clinical types have some significance in terms of treatment. Psychotherapy with a severe catatonic patient is unlikely to be useful, whereas psychotherapy often is an important facet in the treatment program of a patient with a schizoaffective disorder.

Furthermore, the designation of a particular

type of schizophrenia may have significance in terms of the emotional process going on within the patient. For example, the patient with severe catatonic schizophrenia has undergone a profound withdrawal from people because he has found interpersonal relationships devastatingly painful; he protects himself against contacts with people by retiring into muteness and immobility. The paranoid schizophrenic with delusions of persecution has a marked dread of the world, which, because of experiences during his formative years, he views as malevolent, malicious and menacing; he also may be struggling with hostile impulses within himself which he is projecting onto other people, whom he then perceives as threatening toward him.

The clinical types most commonly used by psychiatrists today in discussing their patients are (1) paranoid type, (2) catatonic type, (3) schizoaffective type, (4) simple type and (5) childhood type. The standard nomenclature also contains five other types (hebephrenic type, acute schizophrenic episode, latent type, residual type and chronic undifferentiated type), but, except in hospital and clinic statistical tabulations of patients, these terms are much less used in day-to-day psychiatric work; we shall define these five less used terms briefly in a final part of this section.

Paranoid Type

The predominant clinical features of the patient with paranoid schizophrenia are delusions and hallucinations. Persecutory delusions are the most common kind, and grandiose delusions are second in frequency. Auditory hallucinations are present in most cases, and other types of hallucinations also are present occasionally. The onset of this type may be gradual or sudden. Though some psychiatric writers state that paranoid schizophrenia occurs most frequently between the ages of 30 and 35, I have found it equally common from late adolescence to the early forties. Patients with ingrained paranoid schizophrenic disorders who are seen in public psychiatric hospitals often are between 30 and 35, but patients with acute fulminating paranoid schizophrenia and patients in the early stages of insidious paranoid schizophrenia are seen equally from late adolescence to the early forties in other kinds of psychiatric practice.

The patient with a paranoid schizophrenic disorder of insidious beginning often was a tense, sensitive person before the onset of his schizophrenic process. It begins so gradually that it may be difficult to say when, over a period of many months or several years or more, his psychosis started. Often he begins with ideas of reference in which he feels that casual remarks that he overhears have special reference to him. He feels that people are gossiping about him, are talking depreciatingly about him, or are ridiculing him. Slowly he beings to feel that various persons or groups are trying to injure him or deceive him. He may feel that his enemies are plotting to rob him, to have him dismissed from his job, to disgrace him in his neighborhood or to seduce the affection of his wife away from him. As months pass, these ideas may become more elaborate and more bizarre. He becomes convinced that his persecutors are tapping his telephone wires and are implanting secret microphones in his house to gather information about him, and he may feel that government agencies and prominent public figures have been drawn into the conspiracy. In time he may feel that his enemies are attempting to kill him with x-rays and deadly electrical impulses emanating from his television set, from neighbors' houses or from automobiles he sees in the street. In some instances the paranoid patient becomes assaultive or even homicidal in his attempts to defend himself against his persecutors.

Auditory hallucinations are common. At first the patient may feel that things being said on his television set refer to him and he may feel that automoboile horns are carrying special messages to him. He then begins to hear voices emanating from the walls, ceilings, windows, electrical appliances or from "inside my head." The voices may curse him, give him orders, accuse him of crimes and sexual misdemeanors, or warn him of impending dangers. He may have gustatory hallucinations in which he tastes poisons or sedatives in his food, or he may have olfactory hallucinations in which he smells noxious or foul gases his tormentors are pumping into his room.

The paranoid schizophrenic patient may develop grandiose delusions that appear gradually or suddenly. He may feel that he is a divine religious figure with a world-saving mission, and in his auditory hallucinations he hears religious messages and commands. He may feel that he is an omnipotent military, political or scientific figure with the ability to manipulate large numbers of people or to perform bizarre scientific feats. Visual hallucinations are somewhat more common in patients with grandiose delusions than in patients with persecutory delusions.

In many instances, paranoid schizophrenic disorders develop abruptly. Persecutory or grandiose delusions accompanied by florid hallucinations may develop over a period of a few days or a few weeks. In may experience, about half of all paranoid schizophrenic illnesses develop acutely and the other half come on gradually.

It should be noted that in psychiatry the term paranoid is used in two ways. Firstly, it is used to designate the type of schizophrenia in which delusions and hallucinations are the predominant symptoms. Secondly, it often is used in a more restricted sense in referring to persecutory delusions, as indicated earlier; it is employed as a synonym of persecutory. Thus, a patient with persecutory delusions may be said to have paranoid delusions, regardless of whether these delusions occur as a feature of a schizophrenic illness, a depressive psychosis, an organic brain disease, or any other type of psychiatric illness.

Catatonic Type

The predominant symptoms in catatonic schizophrenia are disturbances of physical movement. Catatonic schizophrenia characteristically begins abruptly; a full-blown catatonic schizophrenic disorder frequently develops over a several day period, though in some instances it may gradually develop during a period of several months. The patient with catatonic schizophrenia may have diminished or excessive physical activity; thus, in the standard nomenclature catatonic schizophrenia is divided into *excited* and *withdrawn* types, and a catatonic patient may pass, sometimes abruptly, from one type into the other, and back again, during a period of from a few hours or less to several weeks or months. In either instance, the physical symptoms are indicative of a profound withdrawal from people and resistance to re-establishing interpersonal contacts.

The catatonic patient with diminished physical activity may withdraw into a state of mute immobility, and he may sit, crouch or stand for days or weeks in the same position. He may require spoon feeding or tube feeding to maintain nutrition, and he may not exercise control over his feces and urine. In other instances, urinary retention may occur and the patient must be catheterized periodically during an acute catatonic episode. The patient sometimes allows his limbs to be placed in any position the examiner chooses and holds them there for from a few minutes to several hours; this is termed waxy flexibility. In other instances the patient is rigidly resistant to efforts to change his position in any way; he holds all his muscles clenched in brittle immobility. He neglects his grooming and his clothing, and in time he becomes a shabby, gaunt statue sitting on a bench and staring blankly into space. Though he seems to pay no attention to events around him, after recovery he may reveal that he was acutely aware of the things that went on in his environment and remembers them accurately.

Hyperactive catatonic symptoms include physical agitation, combativeness, destructiveness, mannerisms, repetitive stereotyped movements and aimless pacing. Hyperactive catatonic symptoms may erupt abruptly in a patient who previously was immobile or they may be the initial manifestations of an acute catatonic reaction of sudden onset. The catatonic patient often has auditory hallucinations and delusions, but he usually does not speak of them. His acute agitation, combativeness and destructiveness often are in response to the commands of auditory hallucinations or the fear engendered by delusions of persecution, and his rigid immobility in a sky-gazing posture may be in response to grandiose, religiously tinged delusions.

Schizoaffective Type

When a schizophrenic illness has strong depressive features or manic features it is classified as schizoaffective schizophrenia. The diagnosis should contain an appended phrase specifying whether depressive or manic features are present. For example, a diagnosis might read "schizoaffective schizophrenia, with depressive features." In the official nomenclature this type of schizophrenia is termed "schizophrenia, schizoaffective type, excited" and "schizophrenia, schizoaffective type, depressed."

The schizoaffective patient with depressive features has, in addition to his schizophrenic symptoms, strong feelings of sadness, guilt and worthlessness. His delusions deal with the crimes, sexual misdemeanors and heinous acts he believes he has committed, and his auditory hallucinations bombard him with curses, accusations and depreciating remarks. He feels he has failed at everything and that everyone is talking about his failures and worthlessness. Schizoaffective patients with depressive features often are suicidal risks; they sometimes commit suicide in response to commands from auditory hallucinations to destroy themselves.

In addition to his basic schizophrenic features, the schizophrenic patient with manic features is exhilarated, hyperactive, optimistic and joyful. He often has grandiose delusions of great accomplishments and omnipotent powers. His auditory hallucinations frequently deal with religious topics, and he has bizarre, world-saving plans. His manic exhilaration may alternate with brief bursts of belligerence or sobbing despair.

Simple Type

In simple schizophrenia the basic symptoms of withdrawal from people and flatness of emotional responsiveness are marked. Fragmentation of thought processes is present, but may not be obvious to the casual observer. Delusions, hallucinations, disturbances of speech and disturbances of physical movement are minimal and may not be present at all.

Simple schizophrenia always is insidious in onset. It develops so slowly over a period of years that the patient's relatives and friends may not be aware that he is psychiatrically ill until his disorder is far advanced. Simple schizophrenia usually begins in adolescence or during the early 20's. The patient gradually loses interest in people and in his usual activities as he withdraws from interpersonal relationships into a world of fantasies and self-preoccupation. He never shows pleasure, anger, sadness or alert interest; his facial expression becomes vacant and wooden, and his eyes stare blankly or wander aimlessly when people address him. He may say odd things occasionally and he often has eccentric habits; he does not talk a great deal and he is seclusive. In most cases he cannot hold a job, but at times he has a menial job or a routine one requiring little contact with people. Many vagrants, shiftless wanderers and odd, dependent people who live marginally off the generosity of others are simple schizophrenics. The diagnosis usually is made after the process has been present for years, and attempts at therapy are almost always fruitless.

Childhood Type

Though schizophrenia is a relatively uncommon illness in children under the age of 12, a busy child guidance clinic or individual child psychiatrist usually sees two or three new cases each year. Schizophrenia may begin at any age during childhood, and early infantile autism, which is probably a variant form of childhood schizophrenia, may begin during infancy. Some schizophrenic children withdraw into mute seclusiveness and have no communication with people, but many other schizophrenic children maintain partial contact with those around them, while at the same time they are preoccupied with a delusional inner fantasy life. Some schizophrenic children are agitated and talk a great deal in obscure language with many coined words and symbolic phrases, which have special meanings for themselves. The facial expressions of schizophrenic children may show vacant flatness of emotional responsiveness, tense agitation or inappropriate grimacing and smiling.

The schizophrenic child may have hallucinations, but he talks about them less frequently and less clearly than the adult schizophrenic. Delusions may occur in schizophrenic children, but the subjects of their delusions usually are not as specific as in adult schizophrenics; their delusions are directed toward vague powers of evil or omnipotence which they cannot define distinctly. Grandiose delusions also may occur.

The onset of childhood schizophrenia tends to be insidious over a period of several years, and the first signs of withdrawn, disturbed behavior may begin at any time from infancy to late childhood. The diagnosis usually is made when the child is in the first two years of grade school, and his schizophrenic behavior is causing increased social problems. However, in a few instances the onset of childhood schizophrenia may be abrupt and is sometimes clearly related to a specific precipitating stress. The prognosis of childhood schizophrenia is much poorer than the prognosis of adult schizophrenia. About 5 per cent recover entirely by late adolescence, and another 20 per cent become shy, tense people who can make a minimally adequate social adjustment. The other 75 per cent continue as severely disturbed schizophrenics throughout their adolescent and adult years. The results of treatment of children with schizophrenia are much poorer than treatment results with adults; in fact, there is no generally accepted evidence that the results of any kind of treatment (psychotherapy, medications or other means) are better than the natural course of the disease process.

Early Infantile Autism. This is a well differentiated psychotic disorder that begins in infancy or early childhood. It is probably a variant form of schizophrenia. The dominant feature of early infantile autism is a profound withdrawal from interpersonal communication. Beginning as early as the fourth or fifth month of life, some autistic children are noticed to be unresponsive to the attentions of the people around them. They lie apathetically and seem, as it were, to be withdrawn within themselves. They do not have the usual responsiveness or fretfulness of other infants, and they seem oblivious to the words and actions of the people who are caring for them. During the first three years of the child's life, as more interpersonal activity is expected of him, the withdrawal from people becomes more apparent. The emotional apathy of these children sometimes is so marked that the diagnosis is suspected during the first 18 months of life and may be made with fair conviction during their third and fourth years.

In contrast with their lack of interest in people, these children as they grow older have marked preoccupation with the inanimate things around them. They are very concerned with the places and positions of things and may become agitated if the least change is made in the arrangement of furniture, toys and decorations in their bedrooms and playrooms. Children with early infantile autism seem to have fled from the world of people into a meticulous, all-consuming preoccupation with the world of inanimate objects.

Some autistic children have remarkable memories for things. For example, they may be able to sing long selections of music or to recite extensive passages of poetry at the age of four or five. These memory feats probably are a function of the child's intense preoccupation with things, as opposed to people, rather than evidence of superior intelligence.

Children with early infantile autism often have language disturbances. One third of them never develop speech; they make grunting and whining noises, but they do not use words. Such children may be incorrectly diagnosed as mentally retarded, deaf-mute, aphasic or grossly brain damaged. Some autistic children repeat the same phrases over and over again, and others parrot back whatever is said to them in an echoing fashion. Some autistic children have a peculiar difficulty in learning to use the word "yes," almost as if an affirmative response represents too much of an acceptance of communication with people. Other children with early infantile autism have a peculiar inability to use the pronouns "I" and "you" correctly; their comprehension of interpersonal relationships seems so poor that the meaning of these pronouns is difficult for them to grasp. Autistic children often have abnormalities of physical movement. They sometimes engage in simple repetitive physical activities for long periods of time. Others remain motionless for an hour or two at a time. Autistic children often walk in stiff, wooden ways and may characteristically hold their arms in rigid, abducted postures.

Though these children appear unresponsive to the events and people around them, closer observation reveals that they actually are quite aware of what is going on in their environment. For example, they often have an insensitivity to noises near them but are quite attentive to background noises. One can shout behind them, almost in their ears, and they seem to have heard nothing. However, they may start and listen attentively to the noise of a typewriter in a room at the end of a corridor or pay close attention to the sound of a truck passing in front of the clinic building.

Enough time has now elapsed since early infantile autism was first described in the early 1940's to begin to evaluate the long-term course of these children. About 5 per cent of them eventually make a good interpersonal adjustment in adult life and 20 per cent more of them are able to lead independent adult lives, but remain timid, insecure people. The remaining 75 per cent of them in adulthood resemble profoundly withdrawn schizophrenics, though, as a rule, delusions and hallucinations are not apparent. All methods of treatment seem to give no better results than would be statistically expected from the general course and outcome of this disorder.

Other Types of Schizophrenia

The standard nomenclature contains five other types of schizophrenia, but these five types are much less employed by psychiatrists in talking and writing about patients; their use also varies somewhat from one region of the United States to another. Furthermore, these terms overlap each other and the preceding schizophrenic types we have described in detail. We shall, therefore, define these types briefly. They are (1) hebephrenic type, (2) acute schizophrenic episode, (3) latent type, (4) residual type and (5) chronic undifferentiated type.

Hebephrenic Type. In the historical development of the concept of schizophrenia, hebephrenia, or hebephrenic schizophrenia as it was later to be called, was one of the first types to be delineated; however, this term is now little used in American psychiatry. Hebephrenic schizophrenia is characterized by onset in adolescence and profound emotional withdrawal. The patient is prone to have facial grimaces, giggling and inappropriate smiling. Hallucinations often are present and the patient's speech frequently deteriorates into an incoherent chain of fragmented phrases. Delusions, though occasionally present, are not prominent. The hebephrenic patient, by definition, has a poor prognosis and in most cases becomes chronically psychotic despite treatment.

Acute Schizophrenic Episode. The standard nomenclature describes this type as a schizophrenic illness of abrupt onset with perplexity, emotional turmoil, ideas of reference, trance-like behavior and excitement or depression. By definition, the patient often recovers within several weeks, but if he does not he usually acquires catatonic or paranoid features; in the latter case, the diagnosis should be accordingly changed.

Latent Type. The official nomenclature includes this somewhat vague category to embrace those schizophrenics who do not have the classical symptoms of schizophrenia but who nevertheless are felt to be clearly schizophrenic. It includes schizophrenics whom various authors have described as having incipient, or borderline, or pre-psychotic, or pseudoneurotic, or pseudopsychopathic schizophrenia. The descriptions of these states by different psychiatrists are so diverse that general characteristics cannot be given.

Residual Type. This category is used to designate schizophrenics who have largely recovered from a schizophrenic illness but yet have some signs of a lingering schizophrenic process.

Chronic Undifferentiated Type. Patients with long-standing schizophrenic illnesses who do not have clinical characteristics of sufficient clarity and prominence (such as paranoid or catatonic features) to justify putting them in other types, may be classified under this heading.

INTERPERSONAL CAUSES OF SCHIZOPHRENIA

Harry Stack Sullivan's Tripartite View of Schizophrenia. Harry Stack Sullivan devoted a large part of his career to the study and treatment of schizophrenics; in this, he differed markedly from Freud, who had almost no experience with psychotic patients, but spent his long professional life treating mainly patients with neuroses and personality disorders. Since an important part of Sullivan's writings deal with schizophrenia we shall give particular attention to his concepts about it.

For purposes of easy exposition, Sullivan distinguished three basic processes in schizophrenia; he called it the tripartite (or threefold) view of schizophrenia.

1. Sullivan felt that each person maintains his contact with reality only by virtue of his ability constantly to check and recheck his feelings, thoughts and actions against the standards of social conformity, *as perceived in vibrant interpersonal relationships.* That is, each individual is continually taking bearings to verify where he is, what he is doing, and how he is relating to people; this process may be compared to that of a ship which can stay on course only by continually taking readings of its position and noting the available landmarks, and when it can no longer do this it wanders erratically off its course. *A person does the same thing in interpersonal relationships.* The schizophrenic loses this ability to evaluate and constantly correct his feelings, thoughts and actions against the landmarks of reality; as a consequence, he ceases to think and feel in logical, reality-oriented ways.

Sullivan employed the term *consensual validation* (which we discussed in Chapter 1 from the viewpoint of personality development) to designate this basic process by which each person maintains his hold on reality; in this process an individual at all times is viewing everyone and everything in his environment from multiple vantage points, and only by this activity can he see things in their true perspectives. This all-important feature of emotional functioning may be made clearer by a simile: If we see a statue only from one side, and perhaps in semidarkness, we get a limited, distorted concept of what the statue represents. However, if we can view the statue in clear light, can go round it and examine it carefully from all sides, and perhaps pass our hands over it and feel its texture, we get an accurate, realistic concept of the statue. The schizophrenic sees the statue from one angle, and in the dusk; hence, his view of his environment, other people and himself becomes unrealistic and warped, and from his erroneous information he draws conclusions which are delusional, hallucinatory and greatly deviant from the data of the logical, workaday world.

The primary defect in schizophrenia, Sullivan says, is not that the patient sees things wierdly, but that he sees and feels them in fragmentary, incomplete ways and has lost his capacity to correct his concepts by multiple, constant checking and rechecking from various viewpoints, the process which allows other people to maintain contact with the ever shifting sets of circumstances we call reality.

The schizophrenic is dimly aware of this defect, and hence he has an eerie, desolated fearfulness which easily passes into terror and disorganized panic in the early weeks and months of his illness. His panic further impairs his capacity to comprehend reality; a terror-stricken person is ill-equipped to evaluate accurately what is going on around him. Thus, a vicious circle is set up, and the schizophrenic process worsens.

As he loses his hold on reality (though this loss is never absolute), the schizophrenic returns to the crude, primitive, chaotic ways of thinking and feeling that characterize an infant. He sees his environment indistinctly and confusedly, and logic and the refined perceptions of later life are lost.

2. In the second process of Sullivan's three-fold view of schizophrenia, the patient no longer can keep out of his awareness a vast mass of abhorrent feelings, thoughts and impulses which he hitherto has been able to push aside from his field of conscious attention. These feelings, thoughts and memories of past, painful experiences sweep in and dominate his emotional functioning. His attention is occupied by guilt-ridden sexual or hostile urges, grandiose infantile fantasies, primitive body preoccupations, and many other things; this emotional turmoil often takes such strong possession of his awareness, and is so divorced from reality that it often assumes the form of delusions and hallucinations which confirm his fears or fulfill his wishes. Thus, the schizophrenic may hear voices that call him foul names or he may feel himself the omnipotent master of the universe.

However, these unleashed feelings and thoughts never assume complete dominance. They coexist in uneasy competition or wavering battle with the forces that seek to draw the schizophrenic back to reality and to sweep out of his awareness the primitive urges and painful memories that characterize, in distorted form, his illness.

3. The third process of Sullivan's three-fold view of schizophrenia occurs when a schizophrenic disorder passes from an acute to a long-lasting phase. If the patient undergoing the first two processes does not recover within a few weeks or months, the crude, infantile ways of thinking and feeling (unrealistic processes) and the refined, logical means of thinking and feeling (realistic processes) become woven into a single fabric, in which it becomes difficult to disentangle them. That is, something new and different is produced in the patient—the ingrained schizophrenic process. Fragmented thought processes, delusions, hallucinations and warped views of himself and his environment become tightly enmeshed with the residuals of logical, reality-oriented thinking and feeling. A classical form of this occurs, for example, in the paranoid schizophrenic who can, in completely realistic ways, operate the complex business machines at his work, but who, at the same time, in very delusional ways feels that his work associates are saying malicious things about him and are putting noxious substances in the water he drinks. If studied carefully, each schizophrenic reveals wide areas of both realistic and unrealistic thinking, feeling and behavior. The problem of therapy is to exploit the patient's contact with reality to draw him completely back into healthy interpersonal life.

This three-fold process, Sullivan says, explains the manifold clinical features of schizophrenia. Because of it, communication with people becomes distorted, as in the paranoid schizophrenic, or stops altogether, as in the mute catatonic. Interpersonal relationships become fragmentary, or threatening, or meaningless. Sullivan emphasizes that the schizophrenic often is a deeply miserable person; he feels panic, loneliness and perplexity, and he is acutely, though confusedly, aware of these things. The schizophrenic with grandiose delusions of power and importance has gone a step further and has found delusions and hallucinations which, with fluctuating success, relieve him of some of his agony. Nevertheless, the schizophrenic tries frequently to contact people, but, frightened or puzzled by each contact with them, flees back into his psychotic morass. He is aware that something is gravely wrong with his personality structure, but he cannot grasp what it is and he does not know what to do about it.

The Interpersonal Causes of the Schizophrenic Process. But why does the schizophrenic undergo this three-fold process of emotional and intellectual disturbance? He does so because, in ways he cannot understand, *he finds interpersonal relationships so painful and devastating that he chaotically flees from them.* Though his schizophrenic illness is painful to him, he suffers much less in it than he did when he was interacting intensely with people.

The production of so severe an illness as schizophrenia requires a combination of marked interpersonal traumas in childhood and painful situational stresses in adult life. During his childhood, the person who later develops schizophrenia usually has unhealthy interpersonal relationships with both his parents, and often with other close persons; daily hammering from damaging cultural and socioeconomic forces may be added to the total of the patient's emotional traumas. The patient does not have during his formative years a comfortable, sound, secure relationship with anyone; his crucial interactions, moreover, are so painful that he develops an ingrained tendency to shrink from them. All relationships with people are contaminated with anxiety, and stresses between him and others push this anxiety toward panic. He therefore tends to form only loose attachments with people and to withdraw into his own fantasy life when interpersonal difficulties arise.

In many cases the mother-child relationship is especially traumatic. The mother's basic attitude toward the child is harsh, rejecting and depreciating, but, in addition, she often has a marked need to dominate him. The mother and child often become locked in a sick relationship in which the mother grapples the child to her with abrasive, loveless dominance, and the child clings to her in frightened, guilt-ridden dependence. The child feels trapped in a torturing relationship he can neither improve nor avoid. As the years of childhood and adolescence grind by, the child's dread of closeness to people increases. He unconsciously fears that every interpersonal relationship in his life will deteriorate into the same kind of grinding pain that characterizes his relationship with his mother and other close people, who also fail him in various ways. The stage is set for a retreat into an inner world of schizophrenic chaos when he faces interpersonal stresses in his adolescence or adulthood. In rare instances the emotional experiences of the child are so devastating that the overt schizophrenic psychosis begins during childhood.

The child also lacks a sound relationship with his father. Often the father is distant and emotionally uninvolved with the child; he abandons the child to the care of the mother, or treats him with irritable indifference. The child finds that the interpersonal suffering of his relationship with his mother is reinforced in his relationship with his father, and he despairs of ever finding anything but pain in his relationships with people. Moreover, the interpersonal life of the future schizophrenic is barren in other areas as well. He does not find in relationships with siblings, other relatives and other close persons the kinds of constructive interactions which would correct the warped view he is forming of interpersonal life. He emerges into adolescence without ever having had a sound, reassuring, intimate relationship with another person; he has no experience with comfortable bonds to the world of people, and he lacks the capacity for developing them.

The severity of this interpersonal trauma varies, of course, from patient to patient. In some instances, the patient's personality structure is so damaged that even the minor day-to-day stresses of adolescent or adult life suffice to precipitate a schizophrenic psychosis. In other instances, the personality structure of the patient is more resistant, and moderate or severe interpersonal stresses are necessary for the production of a schizophrenic disorder. The severity of the schizophrenic patient's basic personality problems also has a marked effect on the success or failure of treatment. The patient who since childhood had only a fragile contact with reality and with people presents difficult therapeutic problems, for he has much unconscious dread of emerging from his inner schizophrenic world and attempting to establish interpersonal relationships. The patient who had a somewhat sounder contact with people before the onset of his illness has a better prognosis, since his dread of a return to interpersonal contact is less severe.

Various emotional features often are said to comprise the *prepsychotic personality* of the patient who later develops a schizophrenic illness. Because of his emotional traumas during his formative years, he is anxious, shy and emotionally insecure. He is sensitive about how people feel toward him, and he often finds hostility and rejection from others very painful. He may have profound feelings of inferiority and inadequacy, and he may feel unable to get along well with people and to establish good relationships with them. He may be socially somewhat withdrawn, but in many instances he camouflages his underlying personality problems with a brittle façade of forced gregariousness and hollow self-confidence. However, one encounters many schizophrenic patients whose prepsychotic personality structures do not fit this clinical picture, despite the emotional turbulence which lurks deep within them.

Various kinds of intepersonal stresses in adolescence or adult life may contribute to the final precipitation of a schizophrenic psychosis; such stresses may occur in the patient's family life, his vocational activities, his social relationships, and other areas. The precipitating stresses often resemble the painful relationships the patient had with his parents and other close persons during childhood and early adolescence. Thus, relationships in which he suffers emotional rejection or a severe assault on his self-esteem may unleash a schizophrenic disorder. A schizophrenic withdrawal may occur when the patient endures much hostility or abrasive competition from others, or when he feels trapped in a painful interpersonal situation, such as a grinding marriage, from which he cannot extricate himself. Job failure, the threat or fear of academic failure in college, or anxiety about his competence in the role of a marital partner or a parent may play a role. Problems of sexual adjustment may contribute; for example, panic when the patient dimly recognizes an upsurge of homosexual feelings within himself may trigger a schizophrenic episode. As a rule, there is no single precipitating stress; multiple stresses combine to cause the final psychotic break, and often the buildup is so gradual and complex that the causative factors cannot be easily identified.

Other Views on the Etiology of Schizophrenia. Some psychiatrists have suggested that, in addition to the interpersonal causes outlined above, various kinds of physiologic or genetic factors may predispose some persons to develop schizophrenia. In general, continental European psychiatrists, and those psychiatrists elsewhere in the world who follow their orientation, are more prone to believe in an organic etiology of schizophrenia than psychiatrists in the English-speaking countries. The areas in which dysfunctions have been suggested include carbohydrate metabolism, lipid metabolism, chromosomal structure, central nervous system biochemistry, endocrinologic functioning, and many others. To date, no organic theory has stood the test of time and the dispassionate appraisal of large numbers of investigators.

Despite much research on possible organic causes of schizophrenia, there is only one body of data which, in my opinion, suggests that there may be constitutional, in addition to environmental, factors in the etiology of schizophrenia. This is the data on the incidence of schizophrenia in identical (monozygotic), as opposed to fraternal (dizygotic), twins. Early, oft-cited studies indicated that when an adult twin has schizophrenia, the illness will occur in the other twin in 86 per cent of identical twins and in 15 per cent of fraternal twins. In childhood schizophrenia first diagnosed between the ages of 5 and 11, the incidence of schizophrenia in both twins is 71 per cent in identical twins and 17 per cent in fraternal twins. Other studies have indicated that the siblings of a schizophrenic have a decidedly higher chance of developing schizophrenia than persons in the general population. More recent studies designed to reduce selective bias and diagnostic errors in sampling have yielded much lower concurrence rates in identical twins.

These studies have been much attacked on both clinical and statistical grounds, and many psychiatrists feel that twin studies give misleading results. They point out that adequate studies have not been made of parental attitudes toward twins; they feel that identical twins are likely to be treated alike and that they have strong empathy with each other. On the other hand, parental attitudes toward fraternal twins may be quite different, especially if they are of opposite sexes or are very unalike in physical appearance; moreover, fraternal twins are less likely to feel the intimate sameness and affinity that identical twins are said to have toward each other. The available genetic and interpersonal data on schizophrenia in twins who were reared in separate households is similarly controversial at this time; such studies are difficult to conduct and to interpret.

TREATMENT OF SCHIZOPHRENIA

The basic task of therapy in schizophrenia is to draw the patient out of the inner schizophrenic world into which he has withdrawn, and to help him reestablish comfortable ways of feeling and thinking about himself and other people. The goal of therapy is for the patient to form sound interpersonal relationships and a firm contact with reality. The treatment methods employed in schizophrenia to accomplish these ends may be grouped under three categories: (1) interpersonal methods, (2) pharmacologic therapy and (3) physical treatments.

In most instances, more than one treatment technic is employed in working with a schizophrenic patient. For example, a patient may be treated simultaneously with a phenothiazine medication, hospital therapeutic milieu therapy and group psychotherapy. The vast majority of schizophrenic patients begin their treatment on an inpatient basis, and continue under outpatient psychiatric management after they are well enough to leave the hospital. However, many psychiatrists treat some carefully selected schizophrenic patients on an outpatient basis during their entire courses of treatment.

We shall now consider in detail each of the three major categories of treatment used in schizophrenia.

Interpersonal Methods

The three interpersonal methods used in treating schizophrenic patients are (1) creation of a hospital interpersonal milieu that encourages patients to reach out and reestablish contacts with the people around them, (2) individual psychotherapy and (3) group psychotherapy.

Hospital Interpersonal Milieu Therapy. The psychiatric hospital environment should be organized to provide healthy interpersonal contacts between schizophrenic patients and the hospital personnel and other patients. The psychiatrists, psychiatric nurses, occupational therapists, recreational therapists and aids should offer friendly, warm opportunities for the patients to begin their efforts to come back across the psychotic gap separating them from reality and interpersonal life. The hospital ward should have a well planned program of group activities, occupational therapy and recreational therapy that encourages the patients to begin to interact with each other and with the hospital staff.

Each patient's program of interpersonal activities should be tailored to his capacity to engage in group relationships at each particular stage of his treatment and recovery. Case conferences should be held periodically in which all hospital personnel who work with the patient can be briefed on the patient's emotional needs and can exchange observations about his ward behavior. The patient should not be pushed prematurely into interpersonal activities that threaten him emotionally and cause him to draw back from the contacts the staff offer him. (The operation of a therapeutic hospital environment is further discussed in Chapter 21.)

Individual Psychotherapy. Psychiatrists differ in their opinions about the role of individual psychotherapy in the treatment of schizophrenia. Some psychiatrists feel that the therapist should restrict his psychotherapy to friendly, encouraging contacts in which he and the patient discuss day-to-day events in the patient's life; they feel that only occasionally should the therapist and the patient discuss painful interpersonal events in the patient's past or current life. These psychiatrists feel that discussion of emotionally painful topics often causes the schizophrenic patient to draw back into his psychotic shell, and that the psychiatrist's task is to deal in a supportive way with everyday topics about the patient's activities and minor current interpersonal stresses. They feel that this kind of supportive counseling is all that can be safely endured by the fragile personality structure of an acutely ill schizophrenic patient. In this way, the psychiatrist uses his personality as an instrument to bridge the psychotic gap that separates the patient from people, and he helps the patient back to healthy interpersonal relationships. After the patient has experienced an accepting, comfortable interpersonal relationship with the therapist, he is able to begin to reach out for similar relationships with other people.

Other psychiatrists feel that some schizophrenics can benefit from deeper psychotherapy to help them understand and resolve some of the emotional causes of their illnesses. Exploratory psychotherapy usually is reserved until the patient has improved significantly on a regimen of phenothiazine antipsychotic medication, hospital interpersonal milieu therapy, and supportive counseling; however, a few psychiatrists advocate beginning exploratory psychotherapy during the acute stage of the patient's illness. Exploratory psychotherapy that begins during the patient's hospital stay is usually continued on an outpatient basis after the patient leaves the hospital. The psychiatrist who carries out exploratory psychotherapy with a schizophrenic must proceed with alert sensitivity to the patient's emotional responses to each topic discussed, because the patient's tolerance to emotional pain is slight. The aim of psychotherapy in schizophrenia is to reintegrate a shattered personality structure that cannot tolerate great amounts of interpersonal tension. To discuss prematurely the painful interpersonal relationships that caused his psychosis may be too great a burden for the brittle personality structure of a schizophrenic patient struggling to reestablish contact with reality.

Every schizophrenic needs careful discharge planning when he is ready to leave the hospital. The psychiatrist, often working in collaboration with a psychiatric social worker, should carry out counseling with the patient's relatives to attempt to remove any obvious emotional stresses in the patient's interpersonal environment. At times, the unhealthy attitudes of the relatives and other close persons toward the patient make such counseling difficult, but in some instances the patient's marital partner, or parents, or other close persons can make some important environmental changes which contribute to the patient's sustained recovery. For example, I often have urged a marital partner to restrict a patient's contacts with difficult relatives, or I have arranged for a part-time housekeeper to be employed to help a convalescent schizophrenic mother with her children for several weeks or a few months after she comes home from the hospital. Such environmental changes often are useful in helping the recovered schizophrenic patient to reintegrate himself gradually into life outside the hospital. In addition, extensive counseling with the relatives sometimes helps them to change unhealthy attitudes toward the patient; such counseling may help the relatives establish better interpersonal relationships with the patient and reduce the amount of emotional tension in the home.

Group Psychotherapy. Group psychotherapy with schizophrenics is employed in some psychiatric hospitals. Many schizophrenic patients who cannot talk well in individual psychotherapy are less inhibited in a group, and can discuss topics in the group that they could not bring up in individual sessions. The patient does not have to engage in an intense one-to-one relationship with a therapist, but can participate in more diluted relationships with the various members of the group; this is less threatening to many schizophrenics. In a sense, the group is a small interpersonal setting where the patient can begin to experiment with relationships with people. The group also enables him to set his own pace; he may talk or be silent, depending on his degree of comfort with the topic at hand. In addition, the therapist working in a large psychiatric hospital can engage many more patients in group psychotherapy than he could reach in individual sessions. Some psychiatrists combine group psychotherapy with occasional individual sessions with each member of the group. (Group psychotherapy is discussed at length in Chapter 21.)

Pharmacologic Therapy

The phenothiazines are the drugs of choice in schizophrenia. The other types of antipsychotic medications (which are chemically related to the phenothiazines, but do not properly fall in the phenothiazine group) are, in my opinion, much less effective and have higher incidences of undesirable side effects. In terms of statistical recovery rates, the phenothiazine medications have had a much greater effect on improving the prognosis of schizophrenia than any other treatment modality that has yet been developed. Between the middle 1950's, when the phenothiazines were first widely used, and the early 1970's, the recovery and improvement rates of schizophrenic patients rose dramatically. Since the early 1970's these rates have tended to level off to their present figures. In addition, by decreasing the intensity of the psychotic process in schizophrenics, the phenothiazine medications have made these patients much more accessible to hospital milieu therapy and individual and group psychotherapy.

The first phenothiazine introduced was chlorpromazine, and it still is probably the most commonly used medication in treating schizophrenia, although many of the other phenothiazines which were later developed are probably of equal efficacy. Most psychiatrists feel that in virtually all instances, a schizophrenic should be placed on a phenothiazine as an initial step in therapy, and that the medication should be continued throughout the patient's treatment. Improvement from phenothiazine therapy may occur within a few days after the patient begins to receive the medication, but it usually requires from 10 days to a few weeks for decisive improvement to be evident. In many instances the patient continues to improve gradually for three to six months after phenothiazine therapy begins.

The initial total daily dose of chlorpromazine (using it as a prototype of the general group of phenothiazines) usually is 300 mg., and the amount of medication is then increased or diminished depending on the patient's reaction to it. The medication may be given in prolonged release capsules covering 12-hour periods, or it may be administered in tablet or syrup preparations given four times each 24 hours. Chlorpromazine, and various other phenothiazines, also may be injected intramuscularly in acutely agitated or uncooperative patients. (The dosages and precautions for the intramuscular use of chlorpromazine are detailed in Chapter 22.) The daily total amount of chlorpromazine varies much from one patient to another. Although it usually ranges between 150 mg. and 450 mg. per day, it may be as low as 75 mg. or as high as 1200 mg., or more.

Although extensive research has been done, and many theories have been advanced, the precise ways in which phenothiazine medications, and other antipsychotic drugs, exercise their therapeutic effects are not known. Phenothiazines were developed as potentiators of anesthetic agents, and their antipsychotic effects were discovered accidentally. However, it is clear that, in contrast with the sedative-hypnotics and most of the antianxiety medications, the phenothiazines and other antipsychotic drugs exert their main effects on lower brain centers rather than on the cerebral cortex. Presumably, by this action on lower brain centers they decrease the patient's emotional turmoil and allow him to integrate his personality functioning once more on a healthy level. Their calming action permits the patient to reach out for interpersonal relationships and gradually to regain firm contact with reality. Nevertheless, the rationale for using phenothiazines and all other antipsychotic drugs rests on clinical experience rather than on knowledge of their physiological modes of action.

The widely used phenothiazines include chlorpromazine (Thorazine, Chlor-pz), trifluoperazine (Stelazine), perphenazine (Trilafon), thioridazine (Mellaril) and various others. The daily dosages of these drugs are quite different, depending on their chemical structures. (The dosages, pharmacologic properties, side effects and complications of the phenothiazines are covered in more detail in Chapter 22.) Although some psychiatrists feel that certain phenothiazines are better for acute schizophrenic disorders and others are better for chronic schizophrenic illnesses, I agree with those psychiatrists who feel that the various phenothiazine drugs may be used interchangeably in all kinds of schizophrenic states with about equal effectiveness.

Most psychiatrists feel that a schizophrenic patient should stay on a daily maintenance dose of a phenothiazine for from several months to a year after his recovery. Such maintenance medication reduces the chance of a relapse. Moreover, patients who tend to relapse repeatedly, or who have been ill for a long time, often need to be on a maintenance dose of a phenothiazine for several years or more. Some schizophrenic patients begin to relapse after from several days to two or three months each time the medication is stopped.

The phenothiazines are most useful in the paranoid, catatonic and schizoaffective types of schizophrenia. They rarely are useful in simple schizophrenia or childhood schizophrenia. They exercise their greatest benefit in the schizophrenic patient who has been ill for less than two years at the time treatment begins. However, they produce recovery in a significant number of patients who have been ill for several years, but these patients as a rule maintain their recovery only if they remain on maintenance doses for several years or more after their return to a sound level of adjustment. Even when the phenothiazines do not lead to recovery they usually enable the patient to make a better adjustment, though still psychotic, in the hospital or under the supervision of relatives at home.

Physical Methods

Electroshock Therapy. The amount of electroshock therapy given in the treatment of schizophrenia has decreased a great deal in recent years. It has been abandoned altogether in some psychiatric hospitals, though it continues to be used in selected patients in many other hospitals. The success of phenothiazine therapy, coupled with improved interpersonal treatment procedures, has rendered electroshock therapy unnecessary in most schizophrenic patients. However, many psychiatrists feel that electroshock therapy still is useful in many acutely ill schizophrenic patients with paranoid, catatonic and schizoaffective schizophrenia. Electroshock therapy is much less likely to help the patient who has been ill for a year or more, and prolonged phenothiazine administration has largely replaced the use of electroshock in patients who have been ill more than two years. (The details of the technic and mode of action of electroshock therapy are covered in Chapter 23.) A course of electroshock therapy in schizophrenia usually consists of between 6 and 14 treatments, though it may go as high as 20, given at the rate of three each week. Most psychiatrists who employ electroshock use it only for those patients who, after a few weeks or longer, show no signs of improving on phenothiazines, hospital milieu therapy and group or individual psychotherapy.

Insulin Coma Therapy. Very few psychiatrists still advocate the use of insulin coma therapy in schizophrenia, and their number is steadily decreasing. The results of insulin coma therapy were never impressive, and it has a serious complication rate that runs from 10 to 15 per cent in various series of cases. (The details and technic of insulin coma therapy are briefly outlined in Chapter 23.)

BIBLIOGRAPHY

Arieti, S.: An overview of schizophrenia from a predominantly psychological approach. Am. J. Psychiatry, *131*:241, 1974.

Bender, L.: The life course of children with schizophrenia. Am. J. Psychiatry, *130*:785, 1973.

Betz, B. J.: Childhood status and adult schizophrenia. Am. J. Psychother., *27*:27, 1973.

Bleuler, E.: Dementia Praeox, or the Group of Schizophrenias. New York, International Universities Press, 1950.

Bleuler, M.: Some results of research in schizophrenia. Behav. Sci., *15*:211, 1970.

Brown, G. W., Birley, B. M., and Wing, J. K.: Influence of family life on the course of schizophrenic disorders: a replication. Brit. J. Psychiatry, *121*:241, 1972.

Evans, J. R., et al.: Premorbid adjustment, phenothiazine treatment and remission in acute schizophrenics. Arch. Gen. Psychiatry, *27*: 486, 1972.

Goldfarb, W., Levy, D. M., and Meyers, D. I.: The mother speaks to her schizophrenic child: language in childhood schizophrenia. Psychiatry, *35*:217, 1972.

Grinker, R. R., Sr. and Holzman, P. S.: Schizophrenic pathology in young adults. Arch. Gen. Psychiatry, *28*:168, 1973.

Lidz, T.: The Origin and Treatment of Schizophrenic Disorders. New York, Basic Books, 1973.

Kanner, L.: Childhood Psychoses. Initial Studies and New Insights. New York, John Wiley & Sons, 1973.

Kuriansky, J. B., Deming, W. E., and Gurland, B. J.: On trends in the diagnosis of schizophrenia. Am. J. Psychiatry, *131*: 402, 1974.

Morrison, J. R.: Catatonia. Retarded and excited types. Arch. Gen. Psychiatry, *28*:39, 1973.

O'Brien, C., et al.: Group vs. individual psychotherapy with schizophrenics. Arch. Gen. Psychiatry, *27*:474, 1972.

Sacks, M. H., Carpenter, W. T., and Strauss, J. S.: Recovery from delusions. Arch. Gen. Psychiatry, *30*:177, 1974.

Sullivan, H. S.: Clinical Studies in Psychiatry. Chapter on the schizophrenic dynamism, p. 182. New York, W. W. Norton, 1956.

———: Schizophrenia as a Human Process. New York, W. W. Norton, 1962.

15

Severe Depressions

The patient with a severe depression has profound feelings of sadness, worthlessness and guiltiness, which usually are incapacitating. These depressive feelings often are so marked that they cause a distortion of the patient's contact with reality. Severe depressions form a significant part of the case load of every psychiatric hospital. In this chapter we shall consider the characteristics, courses, interpersonal causes and treatment of severe depressions, and we shall examine the related subject of suicide, which is a major public healthy problem.

The Concepts of Neurotic and Psychotic Depressions. Depressions (as noted in Chapter 10) traditionally have been divided into *neurotic depressions* and *psychotic depressions*, and this distinction is still maintained in the official psychiatric nomenclature. (Accordingly, in Chapter 10, in the section on neuroses, we outlined the characteristics usually attributed to depressive neuroses and discussed their treatment. However, we also noted there that many psychiatrists, including myself, feel that division of depressions into neurotic and psychotic types is artificial and confusing, that depressions occur in a continuous spectrum that stretches from minor to major, and that it is clinically sounder to divide them into *mild* and *severe* than neurotic and psychotic.)

Nevertheless, a systematic coverage of psychiatry should list the criteria which are sometimes employed to distinguish neurotic from psychotic depressions. We shall enumerate seven criteria often employed for the purpose. (1) A neurotic depression is said to be more likely to have an obvious precipitating stress, such as a marital crisis or a vocational failure, than a psychotic depression. (2) A neurotic depression usually does not incapacitate a patient in his usual vocational and social activities, whereas a psychotic one does. (3) The neurotically depressed patient is said to have only mild feelings of guilt and worthlessness, or none at all, whereas the psychotically depressed patient has severe feelings of these kinds. (4) The patient with a neurotic depression has no impairment of his contact with reality, whereas the patient with a psychotic depression often sees himself and his environment in such melancholy, pessimistic ways that his grasp of reality is warped, and at times frankly delusional. (5) The neurotically depressed patient has mild fatigue, insomnia and weight loss, whereas these features are marked in the psychotically depressed patient. (6) The patient with a neurotic depression does not have a history of both manic and depressive disorders, whereas about 20 per cent of patients with psychotic depressions will also have one or more manic illnesses during their lifetimes. (7) A neurotic depression is said to be a means of defending the individual against becoming aware of underlying anxiety, whereas a psychotic depression is rooted in profound feelings of worthlessness and guiltiness, as well as other kinds of marked emotional turmoil.

However, as noted above, the orientation we use in this book is that the distinction between neurotic and psychotic depressions is contrived and artificial. Depressions span a range from *mild* to *severe*, and are better so divided than split into the artificial categories of "neurotic" and "psychotic."

Throughout this chapter, each time we speak of a *severe depression* we are talking about a disorder which in the official psychiatric nomenclature is termed a *depressive psychosis* or some variant depressive illness of *psychotic* proportions, such as manic-depressive illness, depressed type, and others.

CLINICAL CHARACTERISTICS OF SEVERE DEPRESSIONS

The predominant feature of a severe depression is a profound feeling of melancholy and despair. The patient views himself and the world around him through gray-colored glasses. He sees himself as worthless, inadequate and guilty. He feels that his past life is a long train of failures and that the future holds no hope for anything better. He ruminates gloomily over the minor failings of his earlier years, and he is oblivious to the successes of his life. He believes he is beyond moral redemption, and he broods dejectedly over his minor misdemeanors, which he sees as unforgivable sins. He is indecisive, for he fears that all his decisions will be wrong. Often he feels that some undefinable disaster will occur to him because of his failures and wickedness. He may feel financially destitute despite his actual affluence, and the reassurances and arguments of others make little impression on him. He may feel that he has failed in his work despite the encouraging praise of his colleagues and superiors. These feelings often are so overwhelming that he is socially and vocationally incapacitated by them. He sits at home in a melancholy stupor, or wanders about the house in frightened agitation.

The severely depressed patient loses interest in all his activities; everything seems stale, dull, flat and distant to him. In some instances he is anxious, apprehensive and obsessively worried about his health; medical reassurances do not diminish his obsessive fears of such diseases as cancer, venereal disease or heart disease. I recall a patient who in 20 years had three severe depressions; each depression began with a persistent preoccupation about cancer, which lasted until he recovered from each illness. The depressed patient often has impoverishment of thought processes in which his attention becomes riveted on a few gloomy subjects which he slowly pursues in endless circles. The patient's family and friends note the striking change in his behavior. At first, they may feel he is going through a "low spell" or "the blues." However, as his interpersonal adjustment deteriorates and he withdraws into a depressive shell they become aware that he is mentally ill.

The patient's depressive feelings often are so profound that they cause breaches in his contact with reality. His ideas about his worthlessness, sinfulness and failure are so distorted that they may be properly called delusional. The depressed patient's convictions that he has cancer, or that he is financially destitute, or that he has committed heinous crimes may begin as fearful speculations, but they soon become entrenched delusional ideas in some cases. Sometimes these delusions become very bizarre; the patient may feel that his internal organs have "rotted away" or that his body has become grotesquely disfigured. A small percentage of severely depressed patients develop persecutory delusions. The patient may believe that the people around him are talking about his failures and immorality, and in time he may become convinced that they are conspiring to ruin him, to imprison him, or to kill him. Hallucinations are rare in severe depressions. When delusions and hallucinations are prominent in a severe depression, most psychiatrists today are inclined to diagnose the patient's condition as schizoaffective schizophrenia, depressed type.

A patient with a severe depression usually moves slowly. He may complain that his arms and legs feel as if heavy weights were attached to them and that oridnary activity is a laborious exertion for him. His face is set in wooden sadness, his forehead is wrinkled, and he walks in a stooped position. Sometimes he sits in motionless silence for long periods of time and stares with puzzled muteness when questioned. This type of depressed patient is sometimes said to be in a *stuporous depression*. In other instances, the depressed patient wanders about in an agitated manner, cries and wrings his hands. He sits forward in his chair and twists his handkerchief continually. This type of patient often is described as having an *agitated depression*.

The depressed patient feels chronically fatigued. His appetite is poor, and he usually loses weight. Weight losses may run from 5 or 10 pounds to several times that much, and the patient who is first brought to medical attention after several months of severe depressiveness may be emaciated. He neglects his grooming and his personal hygiene, and often he looks shabby and unkempt. The depressed patient loses interest in sexual activity; the depressed man often is impotent, and the depressed woman is sexually unresponsive. In most instances, the depressed patient feels worse in the morning and slightly better in the late afternoon and early evening. He often has much difficulty sleeping; he may have no difficulty going to sleep at bedtime, but he awakes after three or four hours and spends the rest of the night in gloomy ruminations or in wandering about the house.

The majority of patients with severe depressions have suicidal thoughts at some time during their illnesses, and in many patients suicidal risk is a continual problem for long periods. Suicidal attempts are common, and suicide is a leading cause of death in the United States. Because suicide is a major public health problem, all aspects of this subject will be covered in detail in a separate section at the end of this chapter.

The Clinical Types of Severe Depressions

Severe depressions usually are considered under three headings:

1. *Severe depressions in patients who at other times have manic disorders.* The patient who alternately has depressive and manic disorders fits the category of the classical manic depressive pattern. However, only about 20 per cent of patients who have severe depressions also have one or more manic disorders at other times in their lives.

2. *Severe depressions that occur once or several times in the lifetime of the patient who at no time in his life has a manic disorder.* The vast majority of patients with severe depressions fall in this category.

3. *Severe depressions that occur during the involutional period.* Most psychiatrists feel that the so-called involutional depression is basically similar to severe depressions which may occur at other periods in a patient's life. The precipitating interpersonal stresses, of course, may be related to the emotional adjustments of middle age. However, since the concept of the involutional depression still lingers in psychiatric terminology and thinking, we shall consider it as a particular variety of severe depression.

Manic Depressive Pattern. In some instances, both severe depressions and manic disorders occur at various times during the course of the patient's life; this constitutes the classical manic depressive pattern which in the standard psychiatric nomenclature is termed manic depressive illness (or psychosis), circular type. For example, the patient undergoes a severe depression, and several years later he has a manic disorder; during his life he may have further manic and depressive episodes. These illnesses may occur once every several years, or they may occur at shorter or longer intervals. I have seen patients who had intervals of up to 25 years between manic and depressive episodes, and I have seen others who had several manic and depressive illnesses at intervals of several months. Moreover, in some instances a manic disorder occurs immediately after a patient recovers from a depression, or the patient may slip directly from a manic episode into a depressive one. The manic and depressive illnesses most often do not occur in precise alternation. For example, separated by several months or many years, the patient may have two depressions in succession and then a manic episode, or he may have a depression and then two or three manic disorders much later in his life. In some instances the patient continues a manic depressive pattern of periodic illnesses throughout his entire adult lifetime, whereas in other instances the patient has a brief series of such illnesses in his early or middle adult years and remains free of them for the rest of his life.

The patient who has both manic and depressive episodes usually recovers completely from each illness and functions well between them. I recall a patient in her 60's who had a successful career as a teacher despite manic and depressive disorders which occurred at about 5-year intervals for 40 years. Even before the advent of the improved treatment methods that we have today, the manic depressive patient characteristically made a good recovery from his psychotic episodes, though he usually spent from four to six months in each manic episode and from six months to two or three years in each depression. Modern treatment methods have cut the hospital treatment time of both types of disorders to from a few weeks to two or three months.

The person with a manic depressive pattern often is described as gregarious and energetic between his psychotic episodes. His outgoing prepsychotic personality is contrasted with the shy, retiring prepsychotic personality of the patient who develops a schizophrenic psychosis. However, there are so many exceptions to these broad generalizations that it is better to study each patient as a separate individual with his distinct personality features and interpersonal capacities.

Severe Depressions. In about 80 per cent of cases the patient who has a severe depression never has a manic illness at any time in his life. On the other hand, a patient who has a manic illness has about a 40 per cent chance that he will have at least one depression at some time during his adult life span. The patient may have one severe depression in his lifetime, or he may have several, and they may separated by intervals of a few years or two or three decades.

Severe Depressions in the Involutional Period. Severe depressions that occur in women in the involutional period have traditionally been accorded special attention in psychiatric thinking; in the current standard nomenclature they are titled *involutional melancholia*. Originally this special consideration was based on the supposition that the hormonal changes associated with the female menopause played a large role in precipitating depressions during this age period. Most psychiatrists today feel that the hormonal changes of the involutional period play little or no part in the etiology of depressions in this age group. However, the emotional adjustments of women at this time of life may play a significant role in precipitating their depressions, for these women undergo extensive interpersonal changes in their life styles.

Extensive changes often take place in the family environment of a woman during her menopausal period. She frequently loses her parents by death about this time, and similarly she may begin to lose occasional persons in her own age group, such as siblings and close friends. These deaths also remind the middle-aged woman that her own life horizon is closer than when she was younger, and that illnesses increase and the chance of death draws nearer as one proceeds through middle life. The children of the middle-aged woman are arriving at adulthood and are moving out of the home. Much of her time, thought and energy for 25 years were occupied with the care of these children, and there is now a large vacuum in her life created by their absence.

The experience of ceasing to menstruate and undergoing the various physical sensations of the female menopause may have a significant psychological impact. She may interpret it as a sign of loss of femininity and approaching old age. It may signify to her the loss of beauty and attractiveness to men, or the loss of child-bearing capacity and youth. These feelings are not caused by hormonal imbalance; they are the interpretations the woman places on the experiences she is going through. (Other emotional stresses occurring during middle age and contributing to depressions at this time are discussed in Chapter 25, in the section which deals with the emotional adjustments of middle age.)

The so-called involutional depressions are usually defined as occurring between the age of 40 and the late 50's, and the age limit is sometimes extended to 60. Some psychiatrists feel that severe depressions are more common in women at this time than during other periods. However, the definition of the so-called involutional period is so broad that it includes 30 to 40 per cent of the adult life span, and it is doubtful that more depressions occur during this period than would be expected during so broad a stretch of adult life. Some psychiatrists feel that severe depressions occurring during the involutional period have a tendency to be characterized by anxiousness, agitation, bizarre physical complaints and paranoid ideas. Other psychiatrists feel that the clinical features of severe depressions in involutional women do not differ appreciably from depressions in other age groups.

In the past there has been much speculation about an involutional process in men, variously labeled the male menopause or the male climacteric. It is doubtful that such a process exists. Whatever endocrinological changes occur are moderate, and they do not play a significant role in emotional disturbances of men in this age group. Most psychiatrists feel that the clinical features of depressions occurring in men during middle age are no different than the characteristics of depressions at other times of life. However, the particular interpersonal stresses that precipitate depressions in middle-aged men often are different than the precipitating interpersonal causes in younger or older men. (These stresses are considered in our discussion of the interpersonal causes of depressions later in this chapter, and the special emotional adjustments occurring during middle age are covered in Chapter 25.)

The Clinical Course of Severe Depressions

Severe depressions of the kind we are discussing here do not occur in children. Though children may be very depressed, they do not go through illnesses clinically similar to the severe depressions that occur in adults. Severe depressions begin to occur in middle and late adolescence, and they continue to increase in frequency until the late 20's and early 30's. After the early 30's the incidence of severe depressions remains at about the same level for the rest of the adult life span. In recent times it has been recognized that they are about as common in elderly persons as in other adult age groups.

In most instances, a severe depression begins gradually and unfolds over a period of from several weeks to two or three months. In occasional cases, however, a severe depression begins abruptly and becomes full-blown during a several-day period. In most instances, the patient's family and friends cannot describe a precipitating life crisis, but in a minority of patients the severe depression is clearly precipitated by the death of a close relative, a job failure, economic reverses, a marital crisis, or other types of emotional stresses. (The interpersonal causes of severe depressions are covered in the following section of this chapter.)

Psychiatric treatment of severe depressions is successful in 80 to 90 per cent of cases. Treatment returns the patient to his usual level of adjustment in from a few weeks to two or three months. In about 10 per cent of cases the patient goes through a brief period of mild elation or hypomanic behavior as he emerges from his severe depression, and he then evens out at his usual level of emotional functioning.

About 10 per cent or more of severe depressions are not resolved by treatment. A small number of these patients commit suicide, and the others enter prolonged severe depressions. However, the majority of patients who are refractory to treatment and undergo prolonged depressions spontaneously recover after periods ranging from several months to two or three years. A few patients, perhaps 2 per cent or so, remain in chronic severe depressions for many years or for the rest of their adult lives. The patient with a severe depression that stretches out for a prolonged period of time often has persecutory delusions or bizarre delusions of physical deformities, and auditory hallucinations occasionally are present; many psychiatrists feel that such chronic depressions basically are schizophrenic disorders of schizoaffective type.

More than 10 per cent of the American population are over the age of 65, and severe depressions that occur in the aged have attracted more attention in recent decades. The incidence of severe depressions in elderly persons is probably about the same as in other adult years. The majority of these patients do not have outstanding clinical signs of arteriosclerotic or senile brain disease, though in some cases a depression is superimposed on early intellectual deterioration. The precipitants of depressions in elderly persons are usually related to the emotional stresses of this age group. The elderly person often faces social isolation as his friends and relatives, and perhaps his marital partner, are incapacitated by illness and die. His children leave him to establish homes of their own. He often faces economic problems and increased physical illness at a time when employment opportunities decrease for him. Despite these interpersonal and socioeconomic difficulties, the prognosis of a severe depression in an elderly patient usually is favorable.

INTERPERSONAL CAUSES OF SEVERE DEPRESSIONS

The production of a severe depression requires the occurrence of predisposing interpersonal trauma in childhood and precipitating emotional stress in adult life. We shall consider the clinical causes of severe depressions under the headings of childhood interpersonal background and adult precipitating stresses.

Childhood Interpersonal Background

The childhood of the person who later develops a severe depression is characterized by traumatic interpersonal relationships in which (1) he is emotionally rejected, and his needs for affection are not met, (2) his self-esteem is crushed and (3) strong hostility is mobilized within him toward the people who have damaged him, but he feels much guilt about the rage he feels toward them. This emotional trauma usually begins in the patient's early childhood and continues in varying degrees throughout his formative years into his adolescence.

The child's major emotional trauma occurs in his relationships with his parents or with the persons who take the parents' place in rearing him. In some instances the child is rejected openly, but in the majority of instances the parents' emotional rejection is more subtle but nevertheless equally devastating. The child receives irritability, coldness and emotional neglect in place of the affection and warm acceptance he needs. This emotional rejection leaves him permanently with a painful yearning for affection. He has marked sensitivity about whether people accept him or not. When in later years he receives the affection he needs, he has a feeling of well-being and mild elation, but when people around him reject him he feels lost, desolate and depressed. Thus, the child emerges from his formative years with a vulnerability to depressiveness, which hinges on whether or not he receives affection and acceptance from the people around him. Minor rejections precipitate minor feelings of depressiveness, and accumulated or major rejections or failures plunge him into deeper desolation and despair.

Furthermore, the child's self-esteem is badly battered by the emotional rejection he receives. He feels unloved and unlovable, and he feels that he is an inadequate person whose worthlessness prevents people from giving him affection. The child rarely wonders if the emotional rejection and depreciation he receives from his parents arise from the parents' emotional problems and personality defects; he feels that the scorn and lack of love he experiences are caused by his own inadequacies as a person. He feels that he gets no love because he is not worthwhile enough to receive it. These feelings of worthlessness are ground deeply into the child's personality structure, and emotional trauma in adult life easily accentuates them. When in adult life the person has a job failure, scholastic failure, economic reverses or marital difficulties, his old feelings of worthlessness rise and overwhelm him with depressiveness. Any failures of adult life seem to be the final proof that his old feelings of worthlessness are justified. Hence, the feelings of worthlessness and failure that characterize the depressed patient are forged by the traumatic experiences both of childhood and adult life.

In addition, the child has much lingering rage toward his parents and other close persons because of the emotional pain he has received from them. However, he continues to hope that finally they will change and will give him the love and esteem he so desperately craves. These strong mixed feelings of yearning and rage toward his parents and other close persons exist side by side and produce marked conflicts in the child and early adolescent. He is only partially aware of these feelings, and he rarely can put them into articulate expression. As he emerges into adolescence, these conflicts usually become unconscious, but they continue in unresolved turbulence within him. He feels immense guilt about his hostility toward his parents and the other close people who failed him. The pain of this guilt causes his hostility to be submerged out of his awareness, but both his hostility and guilt lurk on throughout adolescence and adulthood ready to emerge and overwhelm him when he faces distressing interpersonal relationships in later life. Many of the guilty feelings of the adult depressed patient are produced by the lingering rage he feels toward his parents, and also toward other persons later in his adult life, which he can neither face consciously nor express in any way. He is squeezed in a vise composed of his yearning for people and the rage he feels when they reject him. He cannot deal consciously with either one of these powerful feelings, and they grind him into depressiveness.

During childhood the patient may have a series of depressive periods which last from a few weeks to several months, but the clinical features of these episodes are different from those of severe depressions in adults. People around the child note only that he is "moody," tired and apathetic; he may spend much time by himself, and people sometimes find him crying alone. The child terminates each one of these episodes by pushing his conflicts back out of his awareness, because they are too painful for him to deal with consciously. In late childhood and early adolescence, as his interpersonal life begins to take him increasingly out of the home and into groups of his own age level, these conflicts recede into a dormant but unresolved state. These unresolved conflicts predispose him to repeated depressions during his adult life when he is confronted by accumulated difficulties or interpersonal crises.

It is doubtful that a traumatic interpersonal relationship with only one parent, in the presence of a sound relationship with the other parent, can produce so overwhelming an illness as a severe depression. Damaging interpersonal relationships with both parents probably are necessary to create the emotional difficulties that predispose the person to a severe depression. For example, hostility and emotional rejection by the mother may be coupled with callous indifference by the father. In some instances, the father abandons the child entirely to the care of a rejecting mother, and in other instances both parents deluge the child with criticism, depreciation and irritability during all his childhood and adolescent years. In addition, in most cases the emotional problems the child has with his parents are compounded by similar traumas at the hands of other close persons (such as siblings, grandparents and other close associates), or he spends his childhood and early adolescence in relative emotional isolation so that he has little opportunity to repair outside the home the interpersonal damage he experiences in it.

In the deeply ingrained self-image that he has of himself, the depressive person basically fears that he is worthless, inadequate and guilty; he manages to flee from awareness of this self-image most of the time, but periodic interpersonal stresses in adult life cause it to rise up at times and disturb him. The periodic reemergence into consciousness of this self-image also explains, in part, the patient's tendency to repeated, severe depressions. Furthermore, when a depressed patient emerges from a severe depression and feels free of his burden of guilt and worthlessness, he may have a feeling of elation and well-being. This feeling of elated relief plays a significant role in the brief manic period which sometimes occurs at the end of a severe depression. A somewhat similar process occurs in manic disorders; in a sense, the manic depressive cycle is composed of periodic descents into depression, which alternate with episodes of desperate flight into euphoric elation in attempts to avoid depressiveness. (We shall consider the emotional causes of manic disorders at more length in Chapter 16.)

Precipitating Emotional Factors in Adult Life

In our discussion of the childhood interpersonal background of the depressed patient, we outlined some of the kinds of interpersonal stresses in adult life that may be joined to childhood traumas in causing a severe depression. These adult stresses are (1) emotional rejections which may occur in marital problems, close social relationships, work situations and other interpersonal areas, (2) events that crush the patient's self-esteem, as in job failures and economic reverses, and (3) interpersonal relationships in which strong hostile feelings are aroused in the patient, which are coupled with much guilt about his hostile feelings and yearnings for affectionate closeness with the persons toward whom the hostility is directed. In a sense, these adult interpersonal stresses repeat basic emotional conflicts that occurred in the patient's childhood; they jab into early wounds that never completely healed.

In some cases, the patient who is predisposed to develop depressiveness unduly inhibits expression of anger and aggressiveness; he stores up these feelings, and they smolder chronically within him. He represses his angry feelings because he has a strong need for acceptance by people and a dread of being rejected by them. He seeks to win esteem, affection and emotional acceptance by repressing any anger that arises in his dealings with people. This slow build-up of hostile feelings plays a significant role in precipitating a depressive illness in some cases, because eventually this pent-up hostility rises to the surface and presses for some kind of expression. The patient feels overwhelmingly guilty about the hostile feelings that flood him, and, in addition, he dreads that they will poison his relationships with people and lead to rejection by them. Some psychiatrists feel that the inhibited rage of the depressed patient is turned inwardly upon himself since he cannot direct it outwardly toward other people. The patient castigates himself with self-criticism and depreciating reproaches in the same way he would castigate others if he could deal consciously with his hostility toward them. The ultimate in inward directed rage is self-destruction by suicide. The depressed patient also is impelled toward suicide to escape the crushing burden of his painful feelings of guilt and unworthiness.

The vulnerability of a patient to a severe depression varies with the degree of emotional trauma he experienced during his childhood and early adolescence. In some instances the patient suffered such marked emotional damage throughout his formative years that moderate stress in adult life, either slowly accumulated or abrupt, may precipitate a severe depression. This type of patient is prone to have repeated depressions during his adult years as he periodically is assailed by new interpersonal difficulties. In other instances the patient requires a great deal of trauma in adulthood, perhaps building up slowly over a period of many years, before a severe depression is precipitated.

Occasionally a severe depression is precipitated by the death of an emotionally close person, such as a parent, or a marital partner, or a sibling, or some other close person. The severe depression may occur soon after the death of the person, but more often there is an interval of several months to a year before the depression develops. When a severe depression is precipitated by the death of an emotionally close person, the patient usually had mixed feelings of hatred and affectionate yearning for the deceased person. The patient is thrown into emotional turmoil, for he feels immensely guilty about his unresolved hostility toward the dead person. He also feels, though he usually is unaware of it, that the person's death left him with unfinished business; he now has no opportunity to resolve his conflict with the deceased and to effect an affectionate reconciliation with him. At first, the patient may feel a sense of relief at the death of the person with whom he was in conflict, but he soon feels overwhelmingly guilty about his sense of relief. These chaotic feelings stir up old conflicts from the patient's childhood, and a severe depression results.

Consideration of the various adult interpersonal stresses that may contribute to depressiveness explains the common occurrence of severe depressions in middle and old age. Then the patient undergoes multiple emotional losses in the deaths of his parents, relatives, close friends and perhaps his marital partner. He suffers the subtle emotional rejection involved in seeing his children leave home and become primarily preoccupied with the pleasures and problems of their own marriages and children. The middle-aged or elderly person suffers continual decreases in self-esteem as he finds his vocational opportunities diminishing and his physical strength declining. The elderly person may find that he is losing some of his intellectual alertness, and he feels a loss of esteem in a society that puts emphasis on youth, vigor and achievement. Such events, when coupled with predisposing emotional trauma in his formative years, may lead to a severe depression in middle or old age.

TREATMENT OF SEVERE DEPRESSIONS

The patient with a severe depression requires psychiatric hospitalization. He needs a hospital interpersonal setting which facilitates his recovery and makes suicide improbable; he needs antidepressant medication in a medically supervised setting and, in carefully selected cases, he may need electroshock therapy. Careful discharge planning when he is ready to leave the hospital and subsequent psychotherapy are advisable in many cases.

The patient with a severe depression requires psychiatric hospitalization because of various factors. In many instances the patient's suicidal urges are so strong that psychiatric hospitalization is a medical emergency, and in most other cases the possibility of suicide is a menacing specter lurking in the shadows. We do not have entirely reliable criteria for evaluating suicidal risk; we have only suggestive guidelines (outlined in the separate section on suicide at the end of this chapter). The need for psychiatric hospitalization is reinforced by the fact that a patient with a severe depression has a good prognosis if his illness is not tragically terminated by suicide.

In addition, the depressed patient should be removed from whatever stresses exist in his usual interpersonal environment. Problems in his family relationships, work situation or social life often have played a significant role in precipitating his depression, and if he remains in his usual environment he often continues to be subjected to interpersonal traumas that retard his recovery. In the hospital his interpersonal environment can be arranged to afford him the least possible stress, and the hospital personnel are trained to offer a milieu that encourages recovery. Whereas outside the hospital he might be subjected to continued irritability, rejection and depreciation by people, the hospital ward personnel are trained to give him understanding care in an environment free of hostility; moreover, they can put reasonable limitations on his behavior (such as measures to decrease the possibility of suicide), when necessary, in a kindly, firm manner.

In addition, antidepressant medications and medications for agitation and insomnia are best administered to a severely depressed patient in a hospital. The depressed patient often feels so hopeless about himself that he does not take a prescribed medication if its administration is put into his hands, and his relatives may be unreliable in its administration. Moreover, there is always the risk of suicide by overdosage with antidepressant or sedative medications when they are kept at home for administration to the patient. In addition, some depressed patients do not eat unless their meals are carefully supervised by the nursing staff, and spoon-feeding is necessary in occasional instances. In the small percentage of cases in which electroshock therapy is necessary, it should be given in a psychiatric hospital. When the physician explains to the patient's relatives the good prognosis of a severe depreison with hospital treatment, and the risk of suicide is pointed out, most relatives agree to hospital care. The patient himself often is too depressed to seek treatment, but he usually will accept the unanimous, firm decision of his family and the psychiatrist. A confirmatory recommendation by his family doctor or internist whom he has known a long time frequently is helpful. When the severely depressed patient refuses to accept hospital care the risk of suicide usually is strong enough to justify the recommendation that his relatives secure hospitalization by legal commitment.

The patient with a depressive psychosis merits careful study to understand the kinds of interpersonal stresses that have led to his illness. In addition to evaluatory interviews with the patient, his relatives should be interviewed by the psychiatrist or by one of the hospital's psychiatric social workers to get a comprehensive view of the patient's interpersonal history and the various old and recent traumas that have contributed to his illness. However, psychotherapy with a patient in a severe depression is not an effective procedure in itself. The profundity of the patient's depression makes him unresponsive to psychotherapy; he cannot talk spontaneously about his problems, and the interpretations of the therapist seem distant and meaningless to him. After he has emerged from his severe depression psychotherapy may be useful to him in resolving his underlying emotional problems, but other forms of therapy must be relied upon to pull him out of his depressiveness.

Antidepressant Medication. The majority of patients with severe depressions get a good result from antidepressant medication. The recovery rates usually run between 60 and 70 per cent, and some psychiatrists report recovery of 80 per cent of well selected patients. Most psychiatrists now agree that, of the two available groups of antidepressant medications, the tricyclic drugs are more effective and have a much lower incidence of serious adverse reactions; the tricyclic drugs include imipramine (Tofranil), amitriptyline (Elavil), desipramine (Norpramin, Pertofrane), nortriptyline (Aventyl) and others. The monoamine oxidase inhibitors constitute the second group of antidepressant medications; they include isocarboxazid (Marplan), nialamide (Niamid), phenelzine (Nardil) and others. Because they give decidedly lower recovery rates and have a significant incidence of serious adverse reactions, the momoamine oxidase inhibitors should be employed only in patients who have a history of having recovered from previous severe depressions on them or who have not responded to tricyclic antidepressants. [In the section on neurotic depressions (mild depressions) in Chapter 10 these drugs are discussed in somewhat greater detail, and they are covered at length in Chapter 22 on medications in psychiatry. Also, *the criteria which enhance the probability of success with these medications, and the factors which decrease the probability of failure, are fully outlined in Chapter 10.* For example, the probability that antidepressant medications will be successful is reduced when bizarre delusions, persecutory delusions or hallucinations are present.]

When agitation is present the patient may be given a daytime tranquilizer until his depressiveness begins to clear. I prefer the phenothizaines for this purpose. For example, chlorpromazine (Thorazine, Chlorpz) in doses ranging from 150 mg. to 300 mg. each day usually gives the patient relief. Occasionally, the psychiatrist may be apprehensive that, despite the most careful precautions against suicide, the patient may kill himself on a psychiatric ward. I have seen about 15 such patients, one of whom hung himself under a bed by a towel suspended from the bottom of the headboard during a several-minute period when the attendant who was detailed to remain constantly with him thought he was asleep and briefly left the room. In such cases the psychiatrist can decrease the chance of suicide by making the patient continually somewhat drowsy with daily doses of about 600 mg. of chlorpromazine, or appropriate doses of other phenothiazines. This type of "chemical restraint" is undesirable in terms of the patient's total ward adjustment and interpersonal activities, but for those occasional patients who seem desperately intent on self-destruction it is better than suicide, while antidepressant medication or electroshock therapy is pulling them out of their depressiveness.

Insomnia is a common problem in severely depressed patients, and one of the common nighttime sedatives may be useful. Amphetamines are not useful for depressed patients; they are not antidepressants and, although they may give the patient more energy, they serve no valid function in the treatment of depressions.

Electroshock Therapy. Electroshock therapy is necessary for some patients with severe depressions. Before the introduction of antidepressant medications electroshock therapy was the only effective treatment for severe depressions, and between 80 and 90 per cent of well selected patients recovered with it. The amount of electroshock treatment given for severe depressions has diminished greatly since the introduction of the antidepressant drugs, but electroshock continues to resolve some severe depressions that do not respond to antidepressant medication. In my experience, about 65 per cent of patients with severe depressions respond to antidepressant medications, and another 25 per cent are unresponsive to antidepressant drugs but recover with electroshock therapy. The remaining 10 per cent of patients with severe depressions are unresponsive to all therapy, but most of them recover spontaneously after from several months to two or three years of depression. When bizarre delusions or hallucinations are present, electroshock therapy is more likely to be necessary.

Electroshock therapy should never be used in treating the neurotic depressions (mild depressions) described in Chapter 10; it should be employed only in the treatment of a minority of the patients whose depressions are severe and fit the general clinical picture described in this chapter. Also, electroshock therapy should never be employed in treating any conditions except some severely depressed patients and a small percentage of schizophrenic and manic patients.

The usual course of electroshock therapy for a severe depression runs between 6 and 12 treatments; the average is 8 to 10. If the patient is not decisively improved at the end of 12 treatments, the probability that he will recover with electroshock therapy is much decreased. Most psychiatrists feel that 20 treatments is the upper limit for electroshock therapy in depressed patients, and some psychiatrists feel that little further benefit occurs after 15 treatments. However, when bizarre delusions, persecutory delusions or hallucinations are present a total of 15 to 20 treatments may be necessary. (The details of the technic, precautions and complications of electroshock therapy are covered in Chapter 23.)

Other Aspects of the Treatment of Severe Depressions. As he emerges from his depression the patient requires daily clinical evaluation. He must remain in the hospital until he is fully recovered; limited improvement must not be mistaken for recovery, and the physician continually must be alert to the problem of suicidal risk during the patient's convalescence. Prior to the patient's discharge from the hospital, the psychiatrist or perhaps one of the hospital's psychiatric social workers, should carry out counseling with the patient's relatives about any possible steps they may take to reduce obvious interpersonal stresses. The psychiatrist should schedule follow-up visits to supervise the patient's progress in the post-hospitalization period and to facilitate his adjustment back into his usual activities.

At the same time the psychiatrist should evaluate the possibility that psychotherapy may help the patient resolve some of his underlying emotional problems. Patients vary much in their motivation for psychotherapy after recovery from depressions. Many patients feel well and have no motivation for psychotherapy; with these patients the psychiatrist limits his follow-up visits to supportive counseling and supervision of any antidepressant medication the patient still may be taking. Other patients have good motivation to enter exploratory psychotherapy to work on their interpersonal problems. Psychotherapy may deal mainly with current interpersonal stresses or it may delve into the unresolved conflicts of the patient's early life. The nature and depth of the psychotherapy depend on the strengths of the patient's personality structure as well as his motivation. Some patients become so frightened and depressed when they begin to face the conflicts of their childhood and early adolescent years that psychotherapy runs a greater chance of damaging them than of helping them. Insensitive probing in psychotherapy occasionally may precipitate further depressiveness. Hence, the advisability of psychotherapy and its proper depth must be carefully considered in each patient and modified to meet his needs and limitations.

SUICIDE: A CLINICAL AND PUBLIC HEALTH PROBLEM

Suicide is a major public health problem and the most common cause of death resulting from psychiatric illness. About 20,000 deaths by suicide are recorded each year in the United States, but it is well known that the actual number of suicides is at least two or three times that number. Many suicides are listed as accidental deaths to spare the feelings of grieving families, and some deaths recorded as accidental (as in solo driver automobile accidents) are disguised suicides. Psychiatrists estimate that the number of unsuccessful suicidal attempts runs from 5 to 20 times the number of suicidal deaths, and some statisticians have estimated that there are now at least two million people in the United States who at some time in their lives made a serious attempt at suicide.

Suicide in children under the age of 10 is extremely rare; it is a clinical oddity that occurs so infrequently that a general description of its clinical features and causes cannot be given. Among the possible reasons for the rarity of suicide before puberty is that young children have vague ideas about death. They view it as a kind of sleep or a somewhat reversible journey. Only after the age of 10 or 11 do children begin to grasp the concept of death as the end of existence. Moreover, though children may have depressive problems, their depressions do not have the devastating, overwhelming impact of severe depressions in adolescence and adulthood.

Beginning at the age of 10, the incidence of suicide begins to rise, and it continues to increase throughout adolescence. In adolescents it is the second most common cause of death. Suicide continues to be a common cause of death throughout adult life. It officially is ranked as the tenth most frequent cause of death in the United States, but if all suicides were truly counted as such it would probably rank as eighth or ninth. Suicide is more common among professional groups, the well-educated and the well-to-do. Ingestion of large amounts of sedatives or toxic substances is the most common method of suicidal attempt; self-inflicted wounds with firearms or sharp instruments and falls from high buildings also are frequent methods of suicide.

Emotional Causes of Suicide

Most psychiatrists feel that in the majority of cases suicide is caused by severe depressiveness. Various features of severe depressiveness impel the patient toward suicide. The depressed patient may find his painful feelings of guiltiness and sinfulness a crushing burden, and he may see death as the one way to free himself from his agony. His guilt feelings make him feel unworthy to be alive, and he sees death as the only possible course for so worthless and inadequate a person as he feels himself to be. He feels isolated from everyone; he feels unloved and unlovable, and he feels he has no warm interpersonal bonds to hold him to the world of living people. He seeks by suicide to leave the world of people, and to cease to be a person by becoming an inanimate thing. We reviewed the causes of such feelings of guiltiness, worthlessness and isolation in our discussion of the interpersonal causes of depressivness earlier in this chapter.

Sometimes the severely depressed person sees suicide as a kind of absolution in which he cancels out his painful guilt by sacrificing his life; he sees suicide as the only way to pay his guilty debts to the people around him, and at the same time he ends his suffering. In a few instances, the depressed person also envisions suicide as a perverted revenge in which he will punish emotionally close persons with whom he is in conflict by making them feel responsible for driving him to suicide. In some cases a suicidal attempt is, in part, a halfhearted gesture in which the depressed person unconsciously is trying to arouse the people around him to take steps to help him in his desperate emotional state.

Some psychiatrists view the suicidal act as the inward turning on the self of hostility the patient originally had toward others but could not express or deal with consciously. For example, pent-up, unconscious hatred toward parents or other close persons in childhood may be later joined by unrecognized hostility toward a marital partner and others; in time, these hostile feelings become turned inward on the patient himself, since he gives them no outward expression, and the ultimate in inward directed hostility is self-destruction.

Some, or perhaps all, of these emotional forces are present in most persons who attempt suicide. Such depressive forces are most powerful in severe depressions and schizoaffective schizophrenic disorders. However, they also may occur in modified forms in patients with neurotic depressions, various kinds of personality disorders and organic brain states.

Suicide also occurs occasionally in response to hallucinations or delusions. A patient sometimes receives commands from auditory hallucinations to kill himself. The hallucinatory voices may accuse the patient of heinous crimes and may command him to kill himself in self-punishment for his sins. In other instances the hallucinatory voices may direct the patient to commit suicide as a means of achieving a mystical reunion with deceased persons. A person with gradiose delusions sometimes envisions suicide as a religious self-sacrificial act in service to some divine figure; in such instances the suicidal act may be preceded by bizarre self-mutilation. Occasionally, in such instances, the suicidal person kills others, such as his children or his marital partner, before his suicide, in order to take them with him on the mystical journey into death which he contemplates. However, suicide-homicide combinations, which are statistically very rare, may occur in severely depressed patients who do not wish to leave their families, or others, behind them in a world which they view as full of misery and suffering. Suicides precipitated by hallucinations or delusions occur mainly in schizophrenics, but they also may occur in acute and chronic organic brain disorders.

Occasionally a terrified patient in an acute or chronic organic brain syndrome accidentally kills himself while attempting to flee from hallucinatory persecutors. Panic states are common during acute organic brain disorders, such as delirium tremens; the patient, for example, may throw himself through a window in efforts to get away from hallucinatory dangers. Such accidental deaths may also occur in panic states in hallucinating schizophrenics. Though such deaths are not suicidal in the strict meaning of the term, they are sometimes recorded as such.

Various other factors may contribute to suicide. A narcotic addict may commit suicide when he faces the agony of abrupt withdrawal from his drug, and occasionally a person with incurable cancer or a progressive disease such as Huntington's chorea commits suicide. Elderly people, particularly those of higher social and educational groups, sometimes commit suicide as they note failing memory and other signs of impending senile brain degeneration in themselves. Middle-aged people facing grave social humiliation or financial disaster, sometimes commit suicide as an alternative course. Persons who have lost all close interpersonal ties and are economically destitute, particularly in middle age and old age, occasionally commit suicide. However, psychiatrists tend to assume, rightly or wrongly, that there is no such thing as "rational suicide," or at least that it is rare, since only a very small percentage of addicts without drugs, early senile patients and others listed above, kill themselves. Psychiatrists, in general, feel that a subtle but strong depressive thread, similar to that described in severe depressions, exists in the small percentages of persons facing these situations who choose suicide as a way out. In some cases suicide comes as a shocking surprise to the patient's family and associates; it seems, on the surface, inexplicable. In such cases careful study of the patient's life history and current interpersonal life reveals emotional traumas which others had not recognized and a strong depressive strain which the patient had hidden.

Criteria for Evaluating Suicidal Risk

There are no invariable rules by which one may evaluate suicidal risk. However, there are certain broad principles which are helpful, and by application of them the physician can sharpen considerably his alertness to this problem.

The deeper the depression, the more probable is a suicidal attempt. The patient with profound feelings of worthlessness, marked convictions of sinfulness and guilt, and a feeling that everyone would be better off without him, is a great suicidal risk. Some psychiatrists feel that suicidal risk increases as the patient begins to improve somewhat and to emerge from the depths of his depression; however, I feel that any increase in suicide at this time is because the vigilance of relatives and physicians may become less alert as the patient shows slight improvement, and the chance of a successful suicidal attempt may increase. Also, occasional patients develop a quiet calmness and apparent improvement once they make a definite decision to commit suicide and decide on the means; they feel that the end of their agony is near, and hence they appear to be coming out of their depression when actually they are not. I have had several such suicides, one of whom wrote me a four-page letter describing her emotional state before she posted the letter and made an almost successful suicidal attempt in a distant city.

The patient who puts his suicidal ideas and plans into writing, as in farewell notes, is more likely to commit suicide, especially if the suicidal note is written in a matter-of-fact way and deals with details such as the distribution of his possessions to relatives and friends. A note that asks his family's forgiveness for the shame he will cause them by the suicidal act is particularly alarming.

If the patient has made suicidal attempts in the past, there is a greater possibility he will try it again. Also, the probability of suicide is greater when there is a history of suicide, or serious suicidal attempts, in the patient's family or in other persons close to him. Such deaths breach the so-called "death barrier." Recent tragic deaths of persons who were emotionally close to the patient, even if not by suicide, increase the suicidal risk in depressed patients. The absence of strong, warm emotional bonds to relatives and friends increases suicidal risk, and the presence of such bonds tends to diminish suicidal risk.

Serious statements of contemplated suicide should never be taken lightly. Most persons who commit suicide tell someone about it beforehand, and some suicidal individuals mention their suicidal feelings a number of times to various persons. However, the physician must be careful to distinguish patients who have an obsessive fear of suicide, but no desire to commit it, from those patients with true suicidal thoughts and urges. (Obsessive fears of suicide, as opposed to urges to commit suicide, are discussed in Chapter 8.)

The suicidal attempts of some patients are facilitated by easy access to sedatives or firearms, and some of these attempts are fatal. In some instances, the patient would not have made a suicidal attempt if a bottle of sedatives or a revolver had not been close at hand. This is particularly true of suicidal attempts in adolescents and in persons who are emerging from depressions but are not fully recovered from them. The highly suicidal patient usually can find means for a suicidal attempt, but many suicidal attempts are made by persons whose suicidal urges are fluctuating, inconstant and less severe.

The prevention of sucide lies in prompt psychiatric care of the suicidal patient. The psychiatric illnesses of most suicidal patients have good prognoses if the patients are psychiatrically hospitalized to receive treatment. Psychiatric hospitals are carefully organized to try to remove all means for suicidal attempts. All physicians and other professional medical workers should be alert to the fact that suicide is a major public health problem, and they should not hesitate to advise psychiatric hospitalization for the suicidal patient. When the family physician is in doubt, he should advise both the patient and his family to seek psychiatric consultation. When the physician is faced with a severely suicidal patient and a delay of from a few hours to a couple of days before psychiatric hospitalization can be arranged, he may use 300 to 600 mg. of chlorpromazine (Thorazine, Chlor-pz) by mouth, or appropriate oral doses of another phenothiazine, to sedate the patient. This usually sedates him to an extent which makes suicide much less likely without significant medical risk to the patient; in addition, of course, marked vigilance by the relatives is necessary.

BIBLIOGRAPHY

Arieti, S.: Anxiety and beyond in schizophrenia and psychotic depressions. Am. J. Psychother., *27*:338, 1973.

Bellak, L., and Berneman, N.: A systematic view of depression. Am. J. Psychother., *25*:385, 1971.

Briscoe, C. W., and Smith, J. B.: Depression and marital turmoil. Arch. Gen. Psychiatry, *29*:811, 1973.

Harrow, M., and Amdur, M. J.: Guilt and depressive disorders. Arch. Gen. Psychiatry, *25*:240, 1971.

Hirsch, C. S., Rushforth, N. B., Ford, A. B., and Adelson, A.: Homicide and suicide in a metropolitan county. J. A. M. A., *223*:900, 1973.

Minkoff, K., Bergman, E., Beck, A. T., and Beck, R.: Hopelessness, depression and attempted suicide. Am. J. Psychiatry, *130*:455, 1973.

Ollerenshaw, D. P.: The classification of the functional psychoses. Brit. J. Psychiatry, *122*:517, 1973.

Paykel, E. S.: Depressive typologies and response to amitriptyline. Brit. J. Psychiatry, *120*:147, 1972.

Peto, A.: Body image and depression. Int. J. Psychoanal., *53*:259, 1972.

Post. F.: The management and nature of depressive illnesses in late life. Brit. J. Psychiatry, *121*:393, 1972.

Scher, J. M.: The depressions and their structure: an existential approach to their understanding and treatment. Am. J. Psychother., *25*:369, 1971.

Shanfield, S., et al.: The schizophrenic patient and depressive symptomatology. J. Nerv. Ment. Dis., *151*:203, 1970.

Shneidman, E. S. (ed.): Death and the College Student: A Collection of Brief Essays on Death and Suicide by Harvard Youth. New York, Behavioral Publications, 1972.

Raskin, A.: A guide for drug use in depressive disorders. Am. J. Psychiatry, *131*:181, 1974.

Winokur, G.: Depression in the menopause. Am. J. Psychiatry, *130*:92, 1973.

16

Manic Psychoses

The feelings and behavior of a patient with a manic disorder are the opposite of those of a patient with a depression. The manic patient is excessively elated and exuberant, and he is overactive in poorly organized ways. Manic psychoses are much less common than depressions, but they nevertheless are frequently encountered in psychiatric practice.

CLINICAL CHARACTERISTICS OF MANIC DISORDERS

The most common time of life for a patient to have his first manic disorder is between late adolescence and his early 30's. In some instances the patient has only one manic episode, but more commonly he has two or more manic disorders during the course of his life. These episodes may be separated by intervals ranging from several months to two or three decades, and they may occur at any time from late adolescence into old age.

The manic patient is buoyant, exuberant and glibly gay. He treats everyone with cheerful, uninhibited familiarity. He talks and laughs excitedly, and he jokes playfully in a continuous stream of jovial enthusiasm. He knows no strangers; he becomes confidentially friendly with everyone upon first contact. His self-satisfaction, assertiveness and self-confidence are boundless, and he incorporates everyone he meets into his plans and activities. He is extravagant with money, makes gifts to friends and strangers alike and confidently chatters about his elaborate schemes for making large amounts of money. I recall a 46-year-old, parsimonious bachelor bookkeeper who had never owned an automobile; his relatives became abruptly aware of his manic psychosis when he bought two expensive Cadillac convertibles.

The manic patient is in constant physical activity. He flits from task to task, completing none of them and leaving a trail of unfinished projects behind him. He dismisses all objections to his wild schemes with a breezy self-confidence. He walks quickly, gesticulates rapidly and cannot remain inactive for even a brief time. Everything moves too slowly for him. He scribbles exuberant, rambling letters to friends and work associates, and immediately afterwards he calls them by long distance telephone to convey his messages more quickly. He sleeps as little as two to four hours each night and gobbles his food rapidly during brief meals. His energy seems endless and he usually presents a picture of ruddy health, but sometimes he works himself into haggard, bright-eyed exhaustion. He feels too busy to pay attention to physical illnesses, the routine tasks of life and his usual responsibilities. His grand plans may at first seem plausible and exciting to the casual observer, but their helter-skelter, impractical nature soon becomes evident. I recall a 32-year-old electrician who in the early stages of a manic episode decided to abandon his work and to go to law school. As his manic disorder increased in severity he soon discarded plans for law school and began to organize a political campaign to seek his election to the United States Senate. A few days later he shifted his exhilarated activity to opening a campaign to secure the nomination of one of the major political parties for the Presidency of the United States. He was engaged in a whirlwind of letter writing, telephone calls and excited conversations about his plans.

The manic patient talks incessantly; about 20 per cent of manic patients become hoarse because of continual talking. He skims over all subjects and delves into none of them. He scarcely takes up a topic when he abandons it and rushes on to the next one. This pell-mell rush of thoughts is called the manic "flight of ideas." The ideas that succeed each other in the patient's chatter may or may not be logically related. Often the patient's rapid transitions from one subject to another are caused by the similar sounds of words (these are called "clang associations") or some other superficial similarity. For example, I recall a manic patient who on admission to the hospital announced that he would reorganize the hospital's *air* conditioning system, then demanded that the staff call the *air*port to have his private *air*plane made ready for a flight, and immediately afterwards instructed a hospital aid to get a ladder and close the *air* vents in his room. The manic patient often sings, whistles and shouts loudly to people around him. I recall a manic patient who accidentally drove his automobile into a tree and suffered multiple fractures of his mandible a few hours before entry to a hospital psychiatric ward. In order to set the fractured mandible his mouth was wired tightly shut for several weeks, with only a small aperture left between two teeth for the insertion of a tube through which he was fed. Despite this hindrance, the patient managed to talk continually in a muffled, garbled manner for three weeks until his manic disorder began to subside with treatment.

The manic patient sometimes is sexually brazen and overactive. A manic man may make obscene remarks and sexual proposals to a woman he met only a few minutes previously, and he may become sexually promiscuous. A woman may become sexually indiscriminate and may vaunt her licentiousness in a crude manner. If unrestrained by psychiatric hospitalization, a manic person may consort sexually with undesirable individuals with whom he would not associate when well. Unfortunate, impulsive marriages or flagrant marital infidelities may cause much grief to the patient's relatives before they fully comprehend that he is emotionally ill.

In many instances the exuberant joviality of the manic patient is interrupted by brief periods of depressiveness. The patient at times breaks into sobbing sadness, which usually lasts for only a few minutes, before he launches back into exhilaration and overactivity. Because of this depressive quality that lies beneath the surface of manic behavior, the gaiety of the manic patient often has a hollow, forced quality.

The manic patient may become belligerent and argumentative if he cannot do as he wishes. Such belligerence may flash forth at infrequent intervals and for only a few minutes at a time, or it may become a prominent feature of a manic disorder. Some manic patients are angry and verbally abusive much of the time, but physical assaultiveness is rare. The patient may shift abruptly from belligerence to docility, and with equal suddenness his hostility flares out again when he is denied a minor request.

Grandiose delusions involving the patient's exuberant plans occur in some manic disorders. For example, I recall a 24-year-old married woman who rushed about the hospital ward busily preparing for her wedding ceremony, which she each morning announced was to take place that day. The patient may feel that his grandiose plans for financial accomplishment, political success or scientific fame already have been achieved. One of my manic patients continually asked the nurses if the newspaper reporters who were to interview him about his new invention had arrived yet. Grandiose religious ideas and feelings form the most common type of delusions in manic patients. The patient may feel that he has achieved superior religious insights and that he has a divine mission to redeem vast numbers of misguided people. For example, I recall a manic bricklayer whose relatives intercepted him as he was attempting to board an airplane to go to Rome to advise the Pope, and I once treated a young mother with a manic psychosis in the postpartum period who felt that her newborn baby was the Messiah. The delusional manic patient sometimes feels that he has ecstatic, mystical experiences or supernatural religious powers; he more often feels himself to be the agent of divine powers than a divine figurehead himself. Persecutory delusions and all types of hallucinations are uncommon in manic disorders. Some psychiatrists feel that a psychiatric illness characterized by manic behavior and prominent delusions should be classified as a schizophrenic psychosis of schizoaffective type.

Manic disorders conventionally are divided into three categories of ascending severity; they are *euphoria, hypomania* and *mania.*

A mild degree of exhilarated behavior is called *euphoria.* It may be a self-limiting state that lasts from a week or so to two or three months, and does not become severer, or it may be the early phase of a full-blown manic psychosis. It also may occur in some types of organic brain illnesses.

A manic disorder of moderate degree is termed *hypomania.* The hypomanic patient is overactive, distractible, buoyant and busily occupied with grandiose plans. However, he does not have the chaotic disorganization that characterizes mania, and his elaborate plans and ideas do not assume frankly delusional proportions. However, the hypomanic patient often is financially extravagant, sexually irresponsible and injudicious in choosing the people with whom he associates. The hypomanic patient often presents a more difficult problem in psychiatric management than the severely manic patient, because the hypomanic patient's relatives, though they are worried about his injudicious behavior, may not recognize that he is emotionally ill. The hypomanic patient may leave his job abruptly in expectation of brilliant success in an unsound venture, and he may carry out financially self-damaging acts. He may enter into a scandalous sexual affair, an unwise marriage, or a rash divorce. The patient does not recognize that he is ill, and his behavior lacks the markedly disorganized or delusional qualities that would make his illness obvious even to a casual observer. Thus, he usually rejects psychiatric care, and his family may flounder in indecision about procuring a commitment so that he can be treated and prevented from engaging in imprudent activities.

The patient with fully developed *mania* has chaotic behavior, grandiose thinking and wild exhilaration, which quickly cause his family to seek psychiatric care for him. His psychotic disorder is soon apparent to anyone who deals with him.

The Clinical Course of Manic Disorders

A manic disorder may be precipitated by an obvious emotional stress in the patient's life, but in many instances there is no clear-cut precipitating event apparent to the patient's family. The precipitating stress often is an event that ordinarily would cause sadness. For example, I have seen manic psychoses preceded by such events as the death of the patient's child, the death of one of the patient's adult siblings, the death of a marital partner, the death by violence of a parent, the birth of an unwanted child, vocational difficulties and severe marital crises. A manic illness often is immediately preceded by a period of mild depressiveness, which may last from a few days to several weeks.

The prognosis for a manic episode is good. Even before the advent of modern treatment, the vast majority of patients with manic psychoses recovered spontaneously in from three to nine months. With early hospital treatment the manic patient today usually recovers in from several weeks to two months. In about 10 per cent of cases a patient goes through a mild depressive period for several weeks after he recovers from a manic episode. In a few cases a manic psychosis is followed immediately, or after a brief interval, by a severe depression which necessitates further hospital care.

A patient may have only one manic episode in his life, but the majority of manic patients have further manic illnesses in later years. Moreover, a large number of manic patients have the classical manic-depressive pattern of both manic and depressive episodes during their life spans; whereas a patient in his first depression has a 20 per cent chance that at some time in his life he will have a manic illness, a patient in his initial manic disorder has about a 40 per cent chance that at some time in his life he will have a severe depression. The intervals between manic and depressive episodes may range from several months to two or three decades. Intervals of from 2 to 10 years are most common. In general, if a patient's first psychotic illness is a manic one, he will have two or three times more manic disorders during his life than depressive episodes. A frequent pattern is for the patient to have two or three manic episodes, and perhaps one depression, between the ages of 20 and 40, and then to have one or two manic illnesses, and perhaps a depression, during the rest of his life. Manic illnesses occur more frequently during the early adult years than in middle age and old age.

A small percentage of manic disorders stretch into prolonged illnesses that last two or three years in spite of treatment. In such cases the patient may shift from a prolonged manic phase to a brief depressive phase once every several months. In rare instances, the patient enters into a chronic manic psychosis that lasts for many years; many psychiatrists feel that these chronic patients have schizoaffective types of schizophrenic psychoses.

Since the introduction of the diagnostic category of schizoaffective schizophrenia there has been a marked tendency in some psychiatric centers to employ the diagnosis of manic psychosis little, and to classify these patients as schizoaffective schizophrenics. Many psychiatrists, including myself, feel this is an error, since the clinical characteristics, courses and long-term patterns of manic patients are quite different than those of schizophrenics. This distinction also has therapeutic implications. For example, if not kept on maintenance doses of a phenothiazine medication for one to two years after recovery, a sizable percentage of schizophrenics relapse, whereas relatively few manics do.

INTERPERSONAL CAUSES OF MANIC DISORDERS

A manic psychosis is a desperate flight from depressiveness into a state of exhilaration, overactivity and grandiose plans. It is an unconscious attempt to deny an upsurge of depressive feelings by fleeing into feelings and behavior which are the opposite of depressiveness. Whereas the depressed patient is melancholy, the manic patient is gay and buoyant. Whereas the depressed patient feels worthless and inadequate, the manic patient overflows with convictions of self-esteem and self-confidence. Whereas the depressed patient is physically slowed down and fatigued, the manic patient is overactive and has boundless energy. Whereas the depressed patient feels guilty and sinful, the manic patient may feel that he has extraordinary religious insights and a mission to redeem others. The patient's flight into a manic disorder to escape depressiveness is, of course, not a conscious or deliberate act. It is an unconscious process over which he has no control and into which he usually has little or no insight.

A strong depressive force always struggles for release behind the brittle, glittering façade of manic gaiety. This explains why the manic patient sometimes breaks into sobbing despair for brief periods in the midst of his manic behavior, and it also explains why manic disorders often begin with brief depressive periods and frequently are followed by mild depressive phases. In addition, it clarifies why manic episodes sometimes are precipitated by events, such as the death of a close relative, which ordinarily would cause sadness.

However, even at the cost of a manic psychosis, the manic flight usually does not entirely accomplish its purpose. A severe depression occasionally erupts immediately after a manic psychosis, or in many instances it occurs after an interval of from several months to a year or two. The seesaw teeter-tottering back and forth between depressive and manic episodes in the life of a manic depressive patient is caused by periodic upsurges of depressiveness and the camouflaging of depressiveness by mania on some of these occasions.

The manic disorder's function as a counteractant against depressiveness explains many of the clinical features of manic behavior. For example, whereas the depressed patient retires from interpersonal relationships, the manic patient reaches out for them in an avid, helter-skelter manner. The manic patient's boundless energy arises from his great relief in escaping the burden of depressiveness, and it also protects him from lapsing into the apathy of a depression. In a similar way, the manic patient's exhilarated buoyancy is both a joyful feeling of escape from depressiveness and a fragile defense against it.

Since a manic disorder is a defense against depressiveness, the interpersonal causes of a manic disorder are basically similar to the interpersonal causes of a depression. In a sense, a manic disorder is grafted onto a basically depressive process. (Hence, the discussion of the interpersonal causes of depressions given in Chapter 15 is equally applicable to the etiology of manic disorders.) The childhood of the person who later develops a manic disorder is characterized by the same kinds of interpersonal trauma sustained by the depressive patient. This childhood trauma (as outlined in Chapter 15) consists of (1) emotional rejection of the patient by crucial persons in his life, (2) crushing assaults upon his personal esteem, and (3) mobilization of strong mixed feelings of hostility, guilt and affectionate yearning toward his parents and other close persons. These childhood traumas are buried deeply in the patient's personality structure and lie simmering there until they are again stirred up by emotional stress in adult life.

The interpersonal trauma of adulthood that precipitates the patient's manic or depressive disorder consists of events in which the patient (1) undergoes emotional rejections or suffers losses of close persons by death or illness, (2) suffers devastating assaults on his self-esteem or (3) has interpersonal experiences in which strong mixed feelings of hostility and guilt are aroused. (These interpersonal traumas are covered in detail in Chapter 15 and do not need repeated examination here.) The significant difference in the manic patient is that the initial upsurge of depressiveness is quelled by a flood of manic feelings and behavior that protects the patient from the painful burden of a depressive illness. The manic disorder is a further development added to a fundamental depressive process.

The prepsychotic personality of the manic patient often conforms to the pattern of the cyclothymic personality structure (described in detail in Chapter 12). As outlined there, the cyclothymic person is gregarious, prefers activities with people and shuns solitary pursuits. Though he is deeply sensitive to how people feel about him and wants their approval and friendship, he nevertheless can express most of his feelings openly and comfortably. He has good capacities for giving and receiving affection; the affection of other people makes him feel buoyant and exhilarated, but their rejection and scorn make him feel hurt, morose and irritable. He often has mild fluctuations between exuberant cheerfulness and mild depressiveness, which vary from week to week or month to month, depending on the gratifications or stresses of his interpersonal relationships. He often has many friends, is well liked and is successful in his vocational pursuits.

TREATMENT OF MANIC DISORDERS

A patient with a manic disorder should be psychiatrically hospitalized. If he is allowed to remain outside the hospital he runs a strong risk of financial imprudence, vocational irresponsibility and sexual delinquency. Moreover, many psychiatrists feel that the patient tends to deteriorate into increasingly overactive, disorganized behavior if he does not have the limiting influence of a well run psychiatric ward to curb him. In addition, it is difficult to make sure that the patient takes the medication he imperatively needs, and to adjust the dosage in advisable ways every several days or so. On the few occasions on which I have attempted to manage hypomanic or manic patients on an outpatient basis, I invariably have regretted it, and usually have ended up urgently recommending hospitalization to the patient and his family. A further problem in the outpatient management of a manic patient is that in occasional instances he lapses abruptly into a severe depressive episode with acute suicidal risk at the end of his manic illness.

In the psychiatric hospital the manic patient should be allowed a moderate amount of activity for release of his abundant energy. The hospital's occupational therapy department can arrange suitable work for him. For example, a hypomanic patient can pound thin metal sheets into ash trays and platters, or he busily can run an upright shuttle loom in weaving a rug. The severely manic patient can only carry out less skilled activities such as tearing cloth into rag strips for weaving rugs. However, both the physical and interpersonal activities of the manic patient must be carefully limited, because the patient tends continually to increase the tempo of his behavior if his physical and interpersonal activities are stimulating. If at all possible, manic patients should not be allowed to associate with each other on a psychiatric ward, since they mutually incite one another to increasingly hyperactive behavior. The staff should treat the manic patient with calm, firm friendliness. His playful pranks may merit a quiet smile, but they should not provoke a boisterous laugh. I recall an elderly psychiatrist who always spoke to his manic patients in whispers; this unusual procedure had a strangely calming effect on some of them.

Most psychiatrists agree that exploratory psychotherapy is not possible during an acute manic or hypomanic episode. The patient's rapid, poorly organized flow of thoughts and his distractible behavior make it impossible to engage him in effective exploratory psychotherapy. However, the daily visits of the psychiatrist and supportive talk between him and the patient are an important aspect of treatment. In most instances, the manic patient, despite his psychosis, can be engaged to a limited extent in meaningful interpersonal relationships, and the patient is much more likely to cooperate in treatment plans when he has a sound relationship with his psychiatrist. The patient should receive enough nighttime sedation to get a reasonable amount of sleep, and his food intake should be kept under surveillance to make sure he remains well nourished.

We shall discuss the specific treatment of manic disorders under four headings: (1) phenothiazine therapy, (2) lithium therapy, (3) electroshock therapy and (4) psychotherapy during the convalescent and posthospitalization period.

Phenothiazine Therapy

Most psychiatrists feel that the medications of choice for manic disorders are the phenothiazines. Phenothiazines and lithium are of equal effectiveness (as will be discussed later), but lithium has a much higher incidence of serious adverse reactions. All other kinds of calming medications, such as sedatives and antianxiety medications, are ineffective and often produce bewildered agitation. Phenothiazine drugs which are commonly employed in treating manic disorders include chlorpromazine (Thorazine, Chlor-pz), trifluoperazine (Stelazine), thioridazine (Mellaril) and others. In my opinion, other antipsychotic drugs outside the phenothiazine group, such as haloperidol (Haldol), give poorer results and have higher incidences of undesirable side effects.

Using chlorpromazine as a typical, widely employed phenothiazine, the usual dose runs between 400 mg. and 600 mg. each day, but the dosage may run much higher or somewhat lower than that. The patient usually has an immediate improvement on chlorpromazine, and in about 75 per cent of cases his manic disorder gradually subsides during a period of from several weeks to two months. As his manic disorder subsides, the doage of chlorpromazine, or other phenothiazine, can be gradually diminished. The patient often is kept on a reduced daily dosage of 75 mg. to 150 mg. of chlorpromazine each day for from several weeks to three or four months after his apparent recovery and discharge from the hospital, since such maintenance medication helps to level out any minor manic fluctuations which occur in the posthospitalization period. (Further details on the pharmacology and complications of the phenothiazine medications are given in Chapter 22.) Although various theories have been advanced, the mode of action of phenothiazine medications is not well understood; presumably they exercise a calming effect on various lower brain centers, which allows the patient to reintegrate his emotional and interpersonal functioning on his previous good levels of adjustment.

Lithium Treatment

Lithium, given orally and usually in the form of lithium carbonate (Eskalith, Lithane, Lithonate), is an effective drug in the treatment of manic disorders. It leads to recovery in about 75 per cent of patients, thus equalling but not surpassing the phenothiazines in efficacy. It does not begin to decrease the patient's manic symptoms until he has been taking it for from 5 to 10 days, and hence a phenothiazine often must be given until the lithium begins to take effect. Lithium is useful only in manic and hypomanic disorders; though some proponents of the drug have suggested that it acts as a therapeutic or preventive agent in depressions, there is no good evidence that this is so. Some psychiatrists advocate maintaining patients who have tendencies to frequent manic illnesses on maintenance doses of lithium for several years or more, but the statistical evidence is not convincing that this is an effective preventive regimen. Lithium is not effective in schizoaffective schizophrenia with manic features.

Most psychiatrists feel that, since lithium does not give better results than phenothiazines and has a much higher rate of serious adverse reactions, phenothiazines are preferable. Lithium replaces sodium, to which it is related chemically, in the blood electrolyte balance and must be kept in the rather narrow blood serum range of 0.6 to 1.2 mEq/liter. Mild adverse reactions begin at serum levels approaching 1.5 mEq/liter and serious, even fatal, reactions can occur at levels of 2.0 to 2.5 mEq/liter. Thus, during the intensive build-up phase of treatment, serum lithium levels must be checked twice weekly, and a patient on maintenance doses of lithium must have blood serum levels checked at least once a month. However, anything that disturbs electrolyte balance, such as marked perspiration, vomiting or increased or decreased salt intake, can cause sudden changes in the serum lithium level, with grave results within 24 hours. The two most serious effects of lithium intoxication are central nervous system depression with somnolence, memory loss, disorientation, convulsions, coma and death, and cardiovascular collapse with vascular shock and death. There are various contraindications to lithium, such as kidney disease and concomitant administration of diuretics, and there is controversial evidence that it may cause fetal defects. There is no antidote for lithium intoxication; however, its excretion may be hastened by administering sodium bicarbonate and by hemodialysis.

The mechanism of action of lithium in clearing manic disorders is not clear, though it has been suggested that it works by its effects on electrolyte balance and catecholamine metabolism in the brain. (The pharmacology, modes of administration, doses and adverse reactions of lithium are covered in more detail in Chapter 22.)

Most psychiatrists, including myself, feel that lithium therapy offers no advantages over other means of treatment of manic disorders which compensate for its complexity of administration and significant rate of serious adverse reactions. Lithium therapy should be considered only when a patient has not recovered on phenothiazine therapy, or combined phenothiazine and electroshock therapy; many psychiatrists would view this as too cautious a position.

Electroshock Thereapy

About 75 per cent of manic patients recover on phenothiazine therapy in from several weeks to two months. The remaining 25 per cent of patients respond less satisfactorily to phenothiazines; if these patients are maintained on phenothiazines most of them recover in time, but their illnesses stretch out for several months or longer, and the span of time they require for recovery often approximates the time by which spontaneous recovery would occur. However, electroshock therapy leads to prompt recovery in well over half the patients who do not respond readily to phenothiazines.

The manic patient who has prominent delusions is more likely to need electroshock therapy than the patient who does not. The patient who was unresponsive to phenothiazine therapy and required electroshock for resolution of a previous manic disorder often needs it in any subsequent manic episodes. In my opinion, the manic patient who does not show significant improvement on three or four weeks of phenothiazine therapy may be considered for electroshock therapy. The patient who does not improve decisively after 5 or 6 weeks of phenothiazines should have electroshock therapy, since without it his illness will probably stretch out for a prolonged period. With intravenous fast-acting barbiturate anesthesia and succinylcholine muscle relaxation, the risks of electroshock therapy are negligible.

The course of electroshock therapy usually runs between 6 and 12 treatments, and the patient frequently recovers promptly with it. Phenothiazine therapy should be continued during the course of electroshock therapy, though at dosages reduced to about half the prior level of administration. A low maintenance dosage of the phenothiazine should be continued during the posthospitalization period. (The details of the administration of electroshock therapy are covered in Chapter 23.)

In my opinion, the small percentage of patients who do not recover on phenothiazine therapy or phenothiazine therapy combined with electroshock therapy, may be considered for lithium treatment. However, I feel that lithium treatment should be carried out in a hospital with twice weekly serum lithium evaluations, and the patient should be transferred to a phenothiazine drug for maintenance medication when he leaves the hospital. My hesitancy about lithium therapy is based on the good prognosis for a manic disorder to resolve spontaneously over a several-month period and the clear risks of lithium treatment.

Psychotherapy During the Convalescent and Posthospitalization Period

Psychiatrists differ in opinion about the usefulness of exploratory psychotherapy in manic patients in the posthospitalization period. Some psychiatrists feel that supportive counseling dealing with day-to-day decisions and careful supervision of the patient's gradual return to his usual activities is the advisable procedure. They point out that many manic patients are not motivated for more extensive interview work than this. Moreover, they feel that in facing the emotional conflicts that produced his illness the manic patient is prone to become upset again. Many psychiatrists feel that psychotherapy after a manic episode does not decrease the incidence of further manic or depressive episodes in later years.

About two thirds of manic patients are motivated for no more than supportive counseling and follow-up visits to regulate medication dosages. They feel well and see no need for more than this. After three or four months of such follow-up visits, their contact with the psychiatrist is terminated; those who continue for longer periods on phenothiazine medication to decrease the probability of a relapse remain in contact with the psychiatrist, though at more widely spaced intervals.

About one third of manic patients, however, are motivated, for exploratory psychotherapy in the posthospitalization period and can engage meaningfully in it; these patients should be given the opportunity of having such treatment. As a rule, the patients who engage in psychotherapy have persistent emotional discomforts after they emerge from their manic disorders. They often go through mild depressive periods with feelings of guilt and inadequacy, and they wish to explore the causes of these feelings in the interpersonal traumas of their early years and their more recent experiences. In other instances, the patients continue to have minor manic fluctuations in the posthospitalization period, which frighten them. They perceive that the underlying emotional problems that produced their manic illnesses yet persist within them, and they seek resolution of these problems to achieve greater emotional stability.

Such psychotherapy may last from a few months to a year or more, depending on the patient's motivation and his capacity to discuss significant emotional material. Many psychiatrists feel that such psychotherapy lessens the probability of further manic or depressive episodes in the patient's life and contributes to a more comfortable emotional adjustment in various areas of his interpersonal living. There are, however, no studies demonstrating conclusively that psychotherapy reduces the incidence of further psychotic episodes. Such demonstration would require a follow-up study lasting two or three decades involving statistically significant numbers of patients who received psychotherapy matched with an equal number who did not.

BIBLIOGRAPHY

Beigel, A., and Murphy, D. L.: Assessing clinical characteristics of the manic state. Am. J. Psychiatry, *128*:688, 1971.

Carlson, G. A., and Goodwin, F. K.: The stages of mania. Arch. Gen. Psychiatry, *28*:221, 1973.

Freeman, T.: Observations on mania. Int. J. Psychoanal., *52*: 479, 1971.

Janowsky, D. S., El-Youself, M., and Davis, J. M.: Interpersonal maneuvers of manic patients. Am. J. Psychiatry, *131*: 250, 1974.

Morgan, H. G.: The incidence of depressive symptoms during recovery from hypomania. Brit. J. Psychiatry, *120*:537, 1972.

Prien, R. F., Caffrey, E. M., and Klett, C. J.:

Comparison of lithium carbonate and chlorpromazine in the treatment of mania. Arch. Gen. Psychiatry, 26:146, 1972.

——: The phenomenology of mania. Arch. Gen. Psychiatry, 29:520, 1973.

Wadeson, H. S., and Fitzgerald R. G.: Marital relationship in manic-depressive illness. J. Nerv. Ment. Dis., 153:180, 1971.

Woodruff, R. A., Jr., Robins, L. N., Winokur, G., and Reich, T.: Manic depressive illness and social achievement. Acta Psychiat. Scand., 47:237, 1971.

17

Other Psychotic Disorders

In this chapter we shall discuss four groups of conditions related to psychotic disorders. Psychiatrists differ in opinion about whether these conditions merit separate classification in psychiatric thinking. Some psychiatrists feel that they should receive separate consideration because of their special clinical features and interpersonal causes, whereas many other psychiatrists feel they are merely variants of other psychotic processes. However, these topics continue to attract attention in psychiatric thinking and they should be laid before the reader.

The topics we shall discuss in this chapter are (1) paranoia, (2) involutional paranoid state, (3) psychoses of association, including *folie à deux* and others and (4) postpartum and postoperative psychoses. The first two of the these topics, paranoia and involutional paranoid state, are treated as individual diagnostic categories in the official psychiatric nomenclature; the official nomenclature also includes a category titled "psychosis of childbirth." The psychoses of association are not considered as a separate diagnostic category in the standard nomenclature, but they continue to attract the attention of psychiatric writers as a subject of special interest; the dominant features of psychoses of association usually are persecutory delusions.

PARANOIA AND INVOLUTIONAL PARANOID STATE

The person with paranoid feelings believes that people are hostile to him and are persecuting him; he may also feel that he is a superior person whose outstanding talents and achievements have aroused the envy of others. In various psychiatric illnesses, such as some severe depressions and some acute or chronic organic brain disorders, paranoid feelings constitute a minor feature overshadowed by other processes. However, in many instances the paranoid feelings of the patient form the dominant feature of his disturbance. In the official psychiatric nomenclature these illnesses are divided into four groups, depending on the degree of the patient's behavioral disorganization. These four paranoid categories, proceeding from the least severely disorganized to the most severely disorganized, are (1) *paranoid personality*, (2) *paranoia*, (3) *involutional paranoid state* and (4) *paranoid schizophrenia*.

Many psychiatrists feel that to break paranoid disturbances into these four categories is artificial and clinically unsound. However, these four categories are firmly entrenched in psychiatric terminology. *Paranoid personality* is customarily considered one of the personality disorders (and is covered in Chapter 12). (*Paranoid schizophrenia* is covered in Chapter 14 on schizophrenia.) In this chapter we shall cover *paranoia* and *involutional paranoid state*.

In my opinion, it is best to consider paranoia and involutional paranoid state merely as two variants of paranoid disorders, more severe than paranoid personality on the one hand and less severe than typical paranoid schizophrenia on the other. However, each paranoid patient should be understood in terms of the past and current interpersonal relationships that have produced his emotional problems, and his particular diagnostic label is of lesser importance.

Paranoia

Paranoia is a rare psychiatric disorder. However, the incidence of paranoia is greater than psychiatric statistics indicate, since patients with paranoia virtually never seek psychiatric consultation voluntarily and resist it obstinately. They feel they are not ill and that psychiatric consultation is merely a further device of their enemies to harm them and to defraud them by proving they are mentally incompetent. Moreover, the social behavior of the patient with paranoia usually does not deteriorate in such a way as to enable his relatives to force psychiatric consultation and care on him against his will.

A psychiatrist more frequently encounters paranoia in the relatives of patients than in patients themselves. Thus, persons with paranoia are encountered as marital partners who come for one or two consultations but will not come for further counseling about urgent marital problems. They are seen occasionally as parents of disturbed children or adolescents in child guidance clinics, and from time to time they are seen as relatives of hospitalized adult patients. However, the person with paranoia presents a striking clinical picture when he is seen, and he sometimes causes much trouble to his family and to other people whom he involves in his problems.

Clinical Characteristics of Paranoia. The patient with paranoia has an elaborate, closely thought out system of persecutory delusions, which may at first seem plausible to a casual observer. His system of persecutory delusions is based on a few fundamental paranoid assumptions. On top of these he builds a complex structure of convictions that various persons or organizations are scheming against him, persecuting him and attempting to defraud him. He advocates the truth of his beliefs with persuasive, detailed arguments, and often he can produce much data that at first glance seems to substantiate his claims. His paranoid system usually is of many years' duration by the time he comes in contact with a psychiatrist.

The patient with paranoia often talks about his "rights" and wants justice done to him. He may instigate lawsuits alleging stolen property, embezzled money, defrauded patent rights, systematic discriminatory practices, defamation of character and financial conspiracies against him. In some instances the patient seeks protection against his enemies or punishment of them for their unjust acts. The patient's paranoid system may have an obsessive quality that causes him to talk about it endlessly to his family and his acquaintances. In other instances the patient talks about it only when he finds a receptive listener or someone whom he feels can help him in resolving his grievances. Grandiose delusions occasionally become woven into the patient's paranoid system. He believes that he has extraordinary intellectual talents that his enemies are attempting to discredit, or that he has made brilliant technological discoveries that his persecutors are attempting to steal, or that he has an important social or religious mission that his defamers are trying to block.

The patient's system of paranoid delusions slowly becomes more extensive as the years roll by. New people are included in the conspiracy and the patient's list of grievances grows longer and more complicated. The patient becomes more insistent in his beliefs; he feels that people who do not accept his views are either callous to the sufferings of injured people or have secret sympathies with his enemies. He often feels that people who attempt to dissuade him from his beliefs are agents of his persecutors. He usually views any psychiatrists who see him as the misguided dupes of his enemies or their bribed servants. The patient with paranoia usually is not seen psychiatrically until he is in his late 30's or older, and by that time he frequently is leading a bitter, emotionally isolated life. He does not develop hallucinations, and he does not have the diffuse disturbances of thought association processes and emotional responsiveness that characterize schizophrenia.

The social and economic adjustment of the patient with paranoia often remains superficially intact. Usually he is a somewhat reserved person, but in some instances he covers his bitter suspiciousness with a genial mask. As one patient told me, "I laugh and joke along with them, but behind it all I'm watching them every minute." His paranoid ideas gradually poison his marital life and his other intimate relationships. The patient and his marital partner go through a period of arguments about his paranoid delusions, and the patient's insistence that if his marital partner does not share his views she must be sympathetic to his enemies often leads to estrangement and divorce. In other instances the patient's family become resigned to his paranoid ideas and they temporize with them from year to year. In rare instances the patient manages to implant his delusional ideas in a close member of his family, and a psychosis of association results (discussed later in this chapter).

As an example of a patient with paranoia, I recall the father of one of my patients. My patient was a 27-year-old single man who lived with his parents; this young man was hospitalized for a depression. I interviewed the father and mother several times in arranging for the patient's hospital care and in later outlining the patient's posthospitalization plans. In the course of these contacts the father talked to me extensively about his paranoid delusions, and I also learned a great deal more about the father in my subsequent psychotherapeutic sessions with the patient. The father at this time was a man of 66 and his paranoid system dated back at least three decades. In his early adult life he had become convinced that his fellow workers in a large railroad corporation did not like him because he was not a member of a well-known, semi-secret fraternal lodge organization. He gradually accumulated a long list of alleged grievances he felt substantiated his belief. He felt that his working hours, vacation schedules and job assignments were arranged to aggravate him and to try to force him out of the company. Despite the fact that he received periodic promotions, he was convinced that all his fellow workers and superiors were involved in a conspiracy to keep him from advancing to better jobs in the company. His paranoid system extended to involve the company's board of directors and president who were in a distant city and with whom he had no dealings.

He could marshal a large amount of data, replete with dates and figures, that seemed to support his contentions. He maintained that every person with whom he had contact in the company during the 35 years he worked for it was a willing member of the conspiracy against him. When his wife or children pointed out that only a very small percentage of the company employees and officials were members of the fraternal lodge that he claimed was persecuting him, he angrily insisted that those who were not open members of the lodge were "secret members" and that they kept their membership secret in order to persecute him more effectively. The patient's delusions never involved any persons except those who were associated with his work situation. He retired from the company at the age of 65 and received the customary recognition and honors for long service. He had always performed well in his work and talked about his paranoid delusions only to his immediate family. After retirement he dwelt upon the contention that the company's final act of persecution would be to defraud him of his pension. He had a large file of data he intended to use in a suit against the company as soon as his pension checks were discontinued. If his pension check arrived in the mail a few days late in any month, he interpreted this as the railroad's first step in agitating him, and he felt that such measures were carefully planned by the railroad's directors.

During the three decades or more in which this man had his paranoid delusions his marriage withstood the stresses produced by his psychotic disorder, and he reared four children. However, he had no friends and his family life was poisoned by his frequent talk about his delusions. Over the years the patient's wife sought relief by busying herself in social activities in church groups, and the patient's relationships with his children were cold and distant. His personality had a damaging effect on his children, one of whom was my patient and another of whom had marked personality problems.

Because of his ability to maintain his social and vocational adjustments despite his psychosis, a talented paranoiac occasionally reaches a high economic, professional or political position. For example, some psychiatrists feel that the available evidence indicates that Adolf Hitler may have suffered from paranoia. Also, there are elaborate psychiatric studies which were made on Rudolf Hess, the third highest man in Nazi Germany, during his long captivity in England during World War II; these studies indicate that he had either paranoia or paranoid schizophrenia. A talented paranoiac may have the tenacity and ability to suffer and drive toward a goal, that many healthy people lack; he drives on in the face of obstacles, disappointments and failures that would discourage a mentally healthy individual. An able paranoiac can be a formidable, and sometimes dangerous, person; I have seen several such individuals during my professional career.

Harry Stack Sullivan's Interpersonal Theories on the Causes of Paranoid Thinking and Feeling. Harry Stack Sullivan spent a large part of his early clinical career studying paranoid disorders. He felt that the various kinds of paranoid illnesses, including paranoia, were caused by three basic emotional and interpersonal processes.

He termed the first of these the "malevolent transformation of personality." During his childhood and early adolescence the future paranoid patient experiences pervasive emotional rejection and humiliation, which are particularly damaging since at those times his needs for tenderness, esteem and encouragement are acute. As a result, he develops (usually in ways of which he is not consciously aware) a feeling of diffuse hostility toward other people as a means of protecting himself against their rejection and scorn; it is as if he were saying, "I shall reject you and thrust you back before you reject and depreciate me." Thus, he gradually develops the ingrained, scarcely conscious view that all interpersonal relationships are hostile, competitive and malicious, and he feels that aloofness and alertness to defend himself against attack constitute the only reasonable attitudes.

Moreover, by his aloofness and his cautious and ever-ready state of defensive hostility, the future paranoid person cuts himself off from healthy, close interpersonal experiences in late childhood and adolescence which might tend to correct his developing paranoid personality warp. Hence, his paranoid processes of feeling and thinking become steadily more ingrained.

This deeply ingrained view of the world as threatening and malicious is what constitutes the "malevolent transformation of the personality." Depending on variables that differ much from one person to another, this basic malevolent personality transformation leads eventually to one of the four kinds of paranoid clinical disorders—paranoid personality disorder (Chapter 12), paranoid schizophrenia (Chapter 14), paranoia, or involutional paranoid state (this chapter).

The nature of the paranoid process also explains why attempts at psychotherapy are so difficult and so often fruitless; paranoia and paranoid personality are very difficult to treat, and paranoid schizophrenia and involutional paranoid state respond much more readily to antipsychotic medication (with electroshock in occasional, selected cases) than to psychotherapy. Any attempts to breach the patient's defenses against interpersonal closeness and a world which he views as deceptive, malicious and hostile, mobilize marked anxiety in him. Closeness to the therapist, or to anyone, threatens the ingrained convictions on which the patient has built his way of life, even though it is a sick one.

The second fundamental process that occurs in a paranoid person is what Sullivan calls a "massive transfer of blame." Because of the pervasive emotional rejection and depreciation which he experienced during his formative years, the paranoid patient has a debased view of himself (though often he is not consciously aware of it) and much rage about how he was treated. In ways that are beyond his scope of awareness, he resolves this turmoil by relegating the blame for these things to others. He says, as it were, "It is not I, but they, who are worthless and hostile, and they will try to expoit or destroy me if I do not always keep my guard alertly up against them." Thus, at the expense of developing paranoid ideas, he resolves his own inner feelings, and the blame for them, by transferring them to people in his environment.

The third thing that occurs in the paranoid person, from Sullivan's point of view, is the personification in other people of the horror, disgust, guilt and terror which the patient feels within himself. In a sense, he feels that these unacceptable, threatening forces take flesh in the form of the people around him.

He rids himself of these turbulent feelings by personifying them in others, saying, as it were, "They are horrible, disgusting, guilty and terror-inspiring, and I fear them for these qualities and what they may try to do against me because of them."

Other Interpretations of the Causes of Paranoid Thinking and Feeling. According to other psychiatric theories, paranoid ideas arise when a person *projects* onto other people unacceptable feelings he has within himself (this concept obviously is related to aspects of Sullivan's viewpoints, but is expressed with somewhat different terms and emphases). The paranoid individual has strong feelings of smoldering hostility, but he cannot come to grips with them. However, these powerful feelings require some kind of release, and the patient therefore *projects* them outward onto other people; he then perceives in others the hostile feelings that actually lurk within himself. He feels that other people hate him and wish to injure him. The patient may extend the process one step further and feel that his persecutors hate him because he has superior abilities and achievements that they envy; in this way a thread of grandiose delusions is woven into his paranoid process, buttressing his paranoid convictions and also reassuring him of his worth and importance. This process is called *projection*, and many psychiatrists feel that it occurs in all types of paranoid illnesses. The patient with paranoia differs from patients with other types of paranoid disorders only in the relative coherence and closely thought out nature of his paranoid system.

Freudian-psychoanalytic theory suggests that unconscious homosexual feelings play a major role in all types of paranoid disorders. In his oft-cited Schreber case, Freud proposed that the patient with paranoid delusions has an upsurge of latent homosexual urges which he cannot consciously acknowledge and which he drastically must banish from his awareness. He avoids facing his latent homosexual attraction for other persons by erecting a delusional system of mutual hatred between himself and them. It is as if the patient were saying unconsciously, "I do not love them. I hate them. By the intensity of my hatred I prove that I have no love for them or attraction for them. But, my hatred of them is justified, because they hate me. Their hatred of me is proved by the ways in which they persecute me." In this way, the patient's paranoid disorder creates a gulf between him and the people to whom he might feel homosexually attracted if this gulf did not exist, and he defends himself against coming to grips with strong unconscious homosexual stirrings within him. The psychiatrists who advocate this theory point out that male patients with paranoid disorders more often suspect persons of their own sex as their persecutors. However, many other psychiatrists, including myself, feel that Sullivan's theories more adequately explain clinical paranoid phenomena and, moreover, can be more easily verified by study of patients' past and present interpersonal relationships.

Most psychiatrists agree that a patient with well-established paranoia does not respond to any form of psychiatric treatment. The patient with a paranoid personality disorder (discussed in Chapter 12) is similarly resistant to treatment in most cases. However, patients with paranoid schizophrenia (discussed in Chapter 14) and involutional paranoid state (discussed in the following section of this chapter) have good prognoses in the vast majority of cases when treated with reasonable promptness.

Involutional Paranoid State

The official nomenclature of psychiatric diagnoses contains a category titled involutional paranoid state, with the term involutional paraphrenia as a synonym of it. The patient with an involutional paranoid state is described as a woman in the menopausal period who has persecutory delusions but lacks the fragmentation of thought processes, auditory or visual hallucinations, and flatness or inappropriateness of affect which would indicate that she is suffering from a schizophrenic illness.

Most American psychiatrists have marked objections to this diagnostic concept, and it is little used in day-to-day clinical practice. It is a holdover from the idea that the hormonal changes of the menopausal period play a role in the precipitation of emotional disorders in this age group, a view long ago abandoned in American psychiatry. (As pointed out in

Chapter 15 in our discussion of severe depressions during the involutional period), the many interpersonal stresses of middle age—exit of the patient's children from the home, the deaths of one or both of the patient's parents, the end of childbearing capacity, and many others—may play roles in precipitating emotional disturbances during this age span, but it is doubtful that hormonal changes have any importance. It is not the cessation of menses and the minor physical discomforts of middle age that may upset a woman, but rather the interpretation that she puts on them, such as fears of loss of feminity and approaching old age.

Moreover (as pointed out in Chapter 12), the menopausal period usually is described as extending, in various women, from 40 to 60, a span that covers about 40 per cent of the adult life of a woman. Most psychiatrists feel that the incidence of paranoid disorders in this age group is no greater than would be expected in so broad an age bracket. They feel, moreover, that all the paranoid disorders of this age period can be classified within the other three types of paranoid disorders—paranoid personality disorder (Chapter 12), paranoid schizophrenia (Chapter 14) and paranoia (this chapter)—and that the creation of a special category for paranoid illnesses in middle-aged women is both unnecessary and clinically unsound. I agree with this point of view.

It is difficult to give a clear picture of the clinical characteristics, course, interpersonal causes and treatment of the so-called involutional paranoid state, since various psychiatric writers differ so much in describing the attributes of this syndrome. In my opinion, most of the women to whom this diagnosis is given are suffering from late-developing paranoid schizophrenic illnesses (and the treatment is that outlined in Chapter 14 on schizophrenia). The remaining number of women to whom this diagnosis is given have, in my opinion, either paranoid personality disorders or paranoia which have long been present but which become somewhat more prominent and are first diagnosed after the age of 40.

PSYCHOSES OF ASSOCIATION

In a psychosis of association two persons who live intimately with each other develop similar psychoses with similar delusions at the same time. The classical psychiatric term for the most common form of this condition is *folie à deux*, but the term "psychosis of association" is preferable. Most psychoses of association involve paranoid delusions.

Psychoses of association do not constitute a separate diagnostic category, since most persons involved in them are suffering from paranoid schizophrenia or schizoaffective schizophrenia. However, psychoses of association are common enough to merit discussion in their own right as problems occasionally encountered in clinical practice. They are more common than is generally appreciated. If cases are carefully investigated, approximately 1.7 per cent of state hospital admissions involve psychoses of association. In my experience, if patients with organic brain disorders are excluded from the total number of psychotic patients seen, the incidence of psychosis of association runs about 2 per cent of all psychotic patients encountered in clinical practice.

The two persons involved in a psychosis of association are members of the same immediate family, and they have lived closely together for many years. Psychoses of association most commonly involve two sisters or a mother and her adolescent or adult child. However, psychoses of association also may involve a husband and his wife, a father and his daughter, or other family combinations. One of the involved persons is dominant and he emotionally controls the other who is dependent and passive. The dominant person becomes psychotic first, and his psychosis acts as a strong precipitating factor in initiating a similar psychosis with similar delusions in the dependent, passive person. The psychotic behavior and delusional talk of the dominant person slowly weaken the dependent person's grasp on reality and he is drawn into a similar psychotic illness. As mentioned above, the most common type of illness involved in psychoses of association is paranoid schizophrenia; delusions of persecution usually are present, and grandiose delusions, especially of religious eminence and power, also occur in some instances.

Both the involved persons usually have a history of much emotional trauma in childhood which left them predisposed to develop schizophrenic illnesses when they encountered interpersonal stresses in their adult years. In the case of a psychosis of association in two sisters or in a brother and sister, both persons were reared in the same unhealthy family environment during childhood and adolescence. In the case of a parent and child combination, the personality problems of the parent led to a traumatic parent-child relationship during the child's formative years that made the child predisposed to schizophrenia in later years. In most instances the prepsychotic personalities of both persons were characterized by seclusiveness and other schizoid personality features. When a husband and wife are involved in a psychosis of association, they usually have long lived a socially isolated life and both had schizoid personality structures prior to their marriage. The interpersonal precipitants in adult life of the psychosis of the dominant person usually lie outside the family circle, but the immediate precipitant of the psychosis of the dependent person is the stress of intimate living with the dominant psychotic person.

In a psychosis of association, the psychosis of the dependent person usually is more easily cured than the psychosis of the dominant person. When the dependent person is removed from contact with the dominant person and receives hospital treatment, he usually recovers in from a few weeks to two months. The prognosis of the dominant person usually is somewhat less favorable; however, he also recovers with hospital treatment in most cases, though his hospitalization often is more prolonged. However, in my experience the relapse rate of one or both of the patients is significant if they return to living with each other. The treatment, of course, is the same as is outlined elsewhere for the type of psychosis the patients have. Although in most instances they suffer from paranoid schizophrenia, I have seen manic psychoses and severe depressions occur as psychoses of association.

POSTPARTUM AND POSTOPERATIVE PSYCHOSES

An experience that clouds the patient's awareness of his environment may precipitate a psychotic episode or a severe neurotic disorder. Thus, undergoing an anesthesia for a surgical operation or an obstetrical delivery, in combination with the emotional stresses accompanying these procedures, may weaken the integrity of the patient's already fragile personality structure. Many postpartum psychoses and postoperative psychoses are precipitated by these factors.

Postpartum and postoperative psychoses formerly were considered as special diagnostic categories. Today most psychiatrists feel that psychiatric disorders that occur in the postpartum or postoperative period do not differ significantly from disorders precipitated by other stresses. Thus, a postpartum psychiatric disorder is precipitated by the patient's emotional turmoil and conflictual feelings over giving birth to a child, in association with the experience of undergoing an obstetrical delivery and its anesthesia. Postpartum and postoperative syndromes caused by organic brain injury during anesthesia and surgery are now rare due to advances in these fields; the one general exception to this is the field of open heart surgery, which sometimes submits the patient to severe physical stress, temporary oxygen deprivation and a difficult postoperative period. Thus, the precipitating causes of almost all postpartum and postoperative psychoses are to be sought in discovering what childbirth or surgical operation means to the patient emotionally. Somewhat more than half of all postpartum and postoperative psychiatric disorders are schizophrenic illnesses. Depressions and severe neuroses of various kinds rank second. Occasionally, manic psychoses and other psychiatric disorders occur in the postpartum and postoperative period.

Postpartum Psychoses. A postpartum psychosis occurs about once in every 700 deliveries, and the occurrence of one postpartum psychosis does not raise the probability that a woman will have similar problems after subsequent deliveries. The experience of having the child and the emotional conflicts this arouses in the mother precipitate the psychosis; past and current interpersonal traumas make her vulnerable to an emotional disorder in the postpartum period. For example, the patient may have much resentment about having a baby at this particular time, often coupled with strong guilt feelings about her resentment, and these scarcely conscious, unacceptable feelings may threaten to break into her awareness. In other cases, the mother feels depressed and overwhelmed about the pregnancy and the problems of coping with still another child, but her depressiveness does not reach its full force until after delivery. In some cases an emotionally immature, or self-centered, or insecure mother may feel unable to assume the burdens of another child, and she may decompensate into a neurotic state, such as an anxiety neurosis or an obsessive disorder. In occasional cases she flees her emotional turmoil into the hollow gaiety and helter-skelter overactivity of a manic disorder.

The interpersonal causes, past and present, of a postpartum psychiatric disorder are illustrated by a 27-year-old patient of mine. She was a passive, anxious woman with strong feelings of inadequacy and worthlessness, camouflaged by a habitual smile and marked religious devoutness. She had been reared by a socially aspiring mother who set stern goals for her and gave her little love, and a father who treated her similarly but, because of absorption in his profession, gave her little time and attention. At 21 her mother steered her into a marriage with a man whom the mother considered desirable, a businessman 10 years older than the patient. Once in the marriage, the patient discovered that she had in her marriage much the same interpersonal relationship she had had with her parents. Her husband was a domineering, cold, ambitious man who gave her little warmth and support. The same passivity which allowed her mother to push her into the marriage locked her into it; she lacked the assertiveness and self-confidence to free herself of it. Moreover, she felt that her own inadequacies and unworthiness were the sources of her marital unhappiness, just as she felt they had caused her parents to reject her and depreciate her.

She had two children and coped with them fairly well, but when she was pregnant with her third child in the sixth year of her marriage she became visibly anxious and depressed as the time for delivery approached. In ways she could not clearly become aware of, she felt that each child nailed her more firmly into a marriage that met none of her emotional needs. Three days after delivery she abruptly developed a florid schizoaffective schizophrenic psychosis with religiously tinged auditory hallucinations and grandiose delusions that her baby was a divine messenger with a supernatural mission. She alternated between manic elation and moaning despair. With hospital treatment she recovered in six weeks and made much progress in a year of psychotherapy after she left the hospital. Her husband refused to participate in either individual or group psychotherapy. When I last saw her she was doing well emotionally, but the future of her marriage was uncertain and she was determined to have no further children.

Postoperative Psychoses. Postoperative psychoses may occur after any kind of surgical procedure, especially those involving a general anesthesia; however, they are somewhat more frequent after certain kinds of operations.

Brief psychotic episodes after open heart surgery are fairly common, but these are organic brain syndromes caused by the physical stress, anoxia and hemodynamic adjustments of the operation (this subject is covered in Chapter 19 on organic brain disorders). Similarly, the edema, bruising and tearing of brain tissue during brain surgery may precipitate organic brain syndromes, with confusion, memory loss, disorientation, hallucinations and panic; the length of these psychoses varies with the extent and locality of the brain trauma (these conditions are also covered in Chapter 19).

However, in other instances postoperative psychoses are caused by emotional and interpersonal stresses. It is somewhat common, for example, that elderly patients who temporarily have poor vision after cataract removals, or other operations, become panicky, agitated, disoriented and paranoid for several days or more if they are not properly informed before the operation and do not have a reassuring relative constantly at the bedside. For this reason, bilateral, simultaneous eye operations, with subsequent bandaging or temporary poor vision, are somewhat risky in old people, especially if they are inclined to slight confusion because of minimal senile brain changes and will become further confused when they are deprived of clear vision in an unfamiliar hospital setting. Also, operations on the lower urogenital tract, such as cystoscopies and transurethral prostatectomies, may precipitate agitated, paranoid psychotic states; they usually last only a few days, but may last much longer. I also have seen paranoid and catatonic schizophrenic illnesses begin in young adults after cystoscopies and other lower urogenital tract procedures. Presumably, operations on the genitals and adjacent areas raise particular anxiety. I also have seen several postoperative psychoses after removals of lumbar discs with subsequent lumbar fusions, but I feel these were borderline psychotic patients before the operations; emotional factors probably played a large part in their low back pain, superimposed on their disc problems.

It is sometimes said that plastic surgical operations on the face and other exposed body parts have a higher incidence of postoperative psychiatric disorders than surgical procedures in general, but I have been surprised to see the improvement in interpersonal comfort and social ease which some patients have after the removal of facial or limb disfigurements. Of course, persons with delusional complaints, such as the belief that a few minor acne scars are causing people in the street to talk about them, should not be operated on. However, when such persons are carefully screened out by inquiring carefully why they want plastic surgery, plastic surgical procedures may give patients greater emotional benefits than might be expected.

Most postoperative psychoses are schizophrenic disorders or agitated depressions (we shall discuss the other general category of postoperative psychoses, delirious organic brain states, in Chapter 19). Manic disorders after surgical procedures are less common. In general, postoperative psychoses have good prognoses if the patient's preoperative adjustment was reasonably sound, and their treatment is that of the particular type of psychosis involved. Postoperative psychoses could probably be somewhat reduced in frequency if hospital routines, anesthetic experiences and postoperative sensations were more carefully explained to patients beforehand, particularly before those operations which have a somewhat greater than average tendency to precipitate emotional disturbances.

BIBLIOGRAPHY

Freedman, N., et al.: On the modification of paranoid symptomatology. J. Nerv. Ment. Dis., *150*:68, 1970.

Freud, S.: Chapter on a case of paranoia, p. 387. Collected Papers, vol. 3. London, Hogarth Press, 1953.

Fried, Y.: Thinking in paranoia. Brit. J. Med. Psychol., *46*: 347, 1973.

Grunebaum, H., and Perlman, M. S.: Paranoia and naivete. Arch. Gen. Psychiatry, *28*:30, 1973.

Hoaken, P. C. S.: Paranoid-depressive relationship. Can. Psychiat. Assoc. J., *18*:427, 1973.

Lasegue, C., and Falret, J.: Folie à duex (Trans. by R. Michaud). Am. J. Psychiatry (Suppl.), *121*: Oct. 1964.

McNiel, J. M., Verwoerdt, A., and Peak, D.: Folie à deux in the aged. J. Amer. Geriatr. Soc., *20*:316, 1972.

More, R. M.: Postoperative delirium: a syndrome of multiple causation. Psychosomatics, *11*:164, 1970.

Rosenwald, G. C., and Stonehill, M.: Early and late postpartum illness. Psychosom. Med., *34*:129, 1972.

Sullivan, H. S.: Clinical Stuides in Psychiatry. Chapter on the paranoid dynamism, p. 145. New York, W. W. Norton. 1956.

Swanson, D. W., Bohnert, P. J., and Smith, J. A.: The Paranoid. Boston, Little Brown, 1970.

Wilson, J. E., Barglow, P., and Shipman, W.: The prognosis of postpartum mental illness. Compr. Psychiatry, *13*:305, 1972.

Part Four

Psychiatric Disturbances Caused by Organic Brain Disorders

The organic brain disorders are disturbances of brain structure or physiology that produce abnormalities in emotional functioning, thinking and interpersonal behavior. For the sake of convenience, we shall consider the organic brain disorders in two chapters. In Chapter 18 we shall cover the four most common categories of organic brain disturbances, which account for 75 per cent, or more, of all organic brain syndromes seen in clinical practice; they are the organic brain disorders associated with (1) cerebral arteriosclerosis and senile brain degeneration, (2) head trauma, (3) brain damage which occurred in the prenatal, the natal or the postnatal period, and (4) chronic alcoholism.

In Chapter 19 we shall discuss all the other types of organic brain disorders; they are the organic brain disturbances associated with (1) intoxication by drugs and chemicals, (2) circulatory disturbances, such as congestive heart failure, (3) intracranial neoplasms, (4) metabolic disturbances, such as uremia and hepatic coma, (5) intracranial infections, such as meningitis and encephalitis, (6) syphilis of the central nervous system, (7) degenerative central nervous system diseases, such as multiple sclerosis and Huntington's chorea, (8) convulsive disorders, and (9) severe general infections, especially with high fever and prostration.

18

The Common Organic Brain Disorders

An organic brain disorder is a psychiatric state caused by physiologic or anatomic insult to brain tissue. The current official nomenclature divides organic brain disorders into *psychotic* and *non-psychotic*; a psychosis is defined as a state in which the patient's capacity to meet the usual demands of life is impaired by a serious distortion in his contact with reality. However, this distinction is very difficult to apply in many cases, for many patients fluctuate between psychotic and non-psychotic states from one day to the next, or even from one hour to the next.

In a previous standard nomenclature organic brain syndromes were divided into *acute* and *chronic*; in an acute organic brain disorder the patient recovered, whereas in a chronic one he had persistent brain damage and permanent deterioration of his emotional and intellectual functioning. This system also was difficult to apply in many cases; the diagnosis often could be made only in retrospect when it became clear after many weeks or months whether the patient would recover.

In this book we shall divide the organic brain disorders according to their pathological causes and clinical characteristics. Thus, in this current chapter we shall discuss organic brain disorders caused by (1) cerebral arteriosclerosis and senile brain degeneration, (2) head trauma, (3) brain damage in the prenatal, the natal and the postnatal periods, and (4) chronic alcoholism. These four categories encompass 75 per cent, or more, of all patients seen with organic brain disorders in day-to-day clinical practice. (In Chapter 19 we shall cover all other causes of organic brain disorders, which, though more numerous in their kinds of pathology and clinical characteristics, account for less than 25 per cent of patients with organic brain disturbances.)

THE BASIC SYMPTOMS IN ORGANIC BRAIN DISORDERS

Before considering the various kinds of organic brain disorders, we shall discuss the basic symptoms that occur in organic brain disturbances. This discussion applies to all the organic brain syndromes we shall cover (both in this chapter and in Chapter 19). Any individual patient may have only a few of these basic symptoms, or he may have all of them, but these symptoms trace the general clinical features of organic brain disorders.

The symptoms that occur in an organic brain disorder include (1) partially impaired consciousness or loss of consciousness, (2) memory loss, (3) disorientation, (4) impaired judgement, (5) impairment of intellectual functions such as general knowledge, comprehension and learned skills, (6) poor control of emotions, often accompanied by inappropriate emotional responses, much anxiety, and at times panic, (7) changes in the patient's usual personality characteristics and (8) hallucinations and delusions.

The nature and severity of these symptoms, and the particular ones the patient has, depend on the intensity of the insult to the brain, its location, and the patient's underlying personality. An organic brain disorder may be so mild as to be barely noticeable or it may produce a severe disturbance in the patient's behavior and emotional functioning.

Impairment of Consciousness. The impairment of consciousness in a patient with an organic brain disorder may consist only of a slight loss of alert understanding of the meaning of events in his environment and a subtle decrease in his sensitivity to the feelings of other people and the niceties of interpersonal relationships. In other cases he has minor or major clouding of consciousness, with gross impairment in his contact with all aspects of his environment. It may vary from confusion to coma, and its degree may fluctuate markedly as the patient struggles to regain contact with his surroundings.

Memory Loss. If a patient has memory loss in an organic brain disorder it tends to be more marked for recent events than for events of the distant past. For example, the patient may be able to remember the names and faces of his family and old friends, but he cannot remember events of the preceding day or tell how he got to the hospital. In severe organic brain disorders with permanent brain damage the patient may remember the details of a neighborhood incident that happened 30 years ago, but cannot recall things that have occurred in recent years. The memory defects often are spotty, with mixtures of recent and distant events being forgotten. However, the general trend is an inability to remember recent things with better preservation of distant memory. In some types of organic brain disorders, such as those caused by cerebral arteriosclerosis and senile brain degeneration, memory loss may be the predominant symptom, whereas in others, such as those caused by viral encephalitis, there may be no clinically discernible loss of memory.

Disorientation. The patient with an organic brain disorder often is disoriented in time and place; occasionally he also is disoriented as to person and does not know who he is. The degree of disorientation varies much from one patient to another, and may also vary much from day to day or from hour to hour as he struggles to establish firmer contacts with his environment.

To a large extent disorientation is secondary to memory defects. The patient cannot remember the month or year. He usually places the time at some point in the past, often many years in the past. He cannot remember the season and often makes a vague guess based on the season that the weather seems to indicate. Frequently, he cannot tell what time of day it is.

The patient with an organic brain disorder may be disoriented in place. He cannot tell what kind of building he is in or what its name is. He may guess vaguely that he is in a hospital or a doctor's office, but he does not know what hospital or what doctor's office. He may be unable to say what city he is in. In severe disorders the patient may not know who he is, or what his name and occupation are.

Sometimes the patient with an organic brain disorder *confabulates*. He attempts to cover up his defects in memory and orientation with elaborate stories. The patient who cannot remember the events of recent days may tell a long story of fictitious social and vocational activities of the preceding day. He forgets it soon after he tells it and may tell another story if asked the same question. A confabulating patient with an organic brain disorder occasionally may deceive an examiner who does not know the facts about his activities, and it may require correlative interviewing of the relatives before the full extent of his memory and orientation defects is evident.

Impaired Judgement. The patient with an organic brain disorder has impaired judgement and he may act in unwise and inappropriate ways. He may not understand that he is sick or why he is in a hospital. He cannot form sound ideas about what is going on around him and what his attitudes and actions should be. He may make poor decisions in vocational and economic activities, and he loses appreciation for the civilities and proprieties of life. His cleanliness and grooming deteriorate and he becomes shabby, unshaven and unkempt. Crude sexual advances and obscene behavior may occur. If the organic brain disorder is not recognized promptly, the patient's behavior may result in embarrassment and legal difficulties for him and his family.

Impairment of Intellectual Functions. The patient with an organic brain disorder is distractible and his span of attention is short. He forgets from moment to moment the details of what he is doing, and his attention wanders. He is bewildered by new things, which he struggles to comprehend. He often has defects of intellectual functioning such as general knowledge, learning and comprehension. His arithmetical skills and manual skills may be partially impaired. His fund of information, particularly for recent events, becomes impoverished. His attention becomes constricted to himself and the familiar things on which he still has a grasp.

Poor Control of Emotions. The person with an organic brain syndrome is emotionally labile. His mood changes abruptly with little provocation. He may suddenly become frightened or belligerent without apparent reason. His response to a minor irritation may be furious rage, or he may react with silly giggling and uncontrolled hilarity to mildly amusing occurrences. Some types of organic brain disorders are characterized by a persistent euphoria, but in many other kinds the patient may become depressed as he dimly perceives that he is losing his intellectual alertness. States of bewildered, desperate panic are common in some forms of organic brain disease. This unpredictability of mood makes the patient unreliable, and in occasional cases he may be dangerous to himself or others.

Personality Changes. The previous personality characteristics of the patient often become markedly accentuated during an organic brain disorder. A domineering person becomes tyrannical and a shy person becomes seclusive. Previously controlled aggressiveness may erupt in angry tirades or combativeness. In an organic brain disorder, underlying fears, daydreams and personality problems are unleashed by impaired cerebral control of his emotional and intellectual functions. His underlying personality gives strong coloring to the kinds of behavioral changes he has in his acute organic brain disorder. The personality of the patient often is more important in determining the clinical picture than the specific agent causing the disorder. Moreover, as Harry Stack Sullivan pointed out, the personality changes of the patient with organic brain dysfunction are complicated by the reactions of other people toward him. They become overprotective, or irritable, or frightened, or puzzled because of the patient's attitudes and actions, and these reactions further alter his interpersonal functioning and emotional adjustment; this is particularly so in patients with cerebral arteriosclerosis and senile brain degeneration, whose day-to-day adjustment is much affected by the attitudes and actions of their families and other close persons.

Hallucinations and Delusions. The incidence of hallucinations and delusions varies much with the nature of the patient's organic brain disorder. Thus, the patient with delirium tremens often has hallucinations and delusions, whereas the patient who sustained brain damage in the prenatal, natal or postnatal periods rarely has them. In general, hallucinations occur most often in acute, fulminating organic brain disorders, as in delirium trements, syndromes due to recent head trauma, intoxication with drugs and chemicals, and others. Hallucinations are uncommon in long-standing organic brain disorders, as in advanced cases of cerebral arteriosclerosis and senile brain degeneration. Delusions occur in only a minority of patients with brain damage, but they may occur in both acute and long-standing syndromes.

When hallucinations occur they usually are visual, though sometimes they are auditory; olfactory, gustatory and tactile hallucinations are rare. The patient often sees insects, reptiles, other small animals, people and cartoon figures. He may be puzzled or frightened by his hallucinations, or he may accept them in a matter-of-fact way. He may pick at his bedclothes as he grasps at hallucinated insects or blotches of dirt. The patient often has illusions, especially at night; for example, he may think that the shadow cast by an open door is a person or that a belt lying upon a chair is a snake. Persecutory delusions may occur in some kinds of organic brain disorders, and the patient may hide or flee to avoid his enemies. Grandiose delusions may occur, but they are less common than persecutory ones.

As mentioned above, the incidence and severity of these eight basic symptoms of organic brain disorders vary immensely from patient to patient, and an organic brain disturbance may be so mild that it is scarcely apparent or so severe that the patient is completely out of contact with his environment. The clinical picture is also influenced by the etiologic process, the areas of the brain involved, the patient's premorbid personality, the patient's age at the time the brain disorder began, and the reactions of other people to him.

The age of the patient at the time his brain damage occurs is important; brain damage in the prenatal, natal or postnatal periods has very different effects on the intellectual, emotional and interpersonal adjustment of the person than brain damage in adolescence, adulthood or old age. The patient's interpersonal environment also has marked effects on his total adjustment. For example, the brain-damaged child who is reared by irritable, negligent parents becomes a much different person than the brain-damaged child who receives conscientious, affectionate care. The elderly person with senile degeneration and cerebral arteriosclerosis who is calm and content in his long-term home becomes frightened and belligerent in a new environment which he cannot understand and whose details he cannot master.

In managing a patient with an organic brain disorder, the physician does not treat a diseased brain; he treats a person who is struggling to make the best possible interpersonal adjustment despite a certain amount of brain damage or temporarily impaired brain physiology. This person has his potentialities as well as his limitations. The interpersonal aspects of the patient's management often are more important than medications and other treatments designed to affect his brain functioning.

The number of patients with organic brain disorders has increased in recent decades. Despite a marked decrease in the number of patients with such disorders as central nervous system syphilis and bacterial infections, the total number of patients with brain damage is steadily increasing. This increase is due to (1) the much larger number of persons who live into old age and develop organic brain disorders due to senile brain degeneration and cerebral arteriosclerosis, (2) the increased percentage of children with chronic brain damage that occurred in the prenatal, natal and postnatal periods who survive the infections and nutritional difficulties of infancy and childhood and live into adolescence and adulthood, and (3) the increased frequency of head injuries due to automobile accidents, motorcycle accidents, athletic mishaps, industrial hazards and other causes.

ORGANIC BRAIN DISORDERS CAUSED BY CEREBRAL ARTERIOSCLEROSIS AND SENILE BRAIN DEGENERATION

The term cerebral arteriosclerosis is loosely used in psychiatry to designate degenerative cerebrovascular disease of the brain in aged patients. As the arteries narrow, the blood supply to the parenchymal cells of the brain is cut down. Degeneration of cells begins and thromboses of small or major vessels may occur. Discrete thromboses of terminal arterioles supplying the cerebral cortex is an important contributant to the clinical picture of organic brain disease due to cerebral arteriosclerosis. There may or may not be thrombosis of large blood vessels with resultant hemiplegia, aphasia and other neurological disturbances.

The term senile brain degeneration (or senile dementia) is employed in psychiatry to designate organic brain disorders in aged persons caused by gradual biological degeneration of cerebral cortical cells, which presumably is a function of old age and whose causes are not well understood. The progress of symptoms is gradual, and sudden major changes do not occur, as may happen in cerebral arteriosclerosis when a major vessel abruptly becomes thrombosed.

In day-to-day practice most psychiatrists do not attempt to distinguish clinically from each other these two organic brain processes in aged persons; most psychiatrists refer to them simply as organic brain disorders caused by senile degeneration and cerebral arteriosclerosis. In many cases both senile degenerative and cerebral arteriosclerotic processes are present, and the clinical symptoms of these two processes are so similar that distinction of one from the other on the basis of the patient's mental and physical findings is usually speculative. A definitive statement on the relative importance of senile degenerative factors and arteriosclerotic changes in an elderly person with an organic brain disorder can be made only by histological examination of his brain after death.

Certain features, which we shall discuss in

more detail later, incline the clinician to feel that one or the other of the two pathologic processes is predominant. For example, a slow, insidious organic brain picture in an elderly person who does not have clear signs of major cerebral thromboses and who has little evidence of arteriosclerosis of the peripheral vessels may be interpreted as indicating that the main pathologic process is senile degeneration of cortical cells. On the other hand, the presence of neurological signs of cerebral thromboses, such as hemiplegias or aphasias of abrupt onset, and clinical evidence of arteriosclerosis of peripheral vessels and retinal vessels inclines the clinician to believe that cerebral arteriosclerosis is the major process. However, such signs are, at best, approximate guides and do not rule out the possibility that both pathological processes are present in the patient. Moreover, some pathologists and clinicians feel that senile degeneration is to a large extent secondary to impaired vascular supply and that the two processes thus are intricately interwoven. Hence, in our coverage of organic brain damage in elderly patients we shall deal with both these processes in one general discussion, and we shall point out any pathological or clinical differences as we proceed.

Brain Pathology

In cerebral atherosclerosis lipid substances gradually accumulate at many points in the subintima of arteries; the lipid deposition is followed by proliferation of the intima and the surrounding connective tissue. A plaque is formed and it protrudes into the lumen of the vessel. Subintimal hemorrhage or necrosis with subsequent fibrosis and calcification may occur in the region of the plaque. Arteries may be narrowed or completely occluded depending on the sizes and locations of the atheromatous lesions. Reduction of blood flow to the cerebral cortex leads to degeneration and disappearance of cortical cells. Occlusion of a major cerebral vessel causes gross infarction. In advanced cases the convolutions of the brain are smaller and the sulci are wider, and gross atrophy is present.

In senile brain degeneration there is extensive disintegration and disappearance of cerebral cortical cells. Nerve fibers decrease in proportion to the number of cortical cells destroyed. Both the cortical gray matter and the white matter are thin, and the convolutions of the brain are grossly shrunken.

The degree of destruction of brain tissue in both cerebral arteriosclerosis and senile brain degeneration is not always proportionate to the degree of psychiatric disability in the patient. For example, a patient who at autopsy shows much loss of brain tissue may have had little clinical evidence of organic brain damage during his life. On the other hand, the patient who during life had marked symptoms of senile brain degeneration and cerebral arteriosclerosis may show only mild or moderate brain pathology at autopsy. These facts emphasize that the clinical picture of cerebral arteriosclerosis and senile brain degeneration is produced by an intricate interlacing of the patient's basic personality, his interpersonal adjustment in old age and his brain pathology. Psychiatrists have long observed that the patient with good interpersonal relationships, emotionally satisfying activities and a sound basic personality structure tends to withstand the effects of the organic brain deterioration of age much better than the emotionally unstable person with a barren interpersonal life.

Clinical Characteristics

One of the earliest signs of senile and arteriosclerotic brain damage is the patient's inability to remember the names of new acquaintances and new facts. The patient gropes unsuccessfully for the name of a new acquaintance, calls him by an incorrect name, and then apologizes for his confusion. I recall a clergyman who retired from foreign missionary work in his early 60's and became the chaplain of a small liberal arts college; the earliest sign of what proved to be progressive brain damage was his inability to remember well the names and faces of the students and faculty members of the college. The patient may remain at this level of memory difficulty for months, or years, or decades without further memory impairment. Some elderly people never develop further memory impairment than this type of forgetfulness.

In other instances, the patient's memory loss slowly grows worse. His memory loss is more severe for events of recent months and years, and he talks more about events in his early adult years, which he remembers better. He often develops the rambling garrulousness of elderly people who relate in minute detail the events of vocational activities, friendships, trips, weddings, child rearing experiences and other activities of their early adult years. As the patient begins to discuss a subject he frequently loses the thread of his thought and rambles from one topic to another; after long detours into subjects only vaguely related to the topic at hand, he may or may not finish the narrative he originally intended to tell.

The patient's forgetfulness slowly encroaches on his day-to-day activities. The housewife cannot remember where she put things, and she repeatedly calls persons and stores to leave messages she left an hour or so before. The businessman forgets appointments, luncheons and financial obligations. The patient may begin to make notes to remind himself of things, but his notes soon deteriorate into tangled messes of jottings on pieces of paper, which he tucks into pockets, drawers and wallets. As the organic brain process continues the patient loses track of dates and seasons of the year. He usually places the year from several years to two or three decades prior to the current year, and he gropes confusedly for the names of the current month and the day of the week. If asked about current happenings in the world, he names as president the man who was president from one to several administrations previously, and he does not know of recent important world events. Many elderly people become stabilized at some point along this gradual course of memory deterioration and progress no further, but others gradually suffer such extensive memory losses that they mutter incoherently and ramble in continual confusion. The patient often feels that he is living at some much earlier period of his life. For example, he may feel that he is in his young adult years and he may mistake his adult children for his brothers and sisters. He may fill his memory gaps with elaborate confabulated stories.

As the patient slowly loses his cortical brain cells his control over his emotions and his personality problems diminishes. Passions that formerly were well controlled become unbridled, and long-standing personality characteristics become exaggerated. The person who was always economical with money may develop bizarre miserly habits. The shy patient becomes a social recluse and the irritable patient frequently flies into rages. The sensitive patient who throughout his life tended to worry about how people felt toward him becomes suspicious and may develop paranoid delusions. The domineering person becomes an intolerable autocrat, and the patient who was always somber and pessimistic becomes chronically tearful and depressed. An old psychiatric adage states that the senile or cerebral arteriosclerotic patient often becomes a caricature of his former self.

Slovenliness in grooming and dress is an early sign of senile and cerebral arteriosclerotic brain damage. Dirty shirts, soiled dresses, odd combinations of clothing and personal filthiness may startle the patient's relatives into sudden awareness that the patient's mental condition has been deteriorating slowly before their unobserving eyes. The patient may become sexually forward with persons of the opposite sex, and elderly men may make obscene advances to young women or little girls. If the patient's condition is not recognized by his relatives and friends, he may make bad economic decisions.

The individual with senile and arteriosclerotic brain damage gradually loses his intellectual and manual skills. His ability to do arithmetic deteriorates and his manual agility degenerates. Often he remains able to read unless his mental deterioration is profound, but after a few pages he forgets the thread of the narrative he is reading and cannot keep the characters of a story clearly in his mind. He cannot remember the theme or purposes of a television program, and loses interest in it or asks peevish questions about what has gone on before.

Hallucinations are relatively uncommon in persons with senile and arteriosclerotic brain syndromes, but both visual and auditory hallucinations may occur. I recall an elderly woman who called her adult son to complain about the strange men whom she saw in her apartment drinking whiskey and stealing her money, and she pointed out these hallucinated figures to her son when he rushed to see her. Hallucinations of taste, smell, and touch also may occur in elderly people.

Depressiveness is common in elderly people with progressive brain damage, especially in the early stages of their illnesses. The patient may perceive that he is becoming forgetful and, since he has seen friends and relatives follow the downhill course of senile brain disease, he realizes what is happening to him; suicidal urges sometimes are problems in these patients. The first patient who committed suicide while under my care was a 69-year-old, retired single woman who had had a successful business career and who knew that she slowly was becoming senile. After four weeks of hospitalization she presented a smiling, optimistic façade and cajoled me into discharging her from the hospital. The day following her discharge she committed suicide by leaping from a high bridge. In some instances, the elderly patient who has paranoid delusions is dangerous to other people.

Organic brain degeneration may unleash neurotic symptoms which long were latent but come to the surface only when the patient undergoes personality deterioration; interpersonal isolation in old age also contributes to neurotic decompensation. Acute and chronic anxiety states, phobias, obsessive fears and conversion hysterical disorders are fairly common as the older person struggles to make the interpersonal adjustments of old age with a decreasing number of cortical brain cells at his command.

The intellectual and emotional deterioration of an aged person is not dependent exclusively on the amount of brain tissue he has lost. The richness or barrenness of the elderly person's interpersonal life has a profound effect on whether a certain amount of brain damage causes mild personality changes or marked incapacitation. The elderly person has many stressful interpersonal adjustments to make. He loses many of his relatives and long-time friends by death and incapacitating illnesses, and he may also lose his marital partner. His children leave him to establish independent homes of their own, often in distant cities. The older person usually retires from his job, and his interpersonal circle is further narrowed by loss of contacts with the people with whom he formerly worked. Physical illnesses are more common in the aged, and they further limit the elderly person's ability to maintain his waning interpersonal contacts. His world often becomes barren and narrow, and he may become self-centered, querulous and isolated. In his preoccupation with himself he becomes uninterested in the feelings, activities and problems of other people. These interpersonal problems reinforce the difficulties caused by early senile and arteriosclerotic brain damage. The elderly person who can keep mentally occupied, vocationally busy and interpersonally active with as many people as possible runs much less chance of degenerating into incapacitation when he suffers a certain amount of senile and arteriosclerotic brain damage. (The problems of adjustment to the interpersonal difficulties of old age are discussed in more detail in Chapter 25.)

The brain-damaged elderly patient often is worse at night when darkness obscures the clues that keep him partially oriented. He is restless at night, sleeps poorly, ambles confusedly about his room and may become agitated and noisy. Cardiac decompensation, pulmonary edema or emphysema, renal diseases, hypertension and other illnesses are common in elderly people, and they may add further impairment to brain physiology and aggravate the patient's organic brain syndrome.

Psychiatric symptoms due to cerebral arteriosclerosis and senile brain degeneration usually do not begin until after the age of 60, though in rare instances they may start in patients in their middle or late 50's. The incidence of cerebral arteriosclerotic and senile degenerative syndromes increases progressively during the 60's, the 70's and the 80's, and in advanced age most persons have at least minimal signs of brain damage.

Course and Prognosis

The courses of patients with cerebral arteriosclerosis and senile brain degeneration are variable. Many patients become stabilized at levels of mild or moderate symptomatology and may make a reasonably good interpersonal adjustment at home under the loose surveillance of their families. If the patient's interpersonal environment is good, he may be pleasant and content despite mild to moderate forgetfulness and occasional confused periods. In some instances, the patient at times may show much improvement and may seem to recover some of his lost faculties; such improved periods may last for weeks, for months or for years. In other instances, the patient's behavior after mild to moderate brain damage is so disturbed that institutional life is the only possible course.

However, in many cases the patient's organic brain disease is progressive. Over a period of from several months to 10 or 20 years, he becomes increasingly incapacitated and may become a bedridden invalid who mutters confusedly and fumbles aimlessly with the bedclothes. With skillful nursing and medical care, these patients may remain alive in an incapacitated state for many years, but they frequently succumb to coexistent cardiac disease, pneumonia, complications of diabetes, bacteremia from infected bedsores and other illnesses.

Management

Though there is no specific treatment for the basic brain pathology of cerebral arteriosclerosis and senile brain degeneration, skillful medical management may make an important difference as to whether the patient leads a pleasant life at home or enters a custodial institution. When the patient has early brain damage the physician should discuss his condition with members of his family. He should point out that the patient's memory defects are more marked for recent events than for long-term, familiar things, and that the patient will tend to do better if he remains in his long-time home in association with people whom he has known for many years. An abrupt change to a strange environment where he meets new people whose names and faces he cannot remember often causes a rapid deterioration of the patient's adjustment. He cannot remember where the closets, drawers, toilet, kitchen and steps are, and he degenerates from confusion into panic and agitation.

Many small changes in the home may reduce the incidence of accidents in elderly patients and aid their general adjustments. Low beds are better than high ones, small throw rugs should be removed, and ramps should replace small flights of steps when feasible. Handrails should be installed on both sides of ramps and stairs, and they are useful beside toilets and bathtubs or shower stalls. Bathtub and shower floors should have ridges to prevent slipping, and bathtubs are available with sidedoors which open and close when not filled. Bedrooms, corridors and bathrooms should be illuminated with fluorescent nightlights to prevent confusion, disorientation, falls and agitation. There are a host of other measures, which fall more in the field of psychiatric nursing than in strictly psychiatric areas, but, in aggregate, they often determine whether the elderly patient with brain damage makes a good adjustment or a bad one, and in some cases (as in the complications after falls) they may determine how long he lives.

As much as possible, the patient should be spared interpersonal stresses and innovations in his life. He needs reassurances, cheerfulness and a tranquil environment. Simplicity in his daily routines is necessary; complexities confuse and frighten him. The patient needs a certain amount of surveillance by his family. He must not be allowed to make extravagant purchases, to do publicly embarrassing things and to be exploited financially by unscrupulous people. His meals, his grooming and the minor details of his daily life may require a certain amount of supervision. In some instances a responsible relative must be appointed legal guardian for the patient to handle his financial affairs and to make various decisions for him.

Medications are of limited value in the management of patients with cerebral arteriosclerosis and senile brain degeneration. Most sedatives, such as barbiturates, meprobamate, glutethimide and chloral hydrate, depress the cerebral cortex and may precipitate increased confusion in the patient. The medications of choice for agitation in elderly patients are the phenothiazines, which exert much of their calming action on lower brain centers and have less effect on the cerebral cortex. Chlorpromazine (Thorazine, Chlor-pz) and promazine (Sparine) are widely used phenothiazines in elderly patients. Small doses of either of these drugs also may be used at bedtime for insomnia. Aspirin has mild sedative properties, which sometimes help an elderly patient to sleep at night, and aspirin does not increase his confusion. Antidepressant medications of the tricyclic series (Tofranil, Norpramin, Pertofrane, Aventyl and others) sometimes are useful for depressiveness, but the dosage must be carefully adjusted to avoid vasomotor side effects, urinary retention and other problems.

When minimal organic brain damage releases a neurotic process or a psychosis in an elderly person, some of the measures outlined in other chapters for the treatment of these disorders may be used. The psychotherapy of elderly persons with neurotic disorders tends to be supportive, with much use of reassurance, advice about helpful changes in daily activities and limited exploration of day-to-day stresses in the patient's life. Counseling with the patient's family should accompany the psychotherapy. Such psychotherapy sometimes is very useful despite minimal organic brain damage. When brain damage is more marked the patient's forgetfulness of his interviews with the therapist renders them of little value, and the therapist must work mainly through the relatives. A few psychiatrists use electroshock therapy for depressions in elderly persons with early chronic organic brain damage, but most psychiatrists feel that forgetfulness, which is a frequent side effect of electroshock therapy, may cause a temporary aggravation of the patient's confusion despite a beneficial effect on his depression, and they rely mainly on antidepressant medications. Psychiatric hospitalization is a necessity in suicidal elderly patients, for even moderate degrees of senile brain deterioration do not prevent self-destructive attempts.

Many patients with cerebral arteriosclerosis and senile brain degeneration are unable to live at home, and institutional care is necessary. The quality of care in these institutions varies much, and providing decent, humanitarian care for elderly persons with chronic brain damage is a major public health problem that should attract the attention of a concerned public and alert government officials. A well-run institutional home for aged, brain-damaged persons should have good nursing and medical care, recreational programs adjusted to the capacities of patients with different degrees of brain damage, and activity programs for patients who can participate in them. Institutional living should be viewed as a special kind of life experience for people who need special circumstances because of their infirmities.

The number of elderly people needing supervisory care is increasing steadily, and the lengthened age span of the population is producing a social change of marked proportions in our society. New experiments in communal living for elderly persons are being carried out, and society must seek various ways to accomodate its elderly, brain-damaged citizens.

Much more attention should be paid to public education of elderly persons on the preventive aspects of psychiatric symptoms due to cerebral arteriosclerosis and senile brain degeneration. It has long been known that the elderly person who remains vocationally active, intellectually interested in things, and interpersonally busy often withstands a certain amount of organic brain damage with little adverse effect on his total emotional adjustment. All too often the physician sees men who retire from work and rapidly deteriorate into senile invalidism when they are deprived of their usual routines of activities and their customary interpersonal circles. Successful adjustment in old age requires careful planning and guidance. (This subject is discussed in further detail in Chapter 25 on the emotional problems of interpersonal adjustments by elderly people.)

ORGANIC BRAIN DISORDERS CAUSED BY HEAD TRAUMA

Organic brain syndromes due to head trauma may occur in automobile accidents, household accidents, industrial injuries, athletic accidents and other mishaps. The rising incidence of such accidents has increased the frequency of organic brain disorders associated with head trauma. We shall discuss the clinical syndromes caused by head trauma under the following headings: (1) traumatic confusional state, (2) traumatic delirium, (3) traumatic amnesic-confabulatory syndrome, (4) posttraumatic syndrome, (5) permanent organic brain damage after head injury and (6) compensation problems.

General Considerations. The damage to brain tissue caused by head trauma is customarily divided into three categories of increasing severity: concussion, contusion and laceration. In *concussion* the brain damage is intracellular, perhaps molecular, without evidence of gross anatomical abnormality. By definition, concussion always produces a brief period of unconsciousness. Some clinicians limit concussion to head injuries in which unconsciousness lasts no more than 10 or 15 minutes; beyond that, they feel contusion or laceration must have occurred. Other clinicians extend the allowable length of unconsciousness in concussion to several hours. In *contusion*, head injury causes extravasation of blood into brain tissue, but there is no gross disruption of the brain tissue. In *laceration*, brain tissue is torn in minor or major ways.

The degree of damage to brain tissue cannot be correlated exactly with the psychiatric syndrome it produces. The location of the brain injury, the patient's basic personality structure, and his general physical state after a head injury all affect his psychiatric state. For example, a concussion may be followed by a severe confusional state, whereas laceration of brain tissue by a perforating injury to a parietal lobe may cause only transient unconsciousness. Though severe head injuries often cause severe psychiatric symptoms and mild head injuries usually cause few psychiatric symptoms, there are frequent exceptions to these tendencies. Moreover, patients with similar head injuries may have widely different psychiatric states. For example, some patients have few psychiatric symptoms after a mild concussion, whereas others have severe problems. The patient's basic personality structure has a marked influence on the nature and severity of his mental reaction to a head injury.

The management of a patient with an acute organic brain syndrome following a head injury requires the services of a psychiatrist and a neurologist or neurosurgeon. In our discussion of the various organic brain syndromes caused by head injury, we shall deal only with the behavior, ideation and emotional state of the patient; other aspects of the management of head injuries lie beyond the scope of this book. Moreover, we shall not attempt to correlate psychiatric disorders with various types of brain injuries, because, as pointed out above, there are so many variations in these correlations that general statements cannot be made.

In addition to the technics given here for the management of each type of head trauma syndrome, the general principles for treating organic brain disorders (outlined at the end of Chapter 19) are in each instance applicable.

Traumatic Confusional State

The patient who develops a traumatic confusional state after a head injury goes through an initial period of unconsciousness which may last from a few minutes to several hours or more. As he emerges gradually from his period of unconsciousness his contact with his environment remains partially clouded. He is disoriented for time and place, but he usually knows who he is. He usually cannot remember his accident, and he has an amnesia which covers from several minutes to several months or more prior to his accident. This amnesia usually clears up as he recovers from his confusional state, and eventually he can recall everything up to the moment the head injury occurred. However, his amnesia will be permanent for his period of unconsciousness and for most of his subsequent confusional state.

During a severe posttraumatic confusional state the patient also may have extensive memory losses, more marked for the recent years of his life than for his distant past. For example, he cannot recollect the names of new people whom he sees in the hospital, but he can remember the names of members of his family and old friends.

The patient's confusional state lasts from several hours to several weeks or more. It fluctuates in intensity, but the general trend is toward gradual improvement. He is dazed and bewildered as he struggles to understand what is going on around him. In many instances the patient feels lethargic and has headaches, and he prefers to rest in bed or to sit quietly in a chair looking vacantly about him. In other cases, the patient is restless and agitated as he struggles to grasp what is going on in his environment; he is frightened or irritated by his inability to comprehend his situation.

The patient's judgement is poor and his intellectual capacities are impaired. Recently acquired skills are lost more frequently than skills learned many years ago. For example, a patient whose native language is not English and who first learned English as an adult may forget English and speak only his native tongue. As he gets well, his ability to speak English gradually returns and he speaks it fluently again when he is fully recovered.

Treatment of Traumatic Confusional States. The patient with a traumatic confusional state should be hospitalized; if he cannot be easily managed on a general ward, psychiatric hospitalization is necessary. In the early stages, when his confusion is most marked, one of his relatives should be constantly at his bedside; he can remember who the relative is, and the relative can calm him and gain his cooperation in medical procedures, whereas he cannot remember who the hospital personnel are, and where he is, and he may resist medical measures. His vital signs are checked regularly and the essential points of a neurological examination should be reviewed daily. Bed rest is advisable when the patient accepts it easily, and as he begins to recover he is allowed moderate activity on the hospital floor. Sedatives should be avoided if possible. If the patient needs sedation for agitation or insomnia, small doses of one of the phenothiazines are preferable, since phenothiazines cause less sedation of the cerebral cortex than other sedatives.

The patient's nutrition and fluid intake are supervised. The physicians, the nurses and the ward aids should reassure the patient when he is upset and should help to orient him as he grapples to reestablish contact with his environment. During the patient's convalescence his physicians should be as optimistic as the clinical facts permit, in order to minimize the chance that fear and self-preoccupation will worsen the patient's symptoms. In general, these patients do far better than might be expected in the early stages of their confusional states. I have seen complete intellectual recovery, except for amnesia for the period of acute confusion, in patients who were completely confused and disoriented for up to four months. Patients who remain in marked confusional states for 30 to 60 days often recover entirely. If the brain tissue is not lacerated or destroyed at the time of the injury, its recuperative capacity is often quite extensive.

Often it is difficult to decide how soon a patient should leave the hospital and how rapidly he should return to work after he has had a traumatic confusional state. On the one hand, the physician wishes to encourage the patient; he wishes to increase his self-confidence and to decrease the chance that his symptoms will be prolonged by anxious self-preoccupation and inactivity. On the other hand, a premature return to physical and intellectual activity sometimes causes the patient to become discouraged as he undertakes tasks for which he is not yet ready. Moreover, posttraumatic headache, vertigo and fatigue sometimes are made worse by a premature return to work. The schedule of each patient must be adjusted to his invididual needs. In general, however, the patient with a mild, several-day traumatic confusional state may return to work a week or two after his confusion clears. The patient with a several-week traumatic confusional state may return to work six to eight weeks after his confusion resolves, and the patient with a still longer traumatic confusional state returns to work in from two to several months after his confusion clears.

Traumatic Delirium

In addition to profound confusion, disorientation and memory loss, the patient with traumatic delirium has hallucinations and delusions. When a traumatic delirium occurs, it usually takes place as the patient emerges from a coma following a serious head injury. The delirium may be mild and last from a few hours to a day or so, or it may be severe and last a month or more. When the patient with delirium has florid visual hallucinations and marked disorientation, he may believe that he is at work or at home and he goes through some of his customary actions in those places.

I recall a patient in a posttraumatic delirium who pushed a hallucinatory power mower up and down the hospital corridor under the impression he was cutting the grass in his back yard.

In some cases the patient has poorly organized persecutory delusions, which make him fearful and combative. He may wander about the hospital ward in perplexity, agitation and panic. He may abruptly laugh, sob or become belligerent without apparent provocation. The depth of the patient's delirium fluctuates much, and he usually is worse at night. The content of the patient's hallucinations and delusions is influenced by his basic personality structure. Underlying fears and repressed hostilities are unleashed by the patient's impaired cerebral cortical functioning.

The treatment of traumatic delirium is the same as that outlined in the preceding section on traumatic confusional state (*with the addition of the management principles discussed in the concluding section of Chapter 19*). However, the patient with a traumatic delirium usually needs larger amounts of chlorpromazine or some other phenothiazine to control his agitated, belligerent or delusional behavior. He sometimes must be protected from accidentally harming himself or committing suicide in his delusional panic states. The majority of patients with traumatic deliriums recover completely, but they have complete amnesia for their delirious periods. A few of them go on to have evidence of persistently impaired brain functioning or chronic traumatic psychoses.

Traumatic Amnesic-Confabulatory Syndrome

The patient with a posttraumatic amnesic-confabulatory syndrome has a mental picture similar to that described for Korsakoff's psychosis in our discussion later in this chapter of organic brain disorders caused by alcohol. However, the term Korsakoff's psychosis customarily is used only in referring to an amnesic-confabulatory syndrome due to alcohol, and an alcoholic Korsakoff's psychosis often is accompanied by peripheral neuritis.

The patient with an amnesic-confabulatory syndrome due to head trauma has profound memory loss and disorientation, which he covers up with elaborate fictitious tales about his daily activities. For example, though he cannot remember what he ate for breakfast or what he did yesterday, he gives fictitious detailed accounts about these activities which at first may sound plausible if they are not checked with the facts. If asked the same questions 15 minutes later he may give equally elaborate but completely different answers. The patient usually is cheerful and talkative, but at times he may be irritable and belligerent. The patient with a traumatic amnesic-confabulatory syndrome may recover in a few days or a few weeks. His prognosis for complete recovery is good, but he has a permanent loss of memory for the period of his amnesic-confabulatory disorder. However, a few patients with amnesic-confabulatory syndromes do not recover. The treatment for them is the same as outlined for other traumatic organic brain disorders.

Posttraumatic Syndrome

The patient who had a blow to the head and had a traumatic confusional state or a traumatic delirium from which he recovered may continue to have various symptoms for several weeks or many months afterwards. This group of symptoms is so commonly encountered in clinical practice that the term "posttraumatic syndrome," or "postconcussion syndrome," customarily is applied to it. Also, it sometimes is called "posttraumatic neurotic state" or "postconcussion neurotic state," since the head injury, its emotional significance to the patient and the patient's basic personality structure all play large roles in causing the patient's symptoms. The syndrome we are discussing here follows a head injury that does *not* cause persistent brain damage. The prognosis is good, though the patient may require up to 1 or 2 years to recover. Posttraumatic syndromes occur in only a small percentage of patients with acute organic brain disorders after head trauma.

The patient with a posttraumatic syndrome usually has headaches, which may be dull or sharp, persistent or intermittent, and diffuse or sharply localized in any part of the head. The patient's headache characteristically is worse when he exerts himself phsyically or when he is under emotional strain. The headache often is worse at night and the patient may complain that it prevents him from sleeping well. Stooping, sudden head movements and climbing stairs may aggravate the headache. The headache often is accompanied by a giddiness which the patient describes as "dizziness," but true vertigo is rare. He also may complain of mild blurring of vision, photophobia and pain in the eyes when he tries to read. He tires easily, sleeps poorly and awakes from sleep unrefreshed. The patient has chronic anxiousness and he worries much about his health; he fears that he may never recover completely from the effects of his head injury. He complains that he cannot concentrate well, that his span of attention on any task is short and that his memory is not as good as it formerly was. He is irritable and depressed, and he may cry easily. His relatives are worried about him, and their concerned faces make the patient more apprehensive and preoccupied with his symptoms. His field of interest narrows; he shuns people and centers his attention mainly on himself.

Some psychiatric writers emphasize that there usually is a symptom-free period between the immediate, acute effects of the head injury and the onset of the posttraumatic syndrome. For example, a patient may have a confusional state lasting several hours or a few days after his head injury, and he then is free of symptoms for several days or a week or two. As he then prepares to go home from the hospital or to return to work, the symptoms of his posttraumatic syndrome begin. This symptom-free period is sometimes called the "incubation period" of the posttraumatic syndrome. However, in my experience the vast majority of patients with posttraumatic syndromes do not have this symptom-free period; their symptoms fluctuate, but they are present consistently after the head injury.

Neurological studies of the patient with a posttraumatic syndrome are normal, and his electroencephalogram is normal or borderline normal. Psychological testing usually reveals anxiousness, obsessive concern over body functions and some depressiveness; signs of organic brain damage in the psychological testing are minimal or absent.

A posttraumatic syndrome is produced by the combined effects of (1) reversible (that is, the patient's brain will return to its normal state) brain damage due to the head trauma, (2) the patient's basic personality and interpersonal life and (3) his emotional attitude about his head injury. Depending upon the severity of disturbances in these three areas, a posttraumatic syndrome may last from several weeks up to two years, and it may vary from a mild annoyance to an incapacitating disability. The patient who was somewhat anxious and emotionally insecure prior to his head injury is more prone to have prolonged posttraumatic symptoms than the patient who was emotionally secure and self-confident. The patient who is bitterly dissatisfied with his job and has much conflict with his work associates and superiors is more apt to have prolonged posttraumatic symptoms after a head injury at work than the employee who likes his job and has good relationships with the people with whom he works. Problems in marital relationships and other interpersonal areas may play roles in posttraumatic syndromes.

The severity and duration of a posttraumatic syndrome also may be somewhat affected by any financial compensation the patient receives because of his head injury or by any litigation that arises because of the accident in which the head trauma occurred. Prolonged, elaborate, repeated medical work-ups also tend to increase the patient's self-concern and may aggravate his posttraumatic syndrome. The head is a region of the body that plays an important role in the patient's concepts of himself and his functioning; injuries to the head are prone to excite anxiousness and self-concern.

Some psychiatrists attempt to divide patients with posttraumatic syndromes into two groups: (1) those patients whose problems are caused mainly by prolonged but eventually reversible brain damage, and (2) those patients whose posttraumatic symptoms are due primarily to basic personality problems and unhealthy attitudes about the head injury. In my opinion, such a division of patients with posttraumatic syndromes is arbitrary and clinically unsound. I feel it is better to study each patient's syndrome as the product of intricately interwoven reversible organic brain damage and interpersonal problems.

Since both the organic brain factors and the interpersonal factors, at least on their highest level of neurophysiologic organization, operate mainly in the cerebral cortex, distinguishing organic factors from emotional factors is clinically difficult and perhaps unsound.

The eventual prognosis of a posttraumatic syndrome is good, but the patient may require from several weeks up to one or two years before he recovers. The average patient probably is much better within several months and is recovered completely in less than a year.

Management of Posttraumatic Syndromes. The patient with a posttraumatic syndrome is frightened and perplexed, and he needs much reassurance and optimistic guidance from the physicians who care for him. This reassuring help should begin as the patient emerges from the acute organic brain disorder precipitating the posttraumatic syndrome. All physicians who deal with the patient with a head injury should be as reassuring as the clinical facts allow. Elaborate, repeated medical workups should be avoided if at all possible, since they frighten the patient and tend to convince him that he is seriously injured and may not recover completely. When neurological studies, skull films and electroencephalograms are normal, the physician should tell the patient so; the patient should not be left to worry about what they may have revealed.

The physician caring for the patient, whether he is a family doctor, a neurologist or a psychiatrist, should talk frankly with the patient about his condition early in the course of a posttraumatic syndrome, and in many instances the physician also should talk with the patient's relatives. He should emphasize that the patient's symptoms have a good prognosis and that they are caused both by the organic brain trauma of the head injury and by the patient's fears and worries about it. When the patient has obvious problems in his vocational life, in his family relationships or in other interpersonal areas, the physician may indicate that these factors also may play a role in determining the severity and duration of the patient's symptoms.

Medications may help to a limited extent. A nightttime sedative may be given to help the patient sleep better. When depression is a prominent feature of the patient's clinical picture, an antidepressant sometimes is useful, and mild daytime sedation may take the edge off anxiousness. However, the physician should emphasize that these medications are not intended to cure any organic brain damage in the patient; they only may assuage some of the emotional distress his injury has precipitated in him.

Relatively few of these patients will participate in systematic psychotherapy with a psychiatrist. Supportive explanations, guidance, reassurance and limited exploration of relevant interpersonal stresses usually constitute the most that the posttraumatic patient will accept. However, in occasional instances the patient can participate in systematic psychotherapy to explore the emotional factors in his problem and may benefit from such treatment.

Determining when the patient should return to work often is difficult. Long idleness discourages the patient and may prolong his invalidism, but a premature return to work that he finds himself unable to do causes alarm and despair. A middle course, with cautious trials of increasing activity, is best. The length of time after the accident at which the posttraumatic patient returns to work varies from several weeks to six months or longer, and cases vary so much in severity that no general rules can be given.

The physician should talk with the patient frankly about any financial compensation and litigation problems that may arise because of his head injury. The doctor may agree that the patient rightfully may seek whatever compensation is justified, but the physician also should point out the hazards of becoming highly involved emotionally in the outcome of litigation and compensation disputes over the head injury. The physician should emphasize that the patient's primary goal is to get well, and that compensation and litigation should be secondary concerns both to him and his family.

Permanent Organic Brain Damage After Head Injury

After a head injury it may not be clear for many weeks or months whether the patient's brain damage will be acute and reversible or chronic and irreversible. Often, the patient improves much during the first several days or few weeks after the injury, but a long observation of the patient may be necessary before the physician knows whether the patient will have permanent brain damage with persistent personality defects. In general, most patients with head trauma do much better than might be expected on the basis of examining them shortly after their injuries, but a small percentage of them have persistent intellectual and personality defects. The severity of the patient's intellectual and personality defects varies greatly, depending on the areas of the brain involved and the amount of tissue destruction. The degree of psychiatric impairment may vary from complete mental incapacitation to subtle personality changes which are difficult to detect clinically.

Of course, some patients after a head injury have neurological damage with paralyses and other disabilities, but do not have intellectual and personality defects. In general, destruction of areas of the cerebral cortex or of the fibers that connect the cerebral cortex with other areas of the brain produce the most striking intellectual and personality changes. For convenience in considering these problems, we shall discuss permanent brain damage caused by head trauma under the headings of (1) intellectual defects and (2) personality changes.

Intellectual Defects. Many of the patient's symptoms are the direct result of the loss of cortical brain tissue. When brain damage is severe and extensive the patient may have persistent clouding of consciousness or grossly impaired contact with his environment. He may wander confusedly about the hospital ward or may lie in mute seclusiveness. In other instances the patient rambles continually in an agitated, restless, aimless manner, sometimes called "organic drivenness," and may talk and shout noisily some of the time. Memory defects in a patient with permanent brain damage may be so mild as to be barely noticeable or so severe that the patient has little awareness of most of his past and current experiences; as in all organic brain disorders, the memory defects tend to be much more marked for recent happenings than for events in the patient's earlier life. Thus, the patient may feel confusedly that his present employment is on a job at which he worked 20 years ago. A patient with mild permanent brain damage after a head injury usually does not have problems of orientation, but severe permanent brain damage may produce disorientation as to time, place and identity of persons, including himself.

Severe brain damage causes a marked deterioration of judgement. However, the most difficult clinical problems often arise in the patient whose brain damage has produced only subtle defects of judgement. This type of patient may appear normal in casual conversation and in many social settings. However, his family and other close persons note that his judgement is not as sound as it was before his head injury. He makes impulsive, unsound decisions in financial matters, in purchases and in the choice of friends. He may show poor judgement in his sexual conduct and may become crude or promiscuous. He may become intemperate in his use of alcohol, and he may drive recklessly and have repeated arrests for traffic violations.

The patient's job efficiency drops and his colleagues and superiors note many mistakes in his work. The patient who works mainly with his hands finds that he has lost the fine coordination and rapidity of movements that he formerly had; he is clumsy and slow in his tasks, and he often damages materials and tools with which he works. I. Q. testing may or may not reveal reduced intelligence. However, psychological testing usually reveals signs of organic intellectual impairment; difficulties in correlating ideas with visual images and muscular actions may be present, and the patient has reduced capacities for comprehending and using symbols, abstract concepts and geometric designs.

Personality Changes. The patient with permanent organic brain damage is trying to adjust to the interpersonal stresses of life with fewer cortical brain cells at his command. His decrease in cortical brain tissue impairs his ability to control his underlying personality problems and his emotional reactions to interpersonal stresses. These changes in personality functioning vary from minor difficulties to incapacitating defects, depending on the severity of the patient's brain damage.

His emotional responses are erratic and unpredictable. On little provocation he becomes tearful, or hilariously amused, or frightened, or belligerent and combative. He loses his capacity to modulate his emotional responses to environmental stresses; minor incidents cause him to fly into rages, whereas he may stare with blank indifference when confronted with situations that ordinarily would excite pity, guilt or anxiety.

Previous personality features often become accentuated after a head injury. The shy person becomes seclusive, the irritable person becomes belligerent, and the sensitive person develops paranoid delusions. When the patient has diffuse cortical brain damage, especially of the frontal lobes, he often becomes callous to the feelings and rights of other people, and he lacks guilt and anxiety about socially undesirable or dangerous activities. He does not learn from experience, and punishment does not cause him to change his behavior. He acts on the impulse of the moment, careless of the eventual consequences of his acts. He may lie garrulously and deceive the people around him, and he may engage in minor thefts and frauds. He has no remorse when apprehended but lies or adopts whatever course may enable him to avoid the consequences of his acts.

The destruction of cortical brain tissue may unleash underlying neurotic problems that the patient formerly was able to keep under control when his cortical brain tissue was intact. The patient may develop phobias, or anxiety states, or hysterical conversion disorders, or dissociative disorders, or obsessive and compulsive symptoms as he struggles to adjust to the turmoil within him and the interpersonal stresses around him. The patient often becomes anxious as he dimly perceives that his intellectual and emotional control is slipping from him; his anxiety occasionally may mount into panic states or periods of aimless agitation.

The destruction of cortical tissue also may release psychotic disorders. Manic disorders, severe depressions and schizophrenic psychoses occur in a small percentage of patients following chronic brain damage due to head injuries. The manic and depressive psychotic episodes usually improve with treatment; the schizophrenic disorders, which usually are paranoid or catatonic, also may improve, but in many instances they become chronic.

In many instances the emotional problems of the patient with permanent brain damage due to head injury are further complicated by the development of posttraumatic convulsive seizures. Posttraumatic epilepsy is much more common following injuries in which penetration of the meninges and brain tissue occurs. The patient with seizures faces the problem of adjusting to unpredictable attacks of loss of consciousness and convulsive movements, which add to his adjustment difficulties in social, economic and family relationships.

Management of Patients With Permanent Brain Damage After Head Injury. Many persons with permanent brain damage due to head injuries can be rehabilitated to levels of economic and social self-sufficiency. They need carefully planned rehabilitation programs to deal with their intellectual, emotional and vocational difficulties. The majority of brain-damaged persons still have enough brain tissue to benefit much from such programs. Retraining should begin during the period of convalescence from the acute brain injury. The patient may begin with simple tasks in the occupational therapy department of the hospital, and gradually he can begin to regain some of his manual and intellectual skills. At each step he needs much cheerful encouragement and reassurance, and he should proceed to tasks of increasing complexity at a rate carefully adjusted to his capacity to perform them. His progress should be fast enough to encourage him and to develop his capacities, but it should not be so rapid that he frequently fails at tasks and becomes discouraged.

Supportive counseling with the patient and his family should accompany this rehabilitative training. In most instances, the brain-damaged patient is not well motivated to engage in systematic psychotherapy to work on the emotional turbulence and the interpersonal maladjustments that his brain damage precipitates, but supportive counseling and guidance are very useful. After a period of rehabilitative training, which lasts from several months to a year or more, the patient may be ready for carefully planned job placement. In many instances rehabilitation can be conducted on an outpatient basis after the patient's convalescence from his acute brain injury is well established. Many cities have rehabilitation centers with specially trained staffs employing special technics for retraining brain-damaged persons. Children who suffer brain damage in accidents of childhood should attend the special schools most cities have for their education.

The prognoses of patients with permanent brain damage syndromes vary much depending on the severity of the patient's brain damage, his pre-existing personality structure and the soundness of his interpersonal relationships. Many patients with mild to moderate organic brain damage eventually become economically and socially self-sufficient and readjust reasonably well with their families. The neurophysiological basis for such improvement is not well understood; presumably, tissues in the extensive "silent" areas of the brain slowly take over functions formerly carried out by brain regions that have been partially damaged or destroyed. The patient may require from one to three years after his accident to reach his best level of adjustment. However, patients with severe brain damage often remain chronically incapacitated. Some of them are able to live outside a hospital under the careful supervision of relatives, but others are so disturbed intellectually and emotionally that institutional care is a long-term necessity.

Many groups work to decrease the number of accidents that produce chronic brain damage due to head trauma. Private and governmental organizations work to reduce the hazards leading to automobile accidents, industrial accidents, household accidents and athletic injuries.

Compensation Problems

We discussed (in Chapter 9) compensation problems associated with neurotic disorders, especially hysterical conversion neuroses; in those cases there was, of course, no organic brain damage. We are here discussing financial compensation problems in patients who have suffered permanent organic brain injury.

When a patient has severe brain damage and gross personality deterioration after a head injury there usually are few medical or legal quandries about whether financial compensation is medically justified. However, when the patient has mild, long-lasting organic brain damage producing subtle disturbances in his intellectual and emotional functioning, many difficult medicolegal questions may arise. This is particularly true when the patient's major problems consist of subtle personality changes, or psychotic disorders, or neurotic symptoms which are unleashed by the tissue destruction of a head injury. These medicolegal and compensation problems arise from the fact that both the head injury and the patient's pre-existing personality influence the nature and severity of the emotional disturbance the patient has. Attorneys, judges, workmen's compensation commissioners and insurance companies want to know exactly how important both the head injury and the patient's pre-existing personality were in causing the patient's current psychiatric problems.

Hence, psychiatrists and other physicians may be asked if the head injury *caused* the psychiatric problems of the patient. Since these problems were caused by both the previous personality of the patient and the subsequent head injury, it is best to say that the changes were *precipitated* by the injury, and to follow this with a detailed explanation of how brain damage and underlying personality structure are interwoven in the patient's present difficulties. Whether or not the patient would have had his trouble if he had not had a head injury should be based on a careful history of his adjustment before and after the injury. Any striking changes in emotional and intellectual functioning may be said to have been precipitated by the head trauma, and it is justifiable to assume that they would not have developed, at least at this time and in this manner, had the head injury not occurred. A statement about the patient's eventual prognosis should not be given until the patient has been observed for several months or more after his head injury, and it should be based on careful psychiatric and neurological study.

ORGANIC BRAIN DISORDERS CAUSED BY BRAIN DAMAGE IN THE PRENATAL, THE NATAL AND THE POSTNATAL PERIODS

Permanent organic brain damage may occur during the prenatal period because of viral infections or systemic illnesses of the mother or because of defective development of the fetal brain; chromosomal abnormalities account for a small percentage of fetal brain maldevelopments. During birth a child may suffer anoxia, mechanical trauma, intracranial hemorrhage or interrupted blood supply to the brain, which produces permanent brain damage. In the postnatal period, brain damage may be caused by anoxic, metabolic or nutritional problems. However, the mechanism of much chronic brain damage that occurs before, during or shortly after birth is not well understood.

The degree of brain damage occurring in the prenatal, the natal or the postnatal period may be so mild that it is scarcely discernible or so severe that it is disabling. It may affect the interpersonal functioning, the intelligence and the neurological state of the child in mild, moderate or severe degrees. These children are sometimes classified under the broad term of cerebral palsy when obvious neurological signs are present.

In former times a large number of brain-damaged children died of nutritional deficiencies and infections during infancy and early childhood. However, the vast majority of these children today survive the illnesses of infancy and early childhood, and their parents seek aid for the emotional, educational and social problems these children encounter. During childhood and adolescence these children must be educated to their best potentials and they must be prepared for whatever social and vocational roles they can carry out. Many of them can lead independent, useful lives, but others require always the protective supervision of their families or institutions.

Emotional and Intellectual Characteristics

Organic brain damage in early life does not always produce personality disorders. Some children with choreiform movements, spastic limbs, athetoid movements and other signs of central nervous system damage have unimpaired personality capacities and good intelligence that have not been significantly influenced by their brain damage.

A careful work-up is necessary to evaluate impairment of personality functioning and defective intelligence in a child with organic brain damage. This work-up should include physical and personality evaluation of the child, interviews with his parents to obtain data about his development and behavior, psychological testing by a clinical psychologist, and any further examinations, such as an electroencephalogram, which may be needed. Children with marked neurologic damage dating from early life may or may not have problems of emotional functioning and defective intelligence. The child with gross brain damage usually has abnormal findings on neurologic examination; in some instances, however, the child with brain damage has personality impairment and defective intelligence without abnormalities on neurologic examination. Such differences depend on the severity and the location of the brain damage. The emotional functioning and the neurologic condition of each child must be evaluated on an individual basis before conclusions can be reached.

The personality features of the child with brain damage throughout his childhood, adolescence and later life are determined by the type of interpersonal environment in which he is reared as well as his brain impairment. When the brain-damaged child has understanding, affectionate parents, and other close persons, who can give him both sound love and reasonable limitations on his behavior, he often makes a good interpersonal adjustment both during childhood and later life within the limits of his intellectual and physical difficulties. However, if he is reared in an atmosphere of irritability, neglect and impatience, or is indulged because of his problems, he may become socially maladjusted, or belligerent, or negativistic, or seclusive.

Some brain-damaged children have normal intelligence, but many others have I. Q.'s in the ranges of low normal intelligence or mental retardation. If he has defective intelligence, he is slow to learn to walk, to talk and to be toilet trained. He performs unevenly on intelligence testing; he characteristically does much better on some parts of the I. Q. test than on others.

In many instances the child with brain damage has various degrees of difficulty in coordinating his visual, auditory, intellectual and muscular functions. The neurophysiological integration of what he sees, what he hears, what he thinks and what he does physically is erratically impaired. He has much difficulty putting all aspects of a thing into a meaningful whole. For example, a child with intact brain tissue sees an automobile, hears the sound of its motor, mentally comprehends it as a vehicle that can carry him to another place, and wants to get into it; this requires a high degree of coordination between visual, auditory, mental and muscular functions. However, a brain-damaged child, because of his defective brain cells and circuits, may have much difficulty putting all this together, or may not be able to do it at all. He does not comprehend the relationships between the appearance, the sound, the use and the purpose of the automobile, and what his attitudes toward it should be. Hence, he may fear it, or bang against it, or run excitedly from one part of it to another without a clear idea of the nature and function of the whole car. These are the visuomotor disruptions that play a large part in the brain-damaged child's problems. These visuomotor difficulties contribute to the child's short attention span (not integrating the parts into the whole, he runs irom item to item), erratic actions, distractibility, hyperactivity and, in occasional cases, pointless destructiveness. Helping the child establish better integrations of his perceptions, concepts and actions is an important aspect of his education.

The child with organic brain damage may have memory problems. He finds it difficult to recall and integrate his memories into sound formulations for present and future actions. His memory defects are uneven and spotty; he remembers some things well and forgets others quickly. His memory problems also contribute to his short attention span and easy distractibility. He wanders from task to task, and the things he learns one day he may forget the next.

The brain-damaged child often has poor control of his emotions. He struggles to moderate his emotional responses and to maintain self-control with less brain tissue than other children have. He may easily become frightened, aggressive, anxious or angry. He often acts impulsively when he encounters obstacles to his desires and needs. His emotional responses often are inappropriate to the interpersonal situations in which he finds himself.

Chronic organic brain damage in a child often causes poor judgement. He has difficulty in understanding the complexities of new problems and in making sound decisions in new interpersonal situations. He acts impulsively, flounders and makes poor choices. He may become belligerent or frightened when his poor judgement leads him into increasing interpersonal problems.

A child with organic brain damage often is physically restless and he is in constant, aimless movement. He starts many things and finishes few of them; he flits quickly from task to task and from toy to toy. The term "organic drivenness" is sometimes applied to the brain-damaged child's aimless hyperactivity. Such hyperactivity tends to diminish, at least in its most obvious physical manifestations, in middle and late adolescence, but the patient's short attention span and distractibility often remain. When the child's clinical picture is dominated by this physical hyperactivity he may, in the current standard medical nomenclature, be classified as having a "hyperkinetic reaction of childhood, or adolescence." However, this term has caused much confusion and is shunned by many clinicians since (1) the nomenclature says that this diagnosis also may be applied to physically restless children who do not have organic brain damage, but are merely anxious and agitated, and (2) it is based on a single symptom rather than a total personality process.

In some instances, a brain-damaged child engages in antisocial acts such as impulsive aggressiveness, lying, stealing, destructiveness and sexual offenses. He may show no remorse when confronted with his erractic antisocial behavior, but he has an attitude of sullen resistance or indifference. Correction and punishment often fail to deter him from repeating his antisocial acts in the future.

Neurotic problems are somewhat more common in brain-damaged children than in children with intact brain tissue. The brain-damaged child has a greater likelihood of decompensating into neurotic symptoms, since he is trying to cope with the interpersonal problems and challenges of life with less cortical brain tissue than the average child. As he struggles with a puzzling world he cannot understand or grasp, he may develop phobias, anxiety states, obsessive worries or hysterical conversion disorders. He is prone to develop brief panic states or withdrawn depressiveness.

When faced with overwhelming emotional problems, the child with organic brain damage may decompensate into periods of social withdrawal, disorganized panic or diffuse combativeness, which some psychiatrists consider psychotic episodes. These states may persist for a day or two or they may last for several months or longer. These episodes occur more often in later childhood and adolescence as the child faces increasingly complex interpersonal demands and he must also adjust to the sexual maturation and physical development of adolescence. There is much disagreement among psychiatrists about whether these episodes should be termed schizophrenic, and psychiatrists also do not agree about whether the incidence of schizophrenia is greater in brain-damaged children than in other children.

The Concept of Minimal Brain Damage as a Cause of Emotional Disorders in Children

The question is sometimes raised as to whether subtle, minimal organic brain damage with only meager clinical evidence to substantiate it is an occasional cause of emotional disorders in children and adolescents. In a typical case a child may be brought for evaluation of sullenness, rebelliousness, lying, evasiveness, poor academic work at school, tenseness and irritability. He is physically restless and his attention span is short. He tests in the low normal range of intelligence, and some aspects of his responses to psychological testing suggest minimal organic brain damage. His electroencephalogram is borderline normal, or perhaps has a few irregularities. The problem is: did this child, at birth or thereafter, suffer subtle organic brain damage which is causing his personality problems, or are his problems caused by interpersonal stresses in his life? Is the doubtful, borderline evidence of brain damage irrelevant to his problems?

The answer is important, for it determines whether the child's parents, physicians and educators see his difficulties as soluble interpersonal problems or as organic brain dysfunction about which far less can be done. It also influences how much emphasis is put on medications in his treatment regimen.

My opinion is as follows: The diagnosis of minimal brain damage in these children requires clear, unequivocal proof, and the burden of proof lies on the side of demonstrating the brain damage, as opposed to interpersonal factors, in causing the child's problems. Statistically, interpersonal factors are immensely more common than brain dysfunction in these children, and equivocal results from psychological testing and electroencephalograms do not settle the matter. Neither psychological testing nor electroencephalograms, in themselves, are diagnostic in these cases, and interpreting them is an art, not a science.

This question has become the center of increasing controversy and confusion in recent years. In the psychiatric and pediatric literature such children are often said to suffer from MBD, minimal brain damage, and some psychiatrists feel that this is a common cause of a wide variety of behavior disorders in children and adolescents. This concept has received, unhappily, a strong impulse from pharmaceutical firms which promote various "psychic energizers" which are said to benefit these children, and these firms make ample funds available for research by clinicians who accept this point of view. The diagnosis "hyperkinetic reaction of childhood," which is discussed earlier in this chapter, has further complicated this controversy.

Many psychiatrists, including myself, feel that 98 per cent of hyperactive, distractible, rebellious, evasive children have interpersonally caused problems and that minimal brain damage is a relatively rare cause of such behavior. Many parents, who can more easily attribute their children's problems to subtle physical defects than to unhealthy interpersonal life at home, report that everything in the child's interpersonal life is "fine;" however, more meticulous study shows clear interpersonal causes for the child's difficulties. Moreover, it is quite possible that minimal organic brain dysfunction in a child is not causing his emotional problems; it may be an incidental finding that would have escaped clinical detection had not interpersonally caused problems led to psychiatric evaluation of him.

Management of the Child Who Suffers Brain Damage in Early Life

A child should be evaluated emotionally, intellectually, interpersonally and neurologically to decide whether or not he has early organic brain damage. The workup should include a careful history of the child's mental and physical development, careful examination by a psychiatrist, testing by a clinical psychologist, neurological examination and any special studies such as electroencephalography. When choreiform movements, spasticity or other neurological abnormalities accompany the emotional and intellectual disturbances, the diagnosis usually is clear. However, when the child has minimal or moderate brain damage, and especially if he does not have abnormal findings on neurological examination and has neurotic symptoms such as phobias, the diagnosis may be difficult. No single test can be accepted as definitive; psychological testing, the electroencephalogram or the clinical history alone cannot be accepted as the basis for making the diagnosis. All diagnostic procedures must be used, and the final diagnosis can be formulated only when all data are considered together. In some instances, the diagnosis can be established in a child with mild or borderline organic brain damage only after an observation period of many months.

The long-term medical management of children with permanent organic brain damage that occurred in the prenatal, the natal or the postnatal periods requires a special kind of understanding, patience and optimism. Physicians and auxiliary therapists who find themselves easily discouraged with the difficult work of managing these children and counseling their parents should refer them to others who specialize in this field or to special clinics that have comprehensive programs designed to meet the needs of these children and their parents. In many instances, the family physician or pediatrician can serve as the long-term counselor of the parents of the brain-damaged child and he can coordinate the services of various specialists. The therapeutic emphasis must be on the comprehensive care of the child, and one specialist should not dominate in the care of the child to the exclusion of others. For example, the orthopedic problems of the child with spastic limbs should not become the sole focus of attention, so that the interpersonal development, speech and special educational needs of the child receive little attention. Some medical centers have special clinics where psychiatrists, psychologists, pediatricians, orthopedists, psychiatric nurses, speech therapists and social workers work in teams in managing the problems of children with brain damage.

The intelligence of the child should be tested, and this examination should be repeated once every two or three years. I. Q. determination helps to guide the physicians, the auxiliary therapists and the parents in setting appropriate educational goals for the child. The child with good intelligence should have special encouragement, and excessive demands should not be made on the child whose I. Q. is low. In addition, I. Q. testing may give information about particular intellectual problems of the child, such as special difficulties in understanding abstract concepts or in coordinating visual images with ideas and manual actions. This kind of information may help teachers to provide the child with an educational program that develops his capacities to their highest potential. The technic of *multiple sensory learning* (described in the last part of Chapter 20) is of use in training brain damaged children, as well as mentally retarded children.

The parents of a child with brain damage sometimes have emotional conflicts in their attitudes toward him. They may have hostile feelings toward the brain-damaged child who gives them fewer pleasures and more difficulties than their other children. They may be partially aware of these hostile feelings, or their hostility toward the child may be largely unconscious. Their hostile feelings may cause them to reject the child openly, or they may cover their hostility with a layer of overpossessive concern by which they try to conceal their resentment from themselves and others.

A psychotherapist often can help the parents resolve some of these conflictual feelings toward the child. He can point out that many parents of brain-damaged children struggle with such feelings, and in counseling the parents often can resolve many of their unhealthy attitudes toward the child. The parents of a brain-damaged child often have guilt feelings. They feel guilty when their hostility toward the child flashes through at times, and the mother may worry anxiously that something she did during her pregnancy caused the child's brain damage. Some parents tend to push the child into social isolation because they feel ashamed of him. Counseling to resolve these problems often helps the parents lead more comfortable lives, and it enables them to do a better job with their child.

In many instances, the parents of a brain-damaged child can talk about their child, their feelings toward him, and his problems more comfortably in group psychotherapy sessions with four to eight other couples who also have brain-damaged children. Hearing other parents discuss their occasional hostile and guilty feelings about their children helps them to resolve their own unhealthy feelings. The parents also can exchange information about methods for rearing and training their children. In many cases a parent can accept viewpoints and advice from another parent that he could not accept from a professional therapist. A parent often feels that someone "can't understand a problem like this unless he's faced it in his own home." Such psychotherapeutic groups for parents are often sponsored by clinics for brain-damaged children and by laymen's organizations that have a special interest in this area. In such settings the child sometimes is referred to as "cerebral palsied" or "exceptional," but "exceptional" at times is also applied to children with mental retardation or other kinds of difficulties.

As noted briefly above, the basic interpersonal needs of the brain-damaged child are the same as those of other children. He needs the devoted love of his parents and he needs reasonable limitations and discipline when he misbehaves. He should be neither excessively indulged nor unduly restricted. His personality development often is more influenced by his interpersonal relationships during his formative years than by the difficulties caused by his brain damage; unhealthy attitudes by parents and other close persons and neglect of his special educational and social needs may cause more difficulties than his damaged brain tissue. Environmental influences frequently determine whether the child functions to the best of his capacities and is well behaved, or whether he is fearful, belligerent and resistant. The child's total behavior is the product of his interpersonal life and his organic brain damage. Though the importance of these two influences varies much from child to child, they both play significant roles in the adjustment of every brain-damaged child.

Medications in Brain-Damaged Children. Psychiatrist disagree much about the value of the various tranquilizing drugs and so-called psychic energizers that have been much used in brain-damaged children. Many psychiatrists feel they are of little value, except in some agitated children in whom a few medications may reduce hyperactivity. The phenothiazines (Thorazine, or Chlor-pz, Sparine, and others) may help to control agitation, anxiety and restless destructiveness in some children with brain damage. The phenothiazines excert their calming effect with less cerebral cortical sedation than other sedatives. Sedatives that affect mainly the cerebral cortex, such as the barbiturates and most of the antianxiety medications, often make a brain-damaged child worse, for they further impair the efficiency of the cerebral cortex in a child whose problems arise mainly from trying to adjust to a complex world with insufficient cortical brain tissue. The phenothiazines act to a large extent on lower brain centers and the child does not develop physical tolerance to them regardless of the dosage or the length of time he takes them.

There is much difference of opinion among psychiatrists about the use of amphetamines (Benzedrine, Dexedrine and others) and methylphenidate (Ritalin) in hyperactive brain-damaged children. Advocates of these drugs propose that, by their action as central nervous system stimulants, they increase the child's alertness and allow him to concentrate longer on tasks. Many studies report improved deportment and learning in some brain-damaged, hyperactive children who take these drugs daily over long periods of time; the children are less restless while taking them. Some children improve on 10 to 15 mg. per day, whereas others take much higher doses. However, the results are quite variable; many children do not benefit from amphetamines, and others improve only temporarily. When a child improves on an amphetamine he may continue to take if for many years, but since hyperactivity tends to decrease during adolescence the drug usually is tapered off at this time. In my opinion, caffeine gives equally good results with fewer side effects and less alarm to parents who read about amphetamine abuse in the public press. Between 200 and 300 mg. of caffeine per day may be given either in tablet form or by drinking two average-sized cups of strong black coffee. Instant coffee has a lower caffeine content, as a rule, and three cups per day give the child somewhat less than 300 mg. of caffeine.

Residential Living for Brain-Damaged Children. The problems of a minority of children with chronic organic brain damage are so severe that they cannot make an adjustment outside an institution. Institutional placement sometimes is in the best interests of the child, his parents and his siblings. Institutional life is a special existence for people who need a special kind of environment. many children with organic brain damage are more content and receive better care in a well-run institution organized to meet their special needs. The complexities of modern urban living are removed and the child is relieved of the burden of making painful decisions. They are protected from people who do not understand them and might exploit them or ridicule them. In a well-run residential school designed to meet the emotional and educational needs of the child, comprehensive programs are organized to develop the child's skills to his best possible level. Many brain-damaged children attend day schools designed to meet their special educational and interpersonal needs, and they return to their homes evenings or weekends.

ORGANIC BRAIN DISORDERS ASSOCIATED WITH CHRONIC ALCOHOLISM

(The emotional problems that lead to chronic alcoholism are discussed in Chapter 13 on personality disorders, and the course and treatment of chronic alcoholism also are outlined there.) In this chapter we shall discuss the organic brain disorders caused by alcoholism. We shall divide our coverage of the alcoholic psychoses into five parts: (1) *pathological intoxication*, (2) *delirium tremens*, (3) *Korsakoff's psychosis*, (4) *alcoholic hallucinosis* and (5) other organic brain disorders associated with alcoholism, such as *alcoholic paranoid state* and *alcoholic deterioration*.

Pathological Intoxication

In pathological intoxication a patient becomes acutely disturbed after drinking only a small amount of alcohol. One cocktail may be sufficient to precipitate severely upset behavior. In some instances the patient becomes confused and disoriented and has visual hallucinations. In other instances he becomes belligerent and assaultive and may have persecutory delusions. Some patients become abruptly depressed and suicidal. The kind of reaction the person with pathological intoxication develops usually is the same each time he drinks alcohol. The disturbance lasts from an hour or two to a day or more.

The person with pathological intoxication has severe underlying personality problems that are unleashed by the minimal sedation of the cerebral cortex caused by a small amount of alcohol. Some patients have suffered previous brain damage that left them only a fragile self-control which alcohol destroys. The person with acute pathological intoxication should be sedated with oral or intramuscular chlordiazepoxide (Libritabs, Librium). Initial doses may be 50 to 100 mg., and the daily total should not exceed 300 mg. in divided doses. He may also need some of the other measures listed below for acute alcoholic intoxication.

The person who develops pathological intoxication should abstain permanently from alcohol. Disulfiram treatment (outlined in Chapter 13) may help the patient to achieve that goal.

Treatment of Acute Alcoholic Intoxication. The patient who is intoxicated from drinking too much alcohol usually does not require special treatment to recover from his bout of alcoholic excess. If he is agitated or assaultive he may be sedated with 50 to 100 mg. of chlordiazepoxide by mouth or intravenously, with a total 24-hour dosage of this drug that does not exceed 300 mg., until he sleeps off his alcoholic bout. If the alcoholic patient is dehydrated he may be given intravenously 1500 cc. of a 5 per cent dextrose solution in normal saline; an ampule of vitamin B complex and ascorbic acid may be added. If the patient is very deeply intoxicated he should be turned from one side to the other each hour and care should be taken to maintain an adequate airway. Other nursing procedures are important; limb restraints are contraindicated, but, in my opinion, a waist strap does not agitate the patient and prevents him from injury in falling from bed. In rare instances, the patient with acute alcoholic intoxication enters vascular shock, and he should receive appropriate treatment for this complication.

Delirium Tremens

Delirium tremens is an acute organic brain syndrome associated with chronic alcoholism. It is a serious illness frequently encountered in clinical practice, and it has a mortality rate of 5 per cent or more. Fatal cases at autopsy show cerebral edema and punctate hemorrhages, and liquifaction and degeneration of nerve cells.

Physicians are divided in opinion about whether delirium tremens is caused by nutritional deficiencies and the direct toxic effects of alcohol, or whether is a withdrawal syndrome in a person who is physically addicted to alcohol; (aspects of this controversy have been covered in Chapter 13). If it were a withdrawal syndrome analagous to withdrawal from narcotics or sedatives, one would expect relief by administration of alcohol to the patient, and the syndrome would not be expected in a patient who is drinking heavily each day; neither of these things occurs clinically. Hence, many clinicians feel that delirium tremens is caused by the marked vitamin, and other nutritional, deficiencies that accompany alcoholism, in addition to possible toxic effects of alcohol on nervous tissue. The chronic alcoholic often has severe vitamin deficiencies, especially of the vitamin B complex, and he also has disturbances of carbohydrate metabolism, protein metabolism and electrolyte balance. In recent years particular attention has been given to abnormalities of magnesium balance, but this is probably only one of various electrolyte difficulties. Irregular diet, gastritis and other factors contribute to these nutritional and mineral abnormalities.

Delirium tremens occurs in a person who has been a chronic alcoholic for several years or more. As a patient passes into delirium tremens he first becomes restless and ill-at-ease. Over a period of from several hours to two or three days he lapses gradually into marked confusion with clouding of consciousness and disorientation. Visual hallucinations crowd upon him. He often sees small animals such as insects, rats and snakes that dart about his room and climb upon his bed. He may pick at his skin to remove them or he may try to brush them from his bed. Persecutory delusions may occur and panic is common. The patient may shirek in terror as he tries to evade hallucinated animals or pursuing enemies. At other times he looks about, dazed, and tries to puzzle out what is going on around him. He sleeps little and fitfully, and his disorder usually is worse at night. His hands, head and tongue are tremulous, and he may shake so badly that he is unable to feed himself. Often his temperature is elevated and his pulse is rapid. Grand mal convulsions are said to occur occasionally, but, strangely, I have never seen them. Dickens in "The Pickwick Papers" gives a classic description of delirium tremens.

The last four-and-twenty hours had produced a frightful alteration. The eyes, though deeply sunk and heavy, shone with a luster, frightful to behold. The lips were parched, and cracked in many places: the dry, hard skin glowed with a burning and there was an almost unearthly air of wild anxiety in the man's face . . . A short period of oblivion, and he was wandering through a tedious maze of low arched rooms—it was close and dark, and every way he turned, some obstacle impeded his progress. There were insects too, hideous crawling things, with eyes that stared upon him and filled the very air around. The walls and ceilings were alive with reptiles—frightful figures flitted to and fro—and the faces of men he knew, rendered hideous by gibbing and mouthing, peered out from among them. . . .

Delirium tremens lasts from 2 to 10 days and leaves the patient debilitated for from several days to two weeks longer. Myocardial disease and pneumonia are common complications leading to death.

Treatment of Delirium Tremens. The patient with delirium tremens should be psychiatrically hospitalized. He should be kept in bed as much as possible. Limb restraints should not be used; a patient who struggles against restraints exhausts himself, and his panic is increased by his inability to move his hands and arms. Most psychiatrists condemn waist restrainst in bedridden patients with delirium tremens, but I feel they do not disturb the patient, prevent falls from bed, and are better than chasing a wildly delusional, panicky patient down the hall. The currently favored sedative is chlordiazepoxide (Libritabs, Librium), preferably given by mouth. The initial dose may be as high as 100 mg., and the 24-hour dosages should not exceed 300 mg. in divided doses. Initial doses can be given intramuscularly. The patient needs diligent nursing care and he should receive calm, but not insistent, reassurances about his hallucinations and delusions. He should not be allowed to exhaust himself in physical agitation. Some physicians give small doses of alcohol to the patient; I do not, since I doubt that delirium tremens is truly a withdrawal syndrome and one is merely giving to the patient the toxic substance which caused his psychosis.

The patient's fluid intake and nutrition need careful attention. The patient who will take fluids by mouth should receive 3000 cc. of fluid each day. He also should receive a bland diet of 3000 calories each day with a high carbohydrate content. Orange juice is a useful beverage for fluid, carbohydrate and vitamin content purposes. The patient should receive large amounts of vitamin B complex, especially thiamine and nicotinic acid, and vitamin C orally, and during the first week vitamin B complex should be given intramuscularly or added to any intravenous fluids the patient receives. When the patient refuses to take fluids or is nauseated, 1500 cc. of 5 per cent dextrose in water, with vitamin B complex and vitamin C added, may be given by slow intravenous infusion twice daily. Depending on the patient's electrolyte status, normal saline or 1/6 molar sodium lactate solution may be used in place of the 5 per cent dextrose in water for some of the intravenous fluid intake. Tube feedings may be used when the patient refuses solid food for more than 36 hours. Electrolyte studies are made and any electrolyte imbalances, including magnesium deficiency, are corrected. In the infrequent instances in which hepatic coma begins to complicate delirium tremens, the dietary and pharmacologic regimens are appropriately modified.

The patient's room remains brightly lighted at all times because his disturbance is worse when it is dark. *All the other applicable measures for organic brain disorders (listed at the end of Chapter 19) are carried out.* After recovery from his delirium the patient needs several weeks of convalescence and treatment for the alcoholism that led to his organic brain disorder. (The treatment of chronic alcoholism is discussed in Chapter 13.) This is one of the rare situations in medical practice where I feel it is legitimate to attempt to frighten the patient into treatment. The physician can portray to the convalescent patient the dire results of more alcoholic excess, and he can be dogmatic in his manner. This approach occasionally succeeds, and the physician has little to lose. The alcoholic who returns to drinking runs a grave risk of serious physical and psychiatric disease.

Korsakoff's Psychosis

The term Korsakoff's psychosis (it is also called the amnesic-confabulatory syndrome) is applied to a relatively uncommon type of organic brain disorder associated with chronic alcoholism in which the patient has an extensive loss of memory, which he covers up with elaborate, confabulated stories. This syndrome is caused by prolonged deficiencies of thiamine and other vitamin B components in chronic alcoholics; direct toxic action by alcohol may be an added factor. Brain syndromes characterized by memory loss and confabulation also may be caused by head trauma, cerebral arteriosclerosis, other types of brain injury and severe vitamin B complex deficiency unassociated with alcoholism. However, the term Korsakoff's psychosis usually is employed only in reference to chronic alcoholics who develop the amnesic-confabulatory syndrome. Peripheral neuritis often accompanies Korsakoff's psychosis.

Autopsy reports on patients with Korsakoff's psychosis are extremely rare, but the few available ones reveal generalized axonal degeneration, neuronal degenerative changes, and abnormal lipid depositions in brain cells, especially in the motor cortex and other frontal lobe regions.

Korsakoff's psychosis sometimes follows an attack of delirium tremens, but in many instances it appears without prior delirium. Over a several-day period the patient gradually develops profound memory loss and disorientation. However, he covers his memory loss with extensive fictitious stories. For example, a patient who has been hospitalized for a week may give a long, detailed account of how he spent the preceding day at his business office or visiting friends at their homes. I recall a 52-year-old socially prominent lady with a Korsakoff's psychosis who spent nine weeks on a psychiatric ward. She felt she was in her home and each day described to me all her social activities of the preceding day. She frequently suggested that we go into the living room to see her married daughter's picture on the grand piano. The patient with Korsakoff's psychosis usually is pleasant and talkative. His memory loss may not at first be apparent to a casual observer, but it soon becomes obvious as the inconsistencies in his confabulated stories are noticed. The thread of the patient's confabulated stories often can be guided by leading questions from the examiner. Peripheral neuritis is present in some cases, with foot drop, wrist drop and other peripheral nerve weaknesses. Most patients with Korsakoff's psychosis recover completely in 6 to 10 weeks, but they have permanent amnesia for the period during which they were ill. In a few cases Korsakoff's psychosis becomes a permanent organic brain disorder due to irreversible changes in the parenchyma of the cerebral cortex.

A patient with Korsakoff's psychosis should be psychiatrically hospitalized and should receive 50 mg. of thiamine intramuscularly each day for two weeks, since gastrointestinal absorption is sometimes defective in chronic alcoholics. He should also receive daily by mouth large amounts of all the vitamin B complex components for the duration of his illness and for several weeks after recovery, since chronic alcoholics usually have multiple vitamin deficiencies. Vitamin C and other vitamins also may be added to his diet in moderate amounts. Good nutrition, adequate fluid intake, correction of any electrolyte deficiencies and diligent nursing care are necessary. Calming medications usually are not indicated. If the patient has peripheral neuritis he should have physiotherapy to the involved areas, passive and active muscular exercises, and orthopedic appliances to prevent permanent deformities from muscle stretching and wasting. After he recovers, effort should be made to convince the patient to accept one of the treatment methods for chronic alcoholism (outlined in Chapter 13) to prevent a return to drinking.

Alcoholic Hallucinosis

We shall discuss alcoholic hallucinosis under the headings of *acute alcoholic hallucinosis* and *chronic alcoholic hallucinosis*, since these two syndromes have somewhat different characteristics, courses and treatments.

Acute Alcoholic Hallucinosis. Psychiatrists differ in opinion about the nature of the syndrome called acute alcoholic hallucinosis. Its clinical features are virtually identical with those of acute paranoid schizophrenia, but its course and prognosis resemble those of an acute organic brain disorder. Most psychiatrists feel that acute alcoholic hallucinosis is a brief episode of paranoid schizophrenia which may occur in chronic alcoholics; it is felt to be precipitated by minimal, reversible organic brain damage that releases a short paranoid schizophrenic reaction in an alcoholic who is emotionally predisposed to develop schizophrenia. In most instances the patient with acute alcoholic hallucinosis recovers in from 1 to 4 weeks, but in some cases the disorder stretches out into a prolonged or irreversible disorder that, depending on the psychiatrist's orientation, may be termed chronic alcoholic hallucinosis or paranoid schizophrenia.

The patient with acute alcoholic hallucinosis remains oriented for time and place throughout his illness and he does not have memory defects. The predominating symptoms are auditory hallucinations, persecutory delusions and panic. The illness usually begins abruptly with the onset of florid auditory hallucinations. Often the voices accuse the patient of heinous crimes, homosexuality or depraved behavior. They also may threaten him with torture and death. Visual hallucinations occur in a small percentage of cases. The patient often fears that vague but much dreaded enemies are plotting to ruin him, to poison him or to shoot him. He may become combative, homicidal or suicidal in the panic states that his hallucinations and delusions precipitate. It is probable that in acute alcoholic hallucinosis strong underlying emotional conflicts erupt in hallucinatory and delusional ways. (The emotional conflicts that may contribute to paranoid disturbances are discussed at length in Chapters 14 and 17 on paranoid schizophrenia and other paranoid psychoses, and these discussions are relevant to understanding the emotional background of acute alcoholic hallucinosis.) Some psychiatrists feel that the frequency of auditory hallucinations that accuse the patient of homosexuality indicates that many patients with acute alcoholic hallucinosis have underlying emotional conflicts over latent homosexual feelings. The patient with acute alcoholic hallucinosis should be hospitalized and adequately sedated with chlorpromazine or one of the other phenothiazines. Vitamin B complex and other vitamins should be given, and adequate nutrition and fluid intake are maintained. After recovery, every effort should be made to convince the patient to accept treatment for his chronic alcoholism, since continued drinking often results in more episodes of acute alcoholic hallucinosis. In those instances in which the patient does not recover from alcoholic hallucinosis in two months or more, the treatment measures (outlined in Chapter 14) for paranoid schizophrenia may be considered.

Chronic Alcoholic Hallucinosis. The clinical characteristics of chronic alcoholic hallucinosis are indistinguishable from those of paranoid schizophrenia. Chronic alcoholic hallucinosis usually begins insidiously in a patient with chronic alcoholism, and persecutory delusions, auditory hallucinations, belligerence, sullen hostility and occasional combativeness dominate the clinical picture. The patient may barricade himself in his room or flee in panic when he feels that attacks by his enemies are imminent. As noted above, most psychiatrists feel that these patients are suffering from paranoid schizophrenic illnesses unleashed by the emotional and physical stresses of chronic alcoholism. However, in some cases the alcoholism may be merely coincidental; both the schizophrenic illness and the alcoholism may be caused by the same underlying emotional turbulence in the patient. The treatment of chronic alcoholic hallucinosis is the same as that for paranoid schizophrenia, but the results of treatment are not as favorable as in schizophrenia. Nevertheless, over a period of several months of hospital care more than half of these patients recover. If the patient returns to drinking after leaving the hospital the relapse rate back to a psychotic state is high and therefore every effort should be made to convince a convalescent patient to accept disulfiram therapy or some other treatment for chronic alcoholism.

Other Organic Brain Disorders Associated with Alcoholism

The standard psychiatric nomenclature lists two other organic brain syndromes associated with alcoholism: *alcohol paranoid state* and *alcoholic deterioration*.

Alcohol Paranoid State. Most psychiatrists feel that alcohol paranoid state (of which *alcoholic paranoia* is a synonym) is merely a variant form of chronic alcoholic hallucinosis in which persecutory delusions are the outstanding clinical feature. In many cases the patient has strong, elaborate delusions of infidelity by his marital partner, and assaultiveness and threats of revenge on both the marital partner and the alleged paramours are common. Many of these patients are seen psychiatrically only after the process has been going on for several months, or at times for years. An ingrained paranoid illness of this type is often quite resistant to all forms of treatment, though some patients recover with several months or more of phenothiazine therapy, group psychotherapy and hospital therapeutic environmental activities. However, many of these patients show few clinical abnormalities except their delusions, which may be limited to two or three areas of their lives, and their marked excitability and belligerence about them; hence, they may be able to resist all efforts to commit them to psychiatric hospitals since they can reason ably in other areas of their lives. Actual homicides by these patients are less frequent than might be expected, but beatings, assaults and chaotic marital and child-rearing histories are common.

Alcoholic Deterioration. (A large number of the persons included in this category are described in the last four paragraphs of the section titled "Clinical Course of Alcoholism" in Chapter 13.) These patients undergo a gradual socioeconomic, emotional and physical deterioration secondary to chronic alcoholism. In these patients the social deterioration and subtle organic brain damage may be so interwoven that it is difficult to disentangle them. The patient is evasive, profoundly self-centered, irresponsible, emotionally indifferent to other people or sullen, and socially isolated. His life seems to have been reduced to alcohol and the oblivion it gives him. Those patients who show obvious organic brain deterioration with spotty memory defects, occasional disorientation, loss of learned skills, grossly defective judgement and emotional lability would be classified in this category. As a rule, they do not have the delusions, hallucinations and confabulation that would cause them to be given some other alcoholic psychotic diagnosis. Many destitute, long-term, physically debilitated alcoholics have sufficient evidence of brain damage because of nutritional deficiencies and the toxic effects of alcohol, to justify this diagnosis.

BIBLIOGRAPHY

Adler, R., and Engel, G. L.: Psychologic processes and ischemic stroke (occulsive cerebrovascular disease). Psychosom. Med., *33*:1, 1971.

Berlyne, N.: Confabulation. Brit. J. Psychiatry, *120*:31, 1972.

Birkett, D. P.: The psychiatric differentiation of senility and arteriosclerosis. Brit. J. Psychiatry, *120*:321, 1972.

Busse, E. W., and Pfeiffer, E. (eds.): Mental Illness in Later Life. Washington, D. C., American Psychiatric Association, 1973.

Feldshuh, B., Sillen, J., Parker, B., and Frosch, W.: The nonpsychotic organic brain syndrome. Am. J. Psychiatry, *130*:1026, 1973.

Gardner, R. A.: Psychogenic problems of brain-damaged children and their parents. J. Amer. Acad. Child Psychiatry, *7*:471, 1968.

Merskey, H., and Woodforde, J. M.: Psychiatric sequellae of minor head injury. Brain, *95*:521, 1972.

Millichap, J. G.: Drugs in the management of minimal brain dysfunction. Int. J. Child Psychother., *1*:68, 1972.

Palestine, M. L.: Drug treatment of the alcohol withdrawal syndrome and delirium tremens. Quart. J. Stud. Alcohol, *34*:185, 1973.

Rice, E.: Organic brain syndromes and suicide. Int. J. Psychoanal. Psychother., *2*:338, 1973.

Rothstein, E.: Prevention of alcohol withdrawal seizures. Am. J. Psychiatry, *130*:1381, 1973.

Russell, W. R.: The traumatic amnesias. New York, Oxford University Press, 1971.

Satterfield, J. H., Cantwell, D. P., Saul, R. E., and Yusin, A.: Intelligence, academic achievement and EEG abnormalities in hyperactive children. Am. J. Psychiatry, *131*:391, 1974.

Schnackenberg, R. C.: Caffeine as a substitute for Schedule II stimulants in hyperactive children. Am. J. Psychiatry, *130*:796, 1973.

Simon, A.: Physical and socio-physiologic stress in the geriatric mentally ill. Compr. Psychiatry, *11*:242, 1970.

Walzer, S., and Wolff, P. H.: Minimal Cerebral Dysfunction in Children. New York, Grune & Stratton, 1973.

19

Other Types of Organic Brain Disorders

In the preceding chapter we covered the four types of organic brain disorders which account for 75 per cent, or more, of the organic brain illnesses encountered in clinical practice. In this chapter we shall cover all other types of organic brain syndromes. They are those that are produced by (1) intoxication by drugs and chemicals, (2) circulatory disturbances, such as congestive heart failure, (3) intracranial neoplasms, (4) metabolic disturbances, such as uremia and diabetic coma, (5) intracranial infections, such as meningitis and encephalitis, (6) syphilis of the central nervous system, (7) degenerative central nervous system diseases, such as multiple sclerosis and Huntington's chorea, (8) convulsive disorders and (9) severe general infections, especially with high fever and prostration.

The basic symptoms common to most organic brain disorders are discussed at length in the beginning of the previous chapter and therefore will not be repeated here. Certain aspects of the treatment of each of these nine types of organic brain disorders will be covered under each category, and in addition this chapter will end with a discussion of measures applicable in the management of most kinds of organic brain disturbances.

ORGANIC BRAIN DISORDERS CAUSED BY INTOXICATION BY DRUGS AND CHEMICALS

Many medications can occasionally cause organic brain disturbances, and a wide variety of substances used in industry and households can produce brief or long-lasting brain disorders. We shall discuss only those medications and toxic substances that are relatively common causes of brain disorders, but the list of agents that less frequently produce mental symptoms is long.

Bromides

The incidence of bromide intoxication varies much from one decade to the next and from one part of the country to another. Bromide intoxication today is caused mainly by long usage of proprietary sedative preparations that contain bromides and can be purchased without a prescription. The amount of such preparations taken by the public depends on local customs and the vigor with which their manufacturers advertise them. Between 1 and 2 per cent of all psychotic patients seen in clinical practice have brain sydromes due to bromides; I often order a routine blood bromide level on hospitalized psychiatric patients.

When a patient takes bromides over a long period of time, the bromide ion gradually replaces the chloride ion in the body fluids. Symptoms of bromide intoxication may begin in from several weeks to several months or more after the patient begins to take the bromide preparation. In elderly patients, debilitated persons and chronic alcoholics, mental disturbances may begin with blood serum levels as low as 75 mg. of bromide per 100 cc. of serum. However, in most instances psychiatric symptoms do not occur until the blood bromide level goes over 150 mg./100 cc. of serum. Most patients who are hospitalized with an organic brain disorder due to bromides have blood levels between 175 mg. and 600 mg. per 100 cc. of serum. Bromide intoxication is sometimes called bromidism, or bromism.

The clinical characteristics of bromide intoxication are extremely varied and they may mimic schizophrenia, stuporous depressions, agitated depressions and severe anxiety neuroses. In elderly patients bromide intoxication may be mistaken for chronic organic brain syndromes due to cerebral arteriosclerosis and senile brain deterioration. The patient often is somewhat confused and disoriented, but he may also be anxious, agitated and depressed. Persecutory delusions may occur and visual hallucinations are common. I recall a 69-year-old woman whose physician felt she was suffering from senile organic brain disease. He requested psychiatric consultation when she one day stated that the hospital authorities should do something about the man sitting beside her bed; she complained that he was made of chicken wire and had a rooster on his head. Her blood bromide level was 210 mg./100 cc. of serum, and she recovered completely when the bromides were removed from her system. Most of the cardinal symptoms of acute organic brain disorders (listed at the beginning of Chapter 18) may occur in bromide intoxication. Other symptoms that may be present are fever, ataxia, tremulousness, slurred speech and hypoactive deep tendon reflexes. A skin rash resembling acne is present in 20 per cent of patients with bromism.

The patient who develops bromide intoxication usually begins to take the proprietary medication for anxiousness, phobias, depressiveness, insomnia or other emotional problems. In time the bromide preparation itself begins to produce psychiatric symptoms and the patient increases his daily dosage of bromides to combat these new discomforts. An organic brain syndrome due to bromide intoxication results, and the patient's underlying emotional problem is obscured.

The diagnosis is made by determining the blood bromide level. Since bromide intoxication may mimic other psychiatric illnesses, the diagnosis is easily missed if bromism is not considered as a possibility. If the patient remains in a psychiatric hospital for several weeks or longer, he no longer takes his bromide preparation and the bromides are slowly excreted in his urine. His consequent recovery may be attributed to psychiatric treatment which actually was irrelevant to his problem, and the fact that he had bromism goes unrecognized.

The patient with bromide intoxication should be given about 1.5 gm. of enteric-coated ammonium chloride four times each day and he should be maintained on a high fluid intake. The chloride ion replaces the bromide ion in the body fluids and the ammonium ion acts as a diruetic. Intravenous sodium chloride solutions may be used for the first few days when the blood bromide level is very high. Dialysis rarely is indicated. Enteric-coated sodium chloride in doses of 1.5 gm. four times each day may be given in addition to the ammonium chloride to speed the elimination of bromides. Elderly patients who receive sodium chloride must be watched carefully to avoid pulmonary edema and the accumulation of fluid in other body tissues. Many elderly patients have a tendency to accumulate body fluid and they should receive a daily diuretic such as 100 mg. of hydrochlorothiazide (Esidrix, HydroDiuril, Oretic) while receivng sodium chloride. The electrolyte status of an elderly patient should be watched to prevent potassium depletion or other electrolye disturbances. If the patient with bromism is agitated, he may be given small daily doses of chlorpromazine (Thorazine, or Chlor-pz) or another phenothiazine. With about two weeks of treatment the patient's bromide level usually drops to the point where he recovers from his organic brain symptoms. The complete elimination of bromides from the body may take several weeks longer, but the administration of ammonium chloride or sodium chloride is not necessary after the blood serum bromide level falls below 50 mg./100 cc.

After the patient recovers from bromide intoxication he should be psychiatrically evaluated to determine the reason why he was taking a bromide preparation. Some patients take them for long periods because of mild anxiousness, and they do not require extensive psychiatric help. Others take bromides to assuage the symptoms of anxiety neuroses, phobias, depressiveness and other psychiatric conditions, and they should receive treatment for these difficulties. The physician should emphasize the danger of bromide preparations to the patient and his family to deter the patient from returning to bromides when he leaves the hospital. Public education on the dangers of self-administered proprietary bromide preparations would be a useful public health measure.

Sedatives and Antianxiety Medications

Most sedatives and antianxiety medications (minor tranquilizers) can cause organic brain syndromes when they are taken in large amounts, either abruptly or gradually over an extensive period of time. (The distinction between sedatives and antianxiety medications is made in Chapter 22, but, since the organic brain disorders they produce are similar, they will treated together here.)

These drugs include all barbiturates, meprobamate (Miltown, Equanil), glutethimide (Doriden), ethchlorvynol (Placidyl), ethinamate (Valmid), methyprylon (Noludar), chlordiazepoxide (Libritabs, Librium), diazepam (Valium), oxazepam (Serax) and many others. All these drugs, when taken in excessive amounts, produce states ranging from drowsy confusion and disorientation to profound coma. Although their manufacturers state that some of them, particularly those designated as antianxiety medications, act mainly on lower brain centers, there is much doubt of this; based on clinical evidence, I feel they exercise their major effects directly on the cerebral cortex. Hallucinations and delusions are rare in organic brain syndromes produced by these medications, but all other symptoms of organic brain syndromes are common. Also, patients who take excessive amounts of these sedatives and antianxiety medications over long periods of time may become physically addicted to them and may undergo withdrawal symptoms with hallucinatory states and convulsions when withdrawn from them. (The problems of addiction to these drugs and management of their withdrawal syndromes are covered in Chapter 13.)

The only widely used, large group of calming medications which do not produce organic brain disorders and addiction are the phenothiazines (Thorazine or Chlor-pz, Mellaril, Stelazine, Sparine and others) and chemically related drugs such as the thioxanthene derivatives (Taractan, Navane) and the butyrophenone derivatives (Haldol). Regardless of size of dosage and length of usage, they do not produce organic brain syndromes or addiction; abrupt, massive doses may produce somnolent states that last two or three days, but even then fatalities are so rare that some authorities consider suicide by these drugs almost impossible. These drugs are usually referred to as the antipsychotic medications, or major tranquilizers.

Overdosage with sedatives and antianxiety medications (minor tranquilizers) may be abrupt or gradual. Abrupt overdosage often is the result of suicidal attempt. In other instances the patient may take a sedative capsule at bedtime, or an antianxiety medication during the day, and a short time later he confusedly forgets he took it and he takes another one. This process may be repeated several or more times during a two- or three-hour period, and it causes an abrupt overdosage of the drug.

In other instances the patient takes excessive amounts of a sedative over a period of several weeks or several months. He usually takes it to assuage anxiety, and he increasingly takes more than is prescribed to quell his rising titer of anxiousness. Although he often gets the drug by prescription for anxiousness or insomnia, he may obtain it from illicit sources. The patient who misuses a sedative or antianxiety medication either abruptly or gradually has emotional problems which led to his access to the drug and his subsequent misue of it.

We shall discuss overdosage with sedatives and antianxiety medications under the headings of *abrupt overdosage* and *gradual overdosage*.

Abrupt Overdosage. In mild, abrupt overdosage with sedatives or antianxiety medications, the patient is drowsy, ataxic, confused and at least partially disoriented. His speech is slurred and often he sees double. He cannot coordinate his movements well in eating, drinking, smoking and writing. His judgement is poor, his actions are impulsive and imprudent, and he may laugh, cry or become angry on slight provocation.

In moderate overdosage the patient sleeps, but he can be partially roused by firmly pinching the Achilles tendon or by shaking him by the shoulder and talking loudly to him. His deep tendon reflexes are depressed and he has nystagmus, but his respiration and blood pressure are normal or only slightly depressed.

In severe overdosage the patient does not groan or move when the Achilles tendon is squeezed, and he does not respond to any kind of stimulus. Respiration is shallow and slow and the blood pressure begins to fall. Deep tendon reflexes and corneal reflexes are sluggish or absent.

The diagnosis of abrupt intoxication with sedatives or antianxiety medications is easily made when the excessive ingestion of the medication is described by the patient or his relatives. In mild or moderate cases the patient may deny taking sedatives, and blood or urine tests for a few of these medications may be ordered. However, these tests are time-consuming; when the intoxication is mild the patient does not need them, and when the intoxication is grave immediate treatment is an urgent necessity. The diagnosis usually must be made on the basis of the patient's physical condition, diligent interviewing of his family, telephone calls to any physicians who may lately have prescribed medications for him, careful search for empty medication bottles, carelessly dropped capsules, and suicidal notes. Abrupt intoxication with sedatives must be distinguished from head injuries, alcoholic intoxication, diabetic coma, insulin shock, hepatic or uremic coma, cerebrovascular accidents and other causes of lethargy or coma of quick onset. Head injury may complicate intoxication with sedatives, since the patient may stumble and fall in his drowsy, ataxic state.

Treatment of Abrupt Overdosage. Central nervous system stimulating drugs are now rarely used in treating overdosages with sedatives and antianxiety medications, since their usefulness is doubtful and their dangers are clear. Gastric lavage should be performed to remove medications from the stomach if the patient has ingested them within four hours before being seen. Patients with mild intoxication do not require specific treatment. Patients with moderate overdosage of sedatives or antianxiety medication require good nursing care and careful observation, but they usually do not require specific treatment. All patients with drug overdosages should be psychiatrically hospitalized, because the underlying problems that led to the overdosage should be carefully investigated.

In patients with severe overdosage, maintenance of an adequate airway is an immediate necessity. Dentures and removable bridges are taken out, the foot of the bed is elevated, and mucus and excessive secretions are suctioned periodically from the mouth and pharynx. An oropharyngeal hard rubber airway is inserted, and in some instances an anesthetist or an otolaryngologist should insert an endotracheal tube. If respiration begins to fail an automatic positive pressure respirator, or other type of respiratory assistance, must be applied. A tracheotomy is advisable if these measures do not remove all respiratory embarrassment.

The patient's blood pressure is carefully watched and plasma or whole blood is administered if circulatory collapse occurs. The patient is turned from side to side every two hours, and diligent nursing care is imperative. An osmotic diuretic such as mannitol (Osmitrol) may be useful in promoting the urinary excretion of some of these drugs, such as barbiturates. Oxygen is usually given, but it must not be applied in such high concentrations that it removes anoxic stimuli to the carotid chemoreceptors. A bronchoscopy should be performed if atelectasis occurs, or the cough reflex should be stimulated mechanically. Three thousand cc. of fluid is administered intravenously each day, and electrolyte balance is carefully maintained. An indwelling catheter is placed in the bladder to prevent urinary retention. Many physicians prophylactically administer an antibiotic to diminish the chance of pneumonia, urinary tract infections and bacteremia. Hemodialysis may be necessary in severe cases.

In some instances the patient was physically addicted to the sedative or antianxiety medication before his sudden overdosage with it, and he undergoes a withdrawal syndrome after he emerges from his acute intoxication. (The clinical features and treatment of withdrawal syndromes from sedatives and antianxiety medications are outlined in Chapter 13.) After recovery from his overdosage the patient needs psychiatric help for the emotional problems that led to his misuse of the medication.

Gradual Overdosage. Some patients gradually take excessive amounts of sedatives or antianxiety medications over periods of from many weeks to several years. These patients often have fluctuating amounts of drowsiness, confusion, disorientation, ataxia, muscular incoordination and emotional lability. They may laugh, cry or become belligerent without apparent provocation. Their judgement is poor, and they become slovenly and irresponsible. Toxic deliriums with panic, hallucinations and delusions may occur in long-term overdosage with sedatives or antianxiety medications, but they are rare. Delirious reactions occur mainly during withdrawal of these medications from patients who are physically addicted to them.

Many patients who chronically misuse sedatives and antianxiety medications deny it vehemently, and they become very astute in hiding medications in their homes, in their clothing and even in their hospital rooms. They may present puzzling diagnostic problems. Psychiatric hospitalization and careful observation may be the only way to clarify the picture and to stop the patient from taking the medications. Many of these patients are physically addicted to the drugs they are taking and should be withdrawn slowly in the hospital (as outlined in Chapter 13). Urine and blood tests for barbiturates formerly were very useful diagnostically in deceptive patients, but the spectrum of abused sedatives and antianxiety medications has become so broad in recent times that such tests have lost most of their value. The patient with chronic overdosage with these medications often is evasive and uncooperative, but whenever possible he should be engaged in psychiatric treatment for the underlying personality problems that led to his chronic misuse of medications.

Permanent Brain Damage. In the vast majority of cases, the patient who recovers from an abrupt, massive overdose of a sedative or antianxiety medication does not have permanent brain damage. However, in a small percentage of cases the patient suffers irreversible brain damage and has permanent mental changes such as memory losses, partial clouding of consciousness, reduced intellectual abilities, poor control of emotions, and personality changes. In some instances the patient is so brain-damaged that he remains in a semistuporous state and is unable to care for himself in any way. Chronic brain damage of this kind is probably caused by poor cerebral oxygenation and blood flow due to respiratory obstruction or depression, or transitory vascular collapse, during the period of acute intoxication.

Some psychiatrists feel that long-term, severe overdosages of sedatives and antianxiety medications may, by direct toxic action or interference with brain biochemistry, cause gradual degenerative changes in cerebral cortical cells and other brain centers. On neurological work-up these patients may show mental signs of permanent brain damage (spotty memory losses, disorientation, and so forth), diminution of brain size on pneumoencephalogram, electroencephalographic abnormalities, and other dysfunctions. Most psychiatrists, however, feel that such findings are rare and that when they do occur they are the results of repeated episodes of embarrassed respiration and impaired cerebral blood flow, perhaps combined with long-term vitamin deficiencies, that took place after particularly heavy overdosages during a span of many years.

Amphetamines

(The personality problems that lead to misuse of amphetamines and emotional dependence upon them are covered in Chapter 13.) We shall here discuss in more detail the organic brain disorders that may be caused by taking excessive amounts of amphetamines.

An amphetamine may contribute to an organic brain syndrome in two ways. Firstly, it may exert direct chemical influence on brain tissue. Secondly, it may cause the patient to be overactive, to eat poorly and to sleep little for many days, weeks or months, and thus it leads to malnutrition and marked physical exhaustion, which contribute to an organic brain disorder.

As a patient passes into an organic brain syndrome due to an amphetamine he goes through a period of disorganized activity, agitation and tremulousness. He then becomes disoriented and bewildered, though he preserves a bright-eyed distractibility and jerky restlessness in the midst of his confusion. Visual and auditory hallucinations and persecutory delusions are common, but they often fluctuate much in intensity from one day to the next. Most amphetamine psychoses subside in from several days to two weeks when the amphetamine is discontinued and mild sedation is given in a psychiatric hospital. (The choice of calming drugs is discussed in Chapter 13.)

However, in some instances the patient with an amphetamine psychosis passes into a prolonged clinical state undistinguishable from paranoid schizophrenia. I have seen patients who required several months of hospital treatment before they recovered from such illnesses. Psychiatrists disagree about whether such prolonged paranoid illnesses are caused by the persistent effects of amphetamines, or whether the amphetamines precipitate paranoid schizophrenic illnesses in persons who are predisposed to develop them. Nevertheless, there seems to be a definite connection between amphetamines and paranoid psychoses in these cases, because the type of schizophrenic disorder precipitated is almost always paranoid in nature with florid delusions of persecution. The treatment of these reactions is the same as for paranoid schizophrenia.

Other Medications

The natural and synthetic *adrenal corticosteroids* in rare instances can produce organic brain disorders. The prolonged use of adrenal corticosteroid medications in high dosages also is associated occasionally with the development of manic and depressive psychoses. These psychoses seem to be precipitated in persons who have personality problems predisposing them to such disturbances, but the mechanism by which adrenal corticosteroids produce these effects is unknown. The incidence of these disorders has decreased in recent years; this may be due to less danger with the more recently developed synthetic corticosteroids, or it may reflect more caution by physicians in prescribing them.

The list of medications that in rare instances produce organic brain disorders is long. It includes chloral hydrate, paraldehyde, belladonna, trihexyphenidyl (Artane, Tremin, Pipanol), quinacrine (Atabrine), chloroquine (Aralen), lithium salts, phenacemide (Phenurone), urea (Ureaphil, Urevert), digitalis preparations, salicylates, levodopa (Dopar, Larodopa) and many others. Children occasionally develop brief organic brain syndromes after instillation of atropine in the eye. All these disorders usually last from several hours to several days.

Lead

The inhalation or ingestion of lead may cause organic brain disorders. Despite safety programs, inhalation of lead-containing vapors and dust still occurs occasionally in industry. Whereas the respiratory route of lead poisoning is most common in adults, lead poisoning in children most frequently is due to gnawing on objects covered with lead-containing paint or eating paint flakes that peel off metal or wood surfaces. Lead inhibits various metabolic processes in the central nervous system and in other parts of the body.

An acute organic brain syndrome caused by lead is characterized by lethargy, confusion, agitation, disorientation and panic. Visual hallucinations and persecutory delusions may occur. Periods of stupor or delirium may alternate with lucid periods, and convulsions and tremors may occur. Diagnostic clues may be obtained by the careful interviewing of parents or inquiry into an adult's vocational activities. Careful physical evaluation, hematologic studies, laboratory tests and roentgenologic studies often are needed to confirm the diagnosis.

Acute lead encephalopathy is a medical emergency. In children the mortality rate may run as high as 25 per cent. The preferred treatment is administration of the calcium salt of ethylene diamine tetraacetic acid (EDTA) which removes lead from the body. Teamwork between the pediatrician or internist, and the psychiatrist may be necessary in the comprehensive management of the delirious, stuporous or confused patient.

In some instances lead poisoning produces irreversible brain damage. Children with permanent brain damage caused by lead have impaired judgement, reduced learning abilities, emotional lability, memory defects and restless hyperactivity. Neurological signs of focal brain damage may be present. Adults with permanent brain damage from lead often have, in addition, blindness and extraoccular muscle paralyses.

Other Toxic Substances

Many other toxic substances occasionally are the causes of brief or long-lasting organic brain disorders (characterized by most of the basic symptoms outlined at the beginning of Chapter 18). *Carbon monoxide* may produce an acute delirious reaction; the patient often goes through a comatose phase and later develops confusion, panic, hallucinations and delusions as he emerges from his coma. In severe cases the patient may develop permanent organic brain damage; other neurological signs, especially basal ganglia syndromes such as Parkinsonism, are occasional concomitants of carbon monoxide brain damage. Exposure to low concentrations of carbon monoxide over periods of many weeks or months may cause slight intellectual confusion, headaches, spotty memory confusion and emotional lability; these symptoms usually clear when the carbon monoxide exposure ceases.

In rare instances pesticides containing phosphorous or other toxic agents may cause transitory or permanent brain disorders, and mercury and manganese are occasional offenders in industrial processes or wastes. Other intoxicants include carbon disulfide, carbon tetrachloride, camphor, turpentine, gasoline, cigarette lighter fluid, and the many industrial and household chemicals that contain benzene or related substances. Rarer causes of organic brain damage include hundreds of other synthetic and natural chemicals and compounds. (The toxic reactions caused by LSD, the other hallucinogens, cocaine and other illicit drugs are discussed in Chapter 13.)

ORGANIC BRAIN DISORDERS CAUSED BY CIRCULATORY DISTURBANCES

Organic brain syndromes may be caused by circulatory disorders that impair blood and oxygen supply to the brain. The most common extracranial circulatory cause of acute organic brain disorders is cardiac decompensation. Severe cardiac decompensation decreases cerebral blood flow and also impairs oxygenation of blood because of pulmonary edema. Such brain disorders are more common in elderly patients who already have borderline or minimal brain tissue damage due to senile brain deterioration and cerebral arteriosclerosis. The patient is confused, disoriented and forgetful. He often does not realize he is in a hospital and attempts to get out of bed to attend to household tasks or to get dressed to go to work. He may have visual hallucinations and panic, and he may ramble erratically in his speech. In describing Falstaff's delirium in King Henry V Shakespeare writes ". . . for I saw him fumble with the sheets, and play with flowers, and smile upon his fingers' ends . . . his nose was sharp as a pen and he babbled of green fields. . ." Acute brain disorders associated with cardiac decompensation fluctuate markedly; the patient may pass in and out of his confused state from one hour to the next, and he is more bewildered at night.

Organic brain disorders also may be caused by other circulatory problems, such as cerebral embolism or insufficiency of cerebral blood flow due to spasm of intracranial vessels or extracranial vessels that supply the brain. Arterial hypertension often is present in these disorders; these disturbances may be transitory, but cerebral thrombosis and hemorrhage frequently produce permanent organic brain deficits. Acute or chronic lung disease, such as lobar pneumonia and emphysema, may decrease the oxygen content of the blood reaching the brain and thus predispose the patient to confusional states. In many elderly patients both pulmonary and vascular diseases are present.

Most of these patients can be managed on a medical floor; they do not need psychiatric hospitalization. All kinds of sedating drugs should be avoided. If possible, a member of the patient's family should remain at his bedside at all times to orient him, to reassure him and to secure his cooperation in treatment. The patient usually can recognize a family member whom he has known for many years, but he cannot remember who the nurses and doctors are, and he becomes frightened and resistant when they approach him. In addition, all the management measures outlined for organic brain disorders (at the end of this chapter) should be carried out.

Acute Brain Disorders Following Heart Surgery. Acute psychotic illnesses following open heart surgery are fairly common. In the early years of major vascular surgery the frequency of these reactions ran as high as 30 per cent in some series. However, that figure is constantly declining as operative technics, anesthestic methods and postoperative care improve, and such disorders probably occur now in less than 10 per cent of cases. Most of these disorders, and all of them that I have seen, are organic brain reactions, with stuporous confusion, disorientation, memory defects, agitation and panic. Hallucinations and delusions have been reported. These disorders almost invariably clear up within several days after the operation and leave no apparent sequellae. Presumably, they are caused by oxygen deficiency and impaired blood supply to the brain during the operation, in addition to the effects of a prolonged anesthesia and a complex, apparatus-filled postoperative period.

However, emotional factors also enter into these reactions. The significant mortality rate, relative newness and seriousness of open heart surgery is known to the patients, and, as they emerge from the operation, panic contaminates the organic confusion they are passing through. Careful, constant nursing attendance, and the presence of a relative whom the patient can recognize and cling to, help. Preoperative explanations of all that is to come, with massive reassurances, also are helpful. I have found mild sedation with a phenothiazine useful in agitated patients, and I feel that a waist restraint is better than a patient struggling to climb over siderails with a nurse and a relative pulling him back; all other types of restraints, such as limb restraints, should not be used.

Some of these patients face rehabilitation problems in the weeks and months following operation. They may have become accustomed to the life style of a cardiac invalid or semi-invalid, and their newly acquired physical self-sufficiency necessitates readjustment from a dependent, demanding role to an independent, giving one. However, all the patients I have seen have made this transition fairly well.

ORGANIC BRAIN DISORDERS CAUSED BY INTRACRANIAL NEOPLASMS

As an intracranial neoplasm slowly impairs the functioning of the cerebral cortex, the patient's ability to control underlying emotional problems may decrease. He attempts to adjust to interpersonal stresses with less cortical brain tissue at his command, and he may develop anxiousness, phobias, depressiveness, obsessions or hysterical conversion symptoms. These neurotic symptoms, which occur in only a minority of patients with brain tumors, may appear many weeks or months before neurological signs occur. I recall a patient whom I treated for three months in weekly psychotherapeutic sessions for anxiety attacks and phobias; craniotomy a short time later showed a frontal lobe astrocytoma. I probably have repressed the painful memories of one or two other such cases.

However, other personality changes are more common than neurotic symptoms in patients with brain tumors. The patient with a brain tumor often becomes irresponsible, slovenly and crude. Long-standing personality difficulties, such as an irrascible temper or painful shyness, may become exaggerated as the patient's brain capacity to control his emotional problems is progressively destroyed. He may become impulsive, sexually brazen and financially improvident. As his intracranial tumor grows larger, he develops signs of intellectual deterioration. He becomes forgetful and his judgement is impaired. Lethargic clouding of consciousness may occur, and the patient gropes in a puzzled way to understand what is going on around him. He becomes emotionally labile with rapid fluctuations between silly laughing, crying and belligerence. Intellectual capacities such as calculation and general fund of information are impaired, and in late stages the patient may become disoriented and have delusions and hallucinations. I recall a 46-year-old certified public accountant whom I saw in consultation who had been treated psychiatrically for one year for personality changes and paranoid delusions; he died on the operating table while a large astrocytoma was being removed from his left parietal lobe.

Neoplasms in particular locations in the brain have tendencies to produce special symptoms. For example, temporal lobe tumors may produce visual hallucinations and hallucinations of taste and smell. Temporal lobe tumors may produce déjà vu feelings and dreamlike trances. Hallucinations of bright flashes of light may occur in occipital lobe tumors, and the patient with a frontal lobe tumor often has social crudeness, irresponsibility and a mild euphoria.

The degree of reversibility of the personality changes caused by an intracranial neoplasm depends on the type of tumor, its location, its duration and its accessibility to removal. For example, the emotional symptoms associated with a meningioma lying over a frontal lobe may be largely reversible if the diagnosis is made early and the tumor is removed. However, the personality symptoms produced by a glioblastoma multiforme cause a chronic organic brain syndrome, which is only partially relieved by operation, and the tumor in time leads to the death of the patient. Even when a brain tumor is completely removed the brain damage caused by it may be permanent, and this damage may be further complicated by brain tissue destruction during neurosurgery.

ORGANIC BRAIN DISORDERS CAUSED BY METABOLIC DISTURBANCES

A large number of metabolic diseases occasionally cause organic brain disorders; in many instances these disorders are transitory and clear up when the metabolic disturbance is successfully treated, but in other cases permanent brain damage results. In most instances the mental state of the patient is clinically overshadowed by overwhelming physical dysfunctions. We shall discuss briefly a few of the metabolic diseases that may cause acute organic brain syndromes.

Uremia. The patient in the early stages of uremia characteristically is fatigued and apathetic. As his uremia becomes more severe, he may become confused, disoriented and restless. Agitation and hallucinations occur in some instances. The patient often has lucid periods interlaced with episodes of delirium. In advanced uremia the patient becomes increasingly drowsy and lapses into coma.

Hepatic Failure. Acute organic brain symptoms often are prominent features of hepatic failure. Early in the course of hepatic failure the patient may be euphoric or may have mild depressiveness. As the hepatic failure increases, the patient becomes confused, disoriented and agitated. Visual hallucinations and paranoid delusions may occur. The patient's delirium fluctuates in intensity, but he becomes increasingly confused and drowsy as he moves toward *hepatic coma.*

Pernicious Anemia. Mental symptoms caused by pernicious anemia are rarely encountered in psychiatric practice since the introduction of specific therapy for this disease. However, mild emotional symptoms are reported in several per cent of new patients with pernicious anemia seen in hematology clinics. Untreated pernicious anemia can produce an acute or chronic organic brain disorder. The patient may have confusion, disorientation, agitation, persecutory delusions and visual hallucinations. Persecutory delusions predominate in some cases and depression may be a prominent feature in others.

Porphyria. Porphyria is an uncommon disease, but it should be considered in the differential diagnosis of the patient with abdominal pain of obscure origin. Dermatologic changes and lesions of the peripheral, central and autonomic nervous systems may be present. Psychiatric symptoms are common, particular in the type of porphyria termed hepatic porphyria, or acute intermittent porphyria. The patient may be irritable, agitated and depressed, or he may have an acute organic brain syndrome with clouding of consciousness, disorientation, memory disturbances, hallucinations and delusions. The psychiatric symptoms usually are intermittent with recovery after an acute attack. Chlorpromazine (Thorazine, Chlor-pz) is useful in porphyria. It calms the patient and decreases the intensity of his abdominal pain, but it does not alter neurological lesions. In divided doses totaling 400 mg. or more each day, it helps to terminate acute attacks of porphyria, though it does not directly alter the basic metabolic disturbance. Barbiturates are contraindicated, because they often precipitate attacks of porphyria.

Vitamin B Deficiencies. Organic brain disorders due to deficiencies of thiamine or niacin are rare in the United States, except in the brain disorders associated with chronic alcoholism (which are discussed in Chapter 18). Deficiency of thiamine may produce a confusional, hallucinatory brain reaction or it may cause an amnesic-confabulatory picture similar to that seen in Korsakoff's syndrome in chronic alcoholics. The term Wernicke's encephalopathy (also called the Wernicke-Korsakoff syndrome, or cerebral beriberi, or acute hemorrhagic polioencephalitis) is applied to the thiamine deficiency syndrome of ocular nerve paralyses, ataxia, peripheral neuritis and acute organic brain symptoms. Niacin deficiency produces pellagra, which has been virtually eliminated in the United States. Besides its dermatologic, oral, gastrointestinal and neurological symptoms, pellagra often produces irritability, depression, intellectual confusion, memory loss and hallucinations.

Hyperthyroidism. Uncontrolled, severe hyperthyroidism may produce an organic brain syndrome with agitation, disorientation, delusions and hallucinations. In modern medical practice such deliriums are rarely seen, since hyperthyroidism usually is treated before it reaches an advanced stage. The particular complication of severe thyrotoxicosis (often called thyroid "crisis" or "storm") is characterized by an acute delirium, but the grave metabolic crisis of the patient overshadows his psychiatric problems. In rare instances, severe hyperthyroidism may precipitate a manic psychosis, and if the patient is not treated psychiatrically for his manic disorder it may last for several months after the thyroid metabolism has been returned to normal limits by antithyroid medications, or radioiodine therapy, or surgery. (The psychosomatic aspects of hyperthyroidism are discussed in Chapter 11.)

Hypothyroidism. In occasional instances, depressiveness, or apathy, or an organic brain syndrome is seen in adult patients with severe hypothyroidism; as a rule, the hypothyroidism must be severe enough to produce the classical picture of myxedema. Though mild or moderate hypothyroidism may be associated with a certain amount of lethargy, it does not precipitate depressiveness or organic brain disorders. In infantile hypothyroidism (cretinism) the child is apathetic and dull, and often is mentally retarded.

Diabetes. The patient in severe diabetic acidosis may pass through a period of confusion, restlessness and disorientation before he passes into coma. The hypoglycemia, or "insulin shock," produced by an excess of insulin in relation to food intake, may produce an acute organic brain disorder with agitation, delusions and disorientation. (The emotional problems of the patient who must adjust to diabetes are reviewed in Chapter 1.)

ORGANIC BRAIN DISORDERS CAUSED BY INTRACRANIAL INFECTIONS

Bacterial Infections. Acute organic brain disorders may be caused by bacterial meningitis. Meningococcal meningitis (Neisseria meningitis) is the most common epidemic cause of this type of acute organic brain syndrome, but meningitis due to hemophilus influenzae, streptococcus pyogenes, escherichia coli and other bacteria also may produce mental symptoms. Clouding of consciousness is an early symptom of bacterial meningitis. The patient becomes drowsy, restless and somewhat disoriented. His drowsy confusion may be interrupted at times by noisy agitation and visual hallucinations. His symptoms usually are worse at night when darkness aggravates his disorientation and increases his misinterpretation of his environment.

Permanent brain damage due to bacterial infection has become uncommon since the introduction of the many kinds of antibiotic and other antibacterial medications. However, permanent organic brain syndromes still occur occasionally in patients in whom therapy was started late or whose illnesses did not respond well to antibacterial medications. Patients who have personality changes caused by chronic organic brain damage after meningitis often have other signs of neurological damage, such as cranial nerve paralyses, deafness and convulsions. Intelligence, memory and learned skills may be impaired, and the patient may be emotionally labile, socially crude and erratically belligerent. These changes may be so mild that they are barely noticeable or so severe that the patient is socially disabled.

The psychiatric symptoms of tuberculous meningitis begin more insidiously. The patient gradually becomes listless, apathetic and irritable. Agitation, disorientation and memory loss may occur later. The patient at times may be fairly clear and at other times he lapses into confusion and hallucinatory states. His fitful sleep may be interrupted by restless agitation. Permanent personality changes occur in patients who do not receive early, effective treatment.

A brain abscess (now a very rare type of disorder) usually is associated with slowly progressive apathy, somnolence and dulling of intellectual abilities. The psychiatric symptoms of brain abscesses frequently are similar to those of brain tumors, and they vary depending on the location of the abscess in the brain. For example, a slowly growing abscess in the frontal lobes may cause personality changes such as irresponsibility, impulsive crudeness and mild euphoria. Hallucinations, delusions and panic states are rare in brain abscesses.

Intracranial infections due to fungi and yeasts, which have attracted increasing attention in recent years, may produce organic brain changes similar to those of tuberculous intracranial infections.

Viral Infections. The epidemic and endemic forms of viral encephalitis may cause acute organic brain syndromes, and in some cases persistent brain damage occurs. Psychiatric symptoms also may occur in encephalitis due to measles, mumps and other childhood viral diseases; childhood viral diseases have become very rare as causes of encephalitis in developed nations, but they are somewhat common causes in some tropical countries, where measles is still the fourth most common cause of death.

The patient with acute viral encephalitis usually is apathetic and drowsy, and often he is somewhat disoriented. In severe cases the drowsy confusion proceeds into coma. In a minority of cases the patient is agitated, and he may have hallucinations, delusions and panic states. The patient with viral encephalitis may recover entirely, or he may go on to develop the symptoms of chronic organic brain damage. With the exception of drowsiness and mild confusion, which are almost always present in viral encephalitis, the incidence of acute organic brain symptoms varies much depending on the particular etiologic strain of virus.

In a minority of cases viral encephalitis produces permanent brain damage and long-lasting personality changes. There is much dispute about whether these persistent post-encephalitic personality problems are caused by residuals of acute encephalitis or whether they are produced by continued activity of the virus in the brain for months or years after the acute attack.

In occasional instances a patient emerges from an attack of acute viral encephalitis with obvious evidence of neurological damage and gross mental changes. He may have memory defects, difficulty in orienting himself in time and place, impaired judgement and loss of learned intellectual and manual skills. He may have poor control of his emotional responses and may become sullen, belligerent or panic-stricken on little provocation. He is socially crude, insensitive to the needs and feelings of other people, and may engage in antisocial acts such as lying, stealing and assaultiveness toward others. Children who have gross organic brain damage after encephalitis often are hyperactive, aimlessly destructive and erratically belligerent. They may have diminished I. Q.'s and much difficulty in schoolwork, and they may engage in such antisocial acts as cruelty to animals, running away and chaotic defiance of their parents and teachers. Some children and adults who have chronic organic brain damage after encephalitis require institutional care on a long-term basis.

The patient with subtle, less obvious chronic organic brain damage after encephalitis often presents difficult diagnostic problems and has personality difficulties that in time cause much trouble to himself, his family and others with whom he associates. As a rule, he does not have clinically discernible defects of memory, orientation and learned intellectual and manual skills. He has impaired, judgement, however, and his emotional responses are erratic and impulsive. He is irresponsible and insensitive to the feelings of others, and he may engage in antisocial activities such as lying, stealing and sexual delinquency. He acts on the impulse of the moment with little regard for its consequences. Punishment, failure and social disgrace do not deter him from repeated dishonest, irresponsible, impulsive acts. The patient has little guilt or anxiety about his acts, and he tries to evade the consequences of his antisocial behavior by lies and deceptions. The child with minimal postencephalitic chronic brain damage rebels against his parents and teachers, runs away, lies, steals and does not change his behavior despite discipline and punishment. He does poorly in school despite an I. Q. which often is in the normal or low normal range; however, in some instances his I. Q. is low enough to place him in the range of mild mental retardation. He may be sullen or he may flit from one misdeed to another with a careless nonchalance. During adolescence he is prone to get into legal trouble because of thefts, sexual delinquency, irresponsible automobile driving, running away and vagrancy. These patterns continue into adulthood and the patient may drift into a life of petty crime and social maladjustment. Broken marriages, neglected children, alcoholism, prostitution and socioeconomic destitution may characterize his adult life. These postencephalitic personality problems are caused by the destruction of cerebral cortical brain tissue, which impairs the patient's capacities for the finer moral and social aspects of interpersonal living. These defects may be mild, moderate or severe. Encephalitis that occurs in adulthood may produce this kind of antisocial personality deterioration in a person who until the time of his encephalitis made a good interpersonal adjustment.

There are marked resemblances (as pointed out in Chapter 12) between an interpersonally caused antisocial personality disorder and the antisocial behavior of the person who has postencephalitic organic brain damage. These similarities sometimes create marked diagnostic problems. When an adult has a clear-cut history of encephalitis with a substantiating hospital record of the actue illness, and his behavior shows a marked change that dates from the time he had encephalitis, the diagnosis of postencephalitic personality change may be made with confidence. Electroencephalographic abnormalities and characteristic findings on psychological testing supplement the diagnosis. However, in many instances the evidence for encephalitis is not clear-cut, and, in addition, it is difficult to determine whether or not the patient had some of his antisocial personality problems before his illness. Moreover, in children it sometimes is difficult to ascertain whether the child's rebellious, deceptive antisocial behavior is due to his encephalitis or due to unhealthy interpersonal relationships with his parents. In some instances the child may recover entirely from his acute encephalitis but have personality problems due to interpersonal damage rather than persistent organic brain damage. These problems cause marked diagnostic difficulties, (which are discussed in the section on antisocial personality disorders in Chapter 12).

The results of psychiatric treatment of the child or adult with postencephalitic permanent organic brain damage usually are unsatisfactory. Many medications, including various antianxiety and antipsychotic drugs, as well as anticonvulsants, have been used, but the evidence that they help these patients is inconclusive. Amphetamines or caffeine are sometimes employed to try to diminish hyperactivity and to increase attention span in postencepalitic children. Some psychiatrists feel that psychotherapy occasionally helps postencephalitic patients who have minimal brain damage and who still have enough intact personality resources to benefit from interview treatment. However, most psychiatrists are pessimistic about the results of psychotherapy in these patients. Often the psychiatrist must restrict his efforts to counseling the patient's family on how best to manage the patient and to prevent him from getting into chronic social and legal difficulties. Long-term institutional care may be the only feasible recommendation in severe cases.

ORGANIC BRAIN DISORDERS CAUSED BY SYPHILIS OF THE CENTRAL NERVOUS SYSTEM

In the first two decades of the 20th Century about 10 per cent of patients admitted to public psychiatric hospitals suffered from organic brain syndromes caused by central nervous system syphilis. The vast majority of these patients had general paresis, the more commonly employed name for meningoencephalitic syphilis. Penicillin radically altered this picture. Today, internists see and treat patients who have asymptomatic involvement of the central nervous system during the early stages of a general syphilitic infection, but patients who develop psychiatric symptoms because of syphilis of the central nervous system have become uncommon in psychiatric practice. In the following discussion of central nervous system syphilis we shall restrict our attention mainly to its effects on emotional functioning and interpersonal relationships; we shall give scant attention to its neurologic features and brain pathology.

General Paresis

The vast majority of patients with organic brain damage due to central nervous system syphilis fall in the category of general paresis, the commonly used term for meningoencephalitic central nervous system syphilis. It consists of a general inflammatory and degenerative process involving the brain parenchyma, the meninges and the cerebral blood vessels. Though it usually appears from 5 to 20 years after the initial infection, it may appear as late as 30 years or more after syphilis is first contracted. In advanced cases it is characterized by extensive personality changes, tremors, muscle incoordination and weaknesses, pupillary changes, convulsive seizures, hyperactive deep tendon reflexes and other neurological signs. In untreated cases the blood serology tests for syphilis are almost always positive. The spinal fluid always shows a positive complement fixation and it usually shows an increase of cells, an elevated protein and a first phase elevated colloidal gold curve. Untreated cases may proceed to death within five years.

The clinical features of general paresis are extremely varied; the patient has evidence of intellectual deterioration and he also has clinical features that may be similar to manic, or depressive, or paranoid, or neurotic illnesses. An old psychiatric axiom states that general paresis may mimic almost all other types of psychiatric illness. Hence, despite the drastic reduction of central nervous system syphilis as a cause psychiatric illness, it is customary that a routine blood serology test for syphilis is done on all psychiatric hospital admissions.

The first evidence of general paresis often consists of a subtle, progressive deterioration in the patient's social behavior and economic responsibility. His personal cleanliness and grooming become slovenly and his table manners become crude. He becomes tactless and offensive in his daily interpersonal contacts. The man who formerly was meticulous in his financial affairs begins to be irresponsible with money and careless in his business dealings. The patient becomes somewhat forgetful and his attention span is short. His judgement in all areas of his life deteriorates, and he may create serious economic and social difficulties for himself and his family if his relatives and friends do not recognize that he is ill until his general paresis is well advanced. He may become obscene in his conversation and sexually brazen. He may become irritable and morose or gregarious with undesirable people. These early symptoms of personality deterioration may go on for many months before neurological signs or bizarre behavior startle his family into the recognition that he is suffering from a serious disease. If the patient does not receive prompt, adequate treatment, his intellectual deterioration may in time produce gross memory losses, disorientation and loss of learned intellectual and manual skills.

As the inflammatory and degenerative process of general paresis attacks diffuse areas of the cerebral cortex, underlying emotional problems which formerly were well controlled may begin to appear. The particular emotional features that develop, such as euphoria or depressiveness, are much influenced by the patient's basic personality structure. In some instances the patient has fatigue, anxiousness, phobias and insomnia, and on superficial examination he may seem to have a neurotic reaction. The domineering person may become belligerent and tyrannical, and the shy patient may become frightened and withdrawn. In each instance, these emotional symptoms develop as the patient attempts to control his personality problems and to adjust to his interpersonal stresses with less cortical brain tissue at his command.

A euphoric reaction, often accompanied by

grandiose delusions, is common in general paresis. The patient has expansive self-confidence and bizarre delusions that he has great wealth, or vast political authority, or omnipotent religious power. For example, he may feel that he owns a vast industrial empire or that he can manipulate the destinies of nations. In other instances, the patient with general paresis is depressed, and he has bizarre delusions of guilt and inadequacy. In some cases, delusions of persecution dominate the clinical picture, and on superficial evaluation the patient's condition may resemble paranoid schizophrenia. Juvenile paresis, which usually begins in late childhood or early adolescence, has become rare since the introduction of penicillin and routine serology tests for syphilis on pregnant women. Juvenile paresis is characterized by marked intellectual deterioration; delusions and mood changes are less frequent than in adult general paresis.

Treatment with penicillin usually stops the progression of general paresis, and in many instances the patient's clinical condition improves immensely. If treatment is begun during the early stages of the illness the patient may improve enough to be able to make a reasonably good socioeconomic and emotional adjustment. When treatment begins after there has been much irreparable degeneration of cerebral cortical tissue, the downhill course of general paresis may be stopped, but the patient remains unable to adjust outside an institution.

The patient with general paresis should receive a total of 12 to 15 million units of benzathine penicillin G in once or twice weekly injections over a 30-day period. Other antibiotics can be employed in patients who are allergic to penicillin. Subsequently, the patient should be evaluated by spinal fluid examinations at intervals of once every six months for three years, and thereafter the spinal fluid examinations should be made once each year for five years more. Failure of treatment or recrudescence of general paresis, as indicated by spinal fluid examination, necessitates a later course of penicillin.

Successful treatment should be followed by careful discharge planning to help the patient make a good interpersonal adjustment after he leaves the hospital. His socioeconomic status and family adjustment may have deteriorated much before his relatives realized he was ill and brought him for medical help. Often the patient and his family need supportive counseling during the patient's post-hospitalization readjustment.

Meningovascular Syphilis

Meningovascular syphilis consists of meningal inflammation and proliferative endarteritis of cerebral vessels in a patient whose initial syphilitic infection usually occurred three to five years before central nervous system symptoms became evident. The clinical picture usually is dominated by gradual or sudden cerebrovascular thromboses in a person under the age of 40. The blood serology test for syphilis usually is positive, but the spinal fluid may or may not show increased cells, increased protein, a positive complement-fixation test and an abnormal colloidal gold curve. When the disease has a large meningeal involvement the spinal fluid tests are positive, but when the process is mainly vascular the spinal fluid findings may be normal. In some instances the patient has neurological signs, such as hemiplegia or cranial nerve paralyses, without significant mental changes. In other cases, the cerebrovascular thromboses cause clouding of consciousness, memory losses, disorientation, impairment of judgement, personality changes and emotional lability. These patients often recover entirely if penicillin treatment is started promptly, but when there has been irreparable brain damage because of interrupted cerebral blood flow the patient may have permanent neurological and mental changes. The treatment regimen with benzathine penicillin G is the same as for general paresis.

ORGANIC BRAIN DISORDERS CAUSED BY DEGENERATIVE CENTRAL NERVOUS SYSTEM DISEASES

Organic brain syndromes may be caused by a large number of degenerative brain diseases. Most of these pathologic processes are rarely seen in clinical practice; the only commonly encountered one is multiple sclerosis. Internists see a fair number of patients with disseminated (systemic) lupus erythematosus, and it may involve the central nervous system, but these patients are infrequently observed in psychiatric work. We shall discuss briefly a few of these conditions; our attention will be restricted to their effects on emotional functioning and interpersonal adjustment.

Multiple sclerosis is often characterized by changes in the patient's personality and behavior. In advanced cases with widespread cortical brain damage the patient may have memory losses, disorientation, confusion and loss of learned intellectual and manual skills. However, other kinds of personality changes are the most common psychiatric findings in multiple sclerosis. The loss of cortical brain cells may unleash underlying psychiatric problems that the patient was able to hold in check when he had an intact cerebral cortex at his command for interpersonal adjustments. Depressions, manic episodes and paranoid states may occur, and I have seen several patients with multiple sclerosis who also had paranoid schizophrenic disorders. Since multiple sclerosis is a common neurological illness, patients sometimes are aware of its long-term unfavorable prognosis; hopeless despair and suicidal attempts occasionally occur. In other instances the patient develops a mild euphoria with nonchalant insensitivity to the serious problems and tasks of life. Emotional instability is common, with silly giggling, abrupt tearfulness or easily aroused anger and belligerence. These personality problems may fluctuate in intensity; the patient may recover from depressions, manic episodes or paranoid schizophrenic syndromes, but his tendency to relapse months or years later is high.

Disseminated (systemic) lupus erythematosus is an inflammatory disorder of connective tissue which occurs mainly in young women; among its protean features are polyarthritis, diffuse myocarditis, pleurisy, pneumonia, lymphadenopathy, splenomegaly, cutaneous lesions and renal involvement. When the brain is involved psychiatric symptoms may occur. Often they mimic other kinds of psychiatric disorders, presenting neurotic symptoms, or personality changes, or delirious confusional states. In the past some of these psychiatric pictures were thought to be caused by corticosteroid therapy given patients with lupus erythematosus, but it now appears that most of these mental disorders are due to lupus itself. Although some psychiatric writers feel that psychiatric symptoms are common in lupus, I have not found this so. Cases of lupus which are seen in university medical centers tend to be selected samples of patients with obscure or complicated features and do not, in my opinion, represent the general range of persons suffering from this condition.

Alzheimer's disease is a rare brain degenerative disease which occurs mainly in persons between the ages of 50 and 60, but may occur occasionally in younger individuals. The patient has a diffuse cellular degeneration of the entire cerebral cortex. Some neuropathologists feel that in Alzheimer's disease there is a characteristic intracellular degeneration with the production of tangled, curled fibrillar material. Other pathologists feel that these intracellular changes also may occur in other kinds of degenerative brain disease and are not characteristic of Alzheimer's disease. The patient with Alzheimer's disease has gradual memory losses, disorientation, confusion, emotional lability and exaggeration of previous personality characteristics. Dysarthrias, aphasias, convulsions and muscular paralyses may occur as the disease slowly proceeds toward a fatal conclusion in from several years to a decade or so. Some psychiatrists feel that Alzheimer's disease is merely an atypical variant of senile brain degenerative disease, which begins in persons in their 40's or 50's rather than in their 60's or 70's.

Pick's disease is another rare form of cerebral cortical degenerative brain disease which occurs in persons between the ages of 45 and 60. Degeneration is most marked in the frontal and temporal lobes, and these areas show cellular destruction and gross atrophy. The patient has marked personality changes; he may become euphoric and irresponsible, or he may become irritable, belligerent and morose. Gross memory losses and disorientation are not marked early in the disease, but the patient's judgement, emotional control and reasoning capacities deteriorate. Aphasias are common, and the disease progresses to a fatal termination in from 3 to 10 years. Some neurologists feel that this illness may have hereditary determinants in some cases. Many psychiatrists feel that distinction of

Pick's disease from Alzheimer's disease on clinical grounds is speculative, and that both illnesses are rare forms of premature senile brain degeneration in middle-aged persons.

Huntington's chorea is a relatively rare degenerative brain disorder which affects the basal ganglia and the cerebral cortex. It is transmitted as an autosomal dominant trait, and elaborate geneological studies have traced its transmission through many generations. Huntington's chorea usually begins between the ages of 30 and 45 and is fatal within 15 years after onset. Choreiform movements and mental deterioration may begin at about the same time, or the choreiform movements may antedate the onset of intellectual deterioration. Personality changes are marked; the patient may become euphoric or he may become depressed and irritable. The patient may commit suicide as he feels himself slipping into the illness which he knows is carried hereditarily in his family. Memory losses, disorientation, confusion, impaired judgement and emotional lability become gradually worse as the disease progresses.

There is no effective treatment for any of the degenerative brain diseases discussed in this section. However, phenothiazine medications are often useful in agitated, or delirious, or delusional states which they unleash, and I have seen schizophrenic episodes in patients with multiple sclerosis clear entirely with phenothiazine therapy. Antidepressant medications also may be useful in depressions which occur in these patients. Measures to prevent suicide are sometimes needed in patients with multiple sclerosis and Huntington's chorea, especially those who understand clearly the grim futures which lie before them.

ORGANIC BRAIN SYNDROMES CAUSED BY CONVULSIVE DISORDERS

Transient Confusional States Following Seizures. In most cases the patient who has an idiopathic grand mal seizure is slightly confused and somewhat sleepy for from a few minutes to several hours following his convulsion. In some instances, however, the patient has marked clouding of consciousness and disorientation after a grand mal seizure. The patient's memory is profoundly impaired and he is unaware of what he is doing or where he is. For example, after a seizure in a public place the patient may believe he is at home and he may begin to undress to go bed. In other instances the patient wanders from the scene of his seizure in a dazed manner and may travel a considerable distance while unaware of his actions. In a postconvulsive confusional state the patient also may have delusions and visual hallucinations, and he may become panic-stricken and combative. Most transient organic brain states after convulsive seizures clear within a few hours or a few days. Postconvulsive confusional states are most apt to occur after several seizures during a short period of time or after status epilepticus. The patient who has postconvulsive confusion that lasts more than a few hours should be psychiatrically hospitalized and he should continue to receive his anticonvulsant medication. Sedatives, other than those which may be part of the patient's usual anticonvulsive regimen, should be avoided. However, if agitation is severe, phenobarbital by oral or intramuscular route is the sedative of choice. Many psychiatrists feel that phenothiazines should not be used since they occasionally increase the incidence of seizures; other psychiatrists feel that, although phenothiazines may accentuate dysrhythmias on electroencephalograms, the evidence that they actually cause more seizures is unconvincing.

Persistent Personality Changes Associated With Convulsive Disorders. Many psychiatrists feel that a limited amount of chronic organic brain damage occurs in a small number of patients with convulsive seizures. We are discussing here those patients whose seizures fall in the category of idiopathic epilepsy due to periodic electrochemical discharges in the brain. That is, at the time of life, usually childhood, in which their seizures begin, these patients do not have clinically discernible organic brain defects. Neurologists disagree about whether patients with such idiopathic epilepsy have microscopic brain lesions causing their seizures, or whether such small brain lesions sometimes found at autopsy are the results of repeated seizures rather than their cause.

An epileptic seizure is accompanied by a

brief period of anoxia, and this anoxia may be prolonged in some instances by respiratory embarrassment due to mucous secretions or inspired vomitus after the seizure. In addition, some neurologists feel that frequent seizures, especially during status epilepticus, may cause discrete punctate hemorrhages in the brain, and that over long periods of time the combined effects of these hemorrhages and repeated anoxic episodes may cause mild chronic organic brain damage. Furthermore, some physicians feel that the prolonged use of large doses of anticonvulsant medications, which may occur in patients whose seizures are poorly controlled on average doses of medications, also may contribute to minimal organic brain damage.

The patient with chronic organic brain damage associated with convulsive seizures is usually described as somewhat forgetful and easily confused; he loses some of his intellectual alertness and manual agility. His I. Q. may be dull normal or it may fall in the range of mild mental retardation. His personal grooming, judgement and emotional control may deteriorate. In some instances the patient becomes a timid, seclusive person who is interpersonally isolated.

However, many psychiatrists feel that this picture of emotional deterioration and interpersonal isolation which occurs in a small percentage of persons with idiopathic epilepsy probably is in most instances caused mainly by the patient's emotional reaction to his epilepsy and only to a small extent by any mild organic brain damage. The patient with frequent seizures may dread to venture from his home for fear of having seizures in public places. He often drops out of school during middle adolescence, cannot find work and shuns contacts with people. Often he may be slightly drowsy from the effects of large amounts of anticonvulsant medications, which he takes to try to reduce the number of his seizures. Thus, he slowly drifts into interpersonal isolation and apathy in which minimal chronic brain damage plays only a small role; in many cases the personality deterioration of the patient is entirely due to emotional and interpersonal factors.

Improved medical care, a better public understanding of epilepsy and comprehensive interpersonal and socioeconomic planning for epileptic patients is resulting in a decreasing incidence of personality deterioration in persons with convulsive seizures. The comprehensive management of an epileptic patient should include careful counseling and educational planning to help him achieve his best possible social and economic adjustment. (This subject is also discussed in Chapter 11 in our consideration of the psychosomatic aspects of convulsive seizures.)

ORGANIC BRAIN DISORDERS CAUSED BY SEVERE GENERAL INFECTIONS

Transient organic brain disturbances may occur in association with severe, prostrating systemic infections in which the infectious agent does not invade the central nervous system. Such illnesses include viral and bacterial pneumonias, severe upper respiratory infections, the common viral illnesses of childhood, typhoid fever and others. Psychiatric symptoms due to severe systemic infections are more common in small children and elderly people.

The ways in which systemic infections cause transient organic brain symptoms are not well understood. In many instances the patient does not have significant electrolyte disturbances, or anoxia from pneumonia or the accumulation of definable metabolic toxins which might account for his mental symptoms. The way in which high fevers produce delirious states is not clear, but it is assumed that they exercise a direct harmful effect on brain physiology. Children and old people have less capacity to adjust to the physical stresses of severe systemic infections and therefore have greater vulnerability to these disturbances.

Febrile and infectious deliriums often begin at night. The patient rambles confusedly in his speech and picks at his bedclothes. He tries to get out of bed to attend to some task he feels he must do, and it may be difficult to keep him in bed. He misinterprets objects and people, and he loses his sense of time. Visual hallucinations, agitation and noisy shouting are common. During the day the patient often is better, but still confused. He stares about him in a bewildered way and tries to puzzle out what is going on. He may become panic-stricken and combative, and occasionally he tries to flee from his room to elude delusional persecutors. On rare occasions the patient may harm himself seriously in falling downstairs or out of a window in his wild efforts to elude hallucinated dangers. His confusion fluctuates much; at times he is clear, and at other times he sinks rapidly back into his delirium.

In addition to proper medical treatment for his systemic infection and the general measures for organic brain syndromes, which are discussed in the next section of this chapter, the patient needs antipyretic medication, wet sponge baths and similar procedures to reduce high fever when it is present. His nutrition and electrolyte balance must be maintained. Children usually can be managed on a pediatric floor, but the child does much better if a member of his immediate family is at his bedside at all times to reassure him and orient him. Adolescents and adults frequently need management in the hospital's psychiatric division, for they may become agitated and combative at night and may try to flee the hospital ward.

SOME BASIC PRINCIPLES FOR THE MANAGEMENT OF ORGANIC BRAIN DISORDERS

(The material of this section applies to the treatment of many kinds of organic brain disorders discussed in both Chapters 18 and 19).

Management of the basic physical disease or removal of the etiologic toxic agent, when this is possible, is the fundamental step in treating an organic brain disorder. The second step is management of the patient's emotional and intellectual problems while he is struggling to remain in contact with his environment despite impairment of part of his brain tissue. We shall list some general principles for the psychiatric management of a patient with an organic brain disorder.

1. Since the patient's memory loss tends to be for recent events rather than for events and people of the distant past, it often is useful for a familiar person whom the patient has known for a long time, such as a sibling or the patient's marital partner, to be at his bedside much of the time. The patient often can recognize a familiar person, but he reacts with fear and mistrust toward doctors, nurses and aids whose faces and names he cannot remember and whose good intentions he does not comprehend. The familiar person helps to reduce the patient's confusion, disorientation, uncooperativeness and panic. He forms a useful link to the environmental world which the patient is struggling to reach.

2. The patient's room should be well lighted at all times. Most organic brain disorders are worse at night when the patient's confusion is aggravated by loss of orienting clues in the darkness. A well lighted room diminishes the patient's confusion and fear.

3. Environmental stimuli should be reduced as much as possible. Loud noises, bustling activities and elaborate medical procedures add to the patient's alarm and confusion. Medical procedures such as venipunctures and blood pressure readings should be accompanied by calm reassurances, and often the patient cooperates better when the relative at the bedside reassures him also. Visual stimuli should be reduced; wall decorations should be removed, brightly colored blankets should not be used, and drapes are best kept drawn. The patient does better if he remains in his room and sees only the hospital personnel and two or three relatives during the acute phase of an organic brain disorder, such as delirium tremens or a reaction to toxic chemicals or drugs.

4. The physicians, nurses and aids who are caring for the patient should reassure him with quiet, brief comments about any delusions and hallucinations he may have. They should offer their reassurances, but they should not press them insistently; they should lay them before the patient, but they should not cram them down his throat. Reassurances given with calm brevity sometimes quiet the patient; reassurances that are strongly pushed on the patient agitate him. For example, the physician or nurse may say to the frightened, delusional, hallucinating patient, "I can understand how a person with your sickness is troubled by such worries and sights, but I think when you are well they will not bother you," or "I know you are terrified by these things, but when you feel better they will be gone." Often, the tone of the nurse's or physician's voice is more important than what he says. The physicians, nurses, aids and relatives should never argue with the patient

about his delusions or discuss them at length with him; arguments and long discussions tend to fix delusions more firmly in the patient's mind.

5. Patients with severe organic brain disorders of sudden onset should almost always be hospitalized. Some of them can be treated on general medical floors. For example, an elderly patient with a mild or moderate delirium caused by congestive heart failure can be cared for on a medical floor, or a child with a transitory organic brain syndrome due to head trauma or encephalitis can be treated in a pediatric section. However, many patients with acute organic brain disorders require psychiatric hospitalization. Patients with delirium tremens and other acute alcoholic psychoses always should be on a psychiatric floor. Most patients who range in age between adolescence and old age should be hospitalized psychiatrically, for in many instances they may become belligerent, combative or suicidal, and for the safety of others and themselves they should have the protective care that only a psychiatric division can afford. In some instances the panic-stricken patient accidently may injure himself while running down a stairs or through a corridor to escape delusional persecutors. Ideally, the patient should be in the psychiatric division of a general medical hospital rather than in a hospital that receives only psychiatric patients. In the psychiatric division of a general medical hospital the patient may best receive the comprehensive medical and psychiatric care he needs.

6. Limb restraints should never be used, and most psychiatrists condemn the use of waist restraints. However, in my opinion a waist restraint often is better than chasing a delusional, aged patient with congestive heart failure down the corridor, and in such patients heavy doses of phenothiazines or other drugs (so-called "chemical restraint") is medically harmful. Side rails are dangerous for many patients; I have seen several patients who tried to climb over them at night and fell to the floor, sustaining severe fractures. Limb restraints frighten, agitate and exhaust patients, but I feel that waist restraints do not disturb or exhaust patients and often are the least of various evils.

7. When a patient has an acute, severe organic brain disorder careful attention must be given to make sure that he has adequate nutrition, good fluid intake and sound electrolyte balance. The patient's general hygiene should be supervised carefully, and in some cases he must be catheterized periodically or have an indwelling catheter to prevent urinary retention.

8. Sedatives and other calming medications that strongly depress the cerebral cortex should be avoided. To try to control the patient's panic and agitation by administering barbiturates, chloral hydrate and other common sedatives may cause more confusion and disorientation by further impairing a cortex already functioning poorly. Medications such as the phenothiazines (Thorazine, Sparine and others), which exercise much of their calming effect on lower brain centers, are preferable. Some psychiatrists feel that chlordiazepoxide (Libritabs, Librium) and related drugs are useful in organic brain disorders, but I have found them little different from the older sedatives such as barbiturates. (The dosages and means of administration of these drugs are discussed in Chapter 22.)

9. The professional staff taking care of a patient with an organic brain disorder should have some information about his personality characteristics before his brain disturbance began. As the patient struggles to adjust to his environment with fewer brain cells at his command, old personality characteristics often become exaggerated. The timid patient becomes a frightened recluse, the irritable person becomes furious, the self-conscious individual becomes paranoid, and the pessimistic patient may become severely depressed. If nurses, aids and other professional personnel, as well as the psychiatrist, know the nature of the patients' premorbid personality, they may be better prepared to deal with him when he is in an organic brain syndrome.

10. In those cases in which the patient recovers from his organic brain disorder, a thorough effort should be made to prevent its recurrence. For example, the physician should try to persuade an alcoholic to accept treatment for his alcoholism, and the patient who has an organic brain disturbance due to bromides or barbiturates should enter psy-

chotherapy to try to resolve the emotional problems that led him to misuse these drugs. Counseling with both the patient and his family is often indicated.

11. During the patient's convalescence the physician should, in relevant cases, take all possible steps to minimize the chance of disability associated with financial compensation, litigation or other secondary gains produced by the illness or injury. The physician sometimes should discuss these problems frankly with the patient and his family. He should point out that litigation, financial compensation for injury, and prolonged inactivity sometimes make it difficult for the patient to engage wholeheartedly in his rehabilitation. The phsyician may point out that the patient is entitled to whatever compensation is just, but that the patient's primary goal is to get well and to return to full, healthy activity.

12. A comprehensive rehabilitation program is needed in some cases to enable patients with permanent organic brain damage to make the best possible social adjustments, and to prepare them for vocational activities, if possible. Such programs may involve multidisciplinary work by psychiatrists, psychiatric nurses, vocational counselors, rehabilitation workers, physiotherapists, social workers, and other medical specialists such as neurologists and orthopedists.

BIBLIOGRAPHY

Andersson, P. G.: Intracranial tumors in a psychiatric hospital autopsy material. Acta Psychiat. Scand., 46:213, 1970.

Bale, R. N.: Brain damage in diabetes mellitus. Brit. J. Psychiatry, 122:337, 1973.

Boll, T. J., Heaton, R., and Reitan, R. M.: Neuropsychological and emotional correlates of Huntington's chorea. J. Nerv. Ment. Dis., 158:61, 1974.

Chrisstoffels, J., and Thiel, J. H.: Delirium acutum, a potentially fatal condition in the psychiatric hospital. Psychiat. Neurol. Neurochirg., 73:177, 1970.

Dewhurst, K.: The neurosyphilitic psychoses today. Brit. J. Psychiatry, 115:31, 1969.

Ellinwood, E. H.: Emergency treatment of acute reactions to CNS stimulants. J. Psychedelic Drugs, 5:147, 1972.

Ganz, V. H., Gurland, B. J., Deming, W. E., and Fisher, B.: The study of the psychiatric symptoms of systemic lupus erythematosus. Psychosom. Med., 34:207, 1972.

Himmelhoch, J., et al.: Sub-acute encephalitis: behavioral and neurological aspects. Brit. J. Psychiatry, 116:531, 1970.

Jenkins, R. B., and Groh, R. H.: Mental symptoms in parkinsonian patients treated with L-dopa. Lancet, 2:177, 1970.

Layne, O. L. and Yudofsky, S. C.: Postoperative psychosis in cardiotomy patients. New. Eng. J. Med., 284:518, 1971.

Mindham, R. H. S.: Psychiatric symptoms in parkinsonism. J. Neurol. Neurosurg. Psychiat., 33:188, 1970.

Morse, R. M., and Litin, E. M.: The anatomy of a delirium. Am. J. Psychiatry, 128:111, 1971.

Rifkin, A., Quitkin, F., and Klein, D. F.: Organic brain syndrome during lithium carbonate treatment. Compr. Psychiatry, 14:251, 1973.

Synder, S. H.: Amphetamine psychosis: a model "schizophrenia" mediated by catecholamines. Am. J. Psychiatry, 130:61, 1973.

Storey, P. B.: Brain damage and personality change after subarachnoid hemorrhage. Brit. J. Psychiatry, 117:129, 1970.

Storm-Mathisen, A.: General paresis. Acta Psychiat. Scand., 45:118, 1969.

Van Putten, T., and Menkes, J. H.: Huntington's disease masquerading as chronic schizophrenia. Dis. Nerv. Syst., 34:54, 1973.

Wintrob, R. M.: Malaria and the acute psychotic episode. J. Nerv. Ment. Dis., 156:306, 1973.

Wolstenholme, G. E. W., and O'Connor, M.: Alzheimer's Disease and Related Conditions. Baltimore, Williams & Wilkins, 1970.

Part Five

Mental Retardation

A variety of disorders characterized by decreased intelligence of the patient are grouped together under the term mental retardation. At present it is conventional to consider them loosely as belonging to one large category of disorders, though they may be caused by widely differing kinds of etiologies. When knowledge of the causes of mental retardation is greater, this group of disorders will probably be broken into entirely separate conditions, according to their specific causes. The causes of mental retardation are known in only a relatively small percentage of cases at the present time. However, a great deal is known about how to rear and educate mentally retarded individuals so that they may lead socially effective, useful lives. Mental retardation is a large public health problem which presents many challenges to physicians and various other professional workers who evaluate, educate, guide and care for mentally retarded persons.

20

Mental Retardation and the Management of Mentally Retarded Patients

Patients whose dominant clinical feature is defective intelligence are customarily grouped under the term "mental retardation." In their consideration of the subject of mental retardation, most psychiatrists do not discuss those patients whose main clinical features are overwhelming neurological disabilities or other diseases to which defective intelligence incidentally is joined. For example, the child whose major disorder is severe permanent organic brain damage due to brain trauma in the prenatal, natal or postnatal periods, and who has defective intelligence as well as neurological evidence of brain damage, is usually considered in the discussion of organic brain syndromes, since mental retardation is not his primary diagnosis. However, this distinction between patients in whom mental retardation is the dominant clinical feature and those in whom mental retardation is a subordinate feature leads to some arbitrary exclusions and inclusions in any discussion of this subject.

In the vast majority of cases of mental retardation the cause of the patient's intellectual defect is not known, and we say that he suffers from idiopathic mental retardation; however, this is merely an elaborate way of saying that we do not know what is causing the patient's intellectual deficit. At present, a clear cause of the patient's retardation is apparent in only several per cent of cases. In the future, when the causes of retardation are better understood, this diagnostic category will probably be abandoned, and these patients will be diagnosed according to specific metabolic, chromosomal, neurochemical, sociocultural, and other, etiologies. This time is probably far off, and for some time we shall continue to consider these persons under the broad designation of mental retardation. Some psychiatrists prefer alternate terms, such as "mental deficiency," "mental subnormality," and others.

About three per cent of children born each year are mentally retarded, and mental retardation is a major public health problem. There are several million mentally retarded individuals in the United States and 1.5 million retarded persons under the age of 18. About 175,000 retarded patients live in special residential schools and institutions. Many thousands of special teachers, psychiatric nurses, rehabilitation workers, vocational counselors and other professional persons devote themselves to helping the mentally retarded.

CLINICAL FEATURES OF MENTAL RETARDATION

Harry Stack Sullivan felt that the basic problems of a mentally retarded person were twofold: Firstly, he is less able to see the *relatedness of things* and to become aware of the features that distinguish one thing, or experience, or idea from another. Secondly, and to a large extent because of this first problem, he has more than average difficulty in *mastering the interpersonal skills* involved in social living.

Sullivan emphasized that emotional and intellectual development involves the gradual assimilation of a vast cultural and interpersonal heritage, and that much of this heritage is bound up in the mastery of *symbols* (such as words, visual signs and others) and *verbal propositions* (such as, it is wrong to lie, it is necessary to work, and endless others). It is in these areas that the retarded person has particular difficulties. He has trouble making the fine, discriminating judgements on which smooth interpersonal adjustments and consequent emotional stability depend. He grasps the concepts and implications of "family," "friend," "right" and "wrong" more slowly than most people, and in some cases he masters them on only a primitive level. In the final analysis, we diagnose and measure his retardation according to his capacity to deal with the complexities of interpersonal existence.

In most instances the mentally retarded child has no apparent abnormalities at birth or during the first several years of life. There are some exceptions, however. The child with Down's syndrome, the modern name for the disorder long called mongolism, has the characteristic coarse black hair, round face and slight tilt to the eyes which prompted the original name of mongolism for this syndrome. A few children have obvious deformities of the head, such as the small head of the microcephalic child or the large head of the hydrocephalic child. Biochemical tests of the blood and urine can identify a few children with metabolic disorders such as phenylketonuria.

However, the first evidence of mental retardation in a child usually appears in his delayed intellectual and motor development. At the age of four or five months he does not follow bright objects with his gaze. He sits up without support at eight or 10 months rather than at six months. He does not stand with support at 10 or 12 months and he does not begin to walk at between 12 and 16 months. He is from several months to a year or two late in learning to say words and to talk. The child is slow in toilet training, in learning to dress himself, in learning to tie his shoes and fasten his buttons, and in learning to feed himself at the table. Some normal children may run several months or more late in learning motor and intellectual skills, but as the general pattern of slow development in a child unfolds, the question of mental retardation arises.

The child's slowness in intellectual and interpersonal development becomes more apparent after he enters school. He does not master some of the simple skills required in preschool or kindergarten, and his speech is less developed than that of other children of his age. His intellectual difficulties begin to come into painful focus in the first and second grades. He has much difficulty learning to read, and he may read poorly or not at all at the end of two or three years of schooling. His progress in arithmetic is slow, and his art drawings are like those of a child two or three years younger than he is. He may be required to repeat the first or second grade, but in a few schools (mainly in small school districts with limited resources) the child is passed along from grade to grade despite his poor mastery of his studies. At some time during the first year of school the child is given an I. Q. test, which reveals his poor intelligence. His low I. Q. score, together with his poor progress in his studies, often leads the school to put him in a special class for retarded children where his abilities are developed to their best level at a rate appropriate to his ability to learn. In securing information from the parents of some mentally retarded children, the physician sometimes gets the history that the child's intellectual and motor development was normal. Many parents of mentally retarded children retrospectively deceive themselves to avoid coming to grips with the painful fact of the child's mental retardation.

The motor development and school progress of a retarded child, as well as his mastery of interpersonal skills and comfort, are much influenced by his relationships with the close people in his life. An emotionally well-adjusted child learns much more readily than a retarded child who has become rebellious and resistant in the atmosphere of a rejecting, hostile family. The child with mild or moderate mental retardation often can learn to read simple material and can perform elementary arithmetic, and the retarded adolescent or adult can acquire various vocational skills adapted to his intellectual level. However, the retarded person's ability to learn is dependent to a large extent on the soundness of his emotional development.

As the mentally retarded child grows through childhood and adolescence toward adulthood he may be emotionally well adjusted or he may suffer personality problems. The attitudes of his parents and other close people around him during his formative years have much influence on his personality development and total life adjustment. Parents who treat the child with love and kindly patience, coupled with reasonable discipline when needed, usually rear a cooperative, affectionate child. On the other hand, hostile, rejecting parents tend to produce a sullen, negativistic child. Traumatic interpersonal relationships may cause neurotic problems or behavioral difficulties in retarded persons, in the same way that interpersonal stresses may cause similar problems in persons of normal intelligence. It is not clear whether neurotic difficulties, disorders of interpersonal behavior and psychoses are more common in mentally retarded persons because of the problems their intellectual limitations create in their relationships with people. Most mentally retarded persons make a reasonably good emotional adjustment, but they need special schooling and vocational training, and many of them require long-term supervision by their families or by the personnel of special residential institutions for the care of severely retarded persons.

The Various Levels of Mental Retardation

Intelligence testing is a basic tool in the diagnosis of mental retardation and in determining the severity of the patient's intellectual limitations. (The various I. Q. tests, their administration and the meaning of I. Q. scores are discussed in detail in Chapter 5 in our discussion of psychological testing. Some of the uses and limitations of I. Q. testing are pointed out there.)

The present official American (and international) medical nomenclature divides mental retardation into five categories of increasing severity, based on the patients' I. Q. scores.

They are:

Mental Retardation	I. Q.
1. Borderline	68–83
2. Mild	52–67
3. Moderate	36–51
4. Severe	20–35
5. Profound	Under 20

However, this system, which is the product of years of haggling among many committees, seems clinically unsound and clumsy to many mental health professional workers, including ourselves. It is odd to use figures such as 52 and 83 as dividing lines, instead of round figures such as 50 and 85, especially when in the next breath we emphasize that parents and educators ought not to pay too much attention to specific I. Q. figures. This system is quaintly bureaucratic rather than clinically practical. Moreover, to say that a person with an I. Q. of 53, who has half the intellectual capacity of the average person, is suffering merely from *mild* mental retardation seems absurd to many clinicians.

Therefore many clinicians, including myself, use a simpler system which seems sounder and more realistic. In it retarded patients are classified as follows:

Mental Retardation	I.Q.
1. Mild	70–85, or 70–80
2. Moderate	50–70
3. Severe	Below 50

However, as mentioned earlier in this chapter, the patient's total life adjustment is crucial in evaluating his social and intellectual functioning. The I. Q. number is merely one piece of information, albeit a significant one, in evaluating a person. The main task is to understand how the patient's low intelligence and his interpersonal environment have led to a relatively good interpersonal adjustment or to a poor interpersonal adjustment within the limits of his intellectual deficit. Each retarded patient must be studied in terms of his lifelong interpersonal relationships and his current emotional strengths and weaknesses.

I. Q. tests are scored on the assumption that a person reaches his full intellectual potential in middle adolescence; some tests are based on full potential at the age of 15 and others at the age of 16. Although this is a quite artificial scheme, it nevertheless provides a rough guide to the eventual level of intellectual performance a child may be expected to reach, and it also gives a rough measuring stick to the probable capacities of a mentally retarded adult. For example, an adult with an I. Q. of 50 would be expected to function in intellectual skills at the level of a child whose age is 50 per cent of 16—that is, eight years. Thus with proper education and a sound interpersonal upbringing the adult with an I. Q. of 50 would be expected to write, to do arithmetic, to carry out household chores and to exercise judgement on the level of an eight-year-old child. Similarly, an adult with an I. Q. of 75 would function on the level of a twelve-year-old child, and so forth. Likewise, a twelve-year-old child with an I. Q. of 50 would function on the level of a six-year-old child in his educational and social development. At best, however, such a use of I. Q. scores is only suggestive and vaguely approximate. A 50-year-old man with an I. Q. of 50, and hence the intellectual capacities of a child of eight, is a far different person than an eight-year-old child with normal intelligence. Nevertheless, I. Q. scores are useful in setting goals for the educational, social and vocational training of mentally retarded persons so long as the limitations of the I. Q. score and the importance of the patient's basic personality structure are kept in mind.

Some Limitations of I. Q. Testing. Intelligence testing has some important limitations. All widely used intelligence tests were developed and standardized using children and adults from urban, white, middle class and professional class backgrounds, and persons from rural, economically deprived and culturally deprived environments often perform less well on them than persons from the groups in which they were developed. For example, at two periods in our professional careers we worked in clinical settings in different cities in which about 20 per cent and 25 per cent of our patients came from poor, white, culturally deprived rural areas. The majority of these persons scored 10 to 20 points lower on I. Q. tests than the other members of our clinic population. After careful study of these rural patients, we merely assumed that their cultural background was causing their lower I. Q. scores; until proved otherwise, we assumed that their true intellectual levels were 10 to 20 points higher than our tests indicated, and several years of clinical experiences with these patients indicated that this assumption was justified.

In recent times a great deal of attention has been focused on the fact that children from urban, culturally deprived, ethnically isolated areas often score lower on I. Q. tests than middle class and professional class children. Most mental health professional workers assume that this is an artefact produced by the nature of I. Q. tests and the populations on which they were standardized. In the final analysis, an I. Q. test merely compares a person with many thousands of other persons on a set of graded verbal and performance skills, and the background of the person decidedly influences his familiarity with the types of thinking involved. A rural or slum child has had much less experience with simple geometrical designs (in everything from wallpaper to the kinds of toys he plays with), and with specifying the differences and similaritives of objects, than an urban, middle class child whose world is much more replete with visual symbols and intricate patterns. This subject is further discussed in our consideration of social and cultural deprivation as a cause of retardation, or pseudoretardation.

Intelligence, Judgement and Interpersonal Adjustment. Although we have talked glibly about intelligence, we have not yet defined it. There is no adequate, generally accepted definition for this elusive quality. However, in our opinion, the best definition of it is one that is based on Harry Stack Sullivan's definition. *Intelligence is the ability to see and feel the relatedness of things*; the word *feel* embraces the nonverbal elements and the factors that lie outside a person's conscious awareness. However, a fuller definition of intelligence is that it is formed of (1) the capacity to see the relatedness of things, (2) the capacity to employ past and current experience to reach new, valid conclusions, (3) the capacity to devise ways for solving problems not formerly encountered, (4) the capacity to use symbols representing both concrete and abstract things, as in speech and writing, and (5) adequate personality stability to use the first four capacities effectively.

However, even the limitations of this definition become apparent if we consider the relationship of *intelligence* and *judgement*. For example, a person with an I. Q. of 72, which puts him in the range of mild or borderline retardation, depending on which system of classification one uses, may drive an automobile carefully, obey traffic regulations and arrive at his destination without difficulty. Another person with an I. Q. of 150, which puts him in the range of very superior intelligence, may speed through traffic at 70 miles an hour, ignore traffic signals and maim or kill both himself and others. Despite marked differences in intelligence, the first person had good judgement and functioned well socially, whereas the second person had bad judgement and functioned disastrously. (The subject of judgement is further discussed in Chapter 5.)

Also, as noted above, there is no predictable relationship between intelligence and interpersonal adjustment. This is well illustrated by a family with whom we have had both professional and social contact over a period of many years. The father is a busy physician who has given little attention to his children and the mother is a socially ambitious woman who has carelessly indulged her children but has given them little affection and time. The oldest of their three children was a girl with grave emotional problems; in her early 20's she was an alcoholic and died in an automobile accident while driving after heavy drinking. The second child, a boy in late adolescence, is a high school dropout who has had two suspended sentences for narcotics usage. The third child is a late adolescent girl with an I. Q. of 65. Because of her retardation her parents and other close persons have given her more attention than her two siblings received and she has had special schooling. Today she is a pleasant, attractive, helpful girl who works as a salesperson in a store owned by a friend of her parents, and an uncle drives her to and from work. She knows she will not marry, and in her parents' older years she probably will be their companion and offer some consolation for the suffering they have had with their other two children, both of whom had superior intelligence. In this family the mentally retarded child obviously has made the best interpersonal adjustment. When considered in a broad interpersonal way a retarded child, or adolescent, or adult is not necessarily inferior to his peers of average or superior intelligence; he may simply have a special set of problems for which he needs special care and education.

EXPECTED LEVELS OF ADJUSTMENT OF MENTALLY RETARDED ADULTS

In this discussion we shall use the second of the two schemes for classifying retarded persons listed in the preceding section. This divides them into *mild, moderate* and *severe*, rather than into the cumbersome five-part division used in the official nomenclature; as pointed out above, many psychiatrists find the five-part classification clinically awkward and of doubtful validity.

Mild Retardation. The vast majority of retarded persons fall in this category. The adult with an I. Q. between 70 and 85 (or between 70 and 80, if one wishes to draw the line at 80) usually is able to make a fairly good social and vocational adjustment. For example, the adult with an I. Q. of 75 can master the intellectual skills exercised by a child of 12. A 12-year-old child can be expected to have many manual skills, to be able to perform simple clerical work or routine household chores and to exercise reasonable judgement in some areas of his life. If his interpersonal adjustment is good, the person with an I. Q. of 75 should be able to lead a constructive life and to work in simple, unskilled jobs.

However, in our opinion, the person with mild retardation should not marry, since he would be prone to have much difficulty as the economic supporter of a family or as a homemaker, and he would flounder in the tasks of rearing children and guiding them through the trials of adolescence. Most mildly retarded persons should live with their parents, their siblings or other close relatives who offer them general surveillance and guidance; without such guidance, mildly retarded individuals are often exploited financially, sexually or vocationally by unscrupulous persons. However, individuals whose I. Q.'s are in the lower 80's, approaching the range of normal intelligence, may make adequate social, vocational and marital adjustments if their basic capacities for interpersonal relationships are good.

Moderate Retardation. When the mentally retarded person has an I. Q. between 50 and 70 he needs the careful surveillance of his family or other responsible adults throughout his life. He can carry out only very limited independent social and economic activities. The moderately retarded person usually can perform simple household chores and may be able to hold simple, unskilled jobs under the guidance of understanding supervisors. Successful marriage and responsible parenthood are not possible for moderately retarded persons. In some instances their families must obtain legal custody of them to prevent unwise marriages and other activities for which they are not intellectually equipped. When he is emotionally well adjusted the moderately retarded person can make an adjustment at home under the guidance of his family, but when he has emotional turbulence and interpersonal difficulties institutional care may be necessary for either short or long periods of time; this is necessary in only a small percentage of cases. The moderately retarded person often becomes the pleasant companion of his elderly parents or the good-natured uncle or aunt who assists around the home.

Severe Retardation. Only about 10 to 15 per cent of all mentally retarded persons have I. Q.'s below 50, and two-thirds of these individuals have I. Q.'s between 30 and 50. Thus, most severely retarded persons can live quietly in the homes of their parents or their siblings, and they may carry out simple tasks about the home and yard under supervision. Their capacities are quite limited and often they spend much time listening to the radio or watching television. However, a small number of patients with I. Q.'s below 50, and an appreciable percentage of those with I. Q.'s below 30, can live only in the protective setting of a well-run institution. Their families may seek such placement of the patient or they may delay it until the patient's adolescence or young adulthood.

Differential Diagnosis of Mental Retardation

A comprehensive psychiatric workup should be carried out in evaluating the intelligence of a child or an adult. This workup should include a careful history from the patient's family about his development since infancy, his school progress, and his intellectual and interpersonal adjustment in childhood, adolescence and adulthood. The psychiatrist's interview with the patient should be followed by psychological testing by a clinical psychologist who should evaluate the patient's personality structure as well as his I. Q. Since I. Q. testing can give falsely low results when the child or adult is emotionally distraught, interpersonally withdrawn, negativistic or confused, it sometimes is advisable to re-examine the patient after an interval of a year or more before arriving at a definite conclusion. In a small percentage of cases chromosomal studies, metabolic examinations (to rule out phenylketonuria and other inborn errors of metabolism), electroencephalograms, tests of hearing and vision and other physical studies are indicated. The physical state of the patient should be at least briefly checked, or reports from the referring physician or clinic should be obtained.

It should never be assumed that mental retardation is self-evident after cursory evaluation and an I. Q. test. A wide variety of conditions can mimic mental retardation, and they often should be systematically excluded. We have seen a fair number of children who have been erroneously diagnosed as retarded, often gravely affecting their education and general management. Some of the conditions which must at times be considered in the differential diagnosis are (1) emotionally caused learning disturbances, (2) severe neurotic or personality disorders, which interfere with learning and give a false impression of intellectual deficit, (3) learning problems due to mixed cerebral dominance, (4) impaired learning due to defective vision or hearing, (5) early infantile autism and childhood schizophrenia, (6) various kinds of organic brain damage in which intellectual slowness is a minor aspect of overwhelming central nervous system defect, (7) petit mal epilepsy, in which many seizures during the day may prevent the child from learning well, (8) grand mal epilepsy and other physical disorders and handicaps which may cause interpersonal withdrawal and emotional blunting in the patient, (9) debilitating physical diseases, such as untreated celiac disease, in which the child suffers chronic physical distress which inhibits his learning processes and interpersonal development and (10) interpersonal neglect and isolation from people, as sometimes occurs in badly run institutions and in cases of gross parental neglect; this may cause an apathy that on casual observation simulates retardation. The term *pseudoretarded* is sometimes applied to persons who, for one of these causes, gives an impression of mental retardation.

(Most of these 10 processes are discussed in detail in other sections of this book; for example, learning disturbances caused by emotional turmoil or mixed cerebral dominance are covered in Chapter 25, and early infantile autism and childhood schizophrenia are discussed in Chapter 14.)

SPECIAL MENTAL RETARDATION SYNDROMES

The standard nomenclature lists 10 categories of mental retardation, according to specific etiologies. They are mental retardation (1) following infection or intoxication, (2) following trauma or physical agent, (3) with disorders of metabolism, growth or nutrition, (4) associated with gross brain disease (postnatal), (5) associated with diseases and conditions due to unknown prenatal influence, (6) with chromosomal abnormality, (7) associated with prematurity, (8) following major psychiatric disorder, (9) with psycho-social (environmental) deprivation and (10) with other, unspecified condition. The nomenclature then proceeds to enumerate 58 separate causes of retardation.

However, a large number of these conditions (such as trigeminal cerebral angiomatosis and Lawrence-Moon-Beidl syndrome) are so rare that most physicians will never see a case during their professional careers, and many others (bilirubin encephalopathy and cogenital toxoplasmosis) are almost invariably considered organic brain syndromes (discussed in Part IV) in which mental defect is merely a minor feature in an overwhelming neurological disorder. Still others of these conditions (Tay-Sach's disease, Gaucher's disease and many others) are fatal diseases in which retardation is an incidental finding. Moreover, at most, all of these conditions, with the exception of the last one (unspecified condition) account for no more than 10 per cent of the total number of retarded children seen in psychiatric work. If the category of psycho-social (environmental) deprivation is deducted from this list, it accounts for no more than three to five per cent of retarded children and adults. As discussed above, in the vast majority of cases the cause of the patient's retardation is unknown, and we say that he suffers from idiopathic retardation, or retardation due to unknown causes.

However, some mental retardation syndromes are sufficiently common, or of such special clinical interest, that they merit separate consideration. We shall discuss some of them.

Down's Syndrome, and Syndromes Due to Other Types of Chromosomal Abnormalities

Down's syndrome is the modern name for the mental retardation syndrome long called mongolism. Down's syndrome occurs in about one out of each 600 births; in the early child-bearing years the incidence is one in each 2,000 births, but the incidence rises to one in every 50 births in mothers over the age of 40. The immediate cause of Down's syndrome is a chromosomal defect in the child. The chromosomal abnormalities that may cause Down's syndrome have been found to be increasingly diverse and complex since the first chromosomal abnormality was noted in 1959. However, in 85 per cent of cases there is an extra chromosome in group G, presumably due to a defect in mosis in the maturation of an ovum in the mother; the child with Down's syndrome develops from an ovum with an extra chromosomal fragment. Though this type of Down's syndrome may occur in mothers of any age, it is more common in older mothers. In this 85 per cent of cases, Down's syndrome is not an inherited condition; the body cells of both parents are normal.

However, a wide variety of other chromosomal abnormalities have been found in about 15 per cent of children with Down's syndrome, and some of these are caused by chromosomal abnormalities in mothers and fathers who show no evidence of mental or physical abnormalities. In these cases Down's syndrome is a recessively inherited condition, but for unknown reasons the chances that such parents will have children with Down's syndrome are much less than would be expected on the basis of generally accepted genetic principles. However, in extremely rare cases there are exceptions to this general rule; for example, translocation in both pair 21 chromosomes of group G results in a 100 per cent certainty of Down's syndrome in the offspring. In still other cases (commonly called mosaics) Down's syndrome is caused by nondisjunction defects in the fertized zygotes.

Once a child has Down's syndrome he in most cases would transmit it as a dominant characteristic to any offspring he might have, but since individuals with Down's syndrome rarely have children the point is of little clinical significance.

The patient with Down's syndrome often can be identified at birth by the characteristic facial and body signs of the syndrome. In doubtful cases these signs become clearer as the child develops. The diagnosis can be substantiated in doubtful cases by examination of the chromosomal structure of cultured blood cells or cells from other tissues. Young parents of a child with Down's syndrome should also have chromosomal studies of their cells so they may be advised on the statistical chances that any further children they have will have Down's syndrome. The child with Down's syndrome is shorter than average and his occiput is flat. His hair is coarse and dark, and his eyes have the almond-shaped, slanting tilt which prompted the original name of mongolism for this condition. The face is flat and the tongue is large and fissured. The hands and feet are small, thick and short, and the child has a characteristic straight transverse line across each palm and a straight crease on each sole which runs from the heel to the space between the first two toes. Hypermotility of the joints is due to general laxity of the ligaments, and the abdomen is protruding. The genitals are small and congenital heart defects are common.

The patient with Down's syndrome usually has an I. Q. between 20 and 50, and the possible upper limit is in the lower 60's. These patients characteristically are placid and quietly good-natured. Since the diagnosis often is made shortly after birth parents sometimes place the child in a residential institution early in life. In many instances, however, the child remains in his parents' home where his placidity and easy good nature often cause the parents to become fond of him, and he may spend his lifetime in the homes of his parents and his adult siblings. These patients rarely have the emotional turmoil and interpersonal difficulties that other retarded patients have as they pass through adolescence and early adulthood.

Mental Retardation Syndromes Caused by Other Types of Chromosomal Abnormalities. Systematic study of the chromosomal structures of mentally retarded children has revealed a large number of chromosomal defects, and more are being discovered as these investigations are continued. We shall list a few of them. All of them are rare and in aggregate account for only a small number of retarded patients; however, refinement of technics of the study of chromosomes and, in time, genes, is a promising field of research.

In the *trisomy E (trisomy 18)* syndrome, which occurs in one out of every 4500 births, the infant is premature and has abnormalities of the head, abdominal organs and hands; survival beyond infancy is rare. Children with *trisomy D_1 (trisomy 13)* mental retardation similarly have multiple physical defects, in addition to retardation.

In the *deletion syndromes* parts of chromosomes are missing. For example, in the *5p—syndrome* there is a deletion of the short arms of chromosome 5. Among many other abnormalities, these retarded children make a characteristic, high-pitched cry which somewhat resembles a cat's mew, during the first few weeks of life. Thus, this syndrome has been called the *cat-cry syndrome*, or *cri du chat syndrome*. A fair number of these retarded patients survive into adulthood. Other deletion mental retardation syndromes are the 4p—syndrome, the 13q—syndrome, the chromosome 18 short arm deletion syndrome, and others.

Mental Retardation Associated with Psychosocial (Environmental) Deprivation

This category is sometimes separated into (1) mental retardation caused by cultural-familial deprivation and (2) mental retardation associated with general environmental deprivation. We shall consider it as a single category, however.

As noted in our discussion of the significance of I. Q. scores, it has for several decades been noted that children and adults from culturally and socioeconomically deprived environments tend to score lower on intelligence tests than persons from middle class and professional class circumstances (on whom intelligence tests were developed and standardized). In recent times some psychiatrists have proposed that the stultifying effects of social and cultural deprivation may cause a lifelong lowering of intellectual capacity, thus producing a particular category of mental retardation. Other psychiatrists feel that it is misleading to include culturally deprived persons in the general group of mental retardation syndromes; they feel that such persons should be considered individuals of normal intelligence who give low results on the kinds of instruments we have for evaluating the elusive quality we call intelligence.

The standard nomenclature contains a special diagnostic category, within the general group of mental retardation syndromes, for persons whose low functioning intelligence is caused by cultural, or psycho-social, deprivation. We shall outline its causes and features.

The majority of these persons come from black or Spanish-speaking slums in inner city districts, but they also may be found in primitive rural areas, geographically isolated regions and other culturally barren situations. We shall list systematically the main problems that may contribute to a culturally deprived person's low intellectual functioning. (1) By the very nature of his deprived, culturally backward situation, he tends to feel inadequate and inferior, as compared with persons in more favored social groups. (2) By middle or late childhood, if not before, he is acutely aware that his capacity for choice and self-determination in his life role (to be a skilled worker, or a professional person, or a businessperson) is much more limited than that of an individual in a more privileged group, and this stunts his motivation for mastering the intellectual skills and life style habits that lead to socioeconomic progress. (3) He has little experience with personal gain through cooperative group activities. He lacks stimulating school experiences, reassuring neighborhood associations and inspiring church and community experiences; instead, his school is a brutal jungle, his neighborhood is crime-infested and drug-ridden, and other areas of his life are barren. (4) He has few incentives for intellectual development and skilled manual achievement. As he looks about him he sees few people benefitting from such accomplishments; instead he sees more material goods and comforts in the hands of the trickster, the thief, the mugger, the narcotics peddler and the fancy prostitute. (5) He is not exposed to the symbols around which so much of middle class, urban, achievement-oriented life is organized; the flag, the grade school report card, the cross, the lapel button, the political emblem, the baseball league or bowling league trophy, the high school annual, and endless other things have little meaning for him. (6) He does not have the small and large day-to-day experiences in which the common intellectual and manual skills are observed and learned. He does not see people reading books, making shopping lists, paying the end-of-the-month bills, filling out income tax returns, making apple pies, repairing home appliances, working in the flower garden, building minor things in the home and yard, and many other things. Moreover, he does not observe and absorb the habits of orderliness, patient industriousness and punctuality which are crucial in intellectual skills; instead, he sees about him disorder and idleness, and punctuality has no meaning for a person who feels that it holds no rewards for him and the people about him. (7) His language is defective; he learns the slum argot with its special words, its peculiar grammatical constructions, and its different cadences, rather than the language technics and styles of the dominant majority. In some instances these language problems are so great that they constitute a severe barrier to education, job training and interpersonal adjustment outside his own group. They also play a larger role in the poor performance of deprived persons on intelligence tests than is generally recognized, in our opinion; testers all too often assume that they and the testees have more common language characteristics than they actually do.

These things, and many more, contribute to low functioning intelligence, at least as far as it is evaluated by conventional I. Q.

tests, the usual demands of school learning, and the technics required in most skilled employment. In our opinion, however, these persons are not mentally retarded in the usual sense of the term if they are evaluated in terms of the craftiness, cunning and agile adaptability they need to survive and acquire minimal comforts and necessities in the blighted environments in which they live. Hence, whether or not they should be termed mentally retarded depends on how the term retardation is defined. In terms of the intellectual capacities they need to comprehend and adjust to the demands of scholastic performance and job proficiency in our urban, industrialized, sophisticated, competitive, majority-dominated society, they are retarded; in terms of basic shrewdness and interpersonal agility in their own environments, especially if they are evaluated in their own argot, they are not retarded. We have had a good deal of experience working with persons in this kind of environment; our initial impression was that they were of lower functioning intelligence than the dominant social groups, but in time we saw that their innate shrewdness and interpersonal adaptability are in no way inferior to that of the majority groups. Some mental health workers would disagree with us on this point.

Most practicing physicians and psychiatrists do not see many of these patients, but mental health professionals who work in inner city psychiatric, educational and welfare situations often encounter them. The solution of their problems requires complex educational, social, economic and cultural changes, many of which are gradually occurring. The informed physician, both as a citizen and as a professional person, can make a contribution.

Phenylketonuria and Other Inborn Errors of Metabolism

Phenylketonuria is the best understood of the rapidly increasing number of mental retardation syndromes due to inborn errors of metabolism. We therefore shall discuss it at length, and list the others briefly.

Phenylketonuria (also called PKU and phenylalanemia) is an inborn error of metabolism in which the metabolism of the amino acid phenylalanine is defective. Severe mental retardation is the dominant clinical feature of this disorder which occurs in one out of each 15,000 births and is present in from 0.5 to 1 per cent of institutionalized mentally retarded patients; however, it is much less common in the total noninstitutionalized mentally retarded population.

Phenylketonuria is caused by a specific gene defect transmitted in a simple recessive manner (that is, an autosomal recessive gene). The phenylketonuric child inherits a recessive phenylketonuric gene from each of his parents, and there is one chance in four that other children born to his parents will have clinical phenylketonuria. There is one chance in two that other children born to his parents will inherit a single recessive phenylketonuric gene and will be asymptomatic carriers. About one per cent of the adult population are asymptomatic carriers of a single recessive phenylketonuric gene. Asymptomatic carriers of a recessive phenylketonuria gene may often be detected by a phenylalanine tolerance test, in the opinion of many investigators.

As in most disorders, long-term, comprehensive investigation has revealed increasing complexities. Some children with elevated phenylalanine blood levels do not develop mental retardation, and a number of variant, or related, conditions have been found with varying degrees of defective phenylalanine metabolism. At present it is best to regard all these patients as belonging to one clinical category, and to recognize that for unknown reasons the clinical course of infants and children with impaired phenylalanine metabolism is variable. Terms which have been applied to these variants are "atypical PKU," "persistent hyperphenylalanemia," "hyperphenylalanemia with PKU," and others.

According to present concepts of gene function, the defective gene in the phenylketonuric patient fails to transmit biochemical information necessary for the activity of a specific enzyme, liver phenylalanine hydroxylase. The deficiency of this enzyme prohibits the metabolism of phenylalanine into its normal metabolic products. Phenylalanine and abnormal phenylalanine derivatives accumulate in the body fluids, and through various biochemical channels (among which are their secondary effects on the metabolism of the amino acids tyrosine and trytophane) they cause an adverse effect on brain metabolism and development. Large amounts of phenylalanine and its derivatives accumulate in the blood and urine.

The diagnosis is made by blood and urine tests. Urine tests are not positive at birth, but usually become positive at some point during the first few weeks of life. Original tests for urinary phenylpyruvic acid (adding ferric chloride solutions to recently excreted urine) have been much refined; urine can now be tested for the presence of various urinary phenylketones and o-hydroxyphenylacetic acid. The simpler tests, such as the ferric chloride one, give a fair number of false positive results, but, if their limitations are recognized, can be useful screening procedures. Definite diagnosis rests on finding elevated phenylalanine levels in the blood (an average level of 35 mg. in each 100 ml. of serum, but with wide variations), in association with normal levels of blood tyrosine. Nevertheless, the infant must be tested several times to make sure that blood elevations are not transitory variants in normal persons. These observations must be carried out with particular care in newborn siblings of a child with proved phenylketonuria.

Between 10 and 20 per cent of children with phenylketonuria will, even if untreated, have normal intelligence or only mildly retarded intellectual functioning. The rest, if untreated, become moderately or severely retarded; since those who will, or will not, become retarded cannot be distinguished in infancy, all children with phenylketonuria should be treated. The intellectual damage due to phenylketonuria apparently occurs only during the first five or six years of life. In addition to moderate or severe mental retardation phenylketonuric patients may have convulsive seizures which begin in infancy and decrease with age, tremors, hypertonic muscles and skin lesions such as eczema. Many phenylketonuric patients have blond hair, blue eyes and lightly pigmented skin; these features are caused by the effects of defective phenylalanine metabolism on the metabolic processes producing body pigmentation.

If a phenylketonuric infant is started on a low phenylalanine diet in the first few weeks of life, he usually achieves normal intelligence; the mean I. Q. of such treated children is 95. When treatment is delayed the patient usually has low normal or mild retardation, and there seems to be little benefit from treatment begun after the age of three years.

Treatment consists of administration of a diet with a low phenylalanine content. Balanced diets supplying all the child's nutritional needs but low in phenylalanine are commercially available in a powdered form, which may be made into a baby formula or a beverage. The diet must be carefully adjusted to the child's body weight and fluctuating individual needs. The diet contains a certain amount of phenylalanine since it is an indispensible amino acid, and if it is not available in the food the body will break down protein tissue to secure it. The diet is regulated by regular measurements of the child's serum phenylalanine level; they at first should be done weekly, but afterwards may be performed monthly. The goal is to maintain the phenylalanine level at between 3 and 8 mg. in each 100 ml. of serum. In most cases treatment can be discontinued after the age of five or six.

Other Mental Retardation Syndromes Due to Abnormal Amino Acid Metabolism. The elucidation of phenylketonuria has caused extensive research on the metabolism of mentally retarded persons. An ever-increasing number of amino acid disorders are being explored. In many of them mental retardation is a major feature, and in others it is present but is overshadowed by other kinds of physical defects. Some cause early death. We shall list a few of the better known amino acid dysfunction syndromes: (1) Hartnup disease, in which there is a generalized amino aciduria; niacin treatment helps patients with this disorder, who also have pellagra-like skin rashes and intermittent cerebellar ataxia. (2) Lowe's syndrome, which is caused by various amino acid metabolism defects, and which also may produce cataracts and hyporeflexia. (3) Methylmalonic aciduria, in which blood and urine methylmalonic acid levels are elevated; treatment is carried out by administration of vitamin B_{12} and a diet low in various amino acids. (4) Carnosinemia, in which myoclonic seizures and retardation are two of the main features of defects in the enzyme carnosinase. (5) Cystathioninuria, caused by a defect in the enzyme cystathionase; vitamin B_6 treatment is employed. (6) Histidinemia, in which a diet low in the amino acid histidine may compensate for impaired functioning of the enzyme histidase. (7) Citrullinuria, in which a low protein diet is useful. (8) Maple syrup urine disease, in which the child has spaticity, mental retardation and a urine odor that resembles the smell of maple syrup; it is caused by a specific enzyme defect and can be treated by a diet low in the amino acids leucine, isoleucine and valine. At the time of this writing about 30 other amino acid dysfunction syndromes are fairly well defined, and the list of these causes of mental retardation is constantly being enlarged. However, it should be emphasized that all of them are relatively rare, and they account for a few per cent, at most, of all cases of mental retardation.

Mental Retardation Syndromes Caused by Defects in Carbohydrate Metabolism. In statistically rare cases mental retardation is produced by inborn errors of carbohydrate metabolism, transmitted as autosomal recessive characteristics. In *galactosemia* the patient lacks the enzyme galactose 1-phosphate uridyl transferase, which may be treated by elimination of milk, milk products and other foods containing lactose and galactose.

(2) *Hereditary fructose intolerance* is a rare disorder in which the patient lacks a crucial enzyme in fructose metabolism; elimination of fructose and sorbitol from the diet constitutes the treatment. There are other somewhat related diseases (gargoylism, the glycogen storage diseases, and others) in which the enzymatic and metabolic processes are less clear, and they do not fall classically in this group; these conditions cause mental retardation, but the mental defect is overshadowed by more prominent physical dysfunctions.

THE MANAGEMENT OF MENTALLY RETARDED PATIENTS

The way in which a mentally retarded child is reared has a large bearing on the kind of interpersonal adjustment he makes in childhood, in adolescence and in adulthood. Judicious upbringing can help him achieve a stable personality structure within the limits of his intelligence, and may decide whether he is a rebellious, socially maladjusted individual or a calm, cooperative person who can lead a pleasant life under appropriate supervision. Children with clear-cut organic brain damage and associated mental retardation often are restless, impulsive and easily angered, and make poor interpersonal adjustments; however, in the vast majority of instances of idiopathic mental retardation the patient's interpersonal upbringing and special education are more important than his intellectual deficit in determining the quality of his eventual social adjustment.

Counseling With Parents of Mentally Retarded Children

How Do You Tell Parents That Their Child Is Retarded? Simple as this question may seem, poor handling of it by pediatricians, family physicians and even mental health professional workers often causes parents to reject the diagnosis for months or years, while the child's special management and educational needs go unattended. In clinical practice one commonly encounters parents who have not accepted the obvious retardation of children who have arrived to late childhood or even early adolescence. The inability of many parents, especially mothers, to accept their children's retardation is due to many factors, but skillful presentation of the situation helps many of them to face their children's problems and to plan constructively for the children's welfare.

First, it must be admitted that, although we have experimented with many ways of approaching this problem, and have read much about counseling the parents of retarded children, and have discussed the issue with other mental health professional workers, we have never found a completely satisfactory way to tell parents that their child is retarded. Nevertheless, we shall outline the method we have found best. After careful diagnostic interviewing of the child, review of his development and school progress, and observation of the child, we tell the parents that all this data raises the question as to whether he is "somewhat slow." We indicate that testing by a clinical psychologist will be useful in giving more information, and if the parents accept this suggestion, we arrange it. If the parents are unwilling to accept this suggestion we do not press it unduly, but advise that, as the months go by, we should consider again the possibility of such testing to arrange whatever special schooling and training the child may need. Parents who at first put off testing usually accept it in time. To push the issue before they are ready is more likely to increase their resistance than to diminish it. The most the physician or mental health professional can do is to indicate that if the child has any problems that require special attention and education, it is important to start them early rather than to deprive the child of the help he needs.

Let us assume that a five-year-old child is tested and that an I. Q. of 60 is found. We then indicate to the parents that the child "came out somewhat slow" on the examination and that we feel it is a valid test result, but that the I. Q. testing should be repeated in six to eight months, or more, to be absolutely certain. We point out that special schooling must be arranged, since the child is going to have trouble grasping school subjects quickly. We say that he has a lot to learn, but that he needs teachers who are trained to aid slow learners. At home, we explain, the child is going to be slower than his siblings in learning the usual self-care, manual and interpersonal skills, but, granted that he will be a couple of years, or so, behind other children of his age, he will in time master most of the essential social skills and many of the academic ones, though to a lesser extent than many other persons.

If the parents ask if he is retarded, we reply that he is somewhat retarded, but that this is not the crucial point. The crucial thing is that he makes a good adjustment and lives a happy life, and that how he is reared is more important than his I. Q. in determining those things. A person of superior intelligence can be a miserable misfit, whereas a person with much lower intelligence can be a happy, constructive member of his family. We point out that an I. Q. number, moreover, is not so precise that it can be relied on solely in charting a child's day-to-day course, and that a child's emotional environment and schooling have such a large influence on his eventual performance that his precise I. Q. can mislead parents a great deal.

Dealing With the Parents' Feelings Toward a Mentally Retarded Child. A mentally retarded child's parents face a difficult emotional adjustment. As the child's retardation slowly becomes apparent and is in time confirmed by medical and psychological examinations, the parents often have a puzzled bitterness and grief about why this happened to their child. Others try to ignore the child's problem for as many years as possible, until the child's diagnosis is at last forced upon them by the child's accumulating social and scholastic problems. Some parents become hostile toward the child and reject him emotionally; later they often feel much guilt about these feelings and actions toward the child. On the other hand, some parents become engrossed in, or even obsessed with, the problems of caring for their mentally retarded child and neglect their other children. Some parents become overprotective and hinder the emotional and intellectual growth of a retarded child by their overpossessiveness of him. As Harry Stack Sullivan once pointed out, the *social adjustment* problems of a retarded person are not primarily caused by factors inside the retarded individual, but by the attitudes and actions of other people toward him. A simple but striking example of this is found in the wooden, expressionless, smileless faces of many long-institutionalized retarded persons; they do not smile because no one ever smiles at them.

In many instances the parents of a retarded child need help in resolving their unhealthy feelings toward him. Some parents find help in group therapy discussion sessions with the parents of other retarded children. Special schools for retarded children and community societies for aiding retarded children often organize regular group therapy sessions for parents. In such settings the retarded child sometimes is called "the exceptional child." In these therapeutic groups the parents can learn that they are not alone in facing the problems of rearing a mentally retarded child; many other parents share these problems with them. Parents can learn that feelings of bitterness, puzzlement, rejection, guilt and overprotectiveness are common as a parent adjusts to his retarded child, and in talking out such feelings with each other they often can resolve them and establish healthier relationships with their retarded children. Parents also can get information from each other and from the group's moderator on ways to handle day-to-day difficulties, such as toilet training, self-grooming, responsibility with possessions, and many others. Solutions and advice often seem more useful and acceptable when they come from other parents who have faced such problems in their own homes. In occasional cases the emotional turmoil of a parent is so marked that individual psychotherapy or counseling is merited.

Dealing with Parents' Expectations for a Mentally Retarded Child. The parents of a mentally retarded child should understand that, adjusted to his intellectual age, the child has the same emotional needs as children of normal intelligence. The child needs the devoted love of his parents, and he needs their firm discipline at times for undesirable acts. Undue friction with his brothers and sisters or unkind actions by neighborhood children must not be allowed. The retarded child needs a certain amount of freedom at each age appropriate to his intellectual level. The physician, or other professional counselor, should explain carefully that the parents' expectations for the child always must be adjusted to his mental age and not to his chronological age. For example, the parents should expect of a 10-year-old girl with an I. Q. of 60 the things they might expect of a 6-year-old girl. The parents should understand that this offers them merely an extremely rough guide, but it helps them avoid either demanding too much or expecting too little. Many psychiatrists feel it is better if the parents do not know the I. Q. score of a child and merely realize that he is retarded; however, the physician, or other professional counselor of the parents, can use the I. Q. figure in guiding the parents in their training of the child if the marked limitations of I. Q. figures are recognized. (The I. Q. score should, of course, be rechecked every two or three years since it often rises to a certain extent; as the child becomes emotionally comfortable and more self-confident he may be able to cooperate better in I. Q. testing and he sometimes achieves a better score).

In counseling parents, the physician should emphasize that a retarded child has his potentialities as well as his limitations, and he should stress the things that the child will be able to do. For example, he should point out that all mildly retarded children, and some moderately retarded ones, should be able to learn to read fairly well, to do the simple arithmetic needed in common day-to-day tasks, and to acquire a reasonable fund of general information. The retarded child can continue his education throughout adolescence in special classes adapted to his needs. The boy can learn simple clerical or manual skills and a girl with mild retardation can learn most of the basic tasks of housekeeping.

The counselor should always be generous with praise and encouragement when he is talking with the parents of retarded children. "You're doing a good job with Frank"; "Lisa is certainly coming along well, thanks to the way you're rearing her"; or "Don is one of the happiest, most relaxed and best adjusted boys that I see in this office; that's the important thing in life and it's your accomplishment," should be frequently on the doctor's lips. He should praise the ingenuities the parents use in training the child.

We think that a philosophical touch sometimes is sound and useful in talking with the parents of mentally retarded children. Mental retardation diminishes or eliminates some of the opportunities of life, but it also diminishes or eliminates some of the pain and trouble of life. This point usually is overlooked. Though the mentally retarded child will not have the vocational opportunities which the child of average intelligence will have in adulthood, he will be spared much of the anxiety and turmoil of today's hurried, harassing life. In later life the retarded person may not have the joys of watching a family grow up, but he will be spared the distress of their illnesses, the anxiety of their adolescent rebellions and the trials of their many other problems. He will lead a simpler life, which has both advantages and disadvantages. In our opinion, this point of view is not shallowness or sophistry. Perhaps in three decades of work in psychiatry we have seen too much misery to allow us unbiased views of the bliss of this world, but experience also has enabled us to see that the simpler life of a retarded person sometimes has its hidden advantages as well as its glaring disadvantages. To many a father we have said, "Your son may not have the joys of entering your business, but he also is not going to have your stomach ulcers," and to many a mother we have said, "Your daughter is not going to have the joys of rearing children, but she is going to be spared the agony of watching their mistakes, suffering and sorrows."

Special Education of Mentally Retarded Persons

The mentally retarded child should be placed in a special class for children of his own I. Q. group early in his school career. If he is left in classes with children of normal intelligence he soon senses his inferiority, as do his classmates. He is neglected by teachers who find their efforts with him unavailing, and often he is subjected to ridicule and taunts by other children. Despair, depressiveness and angry bitterness well up in the child; he may become sullen and negativistic, or he may withdraw from all interpersonal contacts in the school. On the other hand, when he is put in a class with children of his intellectual capacities, the retarded child learns at a rate which is comfortable for him under a teacher who understands his needs. Ideally, a teacher of mentally retarded children should have training in special pedagogical technics for helping these children. Retarded children should be grouped in classes of roughly similar I.Q.'s, for when children ranging from severe to mild retardation are put in the same class neither the teacher nor the children can function at their most productive levels.

The retarded child should engage in all the usual school activities that promote his social development. Supervised games and athletics, school parties, noontime meals in the school cafeteria and attendance at school events are important in helping the child learn social gracefulness and adaptability. The majority of retarded patients can be educated and vocationally trained in special schools while residing at home with their families. However, in some instances the retarded child or adolescent can benefit from periods ranging from several months to several years in a residential school where he lives while receiving his education. A residential school for retarded children and adolescents combines educational and vocational training with a psychiatrically oriented environment which encourages sound personality development. Teams of specially trained teachers and other personnel under the guidance of clinical psychologists, psychiatric nurses who have specialized in this field, and psychiatrists work with the patients in the residential setting, and counseling with the parents also may be carried out while the child or adolescent is in residence. These schools are particularly useful when there are marked tensions between the child and his parents or when the child is developing behavioral problems which necessitate an environment where his emotional difficulties can be dealt with more effectively by an understanding professional staff. Adolescence is a time when mentally retarded persons are somewhat prone to develop emotional turmoil as they face the problems of adjusting to their new sexual urges and their rapid physical maturation. A period of residence in a special school for retarded children and adolescents sometimes is very useful at this time.

Depending on the age of the retarded child, special *nursery schools* for young children and *day centers* for older children and adolescents may be valuable in training and educating him. The child or adolescent may attend such a facility five days each week from after breakfast to late afternoon, or he may go to it only once or twice a week for training in special manual and interpersonal skills. Such centers are a compromise between exclusive home care and residential management. Such centers can be brought within the economic range of all parents if they are staffed, in rotation, by the mothers and fathers of the children under the direction of two or three mental health professionals who have specialized in working with retarded persons.

In adolescence retarded persons should be carefully evaluated to determine the kind of training in manual crafts, or simple clerical work or homemaking skills they are best suited to undertake, and they should be trained accordingly. The retarded person who receives appropriate education often can become economically self-sustaining while living under the general surveillance of his family. When not properly educated the retarded person often is economically unproductive and eventually may become dependent on community funds for support. Hence, the extra money that communities spend in educating mentally retarded persons is not only humanitarian but is economically sound from the total community point of view. A good job placement service to help mentally retarded persons find their economic places in the community is a useful adjunct to comprehensive educational services for them.

Throughout his education the mentally retarded person benefits from application of the technic of *multiple sensory learning,* and in his interpersonal development the principle of *consensual validation* (discussed in Chapter 1) has particular applicability. In multiple sensory teaching the parent or teacher *tells* the child about a thing, *shows* it to him, guides his hands so that he can *feel* its form and texture, and in some cases can have him *smell* and *taste* it. For example, in teaching the child to put on a slip-on shoe, the parent *tells* the child what it is and explains its purpose simply, *shows* him how to put it on his foot, guides his hands through the steps of putting it on so that he may experience both in his hands and on his foot how it *feels* as it goes on, and in some cases the parent can have him *smell* the crisp odor of new leather. Thus, the *multiple senses* of *hearing, seeing, feeling* and *smelling* are employed to reinforce his learning. It has long been observed that when various kinds of sensory experience occur in learning something a much deeper and more lasting impression is made on the learner. More subtle sensory experiences also occur in the learning experience described above; the child has the *kinesthetic* sense of bending his body to put on the shoe and *proprioceptive* sensations of the shoe pressing the deeper structures of his foot and ankle.

In special schools, day centers, and other training facilities for mentally retarded children, adolescents and adults, *sociodrama* is a valuable educational technic. Sociodrama is a variant form of *psychodrama* (which is discussed in Chapter 21). In sociodrama teachers and mental health professional workers act out with the child many kinds of interpersonal situations he will face. For example, the instructor and the mentally retarded person act out situations in which the patient goes to a store make a purchase, applies for a job, asks a bus driver for instructions about where to get off, and endless other daily situations. The teacher plays the roles of both helpful and rude store clerks, pleasant and unpleasant prospective employers, and so forth, and thus the retarded person develops interpersonal skills in meeting many kinds of interpersonal challenges.

Other Aspects of Managing Retarded Persons

Management of Special Emotional Problems of Mentally Retarded Persons. The mentally retarded person, like the person of average or superior intelligence, may develop neurotic problems, or psychosomatic illnesses, or disorders of interpersonal behavior, or psychoses. Though colored by his intellectual limitations, a psychiatric disorder in a retarded person basically is similar to the same type of psychiatric problem in a person of normal intelligence. The principles of management outlined throughout this book for the various kinds of psychiatric disorders are also applicable to retarded patients, so long as the treatment program for a retarded patient is geared to his intellectual age rather than to his age in years. It is clinically unsound and unkind to dismiss lightly the psychiatric problems of a retarded patient and to give him little treatment because of his intellectual limitations.

Institutional Living for Mentally Retarded Patients. Mentally retarded persons who do not have helpful, interested families may require institutional living. Others cannot cope with the complexities of urban life, and if left unprotected may be exploited sexually or economically by unprincipled persons. In addition, some mentally retarded individuals have severe personality problems grafted onto their underlying retardation and may need institutional care for short spans of time, or for extensive periods. In still other cases the parents, for either economic of personal reasons, are unable to give a retarded child or adolescent the kind of interpersonal environment he needs, and institutional care for several years or more is in the best interests of both the child and his parents. In occasional cases severe conflicts between a retarded child and his siblings precipitate periods of institutional care.

Institutional living, like other ways of life, has advantages as well as disadvantages. Though to a large extent it removes freedom of choice and many opportunities from the individual, it also eliminates many of the anxious problems and painful dilemmas of modern life. When institutional living for a short or long period of time is indicated, it should be presented to the parents as a special way of life for people with special problems. The aim of institutional life should be, whenever feasible, to train the individual for eventual return to the community, either with his own family or with a foster family.

BIBLIOGRAPHY

Adams, M.: Mental Retardation and Its Social Dimensions. New York, Columbia University Press, 1971.

Chess, S., and Korn, S.: Temperament and behavior disorders in mentally retarded children. Arch. Gen. Psychiatry, 23:122, 1970.

Conley, R. W.: The Economics of Mental Retardation. Baltimore, Johns Hopkins University Press, 1973.

Hallas, C. H.: The Care and Training of the Mentally Subnormal. Baltimore, Williams & Wilkins, 1970.

Holmes, L. B., et al.: Mental Retardation: An Atlas of Diseases With Associated Physical Abnormalities. New York, Macmillan 1972.

Katz, E. (ed.): Mental Health Services for the Mentally Retarded. Springfield, Ill., Charles C. Thomas, 1972.

Koch, R., and Dobson, J. C.: The Mentally Retarded Child and His Family. New York, Brunner Mazel, 1971.

Menolascino, F. J.: Psychiatric Approaches to Mental Retardation. New York, Basic Books, 1970.

Murray, R. F., Jr., and Rosser, P. L. (eds.): The Genetic, Metabolic and Developmental Aspects of Mental Retardation. Springfield, Ill., Charles C. Thomas, 1972.

Perry, T. L., et al.: Unrecognized adult phenylketonuria. N. Eng. J. Med., 289:395, 1973.

Routh, D. K.: The Experimental Psychology of Mental Retardation. Chicago, Aldine Publishing Co., 1973.

Thompson, T., and Grabowski, J.: Behavior Modification of the Mentally Retarded. New York, Oxford University Press, 1972.

Wortis, J.: Comments on the ICD classification of mental retardation. Amer. J. Psychiatry (Suppl.), 128:21, 1972.

Part Six

Treatment Methods in Psychiatry

In this section we shall cover the various kinds of treatment used to help emotionally upset people. We shall discuss psychotherapy, the major method of treating the interpersonally caused disorders, and we shall consider the use of psychotherapeutic environments in psychiatric hospitals and other settings. The use of medications in treating psychiatric illnesses will be systematically reviewed, and discussion of the physical methods of treatment will occupy a further chapter. A final chapter will deal with the special technics employed in child psychiatry.

21

Psychotherapy and Psychotherapeutic Environments

We shall define psychotherapy as any type of professional interpersonal situation involving one or more therapists and one or more patients, which is designed to help the patient to resolve emotional problems and to improve his interpersonal functioning. This broad definition covers (a) the many forms of individual interview treatment, (b) the various kinds of group psychotherapy and (c) the broad spectrum of psychotherapeutic environments which are employed in psychiatric hospitals and other settings.

This chapter is divided into two major parts: (1) *psychotherapy,* in which the various forms of one-to-one interview treatment and group psychotherapy are covered, and (2) *psychotherapeutic environments,* in which we discuss the professional organization of psychiatric hospitals and other treatment facilities to meet the emotional needs of patients and to encourage their recovery.

Throughout this chapter we shall consider the terms "psychotherapy" and "interview treatment" synonymous and interchangeable. Moreover, our emphasis will be on psychotherapy as an interpersonal process; it always involves the activities of at least two people, a therapist and a patient, and its aim is to help the patient resolve emotional problems.

THE BASIC PROCESSES IN PSYCHOTHERAPY

In analyzing what psychotherapy is, we shall first talk about one-to-one psychotherapy between a therapist and a patient, since this is the basic model out of which other forms of psychotherapy (group psychotherapy, psychotherapeutic environments, and others) have grown; however, the basic processes of individual psychotherapy are, in modified forms, the constituents of other psychotherapeutic technics.

We shall begin by listing and discussing the basic processes that may occur in psychotherapy. The emphases different psychiatrists place on each of these basic processes vary from one therapist to another and, to some extent, from one patient to the next. These basic processes are: (1) Catharsis, the free expression of feelings and ideas in an interpersonal situation in which the patient encounters neither censure nor emotional response, but only an informed willingness to help. (2) Insight by the patient into the nature of his relationships with people in his current interpersonal situation. (3) Insight by the patient into the nature of his relationships with people in his past interpersonal life. (4) Insight by the patient into his own personality characteristics and his ways of handling feelings. (5) Analysis of the patient's interpersonal relationship with the therapist. (6) Unanalyzed aspects of the patient's relationship with the therapist. (7) A corrective interpersonal experience in the patient's relationship with the therapist, in which the patient develops, by both conscious and unconscious channels, new capacities for interpersonal relationships with people in many areas of his life. (8) Consensual validation, Harry Stack Sullivan's term for the process in which the patient, by perceiving many areas of his life from different perspectives and in various sensory ways, gradually corrects distortions of emotional functioning and warped ways of relating to people. (9) Direct behavioral modifications by coupling, both in the therapeutic hour and outside it, various behavioral patterns with rewards and punishments; the many forms of this approach, including desensitization procedures, constitute the type of psychotherapy known as *behavior therapy*. (10) Direction, in which the therapist gives specific recommendations and advice to the patient about the management of problems in his life. (11) Suggestion, in which optimistic, curative implications of an impressive treatment procedure induce a feeling of well being in the patient which may help to remove symptoms and to modify limited aspects of his behavior.

Obviously, some of these 11 processes overlap each other, and dividing the elements of psychotherapy into neat, separate functions is somewhat artificial. *Moreover, the extent to which a therapist selects and employs combinations of these 11 processes depends on his theoretical orientation, his personal style of doing psychotherapy, his goals with a particular patient, and the patient's capacity to engage in these treatment technics.*

(1) **Catharsis.** In psychotherapy the patient can express feelings, anxious thoughts, guilty preoccupations, impulses, and other emotions and ideas without fear of emotional reaction, censure or criticism from the therapist. In all other interpersonal situations the person who unreservedly expresses his feelings and ideas enounters responses of anger, pity, anxious solicitude, indignation, moral censure, bored indifference or other reactions that do not help him solve his emotional problems and understand himself. Moreover, the psychotherapist has professional training to help the patient resolve his emotional problems and gain new insights. These two characteristics, acceptance of what the patient expresses without emotional reactions to it and the professional ability to help the patient resolve emotional problems, make psychotherapy a unique interpersonal experience. Unloading pent-up felings and getting them out into the open where they can be examined is a basic aspect of psychotherapy and a significant part of its therapeutic usefulness.

(2) **Insight by the patient into the nature of his relationships with people in his current interpersonal life.** In psychotherapy the patient usually gains new insights into his current relationships with other persons. For example, the patient may realize that he has unrecognized hostile feelings toward his marital partner or his children, or he may come to grips with unmet yearnings for affection which he did not know he had. He may discover that he is very passive with people because he feels that submissiveness is the only way to gain their affection and avoid their hostility. In other instances, the patient may realize that he is chronically aggressive toward everyone around him for fear that if he does not dominate them they will exploit him and control him.

(3) **Insight by the patient into the nature of his relationships with people in his past interpersonal life.** In psychotherapy a patient may discover how traumatic interpersonal relationships in his past life are affecting his current behavior. For example, he may realize that he has much sniping hostility toward women which arises from the trauma of a chronically hostile relationship with his mother during his childhood and adolescence. He is carrying over into relationships with his wife, his daughters and other women in his current life unresolved conflicts and attitudes from his earlier years. Another patient may discover that he has unmet yearnings for affection and acceptance from his father who always treated him in a cold, distant manner and left in the patient an aching need for warm acceptance from men. The patient in his current life finds himself seeking the approval of his superiors at work, and he is very upset if he is rejected or criticized by them; he is carrying into current life situations the painful interpersonal needs which were unmet during his formative years.

In many instances, until the patient explored his life in psychotherapy he was not consciously aware of many of the painful experiences in his early life; because of their painfulness, many of his early memories were repressed out of his awareness, and he was unable to recall them until he rediscovered them piece by piece in treatment. In other instances, the patient has distorted memories about his past interpersonal experiences; he is unable to come to grips with the painful things that actually happened, and he unconsciously has substituted less painful, unrealistic memories for what happened during his childhood and adolescence. For example, a woman who during childhood and adolescence had a painful relationship with a self-centered, hostile mother may in retrospect repress these painful memories and may idealize her mother as a generous, affectionate person. However, the unresolved conflicts which lurk beneath her unrealistic memories of her mother may contribute to neurotic problems, psychosomatic symptoms or other psychiatric difficulties.

(4) **Insight by the patient into his own personality characteristics and his ways of handling feelings.** In psychotherapy the patient usually gains important new insights into his personality structure. For example, a very compulsive woman who works endlessly to keep her home in immaculate, excessive order and nags her family into compliance with her unreasonable neatness, may realize in psychotherapy that her compulsiveness is not a virtue; it is a personality problem making her home a cold, tense place in which to rear children and it puts a chronic strain on her marriage. A very passive patient who is on an endless treadmill to please everyone and to gain their approval may view himself as an individual who never has interpersonal difficulties; in psychotherapy he may discover that his never-ending quest for approval and acceptance is a personality problem that allows other people to dominate and exploit him. In many instances a patient has a very limited or distorted understanding of his own personality structure, and a better understanding of himself opens the way to resolution of many emotional problems and interpersonal difficulties.

(5) **Analysis of the patient's interpersonal relationship with the therapist.** A patient tends to carry into his interpersonal relationship with the therapist many of his emotional problems and unresolved conflicts. For example, the frightened patient who seeks emotional dependence on other people in order to feel secure tends quickly to become dependent on the therapist and to cling to him for reassurance and guidance. The patient who is irritably resistant to all authority tends to resist the therapist and to evade his efforts to help him. Patients who try to manipulate all persons of the opposite sex with charm and flirtatiousness may similarly attempt to mobilize the sympathies of a therapist of the opposite sex for use as a tool in chronic battles with martial partners and other relatives.

The interpersonal relationship the patient sets up with the therapist often follows the pattern of the patient's relationships with crucial people in his life. For example, the patient who throughout his childhood and adolescence rebelled with hostile negativism against a harsh, domineering father may be defensive and irritable with the psychiatrist whom he unconsciously puts in the position of a father substitute. The phobic patient who throughout his formative years leaned with clinging fearfulness on his mother often clings emotionally to the therapist. Patients with unresolved hostilities, affectionate yearnings or confused mixed feelings toward one or both parents often attach these feelings quickly to the therapist and behave toward him with the same emotional attitudes.

The therapist, unlike all other persons in the patient's life, does not become emotionally involved in the type of relationship the patient unconsciously tries to set up with him. His task is to help the patient understand himself and resolve his emotional problems. The therapist does not become angry and retaliatory at the hostile patient; he does not become solicitously overprotective toward the clinging, fearful patient; he does not become vainly flattered and charmed by the coy, manipulative patient. Instead, the therapist uses the patient's behavior as material to help the patient see how he tends to set up similar unhealthy relationships with many people in his life. The therapist helps the patient gradually to see how he is carrying over unresolved conflicts from his relationships with his parents and other close persons into his relationship with the therapist. The therapist helps the patient to grasp slowly how his interpersonal behavior toward the psychiatrist reveals many of the emotional problems contributing to his symptoms and his personality difficulties.

In individual psychotherapy, the patient and the therapist deal with many interpersonal relationships in the patient's life, but the only interpersonal relationship directly available for their scrutiny is the relationship between the patient and the therapist. Hence, this interpersonal relationship has particular value in the work of the patient and the therapist in resolving the patient's personality problems.

(6) **Unanalyzed aspects of the patient's relationship with the therapist.** Many aspects of the patient-therapist relationship are never put into words, but nevertheless may have a profound effect on the patient. Just as many of the patient's personality problems and symptoms were formed without articulate understanding of the causative interpersonal processes, so emotional problems sometimes are solved with little articulate awareness of the processes causing their resolution. For example, a hostile, rebellious adolescent may in time develop a warm, friendly feeling toward the psychiatrist, and he may gradually take into himself many of the attitudes and behavior characteristics of the therapist. In the therapist he finds someone who does not retaliate harshly, but who accepts him and understands him. The patient forms a warm identification with this understanding person, and he unconsciously wants to be like him. Hence, the socially defiant adolescent slowly takes on many of the socially conforming attitudes and socially acceptable aspirations implied by the psychiatrist's way of life. Few or none of these goals may have been put into words either by the psychiatrist or the patient at any time during the course of treatment. However, these unanalyzed aspects of the patient-therapist relationship may have been a major reason for the success of the treatment.

In a similar manner, a patient may settle various kinds of conflicts left unresolved by traumatic interpersonal relationships during his formative years. The patient who was depreciated by critical, domineering parents and other close persons, and who emerged from childhood with profound feelings of inferiority may gradually acquire self-confidence and a feeling of greater adequacy through the therapist's treatment of him as a capable, worthwhile person. The therapist may never put this feature of treatment into words, but it may have a marked effect on the patient. In some instances the patient is chronically deluged with depreciation by unaffectionate parents and other persons, and he comes out of childhood with the feeling that anyone who gets to know him intimately will recoil with disgust and will reject him; in therapy the patient finds a person who does not reject him because of his problems, and he slowly develops a more self-confident view of himself, even though he may have had little conscious awareness of either the nature of his fears or the methods of their resolution. He only knows that before treatment he felt worthless and inept and that after treatment he feels more worthwhile and capable. Through the unanalyzed aspects of his relationship with the therapist he resolves personality damage which occurred in his relationships with significant people during his formative years.

The kinds of unanalyzed patient-therapist processes that may contribute to the success of psychotherapy are as varied as the many personality problems which patients bring to treatment.

(7) **A corrective interpersonal experience in the patient's relationship with the therapist.** In some instances the patient acquires in psychotherapy, by both conscious and unconscious channels, new capacities for handling his feelings in interpersonal relationships. For example, a passive patient who fears to express hostility may make his first experiments in expressing anger by getting mad at the therapist. The therapist does not lash back or reject the patient. He helps the patient see that getting angry once in a while is a healthy experience, and he aids the patient in resolving the anxious and guilty feelings he has when he gets angry. The schizoid patient who fears to relax and discuss himself freely with anyone may benefit much from the experience of talking intimately about his problems with the therapist. He begins to lose his fear of exposing himself to other people and he can begin

to emerge from his frightened shell. After he has bridged the interpersonal gap between himself and the therapist he finds it easier to do the same thing with other people in his life, and he can begin to develop a healthier interpersonal life. In many other ways patients may have corrective interpersonal experiences in psychotherapy because the therapist has the professional skill to use the patient-therapist relationship as a therapeutic instrument.

(8) **Consensual validation.** Harry Stack Sullivan employed the term *consensual validation* to designate a complex process which he felt was one of the main ways in which emotional problems and personality warps are corrected. Sullivan felt that consensual validation occurs (a) spontaneously, as a basic aspect of personality development in childhood and adolescence (as discussed in Chapter 1) and (b) deliberately, when a therapist works with a patient in psychotherapy. In consensual validation the patient, with the therapist's help, views many aspects of his past and current interpersonal relationships and emotional functioning from different points of view; he repeatedly analyzes his problems from diverse perspectives. (A detailed example of the spontaneous operation of consensual validation in personality development is given in Chapter 1.)

In psychotherapy consensual validation is systematically employed in a professional setting. For example, a therapist may help a passive patient gradually to grasp how his inability to be assertive arose in childhood relationships, cripples him in current life situations, mobilizes anxiety and thus further hinders interpersonal skills, corrupts his relationship with his marital partner and children, limits him in his job, contaminates his interaction in social groups, warps his relationship with the therapist, and invades many other aspects of his life. Thus, in multiple sensory ways *(consensual)* the patient corrects warped ways of feeling and interpersonal behavior *(validation)*. It is obvious that consensual validation, as Sullivan conceived it, overlaps many of the other 10 basic processes we are here discussing as components of psychotherapy.

(9) **Direct behavioral modifications.** In the form of psychotherapy termed *behavior therapy* rewards and punishments are employed to encourage or discourage various kinds of behavior and emotional responses. This may be set up so that it occurs either during the therapeutic hour or outside it. In a very simple example, an adult patient with a phobia of dogs might be given warm praise (reward) when he fondled a stuffed toy dog, or a small electric shock in an electrode strapped to his leg (punishment) when he shrank back from touching the toy dog. Most behavior therapy technics are more subtle and complex than this model suggests. Obviously, behavior therapy is based on very different premises than therapy employing most of the other 10 principles of psychotherapy enumerated here. [Behavior therapy is discussed in more detail later in this chapter, in Chapter 7 on phobic neuroses (in which many therapists feel it has special usefulness), and in Chapter 3.]

(10) **Direction.** In some types of therapeutic situations the therapist gives the patient specific recommendations and direct advice about the management of problems in his life. As a rule, direction is used in counseling relatively well-adjusted persons who are going through situational stresses. The patient must be sufficiently free of personality problems to be able to accept the therapist's advice and act on it. For example, a therapist may suggest to a relatively stable person who is tense over difficulties in his job that he take a brief vacation from work or that he try to talk things over with his employers and work associates.

Direct advice sometimes is used in counseling the parents of children and adolescents, in counseling on mild or moderate marital problems and in talking with the relatives of hospitalized patients. However, before giving direct advice the therapist should be reasonably sure that he is talking to persons who are able to accept direction and use it in constructive ways. In general, direction is of limited usefulness in most psychiatric patients, but it has its occasional role in the total spectrum of psychotherapeutic services.

Although the technics of Masters and Johnson (sometimes called *sexual retraining*) for nonorgasmic dysfunction (frigidity), impotence, premature ejaculation and other sexual maladjustments involve more than simple direction, direction plays a central role in them. These technics are effective in many patients with sexual problems, but the patients must be highly motivated when they come for treatment and must have sufficient personality stability to use the therapist's direction skillfully and enthusiastically. (This subject is further discussed in Chapter 25.)

(11) **Suggestion.** In suggestion, the optimistic, curative implications of an impressive treatment procedure induce a feeling of well being in the patient, which may help to remove minor symptoms and to modify limited aspects of his behavior. Since suggestion does not resolve the emotional problems causing psychiatric symptoms or disturbed behavior, its effects usually are brief and superficial; the symptoms or disturbed behavior often return in a short time after the effect of the suggestion wears off. However, suggestion sometimes is useful for minor psychiatric symptoms in reasonably well-adjusted persons who are in temporary situational stresses. The encouraging words and actions of the physician may remove symptoms by suggestion in such instances. The use of hypnosis, the most elaborate suggestive technic, is discussed later in this chapter.

As pointed out in the beginning of this chapter, the emphases therapists place on these various processes in psychotherapy vary depending on the theoretical views and technics of the individual psychiatrist and the particular needs of the patient.

THE MAJOR TYPES OF PSYCHOTHERAPY

We shall now consider the five most common types of psychotherapy. They are (1) the interpersonal approach to psychotherapy, (2) the Freudian-psychoanalytic approach to psychotherapy and the modified forms of Freudian psychoanalysis, (3) behavior therapy, (4) electric flexible psychotherapy and (5) supportive counseling. In the historical development of psychotherapy a wide variety of different approaches have been advocated, but today most psychotherapeutic practice falls into one of these five broad classifications. After discussing these five types of psychotherapy, we shall discuss the indications and complications of psychotherapy.

The Interpersonal Approach to Psychotherapy

(The historical evolution of the interpersonal approach to psychiatry and psychotherapy is outlined in Chapter 2; it is the product of the work of many psychiatrists, and it has developed by a progressive evolution of theory and technic that began in the first decade of this century. It is based on the material outlined in Chapter 1 on the interpersonal approach to personality development and psychiatric illness. In a sense, with the exception of Chapter 3, in which we covered a broad spectrum of concepts from many psychiatric schools of thought, all the preceding chapters of this book outline the basic points of view forming the interpersonal approach to psychotherapy.)

The interpersonal approach to psychotherapy views the psychiatrist-therapist relationship as a therapeutic channel that can be used in many ways to help the patient resolve emotional problems. The psychotherapist and the patient meet for 50-minute sessions once or twice each week for a treatment program that runs from several months to two years or more; the average time varies greatly from one therapist to another. The therapist and the patient usually talk in a face-to-face situation in comfortable chairs. They engage in a common venture to evaluate the patient's problems, to explore their causes and to help the patient resolve his emotional turmoil and interpersonal difficulties.

In the interpersonal approach to psychotherapy the therapist's role is quite variable. Although in some cases he may say little for long periods of time as the patient unravels his problems, the therapist more often is fairly active in making interpretations, asking questions, offering explanations and suggesting lines of exploration, depending on the needs of the patient and the particular treatment problem in hand. The therapist may, to a large extent, let the patient make the crucial discoveries himself, or he may identify important points and expose them fully as they come into focus. In some instances the therapist may need to reassure the patient or give some direct advice, but he reserves such intervention for frightened, confused patients who need such support in order to function well in the therapeutic process.

Harry Stack Sullivan himself was a quite active therapist, frequently using exclamations ("Well, that must have given you a jolt!"), pointed questions, hints, reassuring statements and other frankly conversational technics. However, Sullivan emphasized that psychotherapy is hard work, the hardest work he knew (and he was reared on a small farm in upstate New York), and that there was no "fun" in it. The therapist is always in a state of intense alertness to note the feelings, thoughts, gestures, body movements and other communicative things in the patient, and to employ them in the therapeutic process. When the therapist does not grasp what is going on, or only partly senses it, he asks specific questions to seek more information for both himself and the patient in their joint therapeutic efforts.

The interpersonally oriented psychiatrist is not rigid in terms of the content of the interviews. The bulk of the treatment process rests on the first eight of the basic principles of psychotherapy outlined in the initial section of this chapter. These processes are: (1) free catharsis of feelings and thoughts, (2) insight into current interpersonal relationships, (3) insight into past interpersonal relationships, (4) insight by the patient into his own personality characteristics, (5) analysis of the patient-therapist relationship, (6) unanalyzed aspects of the patient-therapist relationship, and (7) a corrective interpersonal experience in the patient's relationship with the therapist, all of which, in Sullivanian terms, contribute to the all-inclusive therapeutic process of (8) consensual validation.

However, the importance of these different processes varies immensely from one patient to another, and from one psychiatrist to another. For example, in some instances the therapeutic process rests largely on catharsis and analysis of the patient's relationships with people in his current and past life situations. In other cases, heavy emphasis is placed on both the analyzed and unanalyzed aspects of the interpersonal relationship established with the psychiatrist. In the to-and-fro communication between patient and therapist, moreover, nonverbal aspects of the behavior of both the patient and the therapist are usually important. Facial expressions, small gestures, body movements, nonarticulate vocal sounds, and other nonverbal ways of exchanging data frequently play crucial roles. For example, I recall one patient to whom I often said "tsk, tsk, tsk," to indicate the unrealistic nature of his strong feelings of inadequacy and inferiority when they cropped up in therapy; for this patient, this nonarticulate vocal sound was more effective than paragraphs of verbal interpretations would have been.

In addition, the relative weight given to various ones of these basic processes of psychotherapy varies much at different phases of treatment in many cases. For example, catharsis and insight into the patient's current interpersonal relationships often are the predominant processes during the early phases of treatment. Later, insight into his own personality characteristics and insight into how these personality characteristics developed in the context of crucial interpersonal relationships during his formative years often become important. As treatment deepens, the analyzed and unanalyzed aspects of the patient's relationship with the therapist and a corrective interpersonal experience in the patient-therapist relationship may become the main channels of therapeutic activity. However, therapy is adjustable and does not follow a rigid, preconceived sequence; it flows onward according to the patient's needs, the patient's comfort in exploring various emotional problems, the patient's ability to use the interview time and the therapist's capacity for helping the patient resolve various phases of his difficulties.

Many interpersonally oriented therapists have on open mind about involving other members of the patient's family in the therapeutic process when it can be helpful. As a rule, the therapist treats only one member of a family. For example, if a patient's marital partner needs psychotherapy he usually is referred to another therapist, since when a psychiatrist treats both husband and wife he usually finds each of them becoming less communicative for fear the therapist inadvertently will reveal confidential material to the other marital partner. However, if toward the end of the course of treatment of a patient, or at any other time, the therapist feels that joint marital counseling of the patient and his marital partner may resolve interpersonal difficulties, he may undertake to see them both in joint counseling sessions.

The interpersonally oriented therapist occasionally may use the patient's dreams as material for exploring his emotional problems. He views dreams as disguised expressions of the patient's desires, fears and unresolved conflicts in past and current interpersonal relationships. In dreams these emotional forces are camouflaged in various symbolic ways which sometimes may be unraveled to give significant information about the patient's emotional problems. However, most interpersonally oriented psychiatrists regard dream analysis as a minor technic in the total therapeutic process, and many interpersonally oriented psychiatrists do not use dream analysis at all.

It is implicit in the interpersonal approach to psychotherapy that the patient is unaware of many of the past and current interpersonal experiences that contribute to his psychiatric problems, and that much of the treatment process is devoted to bringing these experiences and emotional forces into the patient's conscious awareness. Many of these memories and conflicts are so painful that the patient cannot remember them and come to grips with them until he has had much psychotherapeutic help. In this sense, they are unconscious, but the interpersonally oriented psychiatrist does not view the unconscious feelings and thoughts of the patient as rigidly enclosed and congealed. He views the interchange between unconscious and conscious memories and feelings as relatively fluid, and he views psychotherapy as the catalyst allowing the patient to become aware of experiences, feelings and personality characteristics of which he formerly was unaware.

Interpersonally oriented psychiatrists, and other mental health professional workers, hold flexible views about the necessity of a psychotherapeutic experience for the psychotherapist as part of his training. Many interpersonally oriented psychiatrists feel that it often is useful for the psychiatrist to undergo a period of psychotherapy to resolve whatever personality problems and emotional blind spots he may have; it also can be a useful educational procedure, since the psychiatric trainee thereby experiences intimately the treatment methods of an experienced therapist. However, when a psychiatrist is basically well adjusted and free of significant personality problems, such a treatment experience is optional and need not be a part of his preparation for psychotherapeutic practice.

A technic of psychotherapy is best understood by reviewing its use in specific cases. (Cases illustrating briefly the use of the interpersonal approach to psychotherapy are given in Chapters 7 and 9.)

The Freudian-Psychoanalytic Approach to Psychotherapy

(In Chapter 3 we reviewed the basic tenets of Freudian-psychoanalytic theory, and, since the concepts and terminology of the Freudian-psychoanalytic point of view cannot be adequately discussed without examining its treatment technics, the therapeutic approach of Freudian psychoanalysis is outlined briefly there; the history of the psychoanalytic movement is covered in Chapter 2 on the historical evolution of modern psychiatry. We shall now reconsider Freudian psychoanalytic treatment from the viewpoint of the basic processes of psychotherapy outlined at the beginning of this present chapter.)

In classical Freudian-psychoanalytic procedure the patient reclines on a couch while the therapist sits at the head of the couch out of the direct view of the patient. This situation is designed to allow the patient to speak as freely as possible without distracting influences of any kind. The therapist indicates to the patient that he should put into words as spontaneously as he can all the thoughts, feelings and fantasies that come to his mind. The patient is directed to express uninhibitedly all succeeding things that come into his awareness. Psychoanalytic theory holds that through this process the patient gradually explores the unconscious conflicts causing his emotional problems. The patient comes for 50-minute sessions three to five times each week, and the average complete psychoanalysis today lasts between three and five years.

The therapist remains silent during most of this process. From time to time he makes an interpretation, but in general he does not do so until he feels that conscious material is near the surface and ready for crystallization into words. Freudian-psychoanalytic theory holds that greater activity on the part of the therapist distorts both the patient-therapist relationship and the nature of what the patient says. This basic format of classical Freudian-psychoanalytic technic remains largely the same throughout the entire course of treatment.

A basic tenet of Freudian-psychoanalytic theory is that the crucial experiences causing psychiatric difficulties occur during the first seven years of life; though subsequent experiences may be the precipitants of psychiatric illness, they are not basic causes. The fundamental causes of psychiatric illness arise in the patient's relationships with his parents during this time. Hence, treatment eventually is directed toward resolving the emotional conflicts that occurred in the first seven years. However, before reaching these critical areas in the patient's childhood, much preliminary work must be done. The patient has strong unconscious resistances about coming to grips with this painful material, and these resistances must be slowly overcome. Psychoanalytic theory holds that most of the emotional turmoil causing the patient's psychiatric problems is locked in the unconscious parts of his mind and can be recovered only with great difficulty.

One of the major avenues of exploration is the analysis of dreams, which Freud called "the royal road to the unconscious." Through analysis of dreams, hidden fears, feelings, fantasies and traumatic experiences are gradually unraveled. (The concepts and terminology used in Freudian dream analysis are outlined briefly in Chapter 3.)

A second major avenue for exploring the patient's crucial interpersonal traumas with his parents during his early years is the elaborate analysis of the patient-therapist relationship. Freudian-psychoanalytic theory holds that the patient transfers to the therapist all the complex conflicts he experienced with one or both parents during the first seven years of life. For example, if the patient was both afraid of his father and hostile to him, he develops both fearful and hostile feelings toward the therapist during various phases of treatment. If a woman had strong, unresolved sexual feelings toward her father during early childhood, she may develop strong erotic feelings toward the therapist. The Freudian psychoanalyst looks upon these feelings of the patient toward the therapist as a form of reliving emotionally the critical interpersonal traumas causing the patient's psychiatric problems. In the patient-therapist relationship the therapist helps the patient resolve these traumas, which were not resolved in actual life. For example, the patient who had fearful and hostile feelings toward his father and never resolved them in his relationship with his father has the opportunity of reliving these emotional traumas in the patient-therapist relationship and resolving them there. The fundamental objectives in Freudian psychoanalysis are the resolution in the patient-therapist relationship of these basic interpersonal traumas and the conscious confrontation and assimilation of the patient's unconscious emotional turmoil.

The process of conducting this treatment work involves many intricate difficulties. Among many possible problems, for example, the therapist must be alert not to allow the strong feelings the patient develops in the patient-therapist relationship to arouse strong feelings in himself. For example, the therapist must be sufficiently free of personality difficulties that he does not become irritable, anxious, oversolicitous or vainly flattered in response to the patient's feelings toward him. Any such feelings in the therapist limit his ability to see the patient's problems objectively and to help.

Classical Freudian-psychoanalytic technic places relatively little emphasis on current interpersonal stress in the patient's life. The Freudian psychoanalyst feels that if the patient resolves his basic personality problems, which originated in childhood trauma, he will be able to deal maturely with any contemporary stresses and solve them spontaneously. The Freudian psychoanalyst rarely has contact with any members of the patient's family; he feels that such contact inhibits the free flow of the patient's speech and distorts the spontaneous directions the therapist-patient relationship may take.

In recent decades Freudian psychoanalysts have developed the concepts of *ego psycho-*

logy and *ego analysis* in their attempts to take into account the roles of broader interpersonal forces and social factors in the person's emotional functioning. However, in the opinion of many psychiatrists, including myself, ego analysis has in fact had little influence on what psychoanalysts *do* in therapy, though it has altered what some of them *say* occurs in therapy. (These concepts are outlined in Chapter 3.)

The Freudian psychoanalyst goes through extensive training before he is accepted as a fully qualified analyst. Such training is conducted under the auspices of the psychoanalytic institutes existing in many major cities. In addition to the usual psychiatric residency training, the psychoanalytic trainee attends seminars and lectures and treats patients under close supervision. An essential part of his training is a thorough psychoanalytic treatment experience for himself. Psychoanalysts feel that the therapist cannot be objective in seeing the patient's problems unless he has had extensive therapy to eliminate any emotional blind spots in his own personality. Moreover, the therapist is felt to be unable to avoid distorted feelings in the patient-therapist relationship unless he has undergone much personal psychoanalytic therapy. The treatment experience of the psychoanalytic trainee also is an educational procedure, since he learns at first hand the treatment technics of an experienced psychoanalyst. Some psychoanalysts advocate a two-part analysis, divided into a therapeutic analysis and an educational, or didactic, analysis.

Only a small minority of American psychiatrists are fully trained psychoanalysts, and, in terms of hours of work, it is probable that orthodox Freudian psychoanalysis accounts for no more than about three per cent of all psychiatric treatment done in the United States. However, modifications of psychoanalytic concepts have had a significant influence on the development of other forms of psychotherapy. For example, some of the concepts of the interpersonal approach to psychotherapy have been influenced by psychoanalytic points of view; however, these psychoanalytic points of view have been extensively modified in the process of their incorporation into the interpersonal approach to psychotherapy.

Modified Forms of Freudian Psychoanalysis. Many psychoanalytically trained psychiatrists have attempted to modify the psychoanalytic treatment procedure because of the serious economic and other practical difficulties involved in carrying out a form of treatment that requires that the patient attend interviews three to five times each week for from three to five years. Moreover, many patients cannot follow the basic rule of prolonged, spontaneous verbalization in a form of treatment in which the therapist is silent most of the time. Indeed, of all patients seen in general psychiatric work, it is doubtful that more than 10 per cent could, without help, talk sufficiently well to engage in classical on-the-couch psychoanalysis, and only a fifth, or so, of them could afford it financially (these figures are much higher in certain sophisticated, well-to-do groups, but they constitute a very small segment of the total population). These grim facts have become increasingly apparent as the first flush of enthusiasm about psychoanalysis has passed and more mature evaluation of it has occurred. In his old age Sigmund Freud himself stated that, in terms of treatment results and economic feasibility, psychoanalysis could not be justified; he felt that it was of primary value only as a research tool and as a training procedure for mental health professional workers.

Those psychoanalysts who shorten and modify psychoanalytic treatment technics while adhering to the basic body of Freudian-psychoanalytic theory are said to practice modified psychoanalysis. Many of them interview patients in face-to-face treatment situations, set limited goals in treatment for some patients, and see patients for periods of time that run from several months to two or three years.

These alterations of psychoanalytic technic vary immensely among therapists who use modified psychoanalysis. In many instances the psychoanalyst modifies psychoanalytic technics only to a limited extent in order to meet the economic comfort and time limitations of the patient. In other instances the psychoanalyst who practices modified psychoanalysis may make such extensive changes in the psychotherapeutic format that his procedures begin to approach those of the interpersonally oriented psychiatrist.

Behavior Therapy

[The principles of behavior therapy (and its theoretical basis, *behavior theory*) were discussed in detail in Chapter 3, and the special application of behavior therapy to phobic neuroses was sketched in Chapter 7. We shall cover here some of the specific technics employed in behavior therapy, and this discussion should be considered as a continuation of the material in Chapter 3.]

In the behavior therapy technic of *desensitization* the patient is exposed, by stages of increasing intensity, to the thing or situation that makes him anxious. In this way his dread of the object or situation is slowly diminished. (This technic is dealt with in detail in Chapters 3 and 7.) In the technic termed *reinforcement*, desirable behavior and attitudes are encouraged by repeated rewards when they are elicited. For example, a child may be given a nibble of candy each time he restrains a tic, or an adult may be praised and reassured each time he desists from carrying out a compulsive movement. In this way the undesirable trait is gradually abandoned. The term *operant conditioning* is sometimes used to indicate the broadest possible implications of this type of stimulus-response molding of behavior and attitudes; however, the term operant conditioning at other times is employed to designate the broad use of various behavior therapy technics for sociological and political, as well as psychiatric, ends.

In *reciprocal inhibition* the patient is trained to overcome (that is, inhibit) an emotional symptom or behavioral pattern by use of a countermeasure. For example, this method may be employed to treat a patient who experiences marked anxiety when he perceives anger in himself, or when other people are angry at him, or when he observes two people who are angry at each other without involving him. By a series of relaxation exercises, this patient is first trained to induce in himself at will a state of marked muscular, and presumably emotional, relaxation. Then, by film slides, or by short stretches of cinema film, or by hostile accusations directed at him, he is exposed to hostility-laden experiences; each time he is thus exposed to experiences that tend to cause anxiety in him, he counteracts the anxiety by use of the relaxation technic he has previously learned. Thus, in time he automatically *reciprocally inhibits* feelings of anxiety when he is exposed in any way to hostility.

In the behavior therapy method termed *extinction* an undesirable symptom, or personality trait, or behavioral pattern is gradually lost when it no longer brings advantages to the patient. For example, a patient who formerly dominated his family and manipulated his work associates by hysterical conversion fainting spells loses this symptom when the people around him ignore his fainting episodes entirely; they pay no attention to him when he faints or complains of giddiness. Thus, this symptom, or behavioral pattern, becomes *extinct*.

In *conditioned avoidance*, revulsion toward some object or situation is induced by associating it repeatedly with a disagreeable experience. In a long-used type of conditioned avoidance therapy, an alcoholic is given an injection of an emetic drug at the same time that he takes a drink of alcohol; he soon vomits. This is done once daily for many days, usually in a hospitalized patient, until the sight, smell and taste of alcohol cause automatic disgust and revulsion in him. An ingenious variety of this technic has been employed to treat male homosexuals. A simple device is attached to the patient's penis to detect erections. Pictures of handsome men, some of whom are in seductive poses, are then projected on a screen in front of the patient, and each time he begins to get an erection he receives a small, unpleasant electric shock in an electrode strapped to his arm. When he no longer is aroused by pictures of men he is shown pictures of attractive, alluring women and given warm praise and other rewards if he begins to get erections. Thus, *conditioned avoidance* is followed by *reinforcement* in a behavior therapy regimen.

In *negative reinforcement* the patient is placed in an unpleasant or mildly uncomfortable situation which continues until the desired behavior or reaction occurs. For example, an adult patient may receive a very low voltage electrical current in an electrode attached to his leg until he touches a model of an animal, such as a dog or a cat, of which he has a phobia. Each time he removes his hand from the toy model the current begins again. Later he may be required to fondle a real animal in order to avoid the mildly distressing sensation.

Obviously, behavior therapy requires a highly motivated patient who is willing to submit to these types of experiences to rid himself of his problem. The results of behavior therapy in unselected, large series of patients with specific kinds of disorders (such as anxiety neuroses, phobic neuroses and others) are not clear at this time. Many psychiatrists and other mental health professional workers shun behavior therapy because it pays relatively scant attention to the patient's past life experiences, interpersonal relationships and deeper emotions and feelings. However, in some types of disorders, in selected, cooperative patients, the results of behavior therapy are better, and more quickly attained, than with other types of psychotherapy. This field is in the process of evolution, and final appraisal must await many more years of experience in it.

Eclectic Flexible Psychotherapy

Until recently "eclectic" was considered a dirty word by many psychiatrists and mental health professional workers. Although in its true sense eclectic designates a method in which the practitioner selects what he considers best and most worthwhile from a number of systems, theories and technics, to older generations of mental health workers eclectic meant a mélange of procedures employed by persons who were anti-Freudian. In recent years, however, the concept of eclectic, flexible psychotherapy has once more become respectable, and even popular, in some psychiatric circles.

The eclectic psychiatrist draws what he considers most valid and workable from other theoretical systems and technics of psychotherapy. Thus, he may choose elements from the interpersonal approach, the Freudian-psychoanalytic approach, behavior therapy and other approaches; also, his technics usually are molded to meet the needs of each individual patient and the patient's capacity to engage in one or another kind of psychotherapy. Those therapists who classify themselves as eclectic feel that, in its present stage of development, this is the only reasonable and practical mode to conduct psychotherapy for any broad spectrum of patients.

The difficulties with eclectic psychotherapy are (1) it varies so much from one therapist to another that it is difficult to describe it and teach it, (2) it gives the therapist so much leeway that liberty can, in unsuitable hands, develop into license or eccentricity and (3) it does not have a standard, generally used literature to guide its practitioners. This last factor is both a strength and a weakness; it allows an experienced, skillful therapist to do whatever the patient needs without worrying about theoretical quibbles, but it leaves the beginning or inexperienced therapist without clear guidelines.

In our opinion, most experienced psychotherapists in their later years are at least somewhat eclectic. For example, if one reviews the experiences of people who wrote down their treatment by Sigmund Freud, even in his mature period when he had extensively developed psychoanalytic technics and had practiced them for many years, one finds that he was quite eclectic in his day-to-day work with patients. Thus, when the orchestra conductor Bruno Walter consulted him in a single session in 1906 about a hysterical paralysis of his hand, Freud carefully examined the hand and urged Bruno Walter to go to Sicily for a vacation; Bruno Walter was so much impressed by Freud's manner that he immediately went to Sicily, recovered and never had a recurrence of this problem. In other instances Freud gave direct advice, urged changes of environment and during the treatment hours discussed topics that today would be considered almost conversational. In practice he was much more eclectic than his writings would suggest. Careful analysis of the available accounts of therapy by Harry Stack Sullivan in his later years reveal a similar flexibility.

In our opinion, eclecticism is best used by the therapist who has at least 10 years of active psychotherapeutic practice behind him and has practical knowledge of various therapeutic methods. He then can adapt his treatment to fit the needs and capacities of individual patients.

Supportive Counseling

Many patients are seen in psychiatric practice who cannot participate effectively in any of the previously described forms of psychotherapy. They cannot talk at length about their feelings or their past and current interpersonal relationships, and are not sufficiently motivated, or otherwise capable, for involvement in behavior therapy or eclectic psychotherapy. Many of these patients have ingrained neuroses and personality problems of long standing, and others have marked emotional blocks to exploring their feelings and life experiences. A small number of these patients are borderline psychotic and have only fragile holds on reality; exploration of their basic emotional problems disturbs them immensely and incurs the risk of precipitating psychotic breaks.

However, the psychotherapist can help some of these patients by supportive counseling. In supportive counseling the therapist sets limited goals since he recognizes that the patient cannot engage in meaningful exploratory psychotherapy. The therapist tries to relieve symptoms, to give the patient more self-confidence, and to advise the patient on ways of making a better life adjustment. By supportive counseling the therapist may render a significant service to the patient and his family. A woman may be helped to function better as a mother and a wife, or a man may be helped to continue as an economic provider, father and husband to his family. A decrease in the patient's symptoms, such as phobias or anxiety states, may enable him to lead a much more comfortable and effective life. In many instances, supportive counseling is adopted only after an unsuccessful trial of some other kind of psychotherapy has demonstrated that the patient cannot participate in more extensive types of interview treatment.

In supportive counseling the therapist may begin by seeing the patient once every week or two, but in time treatment sessions often become stretched out to once a month or once every two or three months. Such supportive counseling, of course, begins only after a more intensive initial diagnostic workup, and perhaps a trial of systematic psychotherapy, has demonstrated that the patient is not capable of participating in anything more than supportive sessions. Once supportive counseling is under way, the sessions often are 20 or 25 minutes long. As a rule, the therapist uses much reassurance, explanation of the emotional nature of the patient's symptoms, and direct advice on how to handle day-to-day situational problems. In some cases, he may also see the patient's relatives to counsel them on measures that may contribute to the patient's emotional comfort and better interpersonal functioning. A small amount of medication sometimes is given, and it may help as much by suggestive effect as by pharmacologic rationale; however, the physician always emphasizes that the purpose of the medication is to assuage symptoms of interpersonal origin and is not designed to correct any physical disorder.

The patient often gets much relief by telling the therapist about his symptoms, his fears and his interpersonal dilemmas. The therapist's calm acceptance of what the patient says, his reassurances and his ability to understand how the patient feels are helpful. The therapist may point out how certain interpersonal tensions seem to exacerbate the patient's symptoms, and occasionally he may point out the importance of past interpersonal relationships.

In supportive counseling the patient-therapist relationship is not analyzed, but the unanalyzed features of the patient-therapist relationship often are major factors that help the patient. The patient often looks upon the therapist as a strong, wise guiding person from whom he gets calmness and confidence to go about his daily tasks. In the same way, the therapist helps to reduce the severity of symptoms, such as phobias or anxiety, but the suppression of symptoms often is dependent on continued periodic contacts with the therapist. The therapist occasionally may explain aspects of the patient's personality to him and point out ways in which the patient can use this information to make a better interpersonal adjustment. For example, he may explain to a compulsive patient certain features of his personality, and he may point out that a compulsive person usually is more comfortable with neatly organized work schedules both at home and on his job and is very anxious when he has idle or unproductive time.

The possibility that the patient may become overly dependent on the therapist is a common problem in supportive therapy, since the patient's symptoms are held in abeyance by the treatment but are not resolved by it. The therapist should be aware of this possible problem from the beginning; often the patient should have planned "vacations" from treatment, or definite time limits and partial goals should be established for the treatment and discussed tactfully with him. In some instances, undue dependency is avoided by spacing the appointments at wider intervals once the patient has made reasonable gains. Successful supportive counseling requires flexibility, patience and continued alertness to the possibility of undue dependence of the patient on the therapist. However, it offers a large measure of relief to many patients who cannot engage in deeper therapy, and it is a service both to them and their families.

THE INDICATIONS AND COMPLICATIONS OF PSYCHOTHERAPY

Indications

As we covered the various kinds of psychiatric illnesses in the preceding chapters of this book, we discussed the role of psychotherapy in the treatment of them. We shall briefly recapitulate the indications for psychotherapy here. Psychotherapy is the treatment of choice for the neuroses and also for the personality disorders. In our discussions of the various kinds of neuroses and the personality disorders, we examined in detail the application of psychotherapy to these problems. Psychotherapy also is the major avenue of treatment for many of the miscellaneous problems of emotional adjustment (discussed in Chapter 25). Psychotherapy may be employed as a major method of treatment in many psychosomatic illnesses, but in most instances it should be combined with general medical measures (in the manner outlined in Chapter 11).

Psychotherapy has a variable, often limited, role in the treatment of many psychotic patients (it is more often of value in the convalescent and postpsychotic stages); most psychotic patients need other methods of treatment such as pharmacological treatment, physical methods of treatment and hospital inpatient environmental procedures. In most psychotic patients psychotherapy plays a secondary role to these other methods. In many instances, psychotherapy may help mentally reatrded patients who have neurotic problems or other emotional difficulties in addition to their mental retardation; it is used mainly in patients with mild or moderate retardation. Counseling of the parents of a mentally retarded child may help them adjust more comfortably and effectively to the challenges of rearing their child. In occasional instances, supportive counseling may be useful to patients with mild organic brain damage who are struggling to adjust emotionally with less cortical brain tissue at their command.

Complications

Psychotherapy is, explicitly or implicitly, sometimes advocated on the ground that it can do no harm and may possibly help the patient. This is not so. Psychotherapy, like most methods of treatment, occasionally can have adverse effects. A patient should be carefully evaluated before a course of psychotherapy is begun, and the risks of psychotherapy should be considered as well as its prospects of aiding the patient.

If psychotherapy plunges too abruptly into painful emotional areas, the patient may become very upset. For example, a person who discovers latent homosexual trends in himself may develop much anxiousness, and even panic. The therapist may approach such a topic only with extreme caution after much preliminary psychotherapeutic work, and when the patient's personality integration is fragile this topic usually should not be explored at all. In other instances, a patient may develop guilt feelings and marked depressiveness when he discovers in himself strong unresolved hostile feelings toward his parents and other close persons; such guilty and depressive feelings tend to be particularly strong if the emotionally close persons are dead. A compulsive patient may become upset if the emotional causes of his compulsive symptoms are explored before he has mature ways of handling the anxiety and guilt which formerly were encapsulated in these symptoms. Psychosomatic distresses, such as gastrointestinal symptoms and muscle tension symptoms, are common in patients as they explore painful emotional areas.

In occasional instances, the probings of psychotherapy may precipitate psychotic episodes. The schizoid person whose hold on reality was weak may have a schizophrenic break when he begins to face the turmoil within himself. Severe depressions may be precipitated by the abrupt exploration of hostile and guilty feelings, and in rare instances manic episodes are produced by the tumult aroused by psychotherapeutic penetrations.

When psychotherapy leads to a decisive change in the patient's personality structure it occasionally may cause difficulties in his interpersonal life. For example, a man with a passive personality disorder may become more assertive as the result of psychotherapy. If he is married to an aggressive woman with a strong need to dominate the people around her, grave marital problems may be precipitated by his personality change. Before psychotherapy, an equilibrium, although an unhealthy one, existed between the passive man and his dominant wife. After he becomes more assertive he cannot tolerate his wife's domination and she cannot tolerate his newly found assertiveness. Ideally, the wife should enter psychotherapy to resolve her unhealthy needs for controllong people, but in many instances the wife refuses psychotherapy or enters it with such strong prior resistances that she does not benefit from it. This change in the marital relationship of the patient and his wife may have a marked influence on the children of the couple as well as on the future of the marriage. Such possible complications should be foreseen early in treatment and all possible steps to assuage them should be taken.

Another problem that may arise in treatment is the acting out of mobilized feelings. For example, as the patient explores his childhood experiences he may uncover much smoldering hostility. As this pent-up hostility comes to the surface he for a time may become diffusely hostile toward his wife, his work associates, his relatives and his friends. This diffuse acting out of mobilized feelings may cause problems in the patient's family life, vocational life and social relationships, and the therapist should strive to conduct treatment in such a way that feelings come to the surface in quantities that the patient can handle with reasonable comfort and without adverse interpersonal results.

A problem which may occur in intensive, prolonged psychotherapy is the persistence of strong, unresolved feelings by the patient toward the therapist; in some instances, such feelings are not worked through even after years of treatment. These feelings may be hostile, or erotic, or dependent. The patient may become embroiled in a strongly emotional patient-therapist relationship that he can neither resolve nor terminate, and therapy stretches out interminably. The management of patient-therapist feelings is one of the most difficult technical problems in psychotherapy, but in the vast majority of instances they can be used as instruments for giving the patient insight into his personality problems and in helping him to resolve them. However, every therapist should be aware of the occasional occurrence of prolonged or insoluble patient-therapist feelings. In most instances, the engagement of these patients in long-term, intensive psychotherapy was an unwise decision that might have been avoided if the patient had been studied more carefully before starting intensive psychotherapy.

A decision to start psychotherapy should be based on a careful psychiatric study of the patient that may last for several diagnostic sessions and may include psychological testing by a clinical psychologist. Equipped with such information, the therapist will be able to select for psychotherapy patients for whom the chance of help is great and the risk of adverse effects is small.

SPECIAL MODIFICATIONS OF PSYCHOTHERAPY

In the history of psychotherapy many modifications have been developed. We shall discuss a few of them that have proved durable or have continued to attract recurrent professional interest.

Group Psychotherapy

Group psychotherapy has achieved a firm position in the spectrum of various methods of psychotherapy. The first experiments with group psychotherapy were made in the first decade of this century, and a large body of psychiatric practice and theory has evolved regarding it. Various technics of group psychotherapy have been developed employing the principles of the interpersonal approach to psychiatry, the Freudian-psychoanalytic approach, supportive approaches, inspirational approaches, and others.

Group psychotherapy has two possible advantages. The first, and from a scientific point of view the lesser, is that it enables a therapist to treat a larger number of patients than he could treat in individual psychotherapy in clinical settings where the demand for services is great and the number of therapists is small. Hence, group psychotherapy has been extensively used in busy outpatient clinics, large psychiatric hospitals, residential homes for disturbed children or delinquent adolescents, treatment centers for alcoholics, drug addiction centers, family and children's service agencies, large child guidance clinics and other types of psychiatric facilities. Group psychotherapy also offers the possibility of reducing the hourly cost of psychotherapy to the patient or to the institution providing him care.

However, the proponents of group psychotherapy feel that a second, and much more valid, basis for group therapy is that some patients may derive special benefits from group psychotherapy that they could not experience in individual treatment. They point out that group therapy offers the opportunity for resolving in an interpersonal setting emotional problems caused by interpersonal trauma. The causes of psychiatric problems lie largely in interpersonal trauma that occurred in family settings and other intimate interpersonal groups. In group therapy the patient can gradually explore his fears, yearnings, hostilities and other feelings toward various members of the group, and he can thus resolve the emotional turmoil that arose in earlier interpersonal relationships in his life. Thus, group therapy becomes a corrective interpersonal experience for exploring and resolving emotional problems.

Group psychotherapy offers shy, withdrawn patients who are fearful of close contacts with people an opportunity to develop interpersonal comfort in a specially designed social setting. In all other groups in life these persons would be ignored, or rebuffed or dominated by others, but in group therapy they can analyze their fears of being intimate with people and can overcome the normal stresses of interpersonal life from which they always retreated in the past.

In addition, group therapy has some advantages in the treatment of certain types of patients. For example, many adolescents feel inhibited, rebellious and ill at ease about discussing their problems in individual psychotherapy, but they can do so in a group of other adolescents who feel as they do and have the same kinds of problems. Some patients have such strong competitive, hostile feelings toward all authoritative figures that they are unable to engage in individual therapy because the therapist represents authority and social conformance to them. However, in a group of patients with similar problems these patients feel a warm acceptance and understanding which enables them to participate meaningfully in treatment.

Moreover, other strong feelings the patient may feel in psychotherapy, such as dependent needs, erotic yearnings or anixety aroused by treatment, are diluted in a group situation. In group therapy these feelings are not concentrated on a single person, the therapist; they are felt diffusely toward the other group members and hence are less threatening to the patient. Group therapy also allows the patient to vary the degree of his participation depending on his comfort at different times and his needs to participate vigorously or to play a less involved role for a while; the patient may remain silent for periods of time and yet benefit from the verbal interaction of others. Group therapy often is useful for groups of patients with similar problems, such as alcoholics, or adolescents, or delinquent children.

In many clinical settings group psychotherapy is conducted by clinical psychologists, psychiatric nurses with advanced training in psychotherapy, and psychiatric social workers, as well as by psychiatrists. Most psychiatrists feel that group psychotherapy by parapsychiatric professional workers is best done in situations where collaboration with psychiatrists is available, as in child guidance clinics, psychiatric hospital wards and psychiatric outpatient clinics.

The Organization of a Group. A group organized for exploratory psychotherapy usually consists of from 6 to 12 members. As a rule, they are of about the same age, the same socioeconomic background and the same intellectual level; however, there are many exceptions to these general tendencies. The emotional problems of the members of a group usually have some thread of cohesiveness. For example, a group may consist largely of patients with neurotic problems, or of personality disorders, or of problems in rearing their children or coping with their adolescent sons and daughters. Too great a diversity of problems leads to a lack of common interests and insufficient grounds for group interaction. The group usually has some patients who are more aggressive than others and some who act as moderating influences on the group as a whole. As a rule, a group cannot accomodate more than two domineering, aggressive persons, and the success of a group is threatened by the inclusion of paranoid patients, patients with manic tendencies, patients with severe antisocial personality disorders and extremely depressed patients. These patients tend to demoralize the group, to disrupt it or to dominate it so that it cannot function therapeutically for most of its members.

Group sessions usually are held once a week for 90 minutes, but in some instances they are held twice each week for somewhat longer or shorter periods. As a rule, patients attend group sessions for from several months to a year or two, and they may attend for much longer periods. From time to time new members may join the group as old members terminate. Each new member undergoes careful psychiatric evaluation prior to admission to the group to make sure he is a good candidate to benefit from group therapy. Moreover, prior psychiatric evaluation also gives the group's therapist a good understanding of the patient's problems and personality structure. In some instances members of the group have individual psychotherapeutic sessions once a week or once every two or three weeks in addition to group sessions.

The role of the group's therapist varies depending on his theoretical orientation and on the personalities of the group's members. Some therapists say relatively little during group sessions, whereas others are active participants. The group members usually sit in comfortable chairs arranged in a rough circle in an informal setting, and the therapist sits with the group in the same manner as the patients.

The Various Types of Group Therapy. Many forms of group therapy have been devised, but they may be grouped under four general headings: (1) *exploratory group therapy*, in which patients explore the interpersonal causes of their problems, (2) *supportive group therapy*, in which major reliance is placed upon reassurance, explanations, educational measures, and counseling on the management of current difficulties, (3) *inspirational group therapy*, in which strong moral or religious persuasion is used and (4) *sensitivity training groups* (also called *training groups, t-groups* and *encounter groups*), in which the group members study intensively the ways in which they relate to each other, develop greater sensitivity to their own feelings and those of others, and examine some particular task or project of the group.

(1) In *exploratory group therapy* the patients explore the interpersonal causes of their emotional difficulties. The basic processes that occur in exploratory group therapy are the same as those outlined for psychotherapy in general at the beginning of this chapter, though they occur in modified forms in groups. In catharsis of his feelings and problems the patient has an opportunity to examine his difficulties in association with other persons who have similar difficulties, and this process occurs in the presence of a therapist who can offer professional understanding and help. Often the patient is relieved to hear other patients describe problems similar to his own; it rids him of much guilt and anxiety to learn that other people have the same thoughts, feelings and im-

pulses with which he struggles. Moreover, in many instances he can grasp his own feelings and problems better when he hears other patients discuss similar difficulties. The patient also develops new insights into his relationships with people in both current and past interpersonal situations as he discusses his problems and exchanges comments and interpretations with other group members and the therapist. The patient begins to get a clearer concept of his own personality and how he handles feelings and relates to people.

In time the members of the group may begin to analyze their feelings toward one another and toward the therapist. They may examine their hostilities, dependent yearnings, affectionate urges, competitive strivings, antagonisms and identifications in the group. In many instances they can see how their interactions in the group are similar to their relationships in their daily lives outside the group, and they can grasp how these modes of interaction are patterned on earlier experiences in childhood and adolescence. Thus, the group becomes a vital social process offering the patient a chance to have a corrective interpersonal experience. He works out old problems, and he develops new ways of handling feelings and relating to people. Exploratory group psychotherapy may be based on either the interpersonal approach to psychiatry, or the Freudian-psychoanalytic approach, or modified Freudian-psychoanalytic points of view, or eclectic viewpoints, (all of which have been discussed earlier in this chapter).

Psychodrama is a special form of exploratory psychotherapy. In psychodrama some of the group members spontaneously act out life situations on a small stage while others watch the drama. The patient-actors often begin with a set problem or situation and spontaneously act out the ways in which they would handle it. Both the patients, and therapists, who engage in the drama and those who observe it have discussions about the interpersonal problems concerned and the feelings of all persons present.

(The special methods of exploratory group psychotherapy for children are discussed in Chapter 24.)

(2) In *supportive group therapy* major emphasis is placed upon reassurance, explanations, educational measures and advice on the management of current interpersonal problems. The group may run from several persons to 20 or so, and the therapist usually plays a very active part in the group proceedings. The therapist reassures the patients strongly about their symptoms, fears and dilemmas, and he fosters similar mutual encouragement by the group members to each other. The therapist may explain to patients how interpersonal trauma can cause symptoms and personality problems, but his aim is to educate the patients rather than to explore their life experiences. In some instances, the group members make reports on assigned topics, or discuss themes chosen by the therapist, or speak in rotation on a specific subject. The therapist gives concrete advice to group members on how to handle the interpersonal problems they face. Little emphasis is put on exploration of early life experiences, and analysis of the patients' relationships with each other and with the therapist is not carried out. However, much of the effectiveness of supportive group therapy is derived from the feelings of warm allegiance the members feel toward the group and its goals.

In general, supportive group therapy is designed for patients who cannot engage in exploratory group therapy. For example, some patients with long-term, ingrained neurotic problems or schizoid patients with a fragile hold on reality, or psychosomatic patients who have immense difficulty talking about themselves may benefit from supportive group therapy; participation in exploratory group therapy would be difficult for these patients, and in some cases, as with schizoid patients who have a weak hold on reality, it might be unwise.

(3) In *inspirational group therapy* the major emphasis is put on a strong, emotionally colored appeal to moral or religious principles. The group members exhort one another to give firm allegiance to the goals of the group and to help themselves and other group members by devotion to the ideals and purposes of the group. The members may be urged to describe their problems to the group and to pledge themselves to strive to solve their difficulties and to aid others in the same aim. The group may have a leader, or leader-

ship may be divided among the members. Alcoholics Anonymous (discussed in Chapter 13) is a good example of inspirational group therapy. Some psychiatrists have used inspirational methods, but in most instances inspirational methods are used by nonmedical leaders in lay settings. When inspirational methods are used in well-organized groups with unity of purpose, such as Alcoholics Anonymous, many persons may benefit. However, the poorly organized use of inspirational methods by untrained leaders who often are self-appointed may lead to exploitation of upset persons amd may harm them.

(4) *Sensitivity training groups* (also called *training groups*, *t-groups* and *encounter groups*) were developed during the 1950's and 1960's and have been extensively used in a wide variety of settings; they are employed mainly for persons who do not have clear-cut psychiatric problems but wish to learn more about themselves and their relationships with people. A group usually consists of about 12 persons, who may be members of an industrial or commercial organization, or a professional group, or a social group, or a civic or religious group. A sensitivity group's prime aim is educational rather than therapeutic, but such a distinction is often artificial and vague. In intensive interaction, which may go on for several hours or more in a single session, or may be limited to 90 minutes, the group members study how they relate to each other in terms of leadership, dominance, competitiveness, dependence, mutual help, subdivision into smaller groups, and other ways. They also may examine in their frank give-and-take interaction how socioeconomic differences, sexual differences, racial differences and other factors affect their relationships. Thus, the group members strive to develop greater *sensitivity* to the workings of interpersonal relationships and the feelings of both themselves and others. This increased sensitivity, in turn, is designed to *train* them to function more effectively in all the various groups of which they are members. Such a group may meet only several times, or it may meet weekly or twice monthly for long periods.

Often the group uses some common purpose or project as the subject matter for their interaction. For example, the professional staff of a psychiatric hospital ward may discuss how to organize a better therapeutic atmosphere on the ward, or a factory group may discuss how to increase production and diminish interpersonal tensions on a production line, or a commercial group may consider how to mount a sales campaign in a new territory.

Some sensitivity training groups have loose supervision by a mental health professional worker (a psychiatrist, or a clinical psychologist, or a psychiatric nurse with advanced training in psychiatry, or a psychiatric social worker) who both participates in the group and moderates it. Other sensitivity training groups are run entirely by the nonprofessional members of the group, often guided by a popular book on psychiatry for laymen. As a result, the psychiatric literature has increasingly recorded cases of persons who became emotionally disturbed in such groups; the crude, frontal assaults on personality structures that occur in some of these groups have precipitated decompensations into neuroses, psychosomatic illnesses and psychoses.

Many psychiatrists have become uneasy about these groups when they are run entirely by their lay participants. They feel that a mental health professional worker should be an active participant and monitor in sensitivity training groups, and that at least superficial screening should be done to exclude persons who might be damaged by them.

(*Family therapy*, in which the members of a single family constitute the group, is considered in Chapter 24 on the special technics used in child psychiatry, since family therapy is often, but not always, used to help children or adolescents.)

Psychotherapy After Inducing States of Altered Consciousness

The technics we shall describe here are not widely used at present in the day-to-day practice of psychotherapy. However, all of them enjoy periodic waves of interest and are intensively employed by a small percentage of therapists.

Narcoanalysis and Narcosynthesis. In narcoanalysis and narcosynthesis the patient is interviewed after the intravenous injection of a small amount of a barbiturate. (The technic for inducing a barbiturate interview is outlined in Chapter 5.) The process of analyzing the patient's problems during a barbiturate interview is termed *narcoanalysis* and the process of making interpretations at this time is termed *narcosynthesis*. However, either term often is used loosely to cover any therapeutic process occurring after barbiturate injection.

In narcoanalysis and narcosynthesis the patient's inhibitions are diminished by the minimal sedation of the cerebral cortex by the barbiturate. In barbiturate interviews the therapist usually plays an active role in questioning the patient and interpreting his problems and experiences to him. In some instances patients talk more freely after barbiturate injection and occasionally may reexperience traumatic past events in a vivid manner. Toward the end of the barbiturate interview or following it, the therapist may discuss the revealed material more fully with the patient.

Most psychiatrists make little use of this technic, for they feel it has no significant advantages over conventional interview methods. The use of the barbiturate may facilitate a flow of speech in some patients, but it grossly alters the patient-therapist relationship and detracts from therapy as a corrective interpersonal experience. Barbiturate interviews have been used for acute emotional upsets following gross stress in military combat or civilian disasters such as explosions and major fires, but most psychiatrists feel other methods of management are better.

Moreover, barbiturate interviews have some dangers. They may precipitate neurotic exacerbations or psychotic breaks in patients whose defenses against such processes are weak. In addition, the occasional occurrence of laryngospasm and other adverse reactions is an added hazard.

Hypnosis and Hypnoanalysis. (In Chapter 5 on special diagnostic procedures we discussed hypnosis as a diagnostic tool and in Chapter 9 we outlined the use of hypnosis in removing hysterical conversion symptoms. In both instances we pointed out the limited usefulness and possible dangers of hypnosis.) We shall now consider the use of hypnosis and hypnoanalysis as exploratory psychotherapeutic technics.

Hypnosis is induced by the progressive narrowing of the patient's field of awareness on the words and actions of the hypnotist. As a rule, the hypnotist uses repetitive commands which persuade the patient to concentrate on what the hypnotist is saying, and to exclude all other stimuli from his attention. The hypnotist often suggests strongly and repetitively that a state of profound relaxation will come over the patient and that he will enter a drowsy state in which he is aware only of the words of the hypnotist. The patient may enter a light trance or a state of moderate or deep hypnosis, depending on the skill of the hypnotist and the ease with which the patient may be hypnotized. As a rule, several training sessions are required before a patient can enter a state of moderate or deep hypnosis. Many patients cannot be hypnotized even with prolonged effort, and others can be led into only light trances. However, patients who are accessible to hypnosis and have been well trained in its induction may be hypnotized rapidly and deeply. The therapist who uses hypnosis should have considerable training in its employment and he should be aware of its limitations and dangers.

Some psychotherapists have advocated hypnosis as a tool in facilitating exploratory psychotherapy, and this use of hypnosis is often termed *hypnoanalysis*. In hypnoanalysis hypnosis is employed to bypass the patient's conscious and unconscious resistances to discussing his feelings, traumatic experiences and emotional conflicts. The therapist makes a careful psychiatric study of the patient before beginning hypnoanalytic therapy. Hence, he is able to direct the hypnotized patient's attention to specific conflicts and traumatic periods of his life; when successful, the patient may have a free catharsis of feelings and he may reexperience vividly forgotten life events. In some instances the patient can be directed to reexperience interpersonal events that occurred at specific periods of his life; this is sometimes termed "hypnotic age regression." Therapists who practice hypnoanalysis often supplement the hypnotic sessions with conventional interview sessions in which they work to integrate into the patient's conscious awareness material revealed during the hypnotic sessions.

Though few psychiatrists practice hypnoanalysis, it continues to attract a certain amount of psychiatric attention. Most psychiatrists feel that hypnoanalysis has some serious drawbacks. Many patients cannot be hypnotized, and even those who can be hypnotized may not be able to recall life experiences and to talk freely about them while under hypnosis. Moreover, the patient in many instances cannot remember well the material which came out during his hypnotic session after he emerges from it, and most psychiatrists feel that this considerably reduces the therapeutic value of the revealed material. Furthermore, in hypnoanalysis the patient-therapist interpersonal relationship is greatly distorted and no longer can serve in the usual psychotherapeutic way as the instrument for a corrective interpersonal experience and consensual validation.

In addition, in hypnoanalysis the therapist assumes unusual powers over the consciousness of his patient, and the patient becomes submissive to him in directing the course of the therapy. This submissive role of the patient may lead him to develop a marked emotional dependence on the therapist, and when the sexes of the therapist and the patient are different this dependency may have strong erotic features. The therapist must be a very stable person, for the power of exercising unusual jurisdiction over the consciousness and volition of his patients can lead to unreasonable feelings of therapeutic power and personal importance. In addition to these factors, most psychiatrists feel that the results of conventional psychotherapy are better and more enduring. Many psychiatrists feel that hypnoanalysis is of most use as an instrument of psychiatric research.

PSYCHOTHERAPEUTIC ENVIRONMENTS

Most of the basic technics of psychotherapy which are discussed at the beginning of this chapter can be applied to the organization and operation of psychiatric inpatient services and other mental health facilities. We shall here consider the major ways in which this is done.

The Psychiatric Hospital and the Concept of the Therapeutic Environment

During the last few decades a significant change has occurred in the concept of what a psychiatric hospital should be. Although some psychiatrists always have known intuitively that the interpersonal environment of the hospital had much to do with whether or not the patients got well, a psychiatric hospital in former times usually was viewed as a place where patients stayed while they received treatment and recuperated from their illnesses. Psychiatrists and other mental health professional workers now view a psychiatric hospital as a place where the interpersonal environment of the patient is carefully organized to facilitate his recovery. The interpersonal environment of the hospital thus becomes a significant instrument of treatment. A psychiatric patient has undergone a breakdown or a distortion of his emotional and interpersonal functioning. The hospital offers him a therapeutic environment in which his interpersonal relationships with the staff and with other patients help him to recover. In the psychiatric literature, hospital environmental therapy often is called *milieu therapy* or the *hospital therapeutic community*.

Harry Stack Sullivan probably was the first psychiatrist to design and operate a hospital interpersonal environment with systematic, clearly conceived therapeutic aims. In the late 1920's he was Director of Clinical Research at the Sheppard and Enoch Pratt Hospital in Towson, Maryland, and during this period he took over one ward in which staff-patient interpersonal relationships constituted the main therapeutic instrument in treating young male schizophrenics. He instituted daily conferences in which all persons working on the ward discussed how all relationships between the staff members and the patients, and among the patients themselves, were either therapeutic or nontherapeutic. Sullivan used only male aides, in addition to himself, in this initial experiment, but his model was clearly applicable to settings in which various kinds of mental health professional workers dealt with patients with an extensive range of psychiatric problems. Sullivan's pilot project attracted wide attention and all modern hospital therapeutic environmental programs probably have grown, directly or indirectly, out of his work.

The Purposes and Organization of a Hospital Therapeutic Environment. Hospital environmental therapy is designed to meet (1) the emotional needs of the individual patient, (2) the group interpersonal needs of the patients who constitute a hospital ward or other administrative unit, and (3) the educational and interpersonal needs of the professional staff working in the hospital therapeutic environment unit.

(1) *The therapeutic interpersonal needs of individual patients* vary much from one patient to another. For example, a frightened, withdrawn patient who is wavering on the brink of a schizophrenic break needs much individual attention by one or two members of the ward personnel who act in reassuring, supportive ways to help assuage the patient's terror and to aid him to establish closer bonds with people. On the other hand, a manic patient needs quiet, firm, occasionally authoritative contacts with people who do not stimulate an increased tempo of interpersonal activity and are able to put realistic limitations on his grandiose, distractible behavior. An acting-out adolescent needs flexible amounts of noncritical understanding, as well as realistic limitations when his behavior goes beyond permissible social limits. Hence, each hospitalized patient has his individual therapeutic needs, and one of the main tasks of hospital environmental therapy is to meet these needs in ways that will help him recover.

(2) In addition, *the therapeutic needs of the patient group as a whole must be met.* Such a hospital group may consist of 10, or 20, or 30 or more patients. The patient usually is in the hospital because his psychiatric disturbance has made it unwise, unhealthy or impossible for him to continue living outside the hospital. The aim of hospital treatment is to resolve his emotional problems so that he can reenter the community and carry on a sound interpersonal life. Hence, the interpersonal group in which he lives in the hospital should help him regain his capacity to live in the broader interpersonal environment he will encounter outside the hospital. The relationships with the staff members all should be directed toward this therapeutic end. Hence, group social activities, group work projects, group excursions off the ward for cultural or entertainment purposes, group athletic games, group parties and encouraging group social interchanges on the ward are all essential parts of a hospital therapeutic environment.

These ongoing interpersonal, diversified activities are important, for example, in the case of the schizophrenic patient who unconsiously has fled from contact with a threatening world he found too painful to endure, into a delusional, hallucinatory inner world of his own fantasies and preoccupations. In the hospital, all his interpersonal contacts and group activities with the hospital staff and other patients should help to lead him back across the psychotic gap to healthy contacts with people. His hospital interpersonal relationships should be reassuring and not threatening, accepting and not rejecting, understanding and not critical. Whether or not the schizophrenic patient finds these therapeutic environmental aids has much influence on the course of his illness.

(3) *The interpersonal and educational needs of the hospital staff who are engaged in this kind of therapy must be met.* All hospital personnel who come in contact with the patients are, to use Sullivan's term, *participant-observers.* Although they are *observing* and studying the problems and needs of patients, they are *participating* directly in therapeutic interpersonal relationships with them; the staff are using their own personalities as therapeutic instruments. As a consequence, various kinds of emotional stresses and reactions may be aroused in the hospital personnel, and to continue to function effectively the hospital staff's emotional, interpersonal and educational needs must be met.

For example, a hostile paranoid schizophrenic or a taunting, provocative, acting-out adolescent may arouse anxiousness and counterhostility in the hospital staff; to the extent that the staff's feelings contaminate their behavior toward the patient, the therapeutic atmosphere of the ward is impaired. The staff, both through their professional understanding of the patient and their personality resources, should not react in unhealthy ways toward such patients; they should be understanding and realistic, and not fearful or punitive. In other cases, the staff members should not become overly solicitous with clinging, dependent patients with severe neuroses, and they should not be swept into contagious hilarity by the pranks and jovial hyperactivity of a manic patient. To maintain a therapeutic level of interaction with difficult patients, the staff need some kind of ongoing help.

Such help is in many cases best given in twice weekly ward conferences in which the staff discuss not only the needs of the patients but also their own perplexities, feelings and opinions about the patients and the way the ward is being run. The staff can discuss how certain patients, or cliques of patients, are producing various kinds of reactions in themselves, in other patients, and in the general ward atmosphere. This kind of continuous examination of what is occurring among the patients and between the staff and the patients constitutes an important part of the process of keeping the hospital environment therapeutic. The psychiatrists, psychiatric nurses, clinical psychologists, student nurses, occupational therapists, recreational therapists, ward aids, ward secretaries and any other staff personnel can participate in various kinds of conferences; these conferences obviously will vary much in number and staff level, depending on the size of the ward and the number of professional persons working on it. They usually are moderated by a senior staff member.

Patients sometimes mobilize conflicts between staff members. For example, a dependent, manipulating patient may excite oversolicitous feelings in one staff member by complaining bitterly and falsely about his treatment by another staff member who does not treat him with similar solicitousness; in this way the patient may cause hostility between the two staff members. Such conflicts between staff members which are mobilized by patients can be resolved at the regular ward staff conferences. Moreover, in resolving such conflicts the staff can understand how patients manipulate and upset other people outside the hospital in their family, vocational and social groups.

Special Kinds of Therapeutic Environments. Some psychiatric hospitals offer partial hospitalization services. In partial hospitalization, the patient may spend his days in the hospital and return home evenings and weekends. In other cases, the patient goes to his regular work or to his home during the day and returns evenings and weekends to the hospital. The terms *day hospital* and *night hospital* are sometimes employed in referring to this type of hospital care. This type of partial hospitalization is useful in helping borderline or convalescent psychotic patients, persons with severe neuroses, and individuals with other kinds of psychiatric problems who need parttime hospital care while reintegrating their personality structures or gradually reentering interpersonal life outside the hospital.

Other types of therapeutic environments are available in some cities. A *halfway house* is a group residence in which patients live for a time while regaining personality stability or reentering full community life after psychiatric hospitalization. Professional mental health workers supervise the running of the residence and are available for counseling and psychotherapy on both group and individual bases. The general atmosphere of the residence (often a large, older house converted for this purpose) is designed to be interpersonally therapeutic.

(Special residential treatment services for children and adolescents are covered in Chapter 24.)

The Concept of Community Mental Health

The marked prevalence of emotional disorders and interpersonal difficulties has led, especially since the 1960's, to attempts to apply the basic psychotherapeutic principles outlined at the beginning of this chapter to broader segments of the public and to many groups and organizations in the general community. This movement has been termed the *community mental health* or *community psychiatry* movement.

The community mental health movement has four broad aims: (1) to offer comprehensive inpatient, outpatient, consultative and referral services to each patient who seeks them, and to render these services to the patient in the community in which he lives, (2) to provide educational services to the general public on mental hygiene and the principles of preventive psychiatry, (3) to offer psychiatric consultation services to private and public social welfare groups, rehabilitative centers, school organizations and other private and public organizations working to solve social, economic and cultural problems, and (4) to offer psychiatric points of view for the resolution of interpersonal problems in industrial groups, business organizations and whatever other groups seek such help.

One aspect of the community mental health movement is the development of the *community mental health center*. A community mental health center offers inpatient and outpatient psychiatric services to both adults and children. Its services are available for psychiatric emergencies, such as acutely suicidal patients, at all times. The center may offer day-hospital services to help rehabilitate patients who are recuperating from psychoses and to aid patients who need some psychiatric hospital help but do not require 24-hour a day inpatient care. The center offers consultation services to social welfare groups, family and children's service agencies, juvenile courts and other groups, and it serves diagnostically as a clearing house for referring patients to vocational counseling services, rehabilitation institutes and other social and medical services. The center gives these services to the patient and his family in his own community and returns him to active life in the community as soon as his condition permits; the patient, and perhaps other members of his family, continue in outpatient treatment until his problems are resolved.

The staff of a community mental health center includes psychiatrists, clinical psychologists, psychiatric nurses, psychiatric social workers and other professional personnel needed to staff outpatient and inpatient services. A community mental health center may be supported by private or governmental funds. It may be part of a private nonprofit medical center, or a state or municipal medical center, or a medical school. A community mental health center desirably houses its various divisions in a single building or a closely integrated group of buildings, but existing facilities in a community that are somewhat distant from each other may be integrated administratively into a community mental health center.

Flexibility and a sense of experimentation are needed for the development of effective technics for public education about preventive mental hygiene and for the introduction of psychiatric points of view to resolve interpersonal problems in industries, business organizations and social groups. Formal lectures have limited value for these purposes. Technics which apply modifications of the principles of group psychotherapy and group discussions are more useful. The persons who need information and orientation on mental hygiene, or who are embroiled in group interpersonal conflicts in vocational or social situations, explore the issues at hand in group discussions moderated by a psychiatrist or other mental health professional. This technic also may be used to present psychiatric insights to groups dealing with child-rearing problems, neighborhood tensions, conflicts between social and ethnic groups and other interpersonal difficulties between groups in communities.

The Broader Tensions. (As pointed out in Chapter 2 and earlier in this chapter), Harry Stack Sullivan was probably the first person systematically to apply the interpersonal point of view both to individual psychotherapy and to the organization and operation of psychiatric hospitals. Late in his life he also was one of the first psychiatrists to urge that the insights of interpersonal psychiatry be employed in meeting problems in the entire spectrum of social groups. He even speculated during the last three years of his life that the insights that had been developed in psychotherapy might be useful in decreasing international tensions; his last paper, published posthumously after his death in 1949, was titled "Tensions Interpersonal and International."

BIBLIOGRAPHY

Balint, M., Ornstein, P. H., and Balint, E.: Focal Psychotherapy: An Example of Applied Psychoanalysis. Philadelphia, J. B. Lippincott, 1972.

Chapman, A. H., and Almeida, E. M.: The Interpersonal Basis of Psychiatric Nursing. New York, G. P. Putnam's Sons, 1972.

Frank, J. D.: Psychotherapy: the restoration of morale. Am. J. Psychiatry, *131*:271, 1974.

Gurel, L.: Dimensions of the therapeutic milieu: a study of mental hospital atmosphere. Am. J. Psychiatry, *131*:409, 1974.

Kaplan, H. I., and Sadock, B. J.: Comprehensive Group Psychotherapy. Baltimore, Williams & Wilkins, 1971.

Lazar, N. D.: Nature and significance of changes in a patient in a psychoanalytic clinic. Psychoanal. Quart,. *42*: 579, 1973.

Lazarus, A. A. (ed.): Clinical Behavior Therapy. New York, Brunner Mazel, 1972.

Mann, J.: Time-Limited Psychotherapy. Cambridge, Mass., Harvard University Press, 1973.

Marmor, J.: The future of psychoanalytic therapy. Am. J. Psychiatry, *130*:1197, 1973.

Ruesch, J.: Therapeutic Communication. New York, W. W. Norton, 1961.

Sager, C. J., and Kaplan, H. S. (eds.): Progress in Group and Family Therapy. New York, Brunner Mazel, 1972.

Scheflen, A. E.: Communicational Structure: Analysis of a Psychotherapy Transaction. Bloomington, Indiana University Press, 1973.

Sifneos, P. E.: Short-Term Psychotherapy and Emotional Crisis. Cambridge, Mass., Harvard University Press, 1972.

Simon, R. M.: On eclecticism. Am. J. Psychiatry, *131*:135, 1974.

Sterba, R.: A case of brief psychotherapy by Sigmund Freud. Psychoanal. Rev., *38*: 75, 1951.

Strupp, H. H.: On the technology of psychotherapy. Arch. Gen. Psychiatry, *26*: 270, 1972.

Sullivan, H. S.: Conceptions of Modern Psychiatry. New York, W. W. Norton 1953.

———: The Psychiatric Interview. New York, W. W. Norton, 1954.

Weiss, E.: Sigmund Freud as a Consultant. New York, Intercontinental Medical Book Corporation, 1970.

Wolpe, J.: The Practice of Behavior Therapy. Elmsford, N. Y., Pergamon Press, 1974.

22

Experimental and Biochemical Aspects of Treatment with Medications

In the various chapters of this book in which treatment of psychiatric disorders has been discussed, we have considered medications from a general clinical, or empirical, point of view; that is, we have outlined the things that most psychiatrists do in their daily care of patients because they have found them most useful. In this current chapter, however, we shall examine the experimental and biochemical bases of the employment of antipsychotic drugs, antidepressant drugs, minor tranquilizers (antianxiety medications), sedative-hypnotics, lithium and other medications. We shall take a closer look at how their success in the various kinds of psychiatric conditions has been verified, while again considering both the ranges of utility and the limitations of medications in specific disorders.

ANTIPSYCHOTIC DRUGS

Phenothiazine, the prototype of modern antipsychotic medications, was initially synthesized in the 1880's but was not utilized until 1934, at which time it was employed as an antiseptic and antihistamine. Several phenothiazine derivatives were found to produce marked sedative and tranquilizing effects. Eventually the behavioral change produced by these drugs (that is, tranquilization with maintenance of consciousness) encouraged Delay and Deniker to use chlorpromazine, synthesized by Charpentier, with mental patients in 1952.

The serendipitous discovery of the antipsychotic properties of the phenothiazine derivatives has had a profound effect on psychiatric practice. For while these agents do not produce a permanent cure in schizophrenics they do benefit many patients in a way no previous treatment has. The clinically significant therapeutic effects produced by these drugs created an atmosphere within which other therapies (milieu therapy, individual and group psychotherapy, and occupational therapy) could be co-applied assiduously. Whereas public mental hospitals had been, historically, custodial institutions, with most patients too disturbed to participate in psychological and social therapies on a regular basis, the advent of pharmacotherapy began to transform them into actual, rather than nominal, treatment centers. Thus the present-day widespread application of social and psychological therapies is indebted to these pharmacological agents. The result has been a wide variety of potential options for the mental patient: discharge and return to home and job; outpatient treatment with no hospitalization for some; decreased duration of hospital stay for many acute and episodic schizophrenics; and finally, for those who must be treated as inpatients, the hospital has become a more humane, hospitable and truly therapeutic place.

Pharmacotherapy has resulted in a major reduction in the number of hospitalized schizophrenic patients. This is especially remarkable because, until the introduction of these drugs, there had been a steady increase in the inpatient mental population. Between 1920 and 1955 the total number of patients in state and county psychiatric hospitals in the United States increased at an almost steady rate from about 225,000 to about 550,000; between 1955 and 1971, despite a marked increase in the population of the United States and much larger numbers of first admissions to psychiatric hospitals, the total number of patients in state and county psychiatric hospitals dropped from about 550,000 to about 300,000. The changed fate of so many human beings and the concomitant availability of facilities for treatment of a larger number of people who require them is, perhaps, the most convincing proof of the efficacy of these agents. The improvement produced by chlorpromazine was and is unlike anything produced by somatic or psychological therapies, and represents a major advance in therapeutics.

Methodological Refinement

One other advance indebted to the discovery of antipsychotic drugs was a significant refinement in methodology. The use of randomized double-blind trials in which a drug under investigation is compared to placebo (or standard comparison drug) has become standard practice in pharmacological investigation. The replacement of the earlier "evaluation by testimonial" by a controlled trial method of assessment has been a major step in objective scientific investigation and evaluation.

The placebo (inert medication form) is used in clinical drug studies to eliminate several phenomena, one or more of which might influence the outcome of a study. The patient may get better because he believes the pill will help him; the placebo treated group may be used as a control which helps reveal spontaneous improvement or improvement due to other treatments (for example, psychotherapy, group therapy); and the placebo can reduce or remove the effects of observer bias (the expectation that the drug must be helping the patient, leading to unwarranted ratings of improvement).

Rigorous evaluation of treatment then, contains the following aspects: use of placebo; random assignment to treatment groups (so that all good prognosis patients are not placed in the drug, or placebo, group); and, double-blind evaluation (so neither evaluators nor patients know which group is receiving drugs and which group placebo).

In a field marked by rapid advances in research and a proliferation of often contradictory findings it becomes essential that the physician develop the methodological sophistication to form independent evaluations of the validity of current research. Physicians who routinely neglect the "methods" sections of current psychopharmacological research in favor of the "results" sections have no real basis for discriminating good findings from bad.

General Consideration of Efficacy. Years of research and hundreds of double-blind studies have confirmed the finding that antipsychotic drugs are clearly superior to placebo in treating both acute and chronic schizophrenia, when adequate dose levels are administered (Table 22–1). Findings suggest that approximately 75 per cent of the phenothiazine treated patients improve, 5 per cent remain the same, and 2 per cent grow worse, in contrast to the placebo treated groups in which 25 per cent improve and 75 per cent fail to improve or become worse. Furthermore, the fact that some of the placebo groups exhibit new schizophrenic symptoms, even while being treated with individual, group or social therapies suggests that antipsychotic drugs have a "psychostatic" effect. That is, they not only suppress existing symptomatology but they also prevent the appearance of new psychotic symptomatology.

While therapeutic gains tend to occur up to the 12th through 18th week of treatment, the *average* patient exhibits the greatest amount of gain within the first six weeks of treatment. Individual differences do exist, of course, and some patients will make startling gains within a few days whereas other patients will show a gradual course of improvement over many months. Thus, while statements about average drug effects provide reasonable guidelines, they must be coupled with the individual physician's clinical acumen and knowledge of his patient.

Quality and Nature of Change

Presently available data support the hypothesis that phenothiazine therapy brings about a cognitive restoration and a concom-

Table 22-1. The Comparative Efficacy of Antipsychotic Drugs

Drug	Percentage of Studies in which Drug Was				
	More effective than placebo	Equal to placebo	More effective than chlorpromazine	Equal to chlorpromazine	Less effective than chlorpromazine
Chlorpromazine	82.00%	17.0 %	—	—	—
Acetophenazine	—	—	0.0	100.0	0.0
Butaperazine	100.0	0.0	0.0	100.0	0.0
Carphenazine	100.0	0.0	0.0	100.0	0.0
Fluphenazine	100.0	0.0	0.0	100.0	0.0
Mepazine	40.0	60.0	0.0	0.0	100.0
Mesoridazine	100.0	0.0	0.0	100.0	0.0
Perphenazine	100.0	0.0	0.0	100.0	0.0
Piperacetazine	—	—	0.0	100.0	0.0
Prochlorperazine	77.8	22.2	0.0	100.0	0.0
Promazine	43.0	57.0	0.0	33.3	66.7
Thiopropazate	—	—	0.0	100.0	0.0
Thioridazine	100.0	0.0	0.0	100.0	0.0
Trifluoperazine	88.9	11.1	0.0	100.0	0.0
Triflupromazine	90.0	10.0	0.0	100.0	0.0
Chlorprothixene	100.0	0.0	0.0	100.0	0.0
Thiothixene	100.0	0.0	0.0	100.0	0.0
Haloperidol	100.0	0.0	0.0	100.0	0.0
Phenobarbital	0.0	100.0	0.0	100.0	0.0
Reserpine	69.0	31.0	—	—	—

itant decrease in psychotic ideation, projection, suspiciousness, perplexity and ideas of reference. In addition, psychomotor behavior in retarded, as well as hyperactive, patients is normalized. Rating scales show a reduction in the fundamental symptoms (thought disorder, blunted affect, indifference, autistic withdrawal, psychotic behavior and mannerism) as well as in the accessory symptoms (hallucinations, paranoid identification, hostility, and resistiveness) of schizophrenia.

Furthermore, specific aspects of schizophrenic thought disorder such as overinclusive thinking and bizarre inappropriate responses have been shown to respond to these drugs, particularly in process schizophrenia. Thus, the phenothiazines reduce symptoms which are typical of schizophrenia in particular and psychosis in general and, while they do have a tranquilizing effect, their overall effects are far greater than "mere" tranquilization. Consequently, the term "tranquilizer" is a misnomer and these drugs should be referred to as antipsychotic drugs.

Comparative Effects. The effectiveness of chlorpromazine as an antipsychotic agent stimulated research for more effective agents and ones with fewer side effects. The result was the development of several new classes of antipsychotic drugs: the thioxanthenes (close structural analogs of the phenothiazines) and the butyrophenones (whose chemical structure is quite different). This variety from which a physician may choose raises several questions. Which, if any, of these drugs is better than chlorpromazine in treating the average schizophrenic patient? Is any particular drug more effective in managing particular schizophrenic symptoms? Is any drug, or group of drugs, more effective with a particular subtype of patient? Do these agents all produce the same quality of improvement in the patient?

Evidence suggests that, excepting promazine and mepazine, all the phenothiazines are clearly superior to placebo. Controlled comparisons have shown promazine and mepazine to be distinctly inferior to chlorpromazine.

In addition, controlled evaluations have shown all other antipsychotic agents to be equal to chlorpromazine in their therapeutic effect (Table 22-1).

Inspection of the changes wrought upon schizophrenic symptoms reveals a striking similarity among the various agents. The drugs consistently produce changes of the same dimensions, thus supporting the hypothesis that they have a common and specific mode of action. Those differences which do exist are primarily differences in side effects: some produce more sedation, some have a higher incidence of extrapyramidal side effects, and so forth. Nevertheless, all antipsychotic agents normalize the psychosis, calming hyperactive and excitable patients while activating and alerting retarded psychotic patients.

Because these agents are of equal therapeutic efficacy, the practicing psychiatrist is presented with a problem: which drug should one choose from among the wide variety available? Studies have failed to shown that a particular class of schizophrenia responds differentially more favorably to one or another drug, or have produced positive results which have subsequently been invalidated upon replication of the experiment. For example, the allegation that chlorpromazine (Thorazine), which is a more sedating drug, is better with hyperexcitable patients while fluphenazine (Prolixin) or trifluoperazine (Stelazine), which are alerting phenothizaines, are indicated with withdrawn patients, is not true. Indeed, some studics have shown the opposite to be true.

Nevertheless, despite the absence of clear differential indications for one or another antipsychotic agent with a particular patient or class of patients, practicing clinicians continually observe that patients who fail to respond to one phenothiazine may occasionally respond favorably to another, or to one of the non-phenothiazine antipsychotics.

One must allow time to find the optimal dosage of any particular drug and, having found this dosage, allow a reasonable time for the drug to exert its behavioral effect. If, however, after a reasonable length of time (a few days in a severely disturbed acute patient, a few weeks in a less dramatically disturbed patient) no observable clinical effect is produced, a trial with a second, ideally maximally different, antipsychotic agent is warranted.

Dosage and Administration

The aim of drug treatment is to achieve the maximum therapeutic improvement in the patient. One must treat the whole patient, including the underlying disease process, not merely a given symptom. This is particularly true when one is treating a depressed schizoaffective or retarded schizophrenic patient. Such patients often respond dramatically to antipsychotic drugs, even though target symptoms such as agitation or aggression are absent. Fortunately, existing antipsychotic drugs produce generalized reduction in a broad range of schizophrenic psychopathology, rather than only on specific symptoms. Thus, the therapeutic goal is always for maximum cognitive reorganization and lessening of the underlying disease process, not merely symptomatic improvement. However, since patients respond differently to widely different dosage levels there is no set dosage for any particular antipsychotic drug. Rather, there are optimal dose ranges within which a statistically large number of patients respond. But statistical averages are certainly not inviolate and cannot always be adhered to in individual cases.

The wide range between effective dose and toxic overdose is demonstrated by the fact that patients have been safely treated with from 10 to 100 times the recommended therapeutic dose with no ill effects. Therefore, the physician should not be unduly concerned about increasing dose levels if reasonable therapeutic cause exists.

Because no standard dose exists, the correct dose for a particular patient must be determined empirically. The following sugguested dosages must be considered as approximate guidelines.

For the *acute* schizophrenic the *average daily dose* is usually between 400 and 900 phenothiazine units (that is, 400 to 900 mg. Thorazine, 20 to 45 mg. Stelazine, 8 to 18 mg. Prolixin, 6 to 15 mg. Haldol). *How rapidly these levels are attained depends upon the patient's age, size, weight, previous history and present behavior.* Older patients usually require less phenothiazine, usually no more than 400 units; small or frail patients will obviously tolerate less; past history of need for and tolerance of large doses will influence current treatment; agitated and assaultive behavior requires more rapid normalization of the psychosis. Nevertheless, the average *acute* schizophrenic requires about 600 mg. per day if otherwise healthy and, *in the absence of unusual circumstances the dosage should be increased gradually until the optimal therapeutic effect is obtained*, or until a serious side effect occurs. However, serious side effects rarely occur and most of them are not dose related. Table 22–2 provides approximate dose equivalencies of the phenothiazines, using Thorazine as the standard. Since chlorpromazine is a sedating phenothiazine, other less sedating antipsychotics such as perphenazine, trifluoperazine, fluphenazine or haloperidol may be used when large doses are necessary. This will prevent oversedation which may result from high doses of chlorpromazine.

The thioxanthenes are structural analogs of the phenothiazines. Studies have shown they possess clinical effects similar to those of the phenothiazines. Thiothixene (Navane) has a high milligram potency. Consequently, 1 to 5 mg. twice each day is an adequate initial dose, with maximum dose being between 15 and 30 mg. per day. Rarely, doses as high as 60 mg. per day have been reported.

The butyrophenones are structurally different than the thioxanthenes and the phenothiazines but have antipsychotic effects equal to chlorpromazine. Haldol is the only butyrophenone available in the United States. Generally, gradual dose introduction with elevation to approximately 15 to 30 mg. per day is indicated, but doses as high as 60 to 100 mg. per day may be acceptable if absolutely necessary. This drug produces minimal sedation and hypotension and is particularly valuable in violent psychotics or other psychiatric emergencies when high doses are necessary, since hypotension and sedation can limit the dose of chlorpromazine used. Conversely, chlorpromazine may be used when sedation is desirable.

Administration. The dosages of antipsychotic agents vary widely depending upon the setting. Crisis oriented facilities usually begin therapy in an emergency room, administer the drug intramuscularly in turbulent or severely withdrawn patients and raise the dosage rapidly to a high level (such as 1200 mg. per day

Table 22–2. Dosage Equivalency (Approximate)

Generic Name	Commercial Name	Dose in mg. (equaling 100 mg. Thorazine)
Phenothiazines		
Chlorpromazine	Thorazine	100
Triflupromazine	Vesprin	30
Acetophenazine	Tindal	25
Fluphenazine	Prolixin	2
Perphenazine	Trilafon	10
Prochlorperazine	Compazine	15
Carphenazine	Proketazine	25
Trifluoperazine	Stelazine	4
Butaperazine	Repoise	10
Thioridazine	Mellaril	100
Piperacetazine	Quide	10
Mesoridazine	Serentil	50
Thioxanthenes		
Chlorprothixene	Taractan	50
Thiothixene	Navane	5
Butyrophenone		
Haloperiodol	Haldol	2

of chlorpromazine or 30 to 60 mg. per day of haloperidol) over two or three days, reducing dosage only after the patient is clearly less agitated or, in the case of withdrawn patients, is responding to his environment. In better staffed, more selective or private facilities there often exists a drug-free evaluation period of several days or weeks, prior to the gradual initiation of medication; 600 mg. per day of chlorpromazine is a common dosage level in such settings. The average acute treatment doses used in well designed and controlled studies are seven to eight times the dosage equivalent per day. There is no evidence suggesting that one or the other of the above approaches leads to better long-term remission, and in either case the therapeutic goal, noted above, remains the same.

It should be recognized that dosage level is sometimes limited by side effects, necessitating a switch to another drug. However, sedation and extrapyramidal side effects, which are the most frequently occurring side effects, do not require a change of drug. Patients generally develop a tolerance to sedation within a few weeks, but, should it persist, the problem is obviated by administering the drug at bedtime. Neurological side effects are more serious and will be discussed fully under the section on side effects. One may deal with neurological side effects either through the administration of antiparkinsonian medication or through dosage reduction.

Once the patient appears to be maximally improved, and has sustained this improvement over time, the dose level is generally reduced for maintenance purposes. Of course, should symptoms recur the dose level is raised again. Also, it is a wise prophylactic procedure to administer a modest elevation in dosage when the patient is about to undergo a special stress, such as starting a new job or initially returning home from hospitalization.

The antipsychotic effects of the phenothiazines are of relatively long duration while their sedative effects last, usually, only a few hours. Therefore, since thrice daily administration may leave the patient oversedated when he could be working, learning, or participating in psychotherapy, a total dose given at bedtime will promote sleep while leaving the patient calm, though unsedated, during the day. This permits the patient to participate in other therapeutic activities.

The cost factor also favors a once a day regimen. A 25 mg. chlorpromazine tablet costs almost as much as a 100 mg. tablet. Administering the largest indicated dose once a day optimizes medication dollars and, additionally, reduces the expenditure of nursing time and cost to the hospital. Finally, an evening dose, once it becomes part of the patient's repertoire, is more difficult to forget and easier for the family to monitor than a thrice daily regimen.

Although spansules or other delayed release forms of medication are available there is no evidence to indicate that these relatively more expensive forms of medication have any therapeutic advantage over standard preparations.

Phenothiazine Blood Levels and Metabolism. Patients exhibit wide differences in blood chlorpromazine levels with comparable doses of the drug, and this may explain differential patient responsivity to different dose levels, as shown in studies by Curry (1970), and by Davis and coworkers (1970). Some patients, receiving a moderate dose, have exhibited extremely high blood levels and appear excessively sedated. A reduction of the dosage often produces marked improvement. Conversely, some patients manifest extremely low blood levels even though they are on high doses of medication.

Problems such as these may well relate to differential metabolization in different patients. The first patient mentioned above may have a metabolic deficit and therefore build up psychotoxically high levels of blood chlorpromazine, while the latter patient may metabolize it so rapidly that even high doses do not permit adequate levels to reach the brain. These individual metabolic differences may be illustrated by the fact that patients on the same dose may have a 20– or 30–fold variation in serum levels.

Chlorpromazine is metabolized principally in the gut. In rapid metabolizers much of what reaches the blood is in the form of an inactive metabolite and is excreted. Thus excessive metabolism causes low blood levels with the result that the patient does not respond to what should be an effective dose.

With such patients intramuscular administration of such medications as depo fluphenazine should prove most effective. Consistent with this hypothesis both Curry and Davis and coworkers found that chronic schizophrenics, exhibiting lower blood levels when their medication was given orally and higher levels when given parenterally, responded favorably to fluphenazine enanthate (Prolixin), a long acting, parenterally administered phenothiazine.

High Dosage Phenothiazine Treatment. Patients who are treatment resistant have engendered the question of the efficacy of high dose (two to three times usual dosages) treatment, or extra high "mega dose" (20 times usual dosages) strategy. Research findings suggest that younger, more acute patients respond to a high dose, such as 2000 mg. of chlorpromazine per day, while the older, chronic, "burned out" schizophrenics exhibit no benefit.

It is important to recognize, however, that such studies show the average or mean effect. It is entirely possible that individual patients in the chronic group responded to the "mega doses" while some of the acute patients responded better to lower doses. Therefore, we emphasize that, while controlled studies present indications of how the majority of patients respond, treatment must always be adjusted to the level which is optimal for any individual patient.

Exploratory studies using massive doses of fluphenazine (300 to 1200 mg. per day) have produced good to excellent response both in chronic and acute schizophrenics. However, a double blind study comparing fluphenazine doses of 30 mg. per day and 1200 mg. per day found little difference in therapeutic outcome between the two groups. Similarly, another study using 600 mg., in contrast with 60 mg., of fluphenazine found little differential improvement.

In sum, equivocal results of controlled studies suggests that undue optimism regarding the use of "mega doses" (20 to 30 times the usual dosages) in treatment of resistant schizophrenics is unwarranted. Nevertheless, since patients can receive "mega doses" of drugs such as fluphenazine without undue toxicity, treatment resistant patients deserve a trial on moderately high dose treatment. Fluphenazine or trifluoperazine, because of the large clinical literature on their use in "mega dose" treatment strategies, should be considered the drugs of choice when such a procedure is to be attempted. Thus, there is some evidence that a modest dose increase (two to three times the usual dosages) will help some patients. However, extension of dosages to 20 times the usual dose levels reaches a point of diminishing return therapeutically, although it is safe. Some modest increase in dose is indicated for the unresponsive patient, although research studies have not defined the amount of increase precisely. Hence, the physician must use clinical judgement, but should increase the dosage to arrive at a successful treatment level with the seemingly unresponsive patient. Results are often good, a rewarding experience for both doctor and patient.

Maintenance Treatment With Antipsychotic Medication. How long should a patient be maintained on antipsychotic medication once substantial improvement has been achieved and the psychosis brought under control? To the best of my knowledge every properly controlled study (with 24 studies reporting such data) has shown that significantly more patients relapse on placebo than on continued pharmacotherapy. Leff and Wing, for example, found in a study of patients who had recovered from an acute schizophrenic illness that 83 per cent of the group placed on placebo relapsed while only 33 per cent of those maintained on drugs relapsed.

A study by Hogarty and Goldberg also provides important information regarding maintenance treatment. In their investigation 374 schizophrenics, recently recovered and discharged from state hospitals, were stabilized on medication for a period of time as outpatients. Subsequent to this, half of the patients were assigned to a drug group and half to a placebo group. Half of each group received psychotherapy, consisting of individual casework and vocational rehabilitation counseling. The results were striking; 73 per cent of the placebo only group relapsed; 63 per cent of the placebo plus psychotherapy group relapsed; 33 per cent of the drug only group relapsed, and 26 per cent of the drug maintenance plus psychotherapy group relapsed. Taken together, 68 per cent of the placebo group relapsed while only 30 per cent of the drug group relapsed. Moreover, if we eliminate from the drug group those patients who spontaneously stopped taking their medication, the relapse rate over 12 months drops to 16 per cent. Patients maintained on placebo relapse at an approximately linear rate.

It should be noted that such studies find, typically, that relapses are largely unpredictable as to their timing. Patients frequently show few signs of schizophrenic symptomatology until their relapse occurs, at which time they become markedly psychotic. Maintenance treatment with phenothiazines markedly diminishes the risk that a discharged patient will relapse. However, while 50 per cent of moderately ill patients do relapse within six months of discontinuance of pharmacotherapy, it is equally true that 50 per cent do not relapse. Thus, while half the patients are prevented from a relapse which has a serious impact on themselves and their families, half are taking drugs they do not need. For this reason, the decision to maintain a patient on drugs must be an individual one, based on a knowledge of the patient's illness and general life situation. In practice, the decision to maintain or to discontinue phenothiazine treatment is based upon clinical common sense. For example, a history of relapse following discontinuation of medication indicates longer maintenance periods. Furthermore, studies such as those noted above demonstrate that psychotherapy does produce beneficial effects which are independent of the drug effect.

It must be emphasized that the allegation that maintenance drugs interfere with psychotherapy is unsupported. Psychotherapeutic and social interventions, during the recovery phase and in post-hospital care, play an important role in the rehabilitative process. However, treatment with psychotherapy, alone, in the absence of medication, appears to produce a nonsignificant statistical difference in the relapse rate between drug and placebo groups. These therapeutic modalities, then, complement each other, producing a summed effect which is greater than the effect any one of them produces alone, although drug therapy seems to consistently produce the greatest effect.

Drug Holidays. Drug holidays are one way of reducing the risk of toxicity which occurs with long-term use of antipsychotic medication. Studies of chronic patients have shown that drugs can be omitted on weekends or on an every other day basis with either no increase in the relapse rate, or a very modest increase. Such drug holidays may also be useful on minimally staffed wards.

Depo Intramuscular Medication. There are two long acting antipsychotics presently available in the United States. They are fluphenazine enanthate and fluphenazine decanoate. The intramuscular depo forms (slow absorbing over periods of up to two weeks) of medication are particularly useful for patients who refuse or forget to take oral medication. In addition, since intramuscular administration bypasses gut metabolism this form of medication may be useful in patients who fail to respond optimally to oral medication. Data available from double blind studies show depo fluphenazine to be at least as effective as the oral form of the drug.

While depo fluphenazine is most specifically useful for outpatients it can also be useful in emergency room and home or hospital treatment of acute psychotics.

ANTIPSYCHOTIC DRUGS IN COMBINATION WITH OTHER THERAPIES

Antipsychotic Drugs and Somatic Therapies. Many claims have been made about the benefit of using electroshock therapy in conjunction with antipsychotic drugs. While the evidence is equivocal, one study found that electroshock therapy in combination with drugs led to a more rapid remission rate than the use of phenothiazine alone. Two months after admission 84 per cent of the drug group remained hospitalized in contrast to 48 per cent of the group in which electroshock had been used in addition to drugs. After six months 40 per cent of the drug group remained inpatients while only 14 per cent of the group that had both drugs and electroshock therapy had not been discharged. However, in the absence of any verification, this study must be interpreted with caution.

Drug Combinations. The therapeutic value of combining phenothiazines has yet to be demonstrated experimentally. When reading literature on drug combinations there is one methodological point which is most important to remember. For any study of drug combinations to be valid all treatment groups must have received an equal amount of antipsychotic medication. Obviously, treatment of the combination group with double the amount of antipsychotic medication used in either of the single groups demonstrates only a dose-response relationship.

Do combinations of antidepressants and phenothiazines help the depressed or the apathetic schizophrenic patient? Does a minor tranquilizer (antianxiety medication) with anticonvulsive activity help a schizophrenic with suspected "psychomotor epilepsy" or one with episodes of violent behavior? Findings suggest that the addition of imipramine or a monoamine oxidase(MAO)inhibitor does not benefit chronic schizophrenics to a greater extent than does chlorpromazine alone, as demonstrated, for example, by Casey and coworkers. In fact, the addition of amphetamine to chlorpromazine may be slightly harmful. Furthermore, one must be aware of the danger of undertreating a patient with the antipsychotic agent when one uses a minor tranquilizer (antianxiety medication). That is, because sedation is a target symptom and because one is adding a sedating minor tranquilizer to an antipsychotic drug, one might administer less of the antipsychotic and therefore not achieve the optimal antipsychotic effect, even though the patient is sufficiently sedated.

Data from studies combining tricyclic antidepressants and phenothiazines suggest that this mixture may benefit certain depressed patients as well as patients with catatonic-like symptoms. However, results are not uniform, and differences, when exhibited, are small.

In the treatment of individual patients a trial and error approach, in order to obtain the maximum effect, is indicated. When working with drug combinations each medicine should be prescribed individually, until the optimal dosage is ascertained, before adding another agent. Certainly, if a proprietary drug exists which contains the optimal ration one could use it for convenience. However, one should not assume that all patients will exhibit a maximal response to such a medication.

Drugs, Psychosocial and Social Treatments. Drug treatments have been assessed more thoroughly than have psychotherapeutic methods. Various studies demonstrate a beneficial effect of neuroleptics when administered in combination with intensive as well as minimal psychological therapies. In one study, a group of chronic schizophrenics who were receiving concurrent drug therapy and psychoanalysis had a placebo substituted for medication (Thioridazine). Subsequently, their behavior began to deteriorate. Thus, not only was there no evidence that drug therapy interfered with psychoanalytically oriented psychotherapy, but rather the evidence indicated that patients on drug therapy were more involved with their psychoanalysts and the outside world in general. Studies of milieu-total push therapy, individual therapy and group psychotherapy indicate the beneficial effect of neuroleptics. The results are summarized in Table 22–3, which is based on studies by May.

One must remember that these therapies are complementary. Social therapies do not produce the antipsychotic activities of the drugs and, conversely, drug therapies do not rehabilitate the patient's social and interpersonal skills. Phenothiazines will reduce the patient's psychotic symptomatology, but they will not necessarily help him get a job, adjust to his family

Table 22–3. **Comparison of Release Rates of Acute Schizophrenia with Four Methods of Treatment (After May)**

	Percentage Release Rate During Study Period
Milieu alone	65%
Milieu plus psychotherapy	70%
Milieu plus neuroleptic drugs	90%
Milieu plus neuroleptic drugs and psychotherapy	95%

Comparison of Symptomatic Improvement Comparing Four Treatments of Chronic Schizophrenia

	Percentage Highly Improved After Six Months of Treatment
Drug plus high social therapy	33%
Drug plus low social therapy	23%
No drug plus high social therapy	0%
No drug plus low social therapy	10%

situation, nor provide him with the motivation and judgement to remain out of the hospital.

Side Effects and Complications

Every physician must, of course, be familiar with the side effects of the drugs he prescribes. In addition, there is a reasonable likelihood that he will find himself diagnosing and treating side effects produced by drugs prescribed by other doctors or taken by the patient on his own initiative.

Antipsychotic drugs share common pharmacological modes of action. Thus we can consider side effects in categories referring to and including most, if not all, of the antipsychotic agents, with few exceptions. We can classify these side effects of the antipsychotic drugs as: *autonomic, extrapyramidal, other central nervous system effects, allergic, endocrine,* and *long-term skin and eye side effects.* A brief discussion of each category follows.

Autonomic Side Effects. The autonomic side effects of the antipsychotic agents are a result of their anticholinergic and antiadrenergic properties, and include dry mouth and throat, blurred vision, cutaneous flushing, constipation, urinary retention, paralytic ileus, mental confusion, miosis, mydriasis, and postural hypotension.

Dry mouth is, perhaps, the most frequently occurring side effect. Patients frequently complain about it. The patient may be advised to rinse his mouth with water frequently, but he should not be advised to chew gum or candy. Sugar from such confections creates a good cultural medium in the mouth for fungal infections such as moniliasis and, in addition, may increase dental caries. Pharmacologically, pilocarpine can be administered to reduce dry mouth, though its effects are often of short duration. Generally, patients will develop tolerance for this side effect as well as to other autonomic side effects.

Orthostatic (postural) hypotension occurs most frequently during the first few days of treatment, particularly when high doses of intramuscular medication are administered. It can be troublesome, the chief danger being that the patient may faint, fall and injure himself. Patients receiving high doses of parenteral medication are particularly susceptible to this problem; thus it may be prudent to take the patient's blood pressure (lying and standing) during the first few days of treatment. This situation often presents a problem for the physician. A patient may be asymptomatic but have a systolic over diastolic blood pressure of 85 over 50 mm. of mercury. Should one worry or change the dose? Not necessarily. In a medically healthy individual asymptomatic blood pressure decreases must be handled differently than symptomatic decreases in those patients who become faint, weak or dizzy when they stand up. Medical judgement is required here. Support hose may provide some relief to patients with chronically mild symptomatic hypotension. Patients should be warned of this side effect and instructed how to deal with it; the patient should rise from bed gradually, sit with legs dangling, wait for a minute, and sit or lie down if he feels faint.

On rare occasions, volume expansion or vasopressor agents may be indicated. Since phenothiazines are alpha-adrenergic blockers, they will block the alpha-stimulating properties of epinephrine, leaving the beta-stimulating properties untouched. Consequently, administration of epinephrine might result in a paradoxical hypotension. For this reason administration of epinephrine is contraindicated in phenothiazine-induced hypotension.

A predrug electrocardiogram, for baseline purposes, is indicated in patients with preexisting heart conditions. Furthermore, in those patients with a history of cardiovascular disease, doses of antipsychotic agents should be increased very slowly while postural hypotension is monitored. An electroencephalographic abnormality, consisting of broadened, flattened, or cloven T-waves, and an increased Q-R interval of uncertain clinical significance has been described in patients receiving thioridazine in doses as low as 300 mg. per day. This abnormality does not seem to be associated with clinical electrolyte disturbances.

Rarely, a case of sudden death is reported in a patient who has been receiving phenothiazines. However, since sudden deaths in hospitalized schizophrenics were reported to have occurred before the discovery of antipsychotic drugs, it is difficult, in cases which occur at present, to make an accurate assessment as to whether the drugs were the causal agent in the death. Mechanisms proposed as the cause of such sudden deaths are: ventricular fibrillation, asphyxia caused by regurgitated food, endobronchial mucus plugs in an asthmatic schizophrenic, shock in patients with acquired megacolon, and convulsive seizures or complications thereof.

Extrapyramidal Side Effects. Although comparative quantitative data on extrapyramidal side effects is imprecise, butaperazine, chlorperazine, fluphenazine, haloperidol, thiothixene, and trifluoperazine seem to produce the greatest incidence of these effects. Acetophenazine, chlorpromazine, and chlorprothixene produce a moderate number and thioridazine produces the fewest neurological side effects.

For our purposes we will divide the extrapyramidal effects into three arbitrary categories: (1) parkinsonian syndrome, (2) dyskinesias and (3) akathisia.

The parkinsonian syndrome involves tremor of resting muscles, masklike face, a slowing of voluntary movements, shuffling gait, and rigidity. Its symptomatology bears much resemblance to idiopathic parkinsonism. Dyskinesia is characterized by a variety of peculiar movements of the neck, face and tongue, such as torticollis, oculogyric crises, opisthotonus, and buccofacial movements with excess salivation. Akathisias are marked by an inability to sit still, semivoluntary motor restlessness (most marked in the lower extremities), and a general fear of sitting down.

Diagnosis of these side effects can be problematical. Parkinsonism can be sometimes mistaken for schizophrenic apathy, particularly when motor retardation is prominent. The dyskinesias can appear to be the bizarre mannerisms of a psychotic, and akathisia closely resembles psychotic agitation.

Obviously, correct diagnosis of these symptoms is important for proper treatment. A therapeutic trial of an antiparkinsonian agent is particularly useful in arriving at an accurate diagnosis; useful antiparkinsonian medications are benztropine (Cogentin), procyclidine (Kemadrin) and diphenhydramine (Benadryl). Dyskinesias, in particular, respond readily to intravenous or intramuscular antiparkinsonian medication. Patients can experience an acute dyskinetic reaction, usually during the first few weeks of treatment, even when they are receiving only small amounts of phenothiazine. This reaction also occurs frequently with children who have been given a dose of prochlorperazine for treatment of nausea. Although such dyskinesias can disappear of their own accord in a brief period of time they are often painful and psychologically distressing to the patient. Consequently, it is usually best to administer antiparkinsonian medication. Those acute dyskinetic reactions which resist treatment with typical antiparkinsonian medication may be treated with caffeine, diazepam, or methylphenidate.

Parkinsonian syndrome and akathisia may appear early in the course of treatment. The diagnosis is generally obvious but not always. That is, parkinsonism can present as a zombie-like appearance or emotional blunting. One must be most cautious not to confuse these symptoms with emotional withdrawal or retardation. Antiparkinsonian medications readily alleviate such symptoms.

The akathisias can often be confused with psychotic agitation, since the patient is driven by a motor restlessness. Antiparkinsonian drugs often create reversal of these symptoms, but cases which resist such treatment can be dealt with by a lowering of the dosage or by changing to another phenothiazine.

The ability of all antipsychotic agents to produce extrapyramidal effects has engendered the hypothesis that the presence of such effects may bear a relationship to the antipsychotic properties of the drugs. There is no correlation between therapeutic improvement and the presence of extrapyramidal effects, nor is there any correlation between therapeutic improvement and the intensity or severity of extrapyramidal effects, when present. Thioridazine, which has only minimal extrapyramidal side effects, has as much therapeutic effect as butyrophenones such as haloperidol, and phenothiazines such as fluphenazine, which produce far more extrapyramidal effects.

There is much debate as to whether antiparkinsonian medication should be administered prophylactically to all patients receiving antipsychotic medication, or only to those patients exhibiting a given side effect. Physicians who oppose routine administration argue: (1) extrapyramidal symptoms never occur in most patients; (2) high doses of antiparkinsonian drugs create their own side effects, such as blurring of vision, dry mouth and very rarely, paralytic ileus or urinary retention; (3) treatment cost rises greatly; (4) no conclusive evidence exists that routine use of antiparkinsonian medication prevents parkinsonian symptoms; and (5) patients can develop an atropine psychosis which, in its most severe form, may present as the "central anticholinergic syndrome," characterized by loss of immediate memory, disorientation, vivid hallucinations and other features.

On the other hand, physicians favoring routine prophylactic administration of antiparkinsonian drugs argue that extrapyramidal effects are most distressing to the patient, especially when he is not in the hospital, and are often interpreted, by the patient and his family, as a medical emergency. The proponents of prophylaxis also note that many clinical manifestations of parkinsonian extrapyramidal effects (apathy, drowsiness, lack of spontaneity, relative inability to participate in social activity, lifelessness) are indistinct and therefore make accurate diagnosis exceedingly difficult. Thus, avoidance of the dramatic and unpleasant side effects which alarm the patient, and alleviation of the more subtle manifestations of the extrapyramidal syndrome are the arguments advanced in favor of prophylactic measures, by those who favor the routine administration of antiparkinsonian medication whenever antipsychotic agents are prescribed.

We do not recommend the routine administration of antiparkinsonian drugs in a hospital situation, since patients usually develop a degree of tolerance of the extrapyramidal side effects. For outpatients, however, judicious use of preventive antiparkinsonian medication may be occasionally useful. In such cases one should begin with the minimum dose and adjust as required. For example, for every 400 mg. of chlorpromazine or its equivalent, approximately 5 mg. of procyclidine (Kemadrin) or an equivalent antiparkinsonian medication can be prescribed. Initially, because of its short-term effect, procyclidine should be given on a thrice daily schedule. Subsequently it can be administered on a twice daily or bedtime basis. Dosage need not be increased beyond a 15 mg. total, given in divided doses four times a day.

After several weeks or months of phenothiazine treatment, the patient may no longer require antiparkinsonian medication and it is suggested that the drug be gradually reduced. Several studies which investigated the systematic withdrawal of antiparkinsonian drugs from chronic patients found that only 20 per cent of the patients exhibited any untoward neurological side effects subsequent to the withdrawal of the medication. The other 80 per cent had been apparently receiving the medication unnecessarily for years.

An extrapyramidal side effect which requires special note, because of its occasional occurrence in the course of very prolonged courses of antipsychotic medication, is tardive dyskinesia, which is also called terminal extrapyramidal insufficiency. It consists of bucco-facial, mandibular or bucco-lingual movements such as smacking of the lips, sucking, lateral or "fly catching" movements of the tongue, grimacing, lateral jaw movements, tonic contractions of the neck and back, and choreic movements of the extremities of the fingers, ankles and toes.

Tardive dyskinesia is prevalent particularly in those cases in which high doses of medication have been used for many years; however, the symptoms may appear at any time during treatment with antipsychotic drugs. If the symptoms first appear while the patient is on medication they may recur, or become intensified, several days or weeks after the drug dosage has been reduced or treatment discontinued. It is also true that the condition may be inapparent while the patient is on medication, appearing first when the drug treatment is discontinued. The cessation of medication often unmasks the disease because dystonic movements can be suppressed by phenothiazine-induced rigidity. Paradoxically, then, if the patient is given high doses of butyrophenones or phenothiazines, the symptoms may be undetectable.

In some patients, symptoms disappear soon after treatment ceases; in other patients symptoms persist at length. Antiparkinsonian medication is not particularly beneficial in treating tardive dyskinesia and, in some cases, aggravates the symptoms. Reserpine-like drugs may prove helpful. Long-term and high dose treatment with antipsychotic drugs should be used only when specifically indicated to prevent tardive dyskinesia.

Other Central Nervous System Side Effects. Most antipsychotic agents lower the threshold for cortical *seizures,* but seizures occur very rarely in patients treated with antipsychotic drugs and only when extremely high doses are used. When they do occur they are, generally, single and isolated in nature. Therefore, phenothiazines are *not* contraindicated in patients manifesting both a seizure disorder and a psychosis. In fact, clinical data support the assertion that psychotic epiletpic patients who are receiving antipsychotic drugs manifest improvement in their seizure disorder, as well as in their behavior disorder.

Obviously, any patient who experiences a seizure should have an appropriate medical work-up performed. However, when a patient who is receiving a phenothiazine has a seizure an anticonvulsant agent such as diphenylhydantoin (Dilantin) can be added to the treatment regimen, and in some cases the antipsychotic dosage can be reduced.

Antipsychotic agents produce *sedation,* particularly during the first few days of treatment. The drugs vary in the degree of sedation they produce; chlorpromazine and thioridazine are the more sedative of the phenothiazines, while fluphenazine, trifluoperazine, haloperiodol (a butyrophenone) and thiothixene (a thioxanthene) produce less sedation. However, patients rapidly develop a tolerance for such sedation and its resulting drowsiness. Nevertheless, outpatients should be warned about driving or operating machinery. Sedation and drowsiness may be combatted in patients by switching to a less sedating antipsychotic, reducing dosage, or by administering the entire daily dose at bedtime.

The side effects which are sometimes grouped under the term *behavioral toxicity* (adverse behavioral changes produced by an antipsychotic drug) are difficult to evaluate, since to do so accurately would require the separation of drug-induced toxicity from nondrug-related exacerbations of the schizophrenic process. Patients being treated with antipsychotic drugs may display symptoms such as somnambulism, insomnia, toxic confusional states, bizarre dreams, hindered psychomotor activity and aggravation of schizophrenic symptoms. Some of these effects may be dose related, and therefore may be treated by changing dosage, switching drugs, adding or deleting a drug, and other technics. For example, intramuscular antiparkinsonian drugs can reverse akathisia or an organic psychosis which occurs as a concomitant of extrapyramidal disorder. Chlorpromazine-induced central behavioral toxicity in hepatic coma is a result of the brain's enhanced respontivity to the drug's sedative properties, rather than to an impairment of metabolism as reflected in blood levels.

For optimal results, empirical variation of dosage, routes of administration and different types of antipsychotic agents are sometimes suggested. Unfortunately, methods for measuring blood levels of antipsychotic drugs remain technically complex, and it will be some time before psychiatrists can routinely check unresponsive patients to make sure that appropriate drug levels have been achieved.

Allergic Reactions. The allergic reactions to antipsychotic drugs can be divided into three categories: (1) phenothiazine-induced jaundice (relatively rare), (2) agranulocytosis and other blood dyscrasias (very rare) and (3) some kinds of skin sensitivities (somewhat common).

The incidence of chlorpromazine-induced jaundice, originally one of the most striking side effects of the drug, diminished greatly after the first two years during which the drug was widely used in psychiatry; the causes of this extraordinary fact are puzzling and unclear. Today jaundice manifests itself in about one patient per 1000. When it occurs it usually develops within the first eight weeks of phenothiazine therapy, generally preceded by several days of flu-like symptoms such as nausea, fever, abdominal pain, vomiting, diarrhea and general malaise; this syndrome often resembles mild gastroenteritis or infectious hepatitis. Clinical factors indicative of this problem are temporal association of the jaundice with the commencement of phenothiazine therapy, lack of a tender, enlarged liver, and chemical evidence of choleostasis, such as increased alkaline phosphatase, reduction of esterified cholesterol, greater increase in direct relative to indirect bilirubin, and a modest increase in SGPT (serum glutamic-pyruvic transaminase) and SGOT (serum glutamic-oxaloacetic transaminase). Eosinophilia can be observed on peripheral blood smears, and liver biopsy shows bile plugs in the caniculi, with eosinophilic infiltration in the periportal spaces. This syndrome usually disappears within several weeks with complete resumption of normal liver function. Plasma bilirubins do not generally exceed 15 mg. per 100 ml. Very rarely, the more prolonged exanthomatous biliary cirrhosis can occur. This reaction eventually clears, but usually follows a chronic course of 6 to 12 months.

Categorization of chlorpromazine jaundice as an allergic reaction results from the facts that its onset is closely associated with commencement of pharmacotherapy, it is frequently associated with other allergic reactions as well as with peripheral eosinophilia and eosinophilic infiltrations of the liver, and prolonged retention of sensitivity is exhibited on the challenge test. The majority of phenothiazine-induced jaundice cases have been associated with administration of chlorpromazine, but the condition has been reported with promazine, thioridazine, mepazine, prochlorperazine and, very rarely, fluphenazine and triflupromazine. There is no evidence that haloperidol causes this side effect.

While baseline liver function tests are useful, in the event that a patient develops chlorpromazined jaundice at some subsequent time, routine weekly or biweekly liver function tests are neither useful nor necessary. When a patient develops chlorpromazine jaundice it is necessary to discontinue administration of the drug.

Agranulocytosis is a very rare disorder, with a mortality rate exceeding 30 per cent; it is the most serious phenothiazine-related side effect. It usually occurs in older female patients who have other complicating systemic diseases. Fortunately, it is quite rare. Onset of the disease is abrupt, usually occurring within the first eight weeks of treatment, and is characterized by sudden appearance of fever, sore throat and ulcerations of the mouth. The patient should be hospitalized at once for reverse isolation procedure, and phenothiazine medication should be immediately discontinued. Rigorous treatment of infection is indicated, but prophylactic antibiotic therapy may be contraindicated due to the danger of propagating drug-resistant organisms. Corticosteroids seem to have no effect. Incidence of the disorder is said to be about 1 per 500,000 patients, and cross-sensitivity to other phenothiazines may occur, but in neither case is reliable concrete data available. Very rarely, cases have been reported with promazine, prochlorperazine, mepazine and thioridazine.

Routine blood counts are of no value in discovering agranulocytosis. The disease develops so rapidly that only daily blood counts could lead to early detection of the complication. Obviously, such a proceedure is not possible. Moreover, it should be noted that it is not uncommon for phenothiazines to temporarily reduce a normal white blood cell count to a modest degree. This, however, is a benign leukopenia requiring no special treatment nor deletion of medication.

Rarely, thrombocytopenic or nonthrombocytopenic pupura, pancytopenia, or hemolytic anemia may occur with patients receiving phenothiazines, generally during the first weeks of treatment. Contact dermatitis may occur in personnel who handle chlorpromazine.

Chlorpromazine treatment may also cause a photosensitive reaction of the phototoxic type, resembling severe sunburn. Patients should be made aware of this possible side effect and should avoid direct, strong sunlight.

Endocrine Side Effects. The clinically important side effects of antipsychotic agents upon the endocrine system of humans are lactation in females and male impotence, the latter presumably of autonomic rather than endocrine origin; however, neither one of these side effects is clinically common. Antipsychotic drugs also may produce shifts in glucose tolerance curves in a diabetic direction and, in females, result in false positive hormonal (not immunological) pregnancy tests. When breast engorgement and lactation among female patients occurs, this difficulty may be managed by changing drugs or reducing dosage. Thioridazine occasionally produces difficulty with delayed ejaculation. This is, potentially, a very disturbing side effect of which the physician should be aware, since patients frequently will be too embarrassed to mention it.

Long-Term Eye and Skin Effects. More than two decades of experience has made us aware of several skin and eye abnormalities resulting from long-term use of chlorpromazine in small percentages of patients. Discoloration of skin areas exposed to direct sunlight is one such effect. Initially the exposed areas tan rapidly and then progressively become slate gray, metallic blue or purple, or even vivid purple. Histological examination of biopsied areas reveals pigmentary granules similar to, but not histochemically identical with melanin.

Eye changes have also been associated with long-term chlorpromazine treatment. These changes appear as whitish brown, granular deposits localized in the posterior cornea and anterior lens, which eventually progress to opaque white and then yellow brown, often stellate in shape. They are visible by slit-lamp examination. Occasionally, the conjunctiva is also discolored by a brown pigment. These opacities are in no way related to senile cataracts. Moreover, patients manifesting these opacities exhibit neither retinal damage nor impaired vision.

The frequency with which such opacities occur, and their severity when they occur, is related to the duration and total dose of chlorpromazine. The dosage level of the majority of the patients who manifest these deposits is reported to be in the range of one to three kilograms of phenothiazine, throughout the course of treatment.

The prevalence of skin and eye abnormalities vary among hospitals which report such data. Estimates range from less than 1 per cent to more than 30 per cent, but the small percentages are much more commonly reported. Statistical data indicate that lens opacities occur more frequently in patients who exhibit skin coloration.

Because eye and skin effects are related to the amount of exposure to direct sunlight as well as a function of total phenothiazine dose, it has been suggested that exposure to the sun be curtailed. Patients requiring long-term antipsychotic medication may be treated with low dose phenothiazines, or with haloperidol. However, this can be counterbalanced by the psychiatric needs of the patient, since both these side effects are benign.

Thioridazine is the only phenothiazine conclusively shown to cause severe ocular pathology. Doses of 1000 mg. per day or more may result in retinitis pigmentosa. This condition causes substantial visual impairment and may result in blindness. The condition does not necessarily remit when the drug is discontinued; hence, doses of thioridazine exceeding 800 mg. per day are to be strenuously avoided.

Side Effects in the Elderly. Elderly patients require and tolerate lower dosages of antipsychotic agents than younger adult schizophrenics. The specific reason for this is unknown but may be related to decreased plasma or tissue binding ability, to impaired brain function, or to generalized arteriosclerosis. Safe doses for elderly patients are lower than for adults, with individual doses as low as, for example, 25 mg. thioridazine or 0.25 mg. haloperidol. A clinically effective total daily dose of thiroidazine may be 100 mg. and a similar total daily dose of chlorpromazine is occasionally as low as 75 mg. or 100 mg.

Caution must be exercised in establishing initial dose levels, as ataxia and hypotension may result from high doses, resulting in increased risk of falls and subsequent hip fractures. Where hyperarousal exists at the modest dose levels suggested above, careful and gradual elevation of dosage, until symptomatic relief is obtained, is indicated. The psychotic geriatric patient may be treated effectively with antipsychotic agents, and without difficulty, as long as extra precautions are taken.

The Employment of Antipsychotic Medications in Manic Disorders, Organic Brain Syndromes and Other Conditions. Antipsychotic drugs also are effective in the treatment of manic psychoses, and they can be useful in the total management plan of an agitated patient with an organic brain disorder; they occasionally are employed to dampen agitation in some other kinds of psychiatric conditions. However, their most striking and common use is in the treatment of schizophrenia, and it is in schizophrenia that they have had their most dramatic impact on psychiatric practice.

(The use of antipsychotic drugs in the treatment of mania is covered in Chapter 16, and their employment in decreasing agitation in organic brain syndromes is commented on in Chapters 18 and 19; their utility in diminishing restlessness in some other conditions is noted elsewhere.) We have dealt mainly with the use of antipsychotic drugs in schizophrenia in this chapter since scientifically valid studies and controlled double blind investigations of antipsychotic medications have been carried out mainly with schizophrenics. The almost invariable good prognosis of a manic psychosis over a several month period, and the secondary nature of antipsychotic medications in management of organically brain damaged patients, make well controlled studies of antipsychotic drugs difficult in these conditions, though their clinical value has been well established.

ANTIDEPRESSANT DRUGS

The treatment of depressive illness was given considerable impetus in the late 1950's by the discovery of two classes of drugs—the monoamine oxidase (MAO) inhibitors and the tricyclic antidepressants (imipramine type drugs). Since their introduction, the MAO inhibitors and the tricyclic agents have achieved wide currency in clinical application. In spite of their therapeutic effectiveness in the treatment of approximately 85 per cent of depressed patients, there remain problems with their use, particularly with regards to the problem of which sub categories of depressive illness should be medicated.

Table 22–4, in addition to listing all the commonly employed antidepressant medications and some of the less often used ones, summarizes the number of controlled double blind studies done to date (in which there were statistically significant differences) on the efficacy of these drugs. It also presents the results of a few studies of treatment with electroshock therapy and other medications.

The Tricyclic Drugs

The principal tricyclic antidepressants—imipramine, amitriptyline, desipramine, nortriptyline, protriptyline—constitute the most effective class of antidepressants and are of benefit to approximately 80 per cent of depressed patients. They have the least risk of side effects and are probably the drugs of choice for most depressive illnesses. In general, it is the severe psychotic depressions (often called endogenous depressions or, in this book, simply severe depressions) that respond best to these agents, while the chronic characterologic depressions (often called neurotic depressions) respond least well. In addition, a few investigators feel that imipramine has been shown effective in the treatment of some cases of phobic anxiety syndrome. The therapeutic response, when it occurs, develops after a lag of 7 to 14 days. Patients who remain unresponsive after three to four weeks of treatment at adequate dosage levels will probably not respond at all and should be shifted to a different drug or receive electroshock therapy. Most investigations show few tangible statistical differences between the tricyclics with regard to efficacy or speed of onset.

Imipramine (Tofranil, Presamine). Combined data from studies of imipramine effectiveness suggest that, as in studies of other tricyclics, approximately 70 to 80 per cent of depressed patients treated were significantly improved. Variables associated with good drug response are principally those associated with the more severe, or endogenous, depressions. There is a tendency for patients with neurotic depressions, whose premorbid personalities show irritable, hypochondriacal, and hysterical features, along with self pity, to respond less favorably to imipramine. However, since some of these latter patients show dramatic response to imipramine and related tricyclics, trial medication may be worthwhile.

A few writers feel, in addition, that imipramine helps to dampen the panic attacks associated with phobic anxiety syndrome. It may stop the massive panic that phobic patients associate with certain situations—traveling alone in open spaces, on bridges, in tunnels, and in other situations. School phobias, one of the childhood versions of this syndrome, are also sometimes helped by imipramine. Imipramine is less helpful for the

Table 22-4. Summary of Controlled Double Blind Evaluations of Antidepressant Drugs*

Drug		Number of Research Studies in which the Effect of Treatment Was			
Generic Name	Trade Name	Greater than Placebo	Equal to Placebo	Greater than Imipramine	Equal to Imipramine	Less than Imipramine

Generic Name	Trade Name	Greater than Placebo	Equal to Placebo	Greater than Imipramine	Equal to Imipramine	Less than Imipramine
Tricyclic Drugs						
Imipramine	Tofranil	26	12	—	—	—
Amitriptyline	Elavil	9	2	2	5	0
Desipramine	Norpramin Pertofrane	3	2	0	6	1
Nortriptyline	Aventyl	4	0	0	0	0
Protriptyline	Vivactil	2	0	0	2	0
Opipramol	Insidon	4	0	0	0	0
Trimipramine	Surmontil	1	0	2	0	0
MAO Inhibitors						
Tranylcypromine	Parnate	2	1	0	3	0
Iproniazid	Marsilid †	4	3	0	1	1
Isocarboxazid	Marplan	2	4	0	2	2
Nialamide	Niamid	0	3	0	0	1
Pheniprazine	Catron †	1	1	0	1	1
Phenelzine	Nardil	4	3	0	4	3
Pargyline	Eutonyl	2	0	0	0	0
Etryptamine	Monase †	1	0	0	0	0
Other Treatments						
Electroshock		7	1	4	3	0
Chlorpromazine	Thorazine	3	0	0	3	0
Thioridazine	Mellaril	0	0	0	1	0
Chlorprothixene	Taractan	0	0	0	1	0

*The figures above include only controlled studies with statistically significant differences.
† No longer available in the United States.

anticipatory anxiety associated with these situations, which is more responsive to the minor tranquilizers (antianxiety medications).

The effective dose for imipramine is 150 to 300 mg. a day.

Amitriptyline (Elavil). Most studies comparing amitriptyline with imipramine indicate that the two drugs are roughly similar in therapeutic efficacy. Some evidence suggests that amitriptyline is slightly superior at lower dosage levels and may be more effective with older, more severely ill patients. In addition, some writers feel that, at least in the early stages of treatment, amitriptyline has more sedative and hypnotic (drowsiness producing) effects than imipramine. The usual dose for amitriptyline is 150 to 250 mg. a day.

However, the dosages for both imipramine and amitriptyline must be monitored flexibly in the manner described in a later part of this discussion.

Desipramine (Pertofrane, Norpramin) and Nortriptyline (Aventyl). Desipramine and nortriptyline are demethylated derivatives of imipramine and amitriptyline. Recent findings clearly negate initial claims that these tricyclics have a shorter lag period than their parent compounds. Therapeutic effectiveness is comparable to imipramine for both agents, although a few investigators find disappointing results with desipramine.

The effective dose for desipramine is 150 to 250 mg. and for nortriptyline is 50 to 150 mg. However, the dosages of these drugs must be flexibly handled, as outlined in later paragraphs of this section.

Doxepin (Sinequan). There is evidence of doxepin's helpfulness in the treatment of mixed anxiety-depression (non-psychotic) syndrome, a common disorder among outpatients. That is, present evidence tends to indicate that this drug is useful in persons having mixed neuroses with anxious and depressive features. The other antidepressant medications discussed in this section are the drugs of choice in clear-cut depressive disorders.

For mixed outpatient anxiety-depression, typical doses of doxepin consist of 150 to 300 mg. a day. Slightly lower doses for anxiety are indicated (100 to 200 mg.). The effect of doxepin on "pure culture" endogenous depression has not been studied with statistically significant controlled double blind investigations at the time of this writing.

Protriptyline (Vivactil). This is reported to be the least sedative of the tricyclic agents. It may be useful in outpatient depression where sedation is not desirable. The effective dose is 15 to 40 mg. a day, divided into three or four doses.

Dosage and Clinical Use of Tricyclic Drugs

Dosage is a particularly important variable in the treatment of depression with drugs. First, it is essential that the physician make a careful determination of the patient's psychiatric and medical status. The rapidity of dosage increase depends on the patient's age, medical status (particularly cardiovascular status), and severity of depression. If the patient is extremely depressed or suicidal, rapid movement to a higher dosage (or to electroshock therapy) may be indicated. A more cautious approach and careful monitoring is required for patients with pre-existing cardiovascular disease; lower dosages, with smaller and less rapid increases, are used. Under ordinary circumstances, the patient is started on a modest dose such as 25 mg. three times a day of amitriptyline or imipramine; within several days, if the dosage is well tolerated, the patient is graduated to 50 mg. three times a day. After one week the dose may be adjusted up to 200 mg. a day or, in some patients up to 250 mg. a day. A critical dosage exists for each individual patient and this number must be reached for clinical response to occur. The monitoring of side effects and therapeutic results, as well as systematic recording of postural hypotension with lying and standing blood pressures, are important in dosage adjustments.

Once the patient is stabilized and has recovered from the depression, the dosage is gradually reduced by 25 to 50 per cent. At this time it is advisable to give the total daily medication at bedtime. Because of the long half-lives of the tricyclics, this procedure proves as satisfactory as divided dosages. It is simpler for the patient to remember and allows the most pronounced side effects to occur during sleep when they are not noticed. In addition, in the case of amitriptyline, the sedative effects of the drug may induce adequate sleep without the necessity of giving a sleeping medication.

Blood Levels. Approximately 20 to 30 per cent of depressed patients are not helped by tricyclic drugs. Undoubtedly some of the non-responders suffer from forms of depression unresponsive to this class of drugs. There are two further possible reasons for non-response, related to abnormalities of metabolism of the tricyclics. Ordinarily, as these medications are administered, blood levels build up until they reach a fairly constant level by about one week. There are wide individual differences in plasma levels between patients. It appears that some patients metabolize the tricyclic drugs very rapidly, fail to develop adequate blood levels and hence have low brain levels. These patients may prove particularly slow in responding and unresponsive to lower dosages. Other patients appear to accumulate high plasma and brain levels as a consequence of defects in metabolism and fail to respond because they are receiving a toxic dose. Because of the substantial differential in the rates at which the tricyclic drugs are metabolized, the physician should make a careful effort to fit the dose to a given patient. At present, in the absence of adequate laboratory predictors of patient response, this must be done on the basis of clinical acumen.

Maintenance. Once remission of the depression is achieved the clinician faces the decision of when to discontinue the antidepressant medication. Depression is a recurrent disorder for many patients. According to recent investigations, clinicians may expect an approximate 50 per cent incidence of relapse among patients in remission whose medication is discontinued. No data are yet available to predict which patients need tricyclic drugs to prevent relapse. Once remission is achieved patients should be continued at full dosage for one month. Subsequently, for up to six months, dosage is reduced by about 50 per cent for maintenance treatment (for example, to 75 mg. of imipramine). Continued treatment with tricyclic drugs or lithium may be indicated for unipolar patients (that is, patients who have in their life histories either depressed or manic episodes, but not both) subject to frequent recurrences. Bipolar patients (that is, patients who have histories of both depressive and manic disorders in their life histories) should obviously receive maintenance tricyclic medication to prevent the recurrence of both aspects of this disorder.

Side Effects and Adverse Reactions of Tricyclic Drugs

The tricyclic drugs produce roughly comparable side effects, although there are slight quantitative differences; for example, amitriptyline is said to be more sedating than imipramine, while protriptyline is less sedating.

Autonomic Effects. As a result of their anticholinergic pharmacological properties, all the tricyclic antidepressants can cause typical autonomic effects such as dry mouth, postural hypotension, palpitations, tachycardia, fainting, dizziness, vomiting, sweating, constipation, edema, loss of accomodation, and aggravation of narrow angle glaucoma. In rare instances, urinary retention (the tendency of tricyclics to delay urinary evacuation is the basis of their use in small doses to treat enuresis, as outlined in Chapter 25) and paralytic ileus have also been observed; these rare complications can have serious or even fatal consequences, particularly if the tricyclic drugs have been combined with other drugs having anticholinergic effects and if the clinician is unaware of the connection between the tricyclic medication and the urinary or gut problem. Prompt treatment with parasympathomimetic drugs such as bethanecol (Myocholine, Urecholine) can clear urinary retention, combined with termination of the tricyclic or reduction of its dose.

In general, dry mouth is the most common of these autonomic effects and patients should be warned that it may occur. Postural hypotension is not a frequent problem, but when it does occur some authors recommend the use of flurohydrocortisone (0.25 to 0.5 mg. twice a day). On the whole, autonomic side effects tend to be mild and to become less troublesome after the first few weeks of medication; in any event they may be effectively controlled by adjusting the dosage of the drug.

Cardiovascular Effects. Until the question of whether there may be some cardiotoxicity associated with the tricyclic antidepressants is conclusively settled, a note of caution must be added in treating the cardiac patient. Although the causative role of these agents remains unclear, cardiovascular incidents have occurred in patients with preexisting heart disease. Predisposed patients should be started at lower doses, with very gradual dose increment and careful monitoring of cardiac function. It must be remembered, however, that normal therapeutic doses of tricyclic drugs may cause prolonged QT intervals, flattened T-waves, and depressed S-T segments in electrocardiograms.

Central Nervous System Effects. Tricyclic drugs may induce a fine, persistent tremor, particularly in the upper extremities and also in the tongue. Insomnia and disturbance of motor function may occur occasionally in elderly patients. Twitchings, dysarthria, convulsions, paresthesia, ataxia, and peroneal palsies have also been noted in rare instances. Abrupt termination of imipramine after several months of treatment has led to mild withdrawal reactions consisting of nausea, vomiting and malaise. These reactions should not present a clinical problem if gradual reduction in dosage is carried out.

On occasion both imipramine and amitriptyline may cause episodes of confusion, mania and schizophrenic excitement. These incidents tend to occur in patients with bipolar (that is, a history of both manic and depressive illnesses) manic depressive disease, predisposition to schizophrenia, or chronic organic brain syndrome, rather than neuroses. After withdrawal of the drug, symptoms usually subside after one or two days, and they can be controlled by administration of phenothiazine medications.

Allergic and Hypersensitivity Effects. Early in therapy, skin reactions are noted and often subside with reduced dosage. Jaundice, which occurs early, is of the cholestatic type, similar to that attributed to chlorpromazine, but is very rare. Agranulocytosis, leukocytosis, leukopenia, and eosinophilia are also very rare complications of these drugs.

Overdosage. A severe overdosage (in most cases the result of a suicidal attempt) of any of the tricyclic antidepressants produces extremely serious life-threatening consequences. Physicians must be able to differentially diagnose this class of poisoning. The clinical picture is characterized by temporary agitation, delirium, convulsions, hyperactive deep tendon reflexes, bowel and urinary bladder paralysis, disturbance of temperature regulation, and mydriasis. The patient then progresses to coma with shock and respiratory depression. Cardiac rhythm may be disturbed, resulting in tachycardia, arterial fibrillation, ventricular flutters, and atrioventricular or intraventricular block. Coma is generally not protracted more than 24 hours.

Treatment should involve gastric aspiration and lavage. Diagnosis should be confirmed by analyzing the gastric lavage material. Intramuscular anticonvulsants such as diazepam should be used to control seizures, and the patient should have all the measures of standard coma care and support of respiration.

Management of cardiac function is critical during coma, as death can result from cardiac arrhythmia. If the patient survives this period, vigorous resuscitative measures, cardioversion, continuous electrocardiogram monitoring, and chemotherapy to manage arrythmias should be applied in an intensive care unit. Physostigmine (0.25 mg. to 4.0 mg. intravenously or intramuscularly) is useful to counteract anticholinergic toxicity and tachycardia. Propranolol is also helpful in preventing arrythmias. Patients must be kept under medical supervision for several days since late cardiac difficulties can occur.

Ingestion of several grams (20 to 40, or more, of the 50 mg. tablets) can be fatal. Thus, care should be exercised that the suicidal depressed patient does not have access to excessive numbers of antidepressant tablets.

Drug Interactions. If the patient is receiving a monoamine oxidase inhibitor, medication should be terminated for a minimum of one week before tricyclic antidepressants are administered. Severe toxic reactions and extreme hyperpyrexia sometimes leading to death can result when these two general classes of antidepressants are used in close conjunction.

Monoamine Oxidase Inhibitors

As a class, the monoamine oxidase (MAO) inhibitors have proved less effective in treating depressions than tricyclic antidepressants in most controlled studies, although tranylcypromine is of comparable effectiveness to imipramine. Evidence suggests these medications may be classified according to their clinical efficacy as follows. Tranylcypromine and iproniazid appear to be the most effective, phenelzine occupies a position somewhere in the middle, and nialamide and isocarboxazid are least effective.

Although tricyclic drugs are the medications of choice in most depressions, the MAO inhibitors may be useful in treating certain patients. Clinical investigations indicate that some patients who do not respond to tricyclics do respond to MAO inhibitors. Consequently, it may prove useful to administer MAO inhibitors to tricyclic nonresponders in a trial basis.

Dosage. The effective dose ranges of the MAO inhibitors are as follow: tranylcypromine (Parnate), 20 to 40 mg. per day, isocarboxazid (Marplan), 20 to 60 mg. per day, phenelzine (Nardil), 45 to 75 mg. per day, pargyline (Eutonyl), 25 to 75 mg. per day, and nialamid (Niamid), 150 to 225 mg. per day.

Improvement with MAO inhibitors is often quite marked at the time of its onset and frequently occurs from four to eight weeks after initiation of treatment.

Side Effects and Adverse Reactions of Monoamine Oxidase Inhibitors

Autonomic side effects are a frequent result of the MAO inhibitors and include dry mouth, orthostatic hypotension, dizziness, constipation, impotence, delayed ejaculation, and delayed micturition.

Hypertensive crisis, occasionally accompanied by intracranial bleeding, is one side effect of particular importance that may result from the use of the MAO inhibitors, especially tranylcypromine. Common prodromal features include sharply elevated blood pressure, severe occipital headache, stiff neck, sweating, nausea, and vomiting. Attacks may be triggered when the pressor effects of sympathomimetic amines in foods and medicinal amines are potentiated. Hence, patients on MAO inhibitors, and especially tranylcypromine, should be warned to avoid high tyramine cheeses (cheddar, edam, camembert, and others), alcohol (beer, wines), chicken liver, broad beans, pickled herring and various other kinds of foods. In addition, epinephrine, the amphetamines, ephedrine, dopamine, phenylpropanolamine and any other drugs containing sympathomimetic compounds must be avoided. Estimates suggest that one death in 100,000 has occurred after such crises in patients treated with tranylcypromine. The likelihood of such side effects as headache, intracranial bleeding, and hypertensive features can be reduced by careful diet and avoidance of pressor drugs and related substances. Treatment of side effects involves administration of short-acting alpha-adrenergic blocking agents, such as phentolamine (Regitine) 5.0 mg. intravenously, or 50 mg. chlorpromazine intramuscularly. Meperidine (Demerol) should not be used.

Hypotensive crises can occur when MAO inhibitors are combined with diuretics.

Hyperpyrexic reactions are an acute danger when MAO inhibitors are combined with imipramine-type tricyclic antidepressant drugs. Hyperpyrexic reactions also may occur if MAO inhibitors are combined with amphetamines or with meperidine in high doses or given intramuscularly. These reactions are characterized by high fevers (104° to 109°), dizziness, tremulousness, muscle twitching, convulsions and excitement that progresses to coma and death. Consequently, a washout period of 7 to 14 days is recommended to permit the MAO enzyme to regain adequate levels before a substitution is made. Thus, it is imperative to obtain a careful history of previous medication with depressed patients before embarking on a new course of drug therapy. Death has occurred after one injection of 25 mg. of imipramine in a newly hospitalized patient whose previous treatment with MAO inhibitors was not known to hospital staff.

With special precautions these drugs can be used together, but due to the potential, grave hazards of their interaction this practice should be restricted to a physician particularly experienced in this technic. The standard, highly advisable practice is always to leave a 14-day interval between the administration of a MAO inhibitor and a tricyclic antidepressant, or one of the other medications listed in the preceding paragraph.

Overdosage (usually in a suicidal attempt)

caused by MAO inhibitors produces agitation that progresses to coma with hyperthermia, tachycardia, an increase in respiratory rate, dilated pupils, involuntary movements (especially in the face and jaw), and hyperactive deep tendon reflexes. Toxic effects occur after an asymptomatic lag period of one to six hours following ingestion of the drugs; the clinician must be careful that this lag period does not mislead him into complacency. Chlorpromazine is a useful agent in the treatment of poisoning with MAO inhibitors, presumably because of its adrenergic blocking action. Vascular tension crises require appropriate treatment. The excretion of tranylcypromine, phenelzine, and amphetamine is markedly hastened by acidification of the urine. Dialysis has also been used with success in tranylcypromine poisoning.

Other Precautions. MAO inhibitors can precipitate acute confusional reactions with generalized mental clouding, disorientation, and illusions. These drugs can also convert a retarded depression into an anxious or agitated one and can occasionally produce an acute schizophrenic psychosis or hypomania. Altered erotic desires, edema, dizziness, muscle tremor, generalized weakness, slurred speech, clonus, hyperreflexia, and increased muscle tone have also been associated with the MAO inhibitors. Peripheral neuropathy, similar to that originating with pyrodoxine deficiencies, and observed in association with isoniazid treatment, can also occasionally occur.

MAO inhibitors potentiate a great variety of drugs including sympathomimetic amines (such as ephedrine), opiates meperidine, procaine, anesthetic agents, barbiturates, methyldopa, chloral hydrate, and aspirin.

Choice of Treatment In the Use of Antidepressant Drugs

The stakes are fairly high in the more serious depressions. Often remission does not occur for six months or more in untreated depressions. Chronic depression leads to much disability and has serious repercussions for the patient's family as well. Furthermore, it is estimated that about 15 per cent of patients with recurrent depressive illnesses eventually commit suicide. Most cases of depressive disease are readily treatable and should be vigorously and quickly treated.

Comparative studies suggest that tricyclic drugs are slightly more effective and slightly safer than MAO inhibitors. Phenothiazine medications, MAO inhibitors, and electroconvulsive therapy may also be of value in selected cases. Table 22–4 presents a summary of the controlled double blind assessments of the antidepressant drugs. In general, it is more advantageous for the clinician to be thoroughly acquainted with the assets and liabilities of a small number of drugs than to be minimally familiar with and experienced in the use of a large number of drugs. However, the recent literature should be periodically examined to see whether newer antidepressant agents have been demonstrated to have advantages over the older drugs. In addition, the physician will want to determine whether more clear-cut differential indications have been developed for the use of specific antidepressants with the different sub categories of depressed patients.

In retarded, endogenous depressions (that is, those depressions often termed severe, or psychotic) the tricyclic antidepressants are the drugs of choice due to their safety and efficacy. With tricyclic drug treatment, about 70 to 80 per cent of these depressive illnesses remit within one month. Improvement rates may be increased to 85 per cent when treatment-resistant patients are transferred, after a waiting period of one week or more, to medication with MAO inhibitors. Alternatively some clinicians suggest that nonresponders be shifted to electroshock therapy, which is effective with 50 per cent of this tricyclic resistant population. Electroshock therapy is, of course, a very effective form of treatment for the severe depression and is an important part of the psychiatric therapies. (Its technic and clinical applications are covered in Chapter 23.)

The mixed anxiety-depression syndrome, which is usually considered a mixed neurotic disorder with anxious and depressive features, has been effectively treated with a number of approaches. Doxepin (Sinequan) has been found useful in treating this condition, as has a phenothiazine-tricyclic combination (such as perphenazine-amitriptyline). In controlled studies of the drug treatment of this type of disorder, doxepin and antipsychotic-antidepressant combinations appear of about equal value.

Some reactive (neurotic) depressions, especially those that are painful but self-limited, often remit within a few days or several weeks, and are best managed through psychotherapy and minor doses of antianxiety agents. Treatment with tricyclic antidepressants and MAO inhibitors is not indicated. Similar approaches are suggested in instances of bereavement and other kinds of grief reactions (as outlined in Chapter 25). In cases of hysteria with secondary depression, many British psychiatrists have found the MAO inhibitors effective; however, these recommendations should be regarded as tentative until more definite investigations are concluded.

In some cases geriatric depression produces symptoms that may be mistaken for organic brain senility; these include confused and uncooperative behavior, irritability, sloppiness, and social deterioration. Frequently this diagnosis is overlooked. The pseudosenile symptoms may disappear when tricyclic antidepressants are cautiously administered on a trial basis. Positive drug responses can save these patients from further deterioration that comes with assignment to chronic wards of state hospitals or nursing homes.

In general, the antidepressants are quite safe. Since these drugs are quite potent, however, and since rare but potentially dangerous side effects do occur, they should be administered only when there are definite indications that such treatment is necessary. Effective psychotherapy may greatly augment the patient's response to antidepressant drugs and prevent relapse. Moreover, patients whose depressions stem from underlying neuroses and personality disorders may respond dramatically to psychotherapy and not respond at all to existing medications.

MINOR TRANQUILIZERS (ANTIANXIETY MEDICATIONS) AND SEDATIVE-HYPNOTICS

Minor Tranquilizers (Antianxiety Medications)

The minor tranquilizers (antianxiety medications) must be sharply distinguished from the antipsychotic major tranquilizers. Minor tranquilizers (the meprobamate type and the benzodiazepine derivatives), like the barbiturates, have antianxiety and hypnotic (sleep-producing) effects; however, minor tranquilizers produce none of the antipsychotic effects and extrapyramidal side effects of the phenothiazines. As with barbiturates, the minor tranquilizers can produce physical dependence, and subsequent withdrawal symptoms, after prolonged use at high dosages.

Glycerol Derivatives: Meprobamate (Equanil, Miltown) and Tybamate (Solacen, Tybatran). Meprobamate, first synthesized in 1950, has been found to be approximately equal in efficacy, as an antianxiety agent, to barbiturates and other antianxiety drugs.

The usual dosage of meprobamate is 400 mg. three or four times a day, totalling 1200 to 1600 mg. per day. Among the antianxiety drugs, meprobamate has a higher risk of physiological dependence than the benzodiazepines and, after sudden withdrawal from excessively high doses, a patient may go through a withdrawal syndrome with anxiety, restlessness, convulsions and delirium. Meprobamate also has a higher suicide potential in comparison with the various antianxiety drugs, such as the benzodiazepines.

Drowsiness occurs as a side effect in about half the patients on meprobamate. Hence, the therapeutic dose should be built up gradually over several days. Patients should be warned against driving and other hazardous tasks requiring alertness. Also, patients should be warned against the use of alcohol and other central nervous system depressants which potentiate the sedative effects of meprobamate.

Tybamate is an effective antianxiety agent, possibly free of the potential for addiction. Tybamate appears to be particularly effective for somatically oriented, hypochondriacal patients and for treatment-resistant neurotic, anxious outpatients. These findings, however, await more definitive confirmation. The commonly used dosage of tybamate is 500 mg. three of four times a day, giving a daily total of 1500 to 2000 mg.

Benzodiazepine Derivatives: Chlordiazepoxide (Librium), Diazepam (Valium), Chlorazepate (Tranxene). Studies find almost uniformly that the benzodiazepines produce a modest benefit in reducing chronic anxiety in psychiatric outpatients and in anxious persons seen in general practice; these medications are found to be more effective than, or equal to, the barbiturates. These drugs may also overcome cases of acute nonpsychotic anxiety when given intravenously; for example, 10 mg. of diazepam infused intravenously reduces anxiety symptoms in 20 to 30 minutes. During acute alcohol withdrawal they prove useful in preventing delirium tremens, tremors and convulsions. Diazepam has been employed successfully in ameliorating the effects of hallucinogenic drugs such as LSD, mescaline and STP (dimethoxy-methylamphetamine) in doses of 10 to 30 mg. by mouth. Diazepam also has been found effective in treating some patients with acute muscular dystonic (athetoid movements, stiff-man syndrome and others) reactions in doses of 20 to 30 mg. by mouth or intravenously.

Customary daily dosages for the benzodiazepine derivatives are: chlordiazepoxide, 5 to 20 mg. three or four times a day, totaling 15 to 80 mg. each day; diazepam, 2 to 10 mg. two to four times a day, totaling 4 to 40 mg. each day; oxazepam, 10 to 30 mg. three times a day, totaling 30 to 90 mg. each day; chlorazepate, 3.75 to 15 mg. four times a day, totaling 15 to 60 mg. each day. Full therapeutic effect typically becomes apparent within several days.

The benzodiazepines have a relatively low abuse risk when compared with other sedative and hypnotic drugs, though physical dependency can result from prolonged use in excessive doses. From the standpoint of suicide these medications are very safe. Like other antianxiety agents the benzodiazepines cause sedation and warrant particular caution on the part of the outpatient with regard to hazardous tasks and the concurrent use of potentiating drugs such as alcohol.

Effectiveness of Minor Tranquilizers (Antianxiety Medications). A primary use of minor tranquilizers is the treatment of anxiety reactions and chronic anxiety states. In general, the benzodiazepine family of drugs (chlordiazepoxide, diazepam, oxazepam, and chlorazepate) are probably the best medications for anxious outpatients and are generally superior in this respect to the barbiturates. Findings indicate that tybamate is also reasonably impressive, while meprobamate is less consistently superior to the barbiturates.

However, anxiety is far from being unitary a symptom and anxious outpatients constitute an extremely heterogenous group. Although many studies suggest that the minor tranquilizers have greater clinical effect in anxiety reduction at equally sedating doses than do the barbiturates, one recent investigation suggests that effectiveness may vary with social class. Barbiturates are preferred by lower class clinic patients who welcome the sedating effect as evidence that the medication is helping them. Conversely, middle class patients frequently dislike being sedated, feeling that it interferes with mental alertness, and hence prefer the more costly, less hypnotic antianxiety medications.

Acute anxiety reactions in patients free from other serious psychiatric symptoms often remit promptly without drugs. If distress is so severe as to warrant medication, these attacks may be aborted by intravenous administration of barbiturates or diazepam.

The acute anxiety, or even panic, which a patient with a phobic neurosis may experience when he must face his phobic object or situation usually does not respond well to minor tranquilizers or phenothiazines, but some investigators have reported effective treatment with the antidepressant imipramine.

In general, patients with anxiety accompanying chronic or acute schizophrenia, depression, or severe personality disorder are not responsive to antianxiety drugs. Psychotic agitation, for which phenothiazines are mandatory as the treatment of choice, may be worsened significantly by inappropriate treatment with minor tranquilizers which have no antipsychotic properties.

Conversely, phenothiazines are too frequently and erroneously applied to neurotic anxiety states. Phenothiazines are extremely potent and produce a wide variety of side effects (blurred vision, parkinsonian states, and considerable sedation and drowsiness) which are undesirable and potentially dangerous in uncomplicated anxiety states. However, in anxious patients with a prior history of psychotic episodes, as well as patients who respond poorly to antianxiety medication, an antipsychotic drug trial may prove useful. Empirically, some patients with anxiety neuroses and some anxious individuals with character disorders, who do poorly on minor tranquilizers, may at times respond dramatically to antipsychotic medication.

Minor tranquilizers have muscle relaxant properties and are useful in easing muscular tension. Also, the anticonvulsant activity of antianxiety agents renders them effective in the treatment of convulsive disorders, myoclonic attacks, status epilepticus, and prolonged seizures; the benzodiazepine drugs, and particularly diazepam, are the most used in this regard.

Sedatives and Hypnotics

This group contains a wide variety of drugs which can exercise a calming effect when given in small daytime doses (and hence are termed *sedatives*) or can induce sleep when given in larger doses at bedtime (and then are termed *hypnotics*); these drugs are sometimes called sedative-hypnotics as a group, but may be referred to as sedatives or hypnotics depending on which of their two possible functions is under consideration.

Sleep disturbance of varying severity may accompany a range of differing psychiatric disorders and stressful situations. Barbiturates, the benzodiazepine type drugs, meprobamate and other non-barbiturate sedatives and hypnotics are extensively used as sleeping medications. The physician should remain alert to the underlying causes of these disturbances as well as to the untoward drug effects of these various medications.

Transitory insomnia is often a presenting complaint of outpatients. Frequently, much more is involved than the presenting complaint, and exploration in a psychotherapeutic setting reveals that underlying psychological problems contribute substantially to this sleep loss. In this instance, though the fundamental avenue of treatment is psychotherapy, the temporary use of a hypnotic agent should be considered to restore a normal sleeping pattern. Use of hypnotics for brief periods can be helpful in forestalling further exacerbations of the basic emotional problem which may occur with chronic sleep loss.

Many patients with severe psychiatric disorders such as schizophrenia, mania and depression have difficulty sleeping. In these cases it is imperative to identify the underlying disorder and treat it specifically, rather than insomnia itself. Other psychopharmacologic agents, such as the tricyclic antidepressants or antipsychotic drugs, have sedative effects, and if they are given at bedtime they may obviate the need for a separate hypnotic drug. For example, when insomnia is caused by depression the tricyclic drug amitriptyline (Elavil), which has considerable sedating properties, can provide ample sedation when administered at bedtime in many cases. In schizophrenia and mania, one can use a more sedating phenothiazine when sleep disturbance occurs and administer two-thirds or all of the daily dose at bedtime. This strategy is usually sufficient to insure a good night's sleep. In unusual cases a separate hypnotic agent may also be required. Chronic sleep loss may play a role in precipitating a psychosis, and restoring normal sleep may be an important aspect of the therapeutic process.

When sleeping medication is clinically indicated, some controlled studies indicate a preference for the more sedative of the benzodiazepine drugs, such as flurazepam (Dalmane); these studies indicate that such medication has hypnotic properties comparable to those of the barbiturates and nonbarbiturate sedatives. The primary advantage of a sedating benzodiazepine, such as flurazepam, over other classes of drugs is its relative freedom from toxicity, in common with all the benzodiazepines; it also has less potential for abuse and is alleged to have less liability for death in overdose situations. In addition, it has less liability for drug-drug interactions mediated by the liver microsomal enzymes. Thus, some clinicians prefer these agents when sleeping medication is clinically indicated.

Barbiturates. The initial medical use of barbiturates occurred with the introduction of barbital (Veronal) in 1903. Since that time practitioners have made extensive use of such barbiturates as amobarbital (Amytal), pentobarbital (Nembutal), phenobarbital (Luminal), secobarbital (Seconal), thiopental (Pentothal) and hexobarbital (Evipan). These agents produce their effect primarily by depressing the activity of the cerebral cortex. In overdose situations they cause major depression of the central nervous system; the respiratory system is especially vulnerable, and respiratory depression is common in barbiturate overdose.

The barbiturates are conventionally divided into four groups according to their duration of action. The long-acting barbiturates (phenobarbital, barbital) have a duration of more than eight hours and are useful as sedatives in chronic anxiety but are relatively poor hypnotics. Medium-acting barbiturates (amobarbital, pentobarbital, hexobarbital) are effective for from five to eight hours and are useful with patients who wake frequently during the night. The short-acting category (secobarbital), which exert their effect over one to five hours, can be given to patients who have difficulty in falling asleep, but sleep soundly thereafter. Medium- to short-acting barbiturates are effective in the treatment of acute and chronic anxiety and are excellent hypnotics. Thiopental is very short-acting, with a duration of less than one hour.

In anesthetic doses, barbiturates produce hypotension. Barbiturates have no analgesic properties and consequently do not cause sleep when insomnia is due to pain. Instead they may produce confusion and restlessness. The untoward drug effects of barbiturates are further considered below.

Nonbarbiturate Hypnotics. For a period of time considerable interest flourished in the development and clinical application of nonbarbiturate hypnotics (such as etchlorvynol, ethinamate, methyprylon and others) on the mistaken assumption that if barbiturates caused death and physical dependence, nonbarbiturates would not. However, further experience has shown that these agents are no more safe from the hazards of suicide overdose and dependence than are the older drugs, and it is difficult to find any special indication for them at the present time. The benzodiazepines are safer and as effective, while the barbiturates are less expensive.

Glutethimide (Doriden) has been used widely as a daytime sedative and hypnotic, and should be prescribed with the same vigilance that is exercised in the prescription of barbiturates. Glutethimide is dependency-producing and is reported to cause stormier detoxification reactions than those of patients dependent on barbiturates. In addition, it can be particularly dangerous in overdose. The patient is more likely to go into shock than is the case with barbiturate poisoning, his level of consciousness may vary erratically, and convulsions sometimes occur. Pupillary dilatation engendered by the drug's anticholinergic properties may cause patients in glutethimide coma to be misdiagnosed as being in atropine coma. Methyprylon (Noludar) is similar in structure to glutethimide and is likewise used as a daytime sedative; it can be lethal in large doses and is addicting.

Other widely used nonbarbiturate sleeping medications include etchlorvynol (Placidyl), ethinamate (Valmid), methaqualone (Quaalude, Sopor, Parest, Somnafac) and the older drug chloral hydrate (Somnos, Noctec, Hydral and others).

The usefulness of the benzodiazepine flurazepam (Dalmane) as a hypnotic agent has been outlined above, as well as the reasons why some investigators now favor it, or another one of the more sedative drugs of the benzodiazepine group, for nighttime sedation.

Untoward Drug Effects of Minor Tranquilizers, Sedatives and Hypnotics

The side effects of the minor tranquilizers (antianxiety medications) are of small importance and do not constitute contraindications for their use. The most frequent side effects are a slight cognitive and behavioral impairment and drowsiness; with diazepam and chlordiazepoxide, the major side effects are drowsiness, dizziness and ataxia. Consequently, patients should not drive or operate machinery until they can accurately gauge their reactions to the drug. These agents do not cause liver toxicity, autonomic side effects, or extrapyramidal effects, and serious side effects are extremely rare.

With meprobamate, the physician may infrequently see anaphylactoid reactions, urticarial, or erythematous rashes, and angioneurotic edema. More rarely, cases of gastrointestinal upsets, dermatitis, blood dyscrasias, and extraocular muscular paralysis have been reported.

Diazepam use has been associated with an increase in suicidal ideation in a small percentage of patients. Hence the clinician should watch for adverse behavioral changes in anxious patients receiving antianxiety drugs; some clinicians feel that relief of anxiety unmasks an underlying depressiveness in some patients.

In general, the barbiturates produce more sedation in proportion to their antianxiety action than do the minor tranquilizers. In addition, they induce liver microsomal enzymes which alter, among other things, the metabolism of anticoagulants, as discussed below. The nonbarbiturate sedatives, such as glutethimide, must be used with the same precautions.

Paradoxical excitement can occur with all these agents, but probably does so more frequently with the barbiturates. This adverse effect is more often observed in organically impaired or elderly adult patients and in hyperkinetic children.

Physical Dependence and Tolerance. Clear physical dependence has been shown to result from prolonged use of the barbiturates, meprobamate, diazepam, and chlordiazepoxide. On the basis of limited available information, a dose of 300 mg. of chlordiazepoxide for a month, or a dose of 3200 mg. of meprobamate a day for 40 days, can cause definite physical dependence. Methaqualone and glutethimide share the same property and it must be assumed that the other nonbarbiturate hypnotics and the benzodiazepines have this liability. It does appear, however, that cases of physical dependence on benzodiazepines are relatively uncommon.

Tybamate, because of its very brief half life in the body, appears at the time of this writing to be the only hypnosedative drug that is free from physical dependence liability. For this reason it has clear advantages in treating anxious patients who have a history of drug dependence or who are judged likely to abuse drugs.

The nightly use of hypnotics is unlikely to induce serious dependence, since it takes relatively high constant blood levels of a sedative drug to result in definite action. For example, 600 mg. of a medium- or short-acting barbiturate each night will not cause marked dependence. However, research data suggest that tolerance to the sleep enhancing effects of hypnotics develops within a week of nightly use. Thus, a long-term use of hypnotics in insomniacs may have little real usefulness other than as a nightly placebo.

Cross-tolerance exists between all the hypnosedatives, so that any one can be used to lessen the early withdrawal symptoms caused by physical dependence on the other. Pentobarbital has long-standing status as a detoxification agent. However, it seems more sensible to use a longer acting agent such as diazepam, a procedure already standard in some clinics for the detoxification of alcoholics.

Drug-Drug Interaction. Interaction between drugs occurs when one drug modifies the pharmacokinetics or otherwise influences the action or side effects of another drug, either quantitatively or qualitatively. With large numbers of patients taking multiple medications, the potentialities for drug-drug interactions are considerable. Consequently, the clinician must anticipate and adopt a vigilant attitude toward this possibility, particularly when obtaining information about the current medications status of a new patient.

Barbiturates can stimulate chlorpromazine metabolism. In addition, they induce liver microsomal enzymes which in turn accelerate the metabolism of anticoagulants. When patients taking oral anticoagulants terminate daily use of barbiturates, the induced enzymes regress and anticoagulants are metabolized more slowly. Hence, blood levels of the anticoagulants are heightened and the patient may begin to bleed.

The nonbarbiturate sedative glutethimide is said to antagonize similarly the therapeutic action of oral anticoagulants. Preliminary evidence suggests that ethchlorvynol may also have this effect. Present data indicates that the benzodiazepines diazepam, chlordiazepoxide, and nitrazepam do *not* do so; flurazepam and oxazepam have not been fully studied in this regard.

The sedative actions of different medications have a cumulative effect which may contribute, among other things, to significant behavioral impairment. Thus, the indiscriminate combinations of minor tranquilizers, hypnosedatives, phenothiazines, and alcohol may potentiate and heighten each drug's sedative effect in a manner that may jeopardize an outpatient's capacity to function in a judicious manner.

LITHIUM AND MISCELLANEOUS OTHER MEDICATIONS

Lithium

Lithium, which belongs to the family of alkali metals and is the lightest metal element in the periodic table, has come into increased prominence as an effective drug in the treatment of acute manic disorders. In addition, a small amount of data suggest that lithium, given on a maintenance basis, prevents cyclic recurrence of both mania and depression in unipolar (depressive illnesses only in the patient's life history) and bipolar (both depressive and manic disorders in the patient's life history) depressive disorders. The beneficial effects of lithium are achieved without sedation and lethargy, and also without impairment of normal mental and emotional functioning; also, it has no known long-term toxic effects. When employed under proper supervision, lithium is a fairly safe drug. However, physicians must be thoroughly acquainted with its potentially dangerous side effects in order to monitor and regulate them through careful dosage and blood level adjustments.

Clinical Use and Dosage of Lithium in Acute Mania. Lithium is a specific and dramatic agent in converting a patient in an acute manic episode to his normal state without the sedative and tranquilizing side effects that accompany the antipsychotics. Therapeutic response occurs in most acute manics within 10 days to two weeks. Because of this lag period, many clinicians prefer to combine lithium treatment with an antipsychotic drug such as chlorpromazine during the first 10 to 14 days to achieve immediately more effective control of the patient's manic behavior. After the mania is controlled the antipsychotic agent is discontinued. However, the therapeutic response to lithium alone yields diagnostic information particularly relevant to the discussion of maintenance treatment with lithium; hence, lithium alone is to be preferred to the combination of lithium plus a phenothiazine when circumstances permit. Lithium alone may be the drug of choice if the patient is hypomanic and there is no urgency to control his behavior.

(It should be noted that in Chapter 16 on manic disorders treatment with phenothiazines is preferred, whereas in this current chapter preference is given to lithium; also a more cautious policy on lithium blood levels is outlined in Chapter 16. This reflects a difference of opinion between the different authors of these two chapters. We feel that such differences of opinion are healthy at this stage of psychiatric development; each regimen, whether with lithium or a phenothiazine, has enough unsatisfactory features to make dogmatism unsound.)

During the acute manic phase a patient requires twice the lithium dosage of a patient on prophylactic maintenance. Medication is given orally three or four times a day. The effective dose range in the healthy young adult is from 1500 to 2500 mg. per day, ordinarily administered in six to twelve 330 mg. tablets. Blood levels should be measured every two or three days and dosage adjusted to achieve therapeutic serum lithium levels of 1.3 to 1.6 mEq/liter. Lithium's half life is prolonged in elderly patients, and hence lower serum doses are typically used with this population.

It is generally agreed that the risk of toxicity becomes high as blood levels approach 2 mEq/liter. However, it is not uncommon for patients (particularly the elderly) to become toxic and develop confusion at customary acute mania lithium blood levels (for example, 1.5 mEq/liter). Such patients generally exhibit excellent therapeutic results with lower dosage and lower blood levels. Because of individual differences in dosage tolerance, clinical judgement is required to balance therapeutic effects, toxicity and blood levels. Clinical signs are of particular importance in the evaluation of toxicity and the adjustment of blood levels. Because there is a considerable peaking of blood levels following an oral dose, it is customary to make blood determinations 10 hours after the last dose (for example, before the morning dose). Failure to do so may give distorted readings. After the acute manic episode subsides, the lithium dosage must be cut in half, to achieve a blood level of about 0.8 mEq/liter. Remission of the manic phase brings an alteration in the patient's tolerance, and failure to reduce the dosage may produce toxicity.

Prophylactic and Maintenance Regimens With Lithium. Lithium should be considered for prophylaxis in any patient with recurrent affective disorders. On a short-term basis, excellent evidence exists that lithium is effective in maintaining remission of acute manic attacks and, on a long-term basis, in preventing recurrent episodes of mania and depression. Chronic lithium therapy does not alter the normal range of emotion or impair mental status, and no long-term toxic effects have yet been demonstrated.

A more conservative strategy is warrented in building up lithium levels for maintenance and prophylactic measures. For maintenance lithium it is useful to start with 300 mg. of lithium administered thrice daily, giving a daily total of 900 mg.; blood levels should be monitored twice a week to permit dosage adjustment until levels of 0.8 to 0.9 mEq/liter are established. In a hypomanic patient, in no acute distress, one may start with 300 mg. of lithium orally three to five times a day, giving daily totals of 900 to 1500 mg.; the blood lithium level is measured two or three times a week until lithium blood levels of 1.0 to 1.4 mEq/liter are achieved. Thus there is no sharp distinction between the high dose and recommended blood levels for the acute, very sick manic (1.3 to 1.5 mEq/liter) and the hypomanic (1.0 to 1.4 mEq/liter), but rather a gradation. When the physician is not clinically pressed, a more conservative strategy is used.

Patients receiving maintenance lithium on an outpatient basis should have blood lithium level determinations on a monthly basis to detect gradual shifts in lithium tolerance and to remind the patient to continue medication. Patients and their families must be made familiar with the symptoms of serious lithium toxicity resulting from acute changes of lithium tolerance. These symptoms include gastrointestinal symptoms and signs of the onset of central nervous system dysfunction such as confusion, sluggishness, lethergy and drowsiness.

Use of Lithium in Acute Depressions and Schizophrenia. No consensus exists concerning the use of lithium as the initial treatment for acute depression. Since the evidence concerning the effectiveness in treating the depressive phase of bipolar depressive illness (a depression in a patient with a history of both manic and depressive disorders) is contradictory, this drug may be considered in cases of treatment resistant depression when other drugs and measures have failed.

Schizophrenic patients prove generally unresponsive to lithium and in some cases manifest severe neurotoxic reactions, characterized by worsening of the psychosis and aggravation of symptoms. Excited schizoaffective patients respond less well to lithium than do manics and some may develop toxic confusional states. When the diagnosis is unclear, a therapeutic trial can be useful. If the response is positive, lithium maintenance might be considered to prevent recurrent disease.

Side Effects and Toxicity of Lithium. When properly administered, lithium is a reasonably safe drug. In the absence of proper clinical and biochemical monitoring by physicians familiar with its toxic potentialities (this includes blood lithium level measurements at recommended intervals), however, lithium may pose potential clinical hazards.

Certain early side effects are common and usually subside within several days after treatment is initiated. Gastrointestinal symptoms are frequent and include stomach cramps, nausea, vomiting and diarrhea. These discomforts can usually be ameliorated by having the patient take the lithium with meals. Other early symptoms include thirst, frequent urination, fatigue, muscle weakness and slight mental confusion. A fine hand tremor which is not alleviated by antiparkinsonian drugs is common; patients can be reassured that the tremor is a usual side effect and not of serious import. Other side effects include weight gain and abnormalities in thyroid metabolism; a later complication may be goiter formation.

Manifestations which begin to indicate a more serious lithium toxic condition, and constitute reasons for discontinuing medication (while taking a final blood sample for a retrospective blood lithium level measurement), include continued vomiting and diarrhea, reappearance of anorexia, dysarthria, more severe signs of neuromuscular disorders such as twitching, and signs of central nervous system toxicity such as coarse tremor, confusion, choreiform movements, slurred speech, and ataxia.

Advanced states of lithium poisoning are

characterized by somnolence, confusion, increased deep tendon reflexes, seizures, impaired consciousness, fasciculations, nystagmus and markedly increased muscle tone with hyperextension of arms and legs. These symptoms are signs of a grave toxic state which can progress to deep coma and death.

This advanced toxic condition is managed by aminophylline, osmotic diuretics such as urea, sodium bicarbonate, and in severe cases, dialysis. Supportive therapy is important to prevent serious pulmonary complications and to regulate kindey functioning, respiration, blood pressure, electrolyte balance, and central venous pressure.

Precautions in the Employment of Lithuim. Relative contraindications for lithium include cardiovascular disease, kidney disease, low salt diets, concurrent use of diuretics, excess sweating, diarrhea, severe debilitation, brain damage and old age.

Lithium is rapidly absorbed from the gastrointestinal tract and quickly excreted by the kidneys. When salt intake is low more lithium is retained; thus, patients on low salt diets or diuretics, and those perspiring excessively tend to have toxic reactions.

Kidney functioning must be adequate to permit efficient lithium excretion. Pretreatment laboratory tests include blood urea nitrogen determination and a creatinine clearance test. However, a lithium excretion test is of particular value in evaluating kidney functioning; this involves timed monitoring of lithium disappearance from serum and its appearance in urine specimens. Particular care must be exercised with elderly patients who excrete lithium more slowly than younger patients, and so should be started on lower dosages. Chronic toxicity in elderly patients on maintenance therapy can be especially troublesome; these patients may gradually develop toxic confusional states that are falsely attributed to organic brain difficulties of old age.

Lithium may be used safely in conjunction with antipsychotic agents or with tricyclic or MAO inhibiting antidepressants.

Lithium should be administered to pregnant women only in unavoidable cases of severe clinical need. Although several limited studies indicate that lithium is probably safe in pregnancy, an extremely conservative approach is warranted until more definite information is available. Lithium occasionally appears to induce a goiter in a susceptible patient; the goiter disappears if lithium is discontinued or if thyroxine is added to the patient's regimen.

Miscellaneous Other Medications

Amphetamines. Amphetamines have a diffuse stimulating effect on the cerebral cortex in addition to their sympathomimetic actions, but psychiatrists differ much in opinion about their use in psychiatric practice. These drugs alleviate fatigue to a certain extent for brief daily spans of time, but they do not have any true antidepressant actions. Although amphetamines may give giddy sensations of well being to a small percentage of insecure people, they also make many patients restless and anxious and leave them with "letdown" feelings when their effects wear off.

Amphetamines have been extensively employed to reduce overactivity in hyperactive, distractible children; some of these children have demonstrable brain damage, whereas others do not, and both groups comprise the category labeled hyperkinetic reaction of childhood. The use of amphetamines in overactive children is based on the concept that these children are hyperactive and distractible because they cannot concentrate their attention on any task or object for more than a brief time. Some psychiatrists feel that amphetamines increase the alertness of these children and help them concentrate on tasks for longer periods of time. (This subject is discussed in greater detail in Chapters 18 and 25. The subject of amphetamine abuse and its consequences is covered in Chapters 13 and 19.)

Methylphenidate (Ritalin). This medication is a mild cerebral cortical stimulant similar to the amphetamines in its clinical actions. It has been much advocated as the drug of choice in hyperkinetic children and in children with gross organic brain damage with much restlessness. The comments under amphetamines, and the chapter references given there, also apply to methylphenidate.

Caffeine. Caffeine has been proposed in

recent years as a substitute for amphetamines and methylphenidate in treating hyperkinetic children and overactive children with gross organic brain damage. It also can be employed to relieve fatigue in grief reactions and other transitory emotional states in which fatigue is a problem. Caffeine can be given either by tablet or by having the patient drink strong coffee. Some psychiatrists feel that caffeine has clinical effects equal to those of amphetamines and methylphenidate without the side effects and hazards of those drugs. (This subject is covered in Chapter 18.)

Other Drugs. [The use of disulfiram (Antabuse) in the treatment of alcoholism is covered in Chapter 13, and the use of insulin in coma therapy for schizophrenia is outlined in Chapter 23. Flurothyl (Indoklon) convulsive therapy is considered in Chapter 23.]

BIBLIOGRAPHY

Appleton, W. S., and Davis, J. M.: Practical Clinical Psychopharmacology. New York, Medcom Press, 1973.

Casey, J. F., et al.: Combined drug therapy of chronic schizophrenics. Controlled evaluation of placebo, dextro-amphetamine, imipramine, isocarboxazid and trifluoperazine added to maintenance doses of chlorpromazine. Amer. J. Psychiat., *117*:997, 1961.

Cole, J. O.: Phenothiazine treatment in acute schizophrenia. Arch. Gen. Psychiat, *10*:246, 1964.

Curry, S. H. et al.: Chlorpromazine plasma levels and effects. Arch. Gen. Psychiat., *22*:289, 1970.

———, et al.: Factors affecting chlorpromazine plasma levels in psychiatric patients. Arch. Gen. Psychiat., *22*:209, 1970.

Goodman, L. S., and Gilman, A. Z.: The Pharmacological Basis of Therapeutics. ed. 4. New York, Macmillan, 1970.

Hogarty, G. E., and Goldberg, S. C.: Drugs and sociotherapy in the aftercare of schizophrenic patients. Arch. Gen. Psychiat., *28*:54, 1973.

Klein, D. F., and Davis, J. M.: Diagnosis and Drug Treatment of Psychiatric Disorders. Baltimore, Williams & Wilkins, 1969.

Leff, J., and Wing, J.: Trial of maintenance therapy in schizophrenia. Brit. Med. J., *2*: 599, 1971.

May, P. R. A.: Treatment of Schizophrenia. New York, Science House, 1968.

Prien, R. F., and Cole, J. O.: High dose chlorpromazine therapy in chronic schizophrenia. Arch. Gen. Psychiat., *18*:482, 1968.

23

Physical Methods of Treatment

The physical methods of treatment employed in psychiatry are (1) electroshock therapy, (2) insulin coma treatment and subcoma insulin treatment, (3) psychosurgery and (4) other technics such as hydrotherapy, inhalation convulsive therapy and others.

The use of all physical methods of treatment has declined greatly in recent years because of the antipsychotic and antidepressant medications, the skillful employment of interview treatment and the widespread use of therapeutic environment programs in psychiatric hospitals. Some of the physical methods listed above, such as psychosurgery, are now so rarely employed in American psychiatry that they are of only experimental or historical interest. The means by which physical therapies exert their action are highly speculative; both organic and psychological theories have been advanced, but none of these theories have been substantiated and none of them have achieved general aceptance.

ELECTROSHOCK THERAPY

Electroshock therapy was introduced in 1938 and during the 1940's became a widely used treatment in the United States. Its use has declined greatly since the middle 1950's because of the introduction of antipsychotic and antidepressant medications and improved technics in creating therapeutic environments in psychiatric hospitals. In my opinion, electroshock still has usefulness in selected patients, but I feel that the number of patients who merit this treatment has declined by 80 per cent or more in recent years.

The Technic of Electroshock Therapy

Electroshock therapy consists of inducing a generalized grand mal convulsion by passing a very small current of electricity for a brief period of time over the brain by means of two electrodes, one of which is placed on each temple. The patient lies on a treatment table or on the firmly supported mattress of a hospital bed. Any dentures or removable bridges are removed. A small pillow is placed under the lumbar section of his back and a small pillow roll is placed under his neck, thus arching the lower back and the neck slightly. The patient is then given an intravenous injection of about 150 mg. of thiopental (Pentothal) or some other short-acting barbiturate in 10 cc. of sterile water, and following this an injection of 20 to 40 mg. of succinylcholine (Anectine) is given from a separate syringe into the same intravenous needle. Atropine, 0.5 mg. is included in the syringe of thiopental, though many psychiatrists prefer to give the atropine as an intramuscular injection 30 minutes before the treatment. Immediately after the injections of thiopental and succinylcholine, a rubber mouthpiece is inserted into the patient's mouth.

The patient is asleep after the thiopental injection, and after the succinylcholine injection the physician waits about 40 seconds before giving the treatment. The action of the succinylcholine usually can be detected by small muscular fibrillations of the face at the time the succinylcholine takes effect. The psychiatrist then gives the treatment without delay.

A psychiatric nurse assistant places an electrode covered with electrolyte jelly on each temple, and two or three hospital aids firmly hold the patient's head, limbs and body against the treatment table. By dialing the appropriate knobs on the electroshock machine the psychiatrist gradually builds up the current of electricity, which passes over the brain during a 10-second period. As soon as the patient enters into the tonic phase of a grand mal convulsion during this 10-second period, the physician discontinues the current or switches it to a very low level. The tonic phase of the convulsion lasts several seconds and is followed by generalized clonic movements for 30 or 40 seconds more. If the thiopental anesthesia and the succinylcholine muscle relaxation have been adequate, the patient feels nothing during the treatment and the physical movements of the convulsion are very weak. Immediately upon conclusion of the treatment the physician administers positive pressure oxygen or air to the patient for two or three minutes through a face mask until the muscular paralysis due to succinylcholine disappears and the patient begins to breathe spontaneously. The patient usually sleeps for 20 to 30 minutes after the treatment and remains confused for half an hour more. During this time an attendant remains with him. An hour or more after the treatment, the patient arises and has his breakfast. Treatments are given in the morning when the patient has an empty stomach after an overnight fast. Treatments usually are given three times each week and a course usually runs between 6 and 12 treatments. The procedure in each treatment is the same.

The amount of current that passes over the brain varies from 300 to 1200 milliamperes at 70 to 130 volts. In earlier technics of electroshock therapy this full current was given for a period of from 0.1 to 0.5 seconds, but most psychiatrists today use electroshock machines that build the current up gradually over a 5 to 10 second period and then stop the current or decrease it rapidly as soon as the tonic phase begins. The thiopental anesthesia is given because without it the patient may be aware of pain in the temples and other unpleasant sensations during the initial passage of current until the convulsion begins. The atropine is given to decrease bronchial and tracheal secretions during the period of thiopental anesthesia; it reduces the chance of respiratory embarrassment due to excessive secretions. The succinylcholine weakens the muscular contractions during the treatment. Without weakening of muscular contractions there is a several per cent incidence of fractures of the vertebrae and long bones during the convulsive movements of the treatment. The arching of the back and neck and the firm holding of the body during the treatment further reduce the chances of fractures or dislocations, and the rubber mouthpiece prevents biting of the tongue or lips during the treatment and helps to secure an adequate airway.

As in all medical procedures, there are differences among physicians in treatment details, but the treatment outlined here is the most widely used form of electroshock therapy. Electroshock therapy should be given only by an experienced psychiatrist, and some psychiatrists have an anesthetist in attendance to handle the thiopental anesthesia, the succinylcholine administration and the positive pressure respiration of the patient.

Indications and Results

Electroshock therapy may be useful in selected severe depressions, schizophrenic disorders and manic psychoses that have proved resistant to other forms of therapy.

In severe depressions a course of between 6 and 12 electroshock treatments resolves the depression in about 80 per cent or more of patients. Occasionally, a course of electroshock therapy will go as high as 20 treatments, but if extensive improvement has not occurred by the 12th treatment, the chance that electroshock will help the depressed patient is greatly reduced. However, since antidepressant medication resolves severe depressions in 60 to 70 per cent of cases, is simpler to administer, and does not produce memory loss so common with electroshock therapy, most psychiatrists first put the patient on a trial of antidepressant medication and reserve electroshock therapy for those cases that do not respond to antidepressant medication. Antidepressant medication is less likely to be effective if a patient with a severe depression has bizarre delusions; this type of patient has a greater likelihood of requiring electroshock therapy. If a patient is highly suicidal, even in a psychiatric hospital setting, some psychiatrists feel electroshock should be started at once rather than waiting to see if antidepressant medication will work. Some psychiatrists give electroshock therapy and antidepressant medication simultaneously in highly suicidal patients. The treatments usually are given on alternate days three times each week.

Electroshock therapy is employed in schizophrenic disorders, but its use has declined greatly since the introduction of the phenothiazine antipyschotic medications. Electroshock therapy is most likely to be useful when the schizophrenic psychosis is of recent origin and has erupted floridly in a patient who previously seemed to be making a fairly good interpersonal adjustment; however, these are the same patients who usually recover on antipsychotic medications. Electroshock therapy is less likely to help a schizophrenic whose psychosis has come on gradually over a long period and whose prepsychotic personality was characterized by seclusiveness and a poor interpersonal adjustment.

Most psychiatrists begin the treatment of a schizophrenic with a phenothiazine, supportive interview work and hospital programs that encourage the patient's emergence from his psychotic shell and his integration into group interpersonal activities. They hold electroshock therapy in reserve until an ample trial of phenothiazine medication, or other antipsychotic medication, and interpersonal work has been used. The number of electroshock treatments and their frequency is about the same as in severe depression, but with schizophrenic patients there is a greater tendency to carry the total number of treatments to about 20 if results are not apparent earlier.

The majority of patients with manic psychoses recover with phenothiazine antipsychotic medications, or lithium therapy, and hospital interpersonal regimens. However, a small number of manic patients recover more quickly if given electroshock therapy in addition to phenothiazines and interpersonal regimens. A few manic patients are resistant to all types of medication, but recover with 6 to 12 electroshock treatments.

Electroshock therapy is given mainly to hospitalized patients. However, some psychiatrists give the last few treatments of a course of electroshock therapy on an outpatient basis if the patient has improved a good deal during the early part of a treatment course in the hospital. For outpatient electroshock therapy the patient must have cooperative, well-instructed relatives to bring him to and from the hospital and to be with him at home. The patient usually has sufficient memory defects at the end of a course of treatment to necessitate staying around his home for two or three weeks after the last treatment until these memory defects disappear. On the morning of an outpatient electroshock treatment, the patient needs a relative by him the entire morning to help him with any postshock confusion. Outpatient electroshock treatment has decreased greatly in recent years.

Side Effects and Complications

Side Effects. Most patients who receive electroshock treatment have spotty memory defects after four or five treatments. In general, the amount of memory difficulty increases as the number of treatments increases, but there is considerable variation among patients. The patient's memory difficulties tend to be for events of recent days or weeks, as opposed to things which happened months or years ago. The memory defects resulting from short courses of six to eight treatments disappear two to three weeks after the last treatment. However, the patient may have permanent spotty losses of memory for some events that occurred during the two to three week period during which he was receiving the treatment, and for the one or two week period preceding the treatment and following it. In longer courses of electroshock treatment, especially when the course goes over 10 or 12 treatments, the memory loss may be greater and the patient may remember little of his hospital stay or of the events of the month preceding the onset of the electroshock treatment or the month following it. In rare instances the retrograde amnesia may cover some events up to several months before the onset of treatment.

The patient's memory for all events that occur two or three weeks after the last treatment is not impaired. The memory defects of electroshock treatment are benign. The psychiatrist should inform the patient and his relatives of the likelihood of their occurrence before they begin, and he should emphasize that memory defects are a harmless side effect of treatment. He also should emphasize that the object of treatment is not to produce memory defects, but that they are an inconvenience that often accompanies it.

Headaches occasionally occur for a few hours following a treatment, and mild muscle soreness in the arms, legs, neck and trunk at times are present. In a small number of cases a patient gets mild first degree burns over the sites of the electrodes, but this can be handled by appropriate soothing salves and by slight variations of the positions of the electrodes on the skin of the temples from one treatment to another. A certain amount of intellectual confusion usually follows an electroshock treatment for an hour or two, but rarely lasts longer. Other side effects from electroshock treatment are uncommon when effective thiopental and succinylcholine preshock medication is given.

Complications. Before the introduction of succinylcholine, fractures and dislocations of the long bones occurred in about 3 per cent of patients receiving electroshock treatment, and compression fractures of the thoracic vertebrae occurred in a considerably greater percentage of patients; dislocations of the jaw occurred occasionally. These fractures were produced by the initial strong muscular contractions of the convulsion. Adequate muscle relaxation with succinylcholine has made such fractures rare; they happen now only when succinylcholine is by error injected outside the vein and the treatment is given without realizing that this has occurred.

Pulmonary complications of electroshock treatment are infrequent. Laryngospasm is an uncommon complication of thiopental anesthesia, but it usually is brief and is eliminated by the subsequent succinylcholine relxation, though tracheal intubation equipment should be available for the extremely rare instances in which persistent laryngospasm occurs. The atropine given before the treatment reduces respiratory tract secretions, and respiratory embarrassment due to excessive secretions is rare. Prolonged respiratory apnea, independent of succinylcholine muscle relxation, has been reported on rare occasions, but can be handled by positive pressure respiration until spontaneous breathing begins again. The only pulmonary complication that occurs with any frequency with modern technics of electroshock therapy is prolonged paralysis of the respiratory muscles after succinylcholine. Some patients are especially sensitive to succinylcholine and have prolonged muscular paralysis after its use. When this occurs, the patient is maintained on positive pressure respiration until spontaneous breathing returns, and there is no harm to the patient. I recall a patient who did not breath on her own for 25 minutes following an electroshock treatment with 30 mg. of succinylcholine. During this period of time the nursing Sister's rosary was in continual use. At the end of 25 minutes everyone, including the patient, began to breathe more easily.

Cardiac complications from electroshock therapy are very rare. Myocardial infarction occurs so infrequently during electroshock treatment that when it happens its relationship is probably coincidental. Patients with impaired myocardial blood supply should be given oxygen just before and immediately after the treatment, and with this precaution usually tolerate electroshock well. Electroshock therapy should be deferred in a patient with cardiac decompensation until the patient is well compensated; such patients then usually tolerate electroshock therapy well. A very rare but serious complication of electroshock therapy is cardiac arrest, presumably due to ventricular fibrillation precipitated by the treatment. Awareness of this rare but possible complication and vigorous prompt use of cardiac resuscitation measures often resolves it. Actually, the thiopental anesthesia is probably more prominent than the electroshock therapy in causing these rare cardiac complications, for the physical exertion during electroshock of a patient who has been well relaxed with succinylcholine is no more than the exertion of getting in and out of bed.

A rare complication of electroshock therapy is the precipitation of a delusional, hallucinatory state in a patient who previously had showed depression without delusional features. Some psychiatrists feel these states are schizophrenic syndromes unmasked by removing an overlying depression. Other psychiatrists, including myself, feel they are organic confusional states. They characteristically begin after several electroshock treatments or several days after completion of a course of electroshock therapy. They last about one or two weeks and recede spontaneously if the patient is given no further electroshock treatment after the delusional symptoms begin.

Contraindications

The routine work-up for a patient who is to receive electroshock treatment should include a general physical examination, a chest x ray and an electrocardiogram. The psychiatrist should know the physical condition of the patient, and any coexisting diseases should be cared for as part of the patient's total management. However, with adequate succinylcholine muscle relaxation and other precautions, there are few contraindications to electroshock therapy.

Although antipsychotic or antidepressant medications usually offer a viable alternate course of treatment when electroshock would involve risks due to concomitant diseases, cases still are seen occasionally when electroshock is considered in a patient with cardiac disease, pulmonary disease, orthopedic problems or other types of physical difficulty. Patients with cardiac decompensation should be compensated before administering electroshock treatment, and electroshock treatment should be deferred several weeks in a patient with a recent myocardial infarction. Patients with impaired cardiac circulation should receive oxygen just before and immediately after a treatment. If a patient with cardiac illness is physically agitated and uncooperative in his medical care because of his psychosis, the cardiac risk from electroshock may be less than the risk from continued psychotic, agitated behavior.

Advanced age is not a contraindication to electroshock therapy, but elderly patients should have careful physical evaluation before receiving it. Electroshock therapy should be deferred in patients with recent fractures, but with adequate succinylcholine relaxation the risk is slight once the healing process is established. Compression fractures of the thoracic vertebrae usually are not considered a contraindication to further electroshock therapy. Active pulmonary tuberculosis causes the psychiatrist to hesitate to give electroshock treatment, but an agitated, psychotic tuberculous patient may have less risk from electroshock therapy than from continued agitation and poor cooperation in his care. Myasthenia gravis is an absolute contraindication to the use of succinylcholine, but the coexistence of psychosis requiring electroshock and myasthenia gravis is immensely rare.

Mode of Action

Both organic and psychological theories have been suggested to explain electroshock therapy, but none of them have been substantiated or generally accepted. Some psychiatrists believe that electroshock therapy causes an alteration of brain physiology, which allows a patient with a psychosis of recent origin to reintegrate his behavior on his former level of better adjustment. Other psychiatrists have suggested that electroshock therapy induces a brief regression to more primitive emotional levels, and out of this experience the patient emerges and readjusts in a better way. However, these theories are merely vague speculations about a form of treatment employed because of its clinical usefulness but whose mode of action is unknown.

INSULIN COMA THERAPY

Insulin coma therapy, which was widely used for schizophrenia from the early 1930's to the early 1950's, has now been abandoned by most psychiatrists. However, a few psychiatrists still advocate it for selected schizophrenics, especially those who have proved resistant to other forms of therapy, and we shall therefore outline its essential details.

The patient who receives insulin coma therapy must be in good physical health, because the treatment is physically strenuous and serious complications may occur in up to 15 per cent of patients treated. The treatments begin at about 7 o'clock in the morning and are given five or six days each week. Insulin coma treatment is given only to hospitalized patients and its use is restricted to schizophrenics. The insulin injections begin with 5 or 10 units the first morning and increase by increments of 10 or 20 units each day until the dose is reached which induces deep comas. The dose necessary for coma usually is between 80 and 200 units, but it may run considerably higher than that.

The insulin coma reaction is traditionally divided into five stages. In Stage I suppression of cortical and cerebellar functions begins, with drowsiness and muscular flaccidity. In Stage II deeper suppression of cortical and cerebellar functions occurs with clouding of consciousness and muscular restlessness or excitement. Stage III is characterized by release of the basal ganglia and hypothalamic centers from higher cortical control, and the patient loses consciousness, has various kinds of uncontrolled physical movements and shows signs of marked autonomic nervous system activity. In Stage IV the midbrain and upper medullary centers are released from higher control and the patient is in continually deepening coma. In Stage V the lower medullary centers are released from higher control and the patient is in profound coma with depression of tendon reflexes and muscular flaccidity.

The time required for the patient to reach Stage III is usually about two hours after the insulin injection, and most workers consider one hour of deep coma in Stage III or Stage IV as the therapeutic goal of each treatment. Each coma is terminated by the injection of glucagon hydrochloride (Glucagon), or by the intravenous injection of a glucose solution, or by the administration of a saturated sugar solution by gavage tube. High carbohydrate feedings are given as soon as the patient is sufficiently awake to drink and eat. A full course of classical insulin coma therapy usually consists of 50 comas, but at present it may run from 30 to 40. Insulin coma therapy requires the constant attendance of a psychiatrist who has experience with this type of treatment and a well-trained team of nurses and aids. Though various physiological and psychological theories have been suggested to explain the action of insulin coma therapy, none of them have been substantiated or widely accepted.

Insulin coma treatment has various risks. The mortality rate of the treatment is about one per cent of the patients treated, and the incidence of serious complications runs as high as 15 per cent in some series of cases. Among the various complications are prolonged coma lasting from several hours to one or two days, edema of the lungs and upper respiratory tract, vascular collapse, delayed hypoglycemic reactions several hours after termination of the treatment, lung abscesses from aspiration of regurgitated food or gavage material, convulsions and other problems.

The results of insulin coma therapy are not outstanding; they are much inferior to treatment with antipsychotic medications, or antipscychotic medications combined with electroshock therapy, especially when they are carried out in a setting where the hospital therapeutic environment also encourages recovery. In the late 1940's and early 1950's I did a great deal of insulin coma therapy (for six months I ran a ward where 50 patients were receiving it daily), and, when the selection of patients for this therapy was taken into account I was skeptical that the results were much better than the natural course of the disease process. Moreover, the technical difficulties of the administration of insulin coma therapy, its dangers, its long duration and the necessity for experienced personnel in its administration limit its usefulness.

Subcoma insulin therapy consists of giving hospitalized patients injections of 10 to 40 units of insulin each morning as a relaxation procedure. It is used for anxiety neuroses and other neurotic states. The patient never progresses beyond mild drowsiness and the treatment is terminated by having the patient drink a sweet beverage such as orange juice with added sugar. This treatment is not widely used. Most psychiatrists feel that any improvement in the patient is due to other aspects of his hospital experience and not to the subcoma insulin therapy.

PSYCHOSURGERY

Lobotomy, the best known form of psychosurgery, was introduced in the middle 1930's and attracted much attention in the following years. In a lobotomy, the fibers which connect the anterior parts of the frontal lobes with the thalamus were cut through bilateral burr holes cut in the frontal, superior part of the skull. A sharp, narrow instrument called a leukotome was introduced through each burr rhole, and the fibers connecting the anterior parts of the frontal lobes and the thalamus were cut by lateral and medial sweeping movements of the instrument. This operation continued to be the focus of much controversy until the early 1950's. Since then, interest in this procedure, and in all forms of psychosurgery, has declined rapidly. Except for some experimental interest, all forms of psychosurgery have been virtually abandoned in the United States; a small amount of sporadic work has continued on it in Europe and other parts of the world.

Lobotomy was based on the theory that the connections of the anterior parts of the frontal cortex and the thalamus play a large role in the emotional responses of a person to his interpersonal problems. However, the operation was essentially empirical and was based originally on the placid behavior of monkeys who had had similar procedures performed. Lobotomy was used in psychiatric patients to decrease agitation and anxiety in severe agitated depressions, agitated schizophrenic disorders, severe obsessive compulsive neuroses and other psychiatric conditions. The terms lobotomy, prefrontal lobotomy and leukotomy were used interchangeably.

Lobotomy was the subject of much controversy. Many psychiatrists cringed at the idea of destroying brain tissue as a means of solving personality problems. Moreover, the results of the operation were poor. Immediately following the procedure, the patients were confused and over a period of several weeks or more had to be retrained for toilet care, personal hygiene and socially acceptable behavior. They did not reach a persistent level of postoperative adjustment until six months to a year after the operation. Though many of the patients were less anxious and less agitated after the procedure, they usually lost their capacities for the more refined aspects of social and economic responsibility and they lacked the capacity for warm, understanding relationships with people. Often they were boisterous, uninhibited and easily angered; however, other lobotomized patients whom I saw in the late 1940's could, at best, be described as grinning vegetables.

Transorbital lobotomy was a modified lobotomy technic in which a sharp instrument of small diameter was inserted into the superior conjunctival sac of the eye and was firmly shoved upward through the thin supraorbital bone plate into the inferior part of the frontal lobe. The instrument was then swept medially and laterally cutting the fibers which connect the anterior parts of the frontal lobes and the thalamus. Transorbital lobotomy usually produced less striking results than lobotomy performed through burr holes, both in degree of placidity obtained and the amount of undesirable personality changes.

Lobotomy stimulated interest in neurosurgical procedures in which various areas of the frontal cortex were removed or undercut. These technics were called topectomy or gyrectomy, depending on the amount of brain tissue involved. Later workers experimented with ultrasonotomy, in which high frequency sound waves were used to destroy small areas of frontal lobe tissue. Both the short-term and long-term results of these operations have been poor, and except for some lingering experimental interest they have been abandoned.

OTHER PHYSICAL METHODS OF TREATMENT

Physiotherapy and *hydrotherapy* are time-honored technics for assuaging anxiousness and reducing emotionally caused muscle tension. Though the precise manner in which they work to relieve tension is not well understood, they help many patients. Physiotherapy and hydrotherapy probably operate through rhythmic muscular movements, increased skin and deep tissue vascularity and a large measure of suggestion. Although these forms of treatment are much less employed today than in former times, they still are useful measures to relieve tension while the patient is working in interview treatment to resolve his emotional problems. The nonmedical practitioners know the value of physiotherapy well and some of their cults have made an entire therapeutic practice of it.

A common form of physiotherapy is hand massage of the large muscle groups of the back, neck and limbs. The patient can do this at home with a small vibrator strapped to his hand. Some physicians advocate relaxation technics in which the patient lies or sits in relaxed positions while concentrating on progressive loosening of specific muscle groups one after another. The physiotherapy departments of some hospitals have special vibratory and massage devices to encourage muscle relaxation.

Hydrotherapy formerly was used widely in psychiatric hospitals to decrease agitation and relieve anxiety. The continuous lukewarm tub bath and other kinds of water baths and sprays were employed. Although these procedures are employed infrequently now, some psychiatrists feel that they still have a place in the management of some agitated or overactive hospitalized patients. For office patients, a continuous warm tub bath can be devised at home by filling a bathtub with lukewarm water and allowing a constant inflow of water from the faucet and a slow outflow through the overflow opening of the tub. The lukewarm tub bath may occasionally be useful for the outpatient who needs something he can do at times when he is especially anxious; hydrotherapy often is a sounder procedure than increasing the dosage, or changing the prescription, of antianxiety medication each time the patient or his relatives telephone the physician.

In *inhalation convulsive therapy* a convulsive seizure is induced by having the patient breath flurothyl (Indoklon) gas. Between 0.5 and 1 ml. of flurothyl is placed in a vaporizer, which is connected on one side to a five-liter oxygen bag and on the other side to an anesthetic face mask. A positive pressure inhalation is given every five seconds until a seizure occurs; this usually happens in about 40 seconds. The procedure is preceded by atropine and intravenous barbiturate and succinylcholine administration, in the same manner employed in electroshock therapy. The other routine measures preceding an electroshock treatment are similarly carried out. The proponents of this form of convulsive therapy feel that the results are equal to those obtained with electroshock therapy and that the patients have a less postconvulsive confusion. However, most psychiatrists who use convulsive therapy prefer electroshock therapy and inhalation convulsive therapy is not widely used.

Continuous sleep therapy is rarely used in the United States, but is sometimes employed in Europe and other places. It is also called hibernation therapy. The patient is kept asleep, or in a semisomnolent state for 10 days or so, by intramuscular or oral administration of sedatives, or antianxiety medications, or antipsychotic medications in large doses. It has been employed for a wide variety of disorders, but there is no evidence that the results are better than the natural course of the conditions being treated. It has various dangers; patients may develop deliriums with visual hallucinations and gross confusion, and pneumonia and other complications may occur. While on a foreign tour I observed patients who, in my opinion, became demonstrably worse because of this treatment; they emerged from it in puzzled, frightened states.

BIBLIOGRAPHY

Abrams, R., and Taylor, M. A.: Anterior bifrontal ECT: a clinical trial. Brit. J. Psychiatry, *122*: 587, 1973.

Bridges, P. K., Gortepe, E. O., and Maratos, J.: A comparative review of patients with obsessional neurosis and depression treated by psychosurgery. Brit. J. Psychiatry, *123*:663, 1973.

Frankel, B. L.: Research on cerebral electrotherapy (electrosleep). Am. J. Psychiatry, *131*: 95, 1974.

Kalinowsky, L. B., and Hippius, H.: Pharmacological, Convulsive and Other Somatic Treatments in Psychiatry. New York, Grune & Stratton, 1969.

Kelly, D., et al.: Stereotactic limbic leucotomy: a preliminary report on forty patients. Brit. J. Psychiatry, *123*:141, 1973.

Murillo, L. G., and Exner, J. E., Jr.: The effects of regressive ECT with process schizophrenia. Am. J. Psychiatry, *130*:269, 1973.

Philpott, W. H.: Sedac treatment, post sedac, response interference and electric shock. Dis. Nerv. Syst., *34*:105, 1973.

Pitts, F. N.: Medical aspects of ECT. Sem. in Psychiatry, *4*: 27, 1972.

Sargant, W., Slater, E., and Kelly, D.: An Introduction to Phsycial Methods of Treatment in Psychiatry. New York, Jason Aronson, 1973.

Weinstein, M. R., and Fischer, A.: Combined treatment with ECT and antipsychotic drugs in schizophrenia. Dis. Nerv. Syst., *32*:801, 1971.

Wells, D. A.: Electroconvulsive treatment for schizophrenia. Compr. Psychiatry, *14*:291, 1973.

24

Special Technics in Child and Adolescent Psychiatry

Child and adolescent psychiatry occupies an important place in the total spectrum of psychiatric services. The treatment of the emotional problems of children is one of the most hopeful avenues for preventing psychiatric problems during adult life. Moreover, a period of experience in child psychiatry is valuable in the residential training of psychiatrists and other mental health professional workers, since in child psychiatry they can see how the origins of later emotional problems arise from unhealthy interpersonal relationships during the formative years of childhood and early adolescence. In addition, the special technics of child psychiatry offer opportunities for research into the interpersonal roots of many kinds of psychiatric disorders.

The evaluation and treatment of emotional problems of children and adolescents require special technics. We shall divide our discussion of these technics into (1) the child guidance clinic approach to the emotional problems of children and adolescents, (2) special technics of treatment in child and adolescent psychiatry, and (3) other treatment services for children and adolescents.

THE CHILD GUIDANCE CLINIC APPROACH TO THE EMOTIONAL PROBLEMS OF CHILDREN AND ADOLESCENTS

The conventional model for treatment in child psychiatry is the child guidance clinic team. The child guidance clinic professional team consists of psychiatrists, clinical psychologists and psychiatric social workers who are organized in a closely knit group to work diagnostically and therapeutically with children and their parents; psychiatric nurses and other mental health professionals are integrated into some child guidance clinic teams. Their approach is to study the child or adolescent and his family to understand the unhealthy interpersonal relationships that have produced the child's emotional problems. In treatment they work with both the child and his parents to resolve the emotional difficulties of the child and his home. A child guidance clinic may have from several to a dozen professional persons, depending on the aims of the clinic, the scope of its services and its financing.

Each member of the child guidance clinic team has special training and functions. Although the psychiatrist is often the clinic's administrative head, all the professional members of the clinic work as colleagues of equal standing. The psychiatrist usually has some administrative responsibilities as well as his diagnostic and therapeutic work with children and parents. In addition to his regular residency in psychiatry, the psychiatrist has had special training in child psychiatry, and often he has certification from the specialty board of child psychiatry in addition to board certification in general psychiatry.

The clinical psychologist administers psychological tests to children and adolescents to evaluate their emotional difficulties and personality structures, and he also may use psychological tests to examine parents. In addition, the psychologist does a fair amount of psychotherapy as a member of the clinic's treatment team, both with parents and with children. The clinical psychologist has either his master's degree or his doctorate in clinical psychology, and he also has had special training in child guidance work.

The psychiatric social worker in a child guidance clinic spends a great deal of his (or her) time in diagnostic interviewing and therapeutic work with parents. He traditionally interviews the parents in their first visit to the clinic to define the kind of problem for which the family is seeking help. The psychiatric social worker, depending on his interests, also may do a fair amount of psychotherapy with children and adolescents as a collaborative member of therapeutic teams. In addition to his master's degree or doctorate in social work, the psychiatric social worker has had special training in child guidance technics.

In some child guidance clinics psychiatric nurses with advanced training in child psychiatry work as members of the clinic team. In a few clinics educators, sociologists and other professional persons with particular interest in children and adolescents participate, both as a learning experience and in the evaluation of patients. Because of the special usefulness of child guidance clinics in training mental health personnel in understanding the interpersonal origins of psychiatric problems, a child guidance clinic often has a few psychiatric residents, student psychologists, student social workers, psychiatric nurses in training for work with children and adolescents, and other mental health professionals working for several-month periods under the supervision of the permanent staff.

Evaluation of a Child or Adolescent and His Parents in a Child Guidance Clinic

When a parent calls a child guidance clinic for an appointment, the call usually is referred to a social worker who spends a few minutes on the telephone obtaining some information about the kind of problem involved, basic information about the family and the name of the physician or other person who referred the family to the clinic. The social worker makes an appointment to see the mother and often suggests that the father come with her if it is convenient for him to do so. In the first interview, which lasts about 50 minutes, the social worker outlines the nature and history of the problem of the child or adolescent, and he seeks information about the interpersonal relationships of the home. He tries to get a brief sketch of the child, his difficulties and his interpersonal world; to complete this information he may schedule a second interview with either parent.

Several days later the social worker presents a short summary of his information to the entire clinic staff at the weekly case intake conference. The case is discussed briefly, and the further workup is planned and specific clinic members are assigned to carry it out. One of the clinical psychologists arranges to do psychological testing on the child, and the psychiatrist makes plans to see the child after the results of psychological testing are known. The social worker may interview one or both parents again to get more information. In some instances, the psychiatrist also interviews the parents to get firsthand information about them.

Although this elaborate workup is primarily diagnostic, it often has therapeutic effects. As parents systematically explore their interactions with their children, and between themselves, they often begin to see some of the unhealthy things that are going on in their homes.

Since children have less ability than adults to put their problems and feelings into words, and early interviews with anxious or rebellious adolescents often give limited information, testing by the clinical psychologist offers special help in understanding the child. The psychologist observes the behavior, the attitudes and the conversation of the child while he is examining him. Although the psychologist routinely administers an intelligence test, his main concern is to evaluate the child's emotional problems and personality structure. He usually administers the Rorschach test, the Thematic Appercention test and a couple of the other personality tests (described in Chapter 5). After scoring these tests he draws his data together into a comprehensive report describing the child's emotional functioning and personality structure.

In his examination of children, the psychiatrist uses different interview technics with children of various age groups. He usually employs a playroom examination technic with children up to the age of 10 or so. In the playroom there are toy cars, modeling clay, a chalkboard, chalk, building blocks, toy airplanes, crayons, drawing paper, dolls, a doll house and other commonly used play materials. The psychiatrist observes the child while he plays and talks with him, or they may engage in some simple games together. The psychiatrist observes what kind of relationship the child establishes with him, and he notes the child's emotional reactions and attitudes. He also may get some ideas about the child's personality structure by the way he handles the play materials; for example, the child may be careless and destructive in his play, or explosively hostile, or timid and restrained, or anxiously meticulous and precise. When interviewing older children the psychiatrist may rely more on conventional interview technics while engaging in some kind of routine game (tossing a baseball back and forth, Chinese checkers and others) with the child. Interviews with adolescents usually are entirely verbal and take place in the psychiatrist's regular office, though the approach is much more informal and casual than with adults; frequently the interview flows better if the examiner and the adolescent have a cola drink or a snack while it is going on.

The diagnostic workup to this point totals six or seven hours of interview time with the child or adolescent and his parents. Each of the three examiners summarizes his material in the child's case folder, and the clinic team is now ready for a joint conference to formulate their opinions about the child's problems, its causes and the treatment that will be needed to help him and his parents. This formulation occurs at the weekly case conference attended by all members of the clinic staff. Each of the staff members who has examined the child or his parents presents his material and impressions. In the general discussion of the case which follows, all members are free to express their opinions about the child's problems and the unhealthy interpersonal relationships which have produced them. Under the general chairmanship of the psychiatrist, treatment plans are made and prognostic expectations are discussed. A treatment plan is formulated, and two or three members of the clinic team are assigned to carry it out.

The Treatment Approach of a Child Guidance Clinic

The treatment methods of a child guidance clinic are based on the principle that resolution of the emotional problems of a child or adolescent requires that both the child and one or both parents are involved in the treatment. The child's problems have been produced by unhealthy intimate interpersonal relationships in his life, and in almost all instances he is still living in the same environment in which his problems arose. Hence, it is of little value to treat the child individually and to leave him in an unchanged interpersonal environment which continues to produce emotional turmoil and personality problems in him.

As a rule, one parent (usually the mother, but not always) brings the child once each week to the clinic, and the total treatment period extends from several months to a year or two. One of the clinic's staff members sees the child in a 50-minute treatment session, and at the same time another member of the clinic staff has a treatment session with the mother. For example, a psychiatrist may see the child in a therapeutic session while one of the clinic's social workers interviews the mother, or one of the clinic's psychologists may see the child in therapy while the mother is seen by one of the clinic's psychiatrists. In many instances, the child's father also is involved in treatment; he may come on alternate visits to be seen jointly with the mother, or he may be seen individually. In some cases, the parents come for group therapy sessions in the late afternoon or evening when both fathers and mothers can come, and the child is brought for his treatment sessions in the morning or afternoon on another day of the week. The possible variations of therapeutic plans are many, but they are all based on the principle that effective treatment requires involvement of both the child or adolescent and his parents.

The type of treatment of the child or adolescent and his parents varies much from case to case depending on the age of the child and the personality structures of the parents. In many instances, the child is engaged in psychotherapy while counseling is carried out with the parents to help them change some emotionally unhealthy attitudes and activities in the home. In other cases, the personality problems of one or both parents are so marked that one of them, or both of them, must be engaged in meaningful psychotherapy to resolve some of their basic emotional difficulties which produce damaging attitudes and actions toward the child. In problems with adolescents, the adolescent often is seen in individual therapy and his parents attend group therapy sessions with the parents of other adolescents to discuss their problems with their sons and daughters. The treatment plan is adapted to fit the needs of each individual case.

The individual therapists involved in a case have periodic conferences to exchange data and correlate their treatment efforts. Many cases also are reviewed periodically at a weekly case review conference which is open to all members of the clinic. The details of treatment technics, such as play therapy, group therapy and others, are discussed later in this chapter.

The case load of a child guidance clinic includes the full range of emotional problems of children and adolescents. It embraces neurotic disorders, situational adjustment problems, behavior disorders, some psychosomatic problems and selected disorders of learning and speech which require psychiatric treatment. The clinic also serves as a center for the evaluation and management of adjustment problems of children and adolescents with mental retardation and organic brain damage, and the clinic staff may manage a few psychotic children on an outpatient basis. Psychotic adolescents over the age of about 14 are usually treated on adult psychiatric wards, but large hospitals may have special divisions for severely disturbed adolescents.

Because of the expense involved in the extensive amounts of time spent with the child or adolescent and his parents in child guidance clinic work, most child guidance clinics are sponsored by a civic group, a philanthropic organization, a medical school or a large hospital center which subsidizes the cost, in addition to fees paid by the patients. A child guidance clinic often provides consultation services to juvenile courts, child welfare agencies, family and children's service agencies and other groups that deal with children.

An important function of a child guidance clinic is to train psychiatrists, clinical psychologists, psychiatric nurses, psychiatric social workers and, occasionally, other mental health professional workers, regardless of the type of work they will do in the future. A child guidance clinic offers a unique opportunity to study psychiatric problems in the process of being created; the causative interpersonal relationships can be directly scrutinized. Many psychiatrists feel that ample experience in a child guidance clinic is an essential part of the training of all mental health professionals.

SPECIAL TECHNICS OF TREATMENT IN CHILD AND ADOLESCENT PSYCHIATRY

The main method of treatment in child psychiatry is psychotherapy; except for some specific problems (such as amphetamine drugs, or caffeine, in hyperactive children and imipramine in enuresis) medications are of little value. Psychotherapy in child psychiatry includes the various technics of (1) play therapy with children in a playroom setting, (2) direct verbal psychotherapy with older children, adolescents and parents, (3) group psychotherapy, both for children and for parents and (4) the treatment of multiple family members in the same session, which is termed family therapy.

Play Therapy

Play therapy was developed as a special technic in child psychiatry to meet the difficulties of communication with children up to the age of 10 or 11. In play therapy a playroom setting is used as the basis for communicating with the child. Games and toys are employed as avenues of interaction between the child and the therapist.

Special rooms for play therapy are organized in a child guidance clinic. The playroom contains a chalkboard, colored chalk, drawing paper, crayons, dolls, a doll house, building blocks, cars, airplanes, molding clay and various other materials. Games such as checkers and simple games played on playing boards are available for use with older children who feel uncomfortable playing with toys. Play therapy sessions last about 50 minutes each and usually are scheduled once a week. In the final stages of therapy, the sessions may be spaced at intervals of two or three weeks.

The two aspects of therapy the therapist can work with and interpret are (1) the nature of the interpersonal relationship which the child establishes with the therapist during play sessions and (2) the things the child does with the play materials and toys.

The therapist observes the type of relationship the child establishes with him; he notes whether the child is outgoing or withdrawn, passive or aggressive, defiant or anxious to please, fearful or self-confident. As treatment proceeds, the therapist begins to interpret the child's feelings and to work through the interpersonal difficulties of the child as they appear in the child-therapist relationship. For example, the therapist may indicate to a defiant, aggressive child that he can understand that the child is testing him by his provocative behavior to see if the therapist really likes him, or if the therapist is going to lash back at him the way the child feels everyone will do who has prolonged interpersonal contact with him. The therapist later may point out that the child does not have to fear interpersonal closeness and prevent it by fighting with everyone. In another case, the therapist may indicate to a frightened, shy child that he hopes the child will learn through the child-therapist relationship that close relationships with people need not be painful.

Toys and other play materials also may be used as an avenue of therapeutic communication with the child. For example, in a frequently used kind of play therapy the therapist sets up in the doll house a family identical to the child's family. The therapist then invites the child to show what happens in the daily lives of the members of the doll family. As the child plays out the activities of the mother doll, the father doll and the children dolls, the therapist makes interpretations about how the child feels about the various situations that arise. The child often portrays many emotionally stressful relationships which occur in his own life as he carries out doll play. From the therapist's knowledge of the child's emotional problems through the diagnostic workup, he can comment on the child's doll play in the same way he would comment on the verbal material of an adult. For example, a small girl may show the parents giving special favors to a little boy doll and harshly criticizing the little girl doll in the family. She may be portraying situations in her own family, and the therapist can verbalize the little girl doll's feelings of rejection and anger; he can then relate the doll play material to the patient's emotional conflicts and interpersonal stresses.

Finger paints often are useful in play therapy with inhibited, overly meticulous children. By his enthusiastic participation in sloshing designs and pictures on paper, the therapist helps the inhibited child to give freer expression to his feelings and he helps to emancipate the compulsive child from pathological preoccupations with meticulousness and order. With passive children who fear to express aggressiveness and anger, the therapist may structure play therapy to help them become more comfortable with their aggressive feelings. For example, the therapist and the child may build houses and forts out of blocks and then destroy them in mock battles. During such destructive play the therapist interprets the reasonableness of expressing a certain amount of one's aggressive urges without feeling guilty and anxious about them. The applications and resources of play therapy are wide, and technics of therapists differ much from one to another.

Verbal Psychotherapy

In child psychiatry conventional psychotherapy is employed mainly with adolescents and parents. The difficulties in conducting meaningful verbal psychotherapy with a small child are marked; although a few gifted psychotherapists have reported success with conventional verbal psychotherapy with selected small children, the vast majority of child psychiatrists rely on play therapy with prepuberal children.

If the therapist adjusts himself to the communication needs of adolescents, he often can engage them in meaningful psychotherapy. A therapist usually must approach an adolescent with casual informality and he must be careful to avoid the impatient, censuring attitudes adolescents often provoke in adults. The interpersonal relationship that grows up between the adolescent and the therapist is crucial; often it is more important than the verbal content of the interviews. The adolescent who is seen in psychotherapy often does not have a sound relationship with his parents or with any other adult. The understanding, the uncritical acceptance and the occasional suggestions that the therapist gives him may assuage some of the adolescent's emotional turmoil and form a bridge back to better social adjustment. In addition to casual informality with an adolescent, the therapist often must use some of the adolescent's special jargon and talk in a free give-and-take on subjects the adolescent likes. The therapist must not explore forcefully topics the adolescent cannot discuss comfortably, and often the therapist must be prepared for a fair amount of hostile, provocative testing out by the adolescent.

Psychotherapy with parents in child guidance work may vary in different cases from counseling on the management of minor emotional problems of a child to individual psychotherapy of a parent to resolve personality problems causing unhealthy attitudes toward the child. In some cases, a parent cannot give his child a comfortable, emotionally healthy relationship until he is freed of some personality problems of his own; in such instances, the psychotherapy of the parent may deal more with the parent's life history and old interpersonal conflicts than with his current difficulties with his child. For example, a parent who emerged from a harsh, cold childhood with much lingering hostility which he is now inflicting on his child often must resolve some of his own personality problems before he can give his child more love and less anger. Therapy with parents occasionally involves counseling to work out severe problems in their marriage. Parents who are embroiled in an unhappy marriage often cannot give their children emotional security and love. Such marriage counseling may be done with the parents in joint or separate sessions.

Group Psychotherapy in Child Guidance Work

(The general principles and technics of group therapy with adults are discussed in Chapter 21.) We shall discuss here the special application of group psychotherapy to child psychiatry.

Group psychotherapy for prepuberal children usually is conducted in a playroom situation. The group may contain from 3 to 10 children who meet for weekly sessions of one and one-half to two hours each. The children attend the group from several months to one or two years. The children interact and play together in a large playroom with one or two therapists participating, depending on the size of the group and the problems of the children. The members of the group are carefully selected to insure good group interaction and to avoid excessive hostile friction. For example, the number of aggressive children in a group must be restricted because three or four aggressive, hostile children often bully the other children or fight among themselves and disrupt the group. Group therapy may be especially effective with shy, frightened children who withdraw from interpersonal relationships. The group may offer a corrective emotional experience in which these children lose their fears of people. The therapist may be a quiet observer who speaks only occasionally, or he may participate actively in the group interaction.

The group situation is in some respects similar to a family setting; the therapist is a parent figure, and the other children are sibling substitutes. Through the previous diagnostic workups of the children, the therapist understands their backgrounds and emotional problems. Thus, he can use the interpersonal conflicts, fears and activities of the children in the group as material for his interpretations. For example, the therapist may point out to the children the hostilities and feelings of rejection that arise in them as they struggle competitively for his attention. He may indicate that he has equal interest in all of them and that the goal of the group is to live in a comfortable, harmonious give-and-take relationship. The therapist may interpret the fears, the anger, the rivalries, the feelings of rejection, the tendencies to withdraw from group activities after emotional stress and other interpersonal relationships.

Group therapy of adolescents is carried on in informal discussions by 4 to 10 adolescents, who may be of one or both sexes. In group sessions adolescents discuss their interests, problems, resentments and conflicts. Many adolescents can talk much more freely in a group with other adolescents than they can in individual psychotherapy with a psychiatrist. Moreover, often they can accept comments and suggestions more easily from their peers than from an adult; an adolescent frequently rebels against all interpretations made in individual psychotherapy, but assimilates interpretations arising from group discussions. In adolescent group therapy, the therapist may be a quiet, informal observer who says little, or he may be an active participant in the group discussions.

Group therapy sessions for parents are held once each week or once every two weeks and last from one and one-half to two hours. The parents usually attend the group sessions from several months to one or two years. Each group has from three to eight couples, and many clinics schedule group therapy sessions in the evenings so both parents can attend the sessions easily. Each group is composed of parents who have children of roughly the same age level and with somewhat similar problems. The therapist acts as moderator while parents discuss the problems they are having with their children and explore possible causes and solutions. The parents may examine the conflictual feelings that various group members have toward their children, and the members of the group may gain much insight in this way.

Family Therapy

In family therapy two or more members of a family are interviewed in each session. For example, family therapy sessions may include a mother and a daughter, or both parents and one of their children, or both parents and two or three children. Such sessions may be held once or twice a week and may last from the conventional 50 minutes to one and one-half or two hours.

Family therapy has both advantages and disadvantages. Among its advantages, it enables the therapist to observe and treat the family as a unit; he can participate directly in correcting their unhealthy relationships as they interact in a lively to-and-fro way before him. The therapist can interpret to all the family members how they handle hostility toward one another, arouse feelings of anxiety and guilt in each other, and pair off in twos and threes against one another. Patterns of domination and submissiveness can be pointed out as they unfold during the treatment session. The therapist does not have to speculate on probable family ways of interaction from information gathered from its separate members; these things are available for his direct scrutiny. In Sullivanian terms, family therapy offers an excellent opportunity for the therapist to be a *participant-observer*.

In addition, family members cannot in their later discussions at home distort and misquote what the therapist says as easily as they may when they have separate sessions. Such misinterpretations, usually unconscious but sometimes deliberate, may occur at home as family members maneuver in patterns of dominance, submissiveness and guilt manipulation among themselves. In family therapy healthy plans of action can be formulated by all members, and they can understand each of their roles in carrying them out. A subtle system of intrafamilial checks and balances often arises during family therapy; this system dampens unhealthy relationships and stimulates healthy ones.

Moreover, the very nature of family therapy emphasizes the need for everyone in the family to participate in correcting the unhealthy relationships that have produced the problems of the child or adolescent. A busy father who has abandoned the rearing of his child to an anxious, floundering mother or a domineering, depreciating one, sees clearly that he must take an active part in the healing process. A bickering marital couple gradually perceives how their marital problems and their child's difficulties are woven together.

Also, family therapy enables a child guidance clinic or an individual therapist to reach more people in his available working time, and the economic advantages are obvious. This is particularly important when a child psychiatric facility has a long waiting list of families whose problems may be worsening while they wait for treatment openings.

Nevertheless, family therapy has some disadvantages. It requires a skillful, experienced therapist who is always alert to the continuing flow of feelings and words between several people; therapists of limited experience usually have much trouble managing the complex processes unfolding before them. It is easy for a family therapy situation to get out of control and deteriorate into a brawl or a subtle tug-of-war which helps no one. One family member may dominate the sessions or may attempt to maneuver the therapist into the role of an ally or an enemy, depending on his personality problems. Both children and parents may try to manipulate the therapist in their efforts to dominate others. Some family members shrink from the vivacious participation in the interview which family therapy requires if it is to be successful. Moreover, family therapy tends to deal with current interactions rather than past ones, and children and adolescents whose emotional difficulties are related more to old traumas than to present ones are less likely to be helped than those whose traumatic experiences are still going on in their day-to-day lives.

However, family therapy has a sound place in the treatment services and technics of all child and adolescent psychiatric facilities; it also lends itself easily to the work of individual therapists. I have used it on a pragmatic basis in selected cases for many years, long before it was well defined as a particular type of therapy. I have found it of most value in treating older children and adolescents in families in which the unhealthy interpersonal patterns are not deeply ingrained. Family therapy also can be used before or after a period of individual therapy for one or more family members, and it may be employed concurrently with individual therapy. It is, in essence, a form of group psychotherapy in which the family is the group.

OTHER TREATMENT SERVICES FOR CHILDREN AND ADOLESCENTS

In meeting the widespread psychiatric needs of children and adolescents, teams of psychiatrists, psychiatric social workers, psychiatric nurses and clinical psychologists work in association with pediatric hospital inpatient and outpatient services, juvenile courts, mental hygiene units in public and private schools, residential homes for delinquent or neglected children, and welfare agencies in underprivileged districts. The family and children's service agencies, both private and public, modify the child guidance clinic format to fit their situations; as a rule, they are staffed mainly by psychiatric social workers who work with psychiatric consultation services and supervision available.

In each situation the case load of the particular child and adolescent services team is determined by the available personnel and their aims. Their activities vary from counseling on minor emotional problems to services that approach the child guidance clinic model in case load and technic. The child psychiatrist in private practice usually modifies the child guidance clinic approach to some extent. In dealing with minor emotional problems he may interview both the parents and the child, and for dealing with more difficult problems he often has a psychiatric social worker who works under his supervision to provide separate interviews with the parents and the child; he usually has psychological testing done by a clinical psychologist who does such work on a private practice basis.

Psychiatric Inpatient Services for Children and Adolescents

In occasional cases the severity of the emotional problems of a child or adolescent requires treatment in an inpatient facility. In some instances the unhealthy interpersonal relationships in the child's home are so ingrained that it is unreasonable to hope that the parents can change their behavior toward the child quickly enough to stem the tide of his personality maladjustment. Sometimes the problems of the child are so severe that intensive help in a specially organized residential treatment center is the only promising course. Psychotic children may require institutional care because of the severity of their psychoses.

Many residential treatment centers function

as special schools where the interpersonal environment is organized to meet the treatment needs of children and adolescents. The children's education continues while the interpersonal environment is directed toward giving the child or adolescent emotionally healthy relationships with people, and each patient also may have individual psychotherapy if the staff size permits it; group psychotherapy is commonly employed in these centers, either alone or in combination with individual psychotherapy. The child remains in the residential treatment center from several months to a year or two. During this time the parents get help to solve their own personality problems so they can offer the child an emotionally healthier home to which to return when his treatment in the residential center is terminated.

In many residential treatment centers children or adolescents of about the same age, and of the same sex, live together in small dormitories or cottages. When the number of children or adolescents in any residential subunit goes above 10 or 12 it is difficult to maintain a therapeutic atmosphere; the interpersonal conflicts of the patients get out of hand. The staffing of residential treatment facilities presents special problems. To staff these centers with adequate numbers of therapeutically skilled persons who can live with children and deal with them in emotionally helpful ways, increases the cost immensely. They thus become too expensive to serve more than a small fraction of the children and adolescents who need their help. The use of graduate students in psychology and the social sciences as resident counselors and adjuvant therapists often is an economically feasible plan. These graduate students can work under the guidance of the fulltime staff of psychiatrists, clinical psychologists, psychiatric social workers and psychiatric nurses.

The staff members of the residential treatment center work as a team in dealing with the emotional needs and problems of the children in the same manner that the child guidance clinic team works in group and individual therapy. The child learns to live harmoniously with adult parent substitutes, the therapists, and with other children who are sibling-substitutes. The school environment is organized to provide an interpersonally healthy setting, and his emotional growth prepares the child for eventual adjustment back in his home.

Some state, municipal and private psychiatric hospitals have special psychiatric divisions for children; in general, these units function as intensive treatment facilities along the same lines outlined above for children's residential treatment centers, but in many of them the children and adolescents stay for shorter (30 to 90 day) periods. In recent decades juvenile court authorities and officials of correctional institutions have realized that detention centers for juvenile offenders should be therapeutically oriented and not be merely custodial and punitive. Hence, many reform schools for juvenile offenders have taken steps toward becoming therapeutic residential centers. These steps often have been halfway measures which have been poorly financed and have included poorly selected patients; the results frequently have been disappointing. However, the general trend in such institutions has been to acquire greater child guidance and psychiatric affiliations and to move nearer to becoming therapeutic residential centers to correct the emotional problems which led the children and adolescents to perform antisocial acts.

BIBLIOGRAPHY

Ackerman, N. W.: Child participation in family therapy, Family Process, 9:403, 1970.
Berkovitz, I. H. (ed.): Adolescents Grow in Groups. New York, Brunner Mazel, 1972.
Brandes, N. S., and Gardner, N. L. (eds.): Group Therapy for the Adolescent. New York, Jason Aronson, 1973.
Chapman, A. H.: Management of Emotional Problems of Children and Adolescents. Philadelphia, J. B. Lippincott, 1974.
Gardner, R. A.: The mutual storytelling technique Am. J. Psychother., 24:419, 1970.
Howells, J. G., (ed.): Theory and Practice of Family Psychiatry. New York, Brunner Mazel, 1971.
Kahan, V. L.: Mental Illness in Childhood: A Study of Residential Treatment. Philadelphia, J. B. Lippincott, 1971.
Maclay, D. T.: Treatment for Children: The Work of a Child Guidance Clinic. New York, Science House, 1971.
Minuchin, S.: Families and Family Therapy. Cambridge, Mass., Harvard University Press, 1974.
Moustakas, C.: Children in Play Therapy. New York, Ballantine Books, 1974.

Orgun, I. N.: Playroom setting for diagnostic family interviews. Am. J. Psychiatry, *130*: 540, 1973.

Proskauer, S.: Focused time-limited psychotherapy with children. J. Amer. Acad. Child Psychiatry, *10*:619, 1971.

Part Seven

Other Aspects of Psychiatry

In this final section we shall deal with various special difficulties of interpersonal adjustment, and we shall cover the legal aspects of psychiatry.

In Chapter 25 we shall consider three broad categories of interpersonal problems which do not fit conveniently elsewhere in this book. They are (1) special problems of adjustment in children, such as enuresis, learning problems, speech problems and others, (2) special problems of situational adjustment in adulthood, such as grief reactions, gross stress reactions, emotional reactions to physical illness and adjustment problems in middle age and old age and (3) special problems of sexual adjustment, such as premature ejaculation, impotence, orgasmic dysfunction (frigidity) and others. Throughout this chapter our emphasis will be on treatment measures for these common problems.

In Chapter 26 we shall discuss the legal aspects of psychiatry. Since psychiatry deals with the intellectual, emotional and interpersonal functioning of people, and the law deals with the socioeconomic arrangements and conflicts which people have with each other and with society as a whole, psychiatry and the law meet at many points. In this chapter we shall consider psychiatric and legal concepts of criminal responsibility, mental competence to enter contracts and to make wills, problems in committing patients to mental hospitals, confidentiality of patient-therapist communications and other areas of confrontation of psychiatry and the law.

25

Special Problems of Interpersonal Adjustment

In this chapter we shall consider a wide variety of emotionally caused problems, and related disorders, which do not fit conveniently elsewhere in this book. In general, they are special problems that individuals have in adjusting to life situations and interpersonal stresses. We shall divide them into three broad categories: (1) *special problems of adjustment in children,* (2) *special problems of situational adjustment in adulthood* and (3) *special problems of sexual adjustment.* In the standard nomenclature the conditions which we shall discuss in this chapter are included in sections titled special symptoms, transient situational disturbances, behavior disorders of childhood, and nonspecific conditions.

SPECIAL PROBLEMS OF ADJUSTMENT IN CHILDREN

In this section we shall cover some common emotionally caused problems of children, and we shall consider some other difficulties that are related to them. The problems we shall discuss are (1) enuresis, (2) encopresis, (3) learning problems, (4) speech problems, (5) acting-out behavior disorders, (6) other adjustment problems of childhood which are listed in the standard nomenclature and (7) tics, which, though they may occur at any age, are particularly common during childhood.

Enuresis

Emotionally caused urinary incontinence is a common problem in children. Most children are toilet trained by the age of three, but an ample margin for error is allowed, and urinary incontinence usually is not labeled enuresis until after the age of four. In most instances, enuresis occurs only at night during sleep, but diurnal enuresis also is seen.

Most enuresis is caused by emotional factors. When an enuretic child has a normal physical examination and a normal urinalysis, the chances are 99 per cent that his urinary incontinence is psychogenic. Urinary incontinence caused by abnormalities of the urinary tract or by neurological defects usually is accompanied by some abnormality in the physical examination or by evidence of infection in the urinalysis (due to residual urine after each urination). Spina bifida occulta, unless it is producing other signs of neurologic dysfunction, rarely is a cause of enuresis. When the physical examination and urinalysis are normal, extensive urinary tract investigations such as cystoscopy and pyelograms almost invariably do not reveal pathology; such examinations usually frighten the child and make treatment of the enuresis more difficult.

Various kinds of emotional problems may cause enuresis. Some enuretic children have minor situational problems and may even fall within the broad group designated as "within normal limits." In other instances, enuresis may accompany mild, moderate or severe emotional problems in children and adolescents. For example, enuresis may occur in passive children who cannot express anger or assertiveness; the child unconsciously expresses a certain amount of anger and devious rebellion in his enuresis and defies his parents' efforts to make him conform to their toilet training demands. Enuresis also may occur as one of many hostile symptoms in children who are chaotically acting out hostile feelings toward their environment. Many psychiatrists feel that enuresis sometimes is caused by anxious or guilty feelings over masturbation and sexual urges. In some instances, enuresis may occur in insecure, tense children whose needs for affection and emotional security have not been met.

Even without treatment, most children with enuresis lose this symptom spontaneously by puberty or early adolescence. However, in a minority of cases it persists into adolescence or early adulthood. Enuresis very rarely persists past the age of 25, except in psychotic or severely mentally retarded patients.

The treatment of enuresis may be considered in two parts: (1) counseling with the parents and the child to resolve emotional tensions in the child's life, and (2) technics for the direct removal of the symptom itself.

When an inventory of the child's emotional state and interpersonal relationships reveals only minor disturbances, the pediatrician or the family physician in many instances can manage enuresis successfully. He can talk with the parents about ways of reducing obvious stresses in the child's life, or he can discuss some of the unmet emotional needs of the child. For example, he can point out that an unduly passive child may be encouraged to express some of his pent-up anger without fears of being shamed for it or rejected by his parents and others. However, when the child or adolescent has extensive other emotional problems and personality difficulties in addition to his enuresis, the pediatrician or family physician should refer the child and his family to a child guidance clinic or a practicing child psychiatrist.

Physicians employ various methods for direct removal of enuresis as a symptom. These technics may be employed with or without counseling on the emotional stresses causing the enuresis. To be rid of enuresis has some beneficial emotional effects on the child; it frees him from the daily embarrassment about his "wet bed," and it removes the ridicule of his siblings and the irritability of his mother that the nightly enuresis sometimes causes. Also, it permits him to spend nights away from home without embarrassment, as at summer camp and in the homes of friends and relatives. Hence, elimination of the symptom by any reasonable means is a worthwhile goal. In my opinion, the removal of the symptom of enuresis without resolving its underlying emotional causes rarely produces a new emotional symptom in its place. When other types of emotional symptoms, such as phobias or compulsions, are removed without correcting the underlying emotional causes, another symptom may appear in the place of the one which was removed; however, in my experience, this is not true of enuresis. Hence, it often is useful to use a direct technic to remove the symptom of enuresis while conducting counseling to resolve its emotional causes.

Direct technics fall in two categories: *medications* and *other kinds of regimens*. It is now generally agreed that the only medications which give reasonably good results are the imipramine compounds. These drugs include imipramine (Tofranil), amitriptyline (Elavil) and desipramine (Norpramin, Pertofrane). Other imipramine derivatives are usually not recommended for children because there are limited data about proper dosages. It is well known that these drugs, which are primarily used for treating severe depressions, tend to retard bladder evacuation. They presumably do so through autonomic nervous system side effects. The usual dosage of imipramine and amitriptyline is 25 mg. at bedtime for children under the age of 11, and 50 mg. for older children. The dosage of nortriptyline is less. Some psychiatrists recommend slightly lower dosages than these, but I have found best results occur with the schedule listed here. A few parents report restlessness in children taking imipramine drugs, but I have not found this a significant problem. Treatment may continue from 30 to 90 days, often in combination with some of the technics listed below.

Many kinds of regimens and direct technics are advocated for enuresis. New technics are developed from time to time, and each new measure has its advocates. The enthusiasm and confidence of the physician in any direct treatment of enuresis undoubtedly plays a large role in the frequency of cure, since enuresis is influenced by strong suggestion in many cases. Among the common procedures that sometimes succeed are prizes for "dry nights," getting the child up to void once during the night, restrictions of evening fluids, electrical devices that are attached to the bed and ring bells to awaken the child when he begins to wet the bed, and others. Our preferred technic is the "bladder training procedure," in which the physician instructs the child to let his urine out in interrupted spurts each time he urinates, and thus exercises and strengthens the muscles around the outlet of the bladder which control micturition. Using a combination of this bladder control training technic and an imipramine drug, we are able to rid the child of enuresis in about 75 per cent of cases. The bladder control training technic is outlined in detail in each of the two publications by us listed in the bibliography of this chapter.

Regardless of the direct technics he uses in treating enuresis, the physician should emphasize to the parents that enuresis is caused by emotional stresses, and that any improvement in the child's interpersonal environment is a contributant. Also, a technic is more likely to be successful if the doctor and the parents present it to the child as a cooperative venture of the patient, the doctor and the parents, rather than as a regimen forced on the child regardless of how he feels about it.

Encopresis

Emotionally caused fecal soiling, often called encopresis, is much less common than enuresis, but it occasionally is encountered in clinical practice. It may occur both during the day and at night, and it can be socially restricting to the child, for the odor of feces prevents a good interpersonal adjustment at school and in other social areas. Except when the child has gross neurological disease or is mentally retarded, fecal soiling usually is caused by emotional factors. However, since the possibility of an organic cause is somewhat greater in encopresis than in enuresis, the child should have an examination of the rectum, roentgenologic study of the lower gastrointestinal tract and a careful physical examination.

Fowler in 1882 described the first case of emotionally caused fecal soiling. He reported a 7-year-old boy whose vain parents pushed him prematurely into a rigorous educational schedule. The child could spout forth large amounts of complex information, which delighted his parents and astonished their friends. "Under such conditions," Fowler wrote, "it is not to be wondered that something gave way and, fortunately for the brain, it was the anal sphincter."

For unclear reasons the vast majority of cases of encopresis are in boys. For example, in 10 consecutive cases of encopresis seen in our practice over a several year period, 9 were in boys. It is, moreover, largely a condition of prepuberal children; in our 10 cases all patients were between the ages of 3 and 11, and the median age was about 7. Encopresis in adolescence is very rare, and usually indicates a severe psychiatric disorder, whereas in prepuberal children it often is the result of mild or moderate emotional stresses.

Encopresis may develop when toilet training deteriorates into a prolonged battle between mother and child. In very passive children encopresis may be a symptom through which they unconsciously express resentment toward domineering, harsh parents. It also may occur in children whose parents worry obsessively about bowel movements and deluge the child with enemas, cathartics and suppositories to "regulate" the child's bowel movements. Encopresis occasionally occurs as one aspect of a regression to more immature behavior by a child who is competing with a newborn sibling for parental attention. Encopresis also may occur in schizoid children who have withdrawn from interpersonal relationships into an inner world of daydreams. The encopretic children who are referred to psychiatrists and child guidance clinics often have severe personality problems, and many articles in the psychiatric literature therefore give the impression that encopresis usually is a sign of a severe emotional disturbance. However, pediatricians and those psychiatrists who work in pediatric clinics see many encopretic children with mild situational problems, and the pediatric literature reflects a less serious view of this disorder. Even when untreated, encopresis usually clears spontaneously by puberty.

When an inventory of the child's emotional state and interpersonal relationships does not reveal profound problems, the pediatrician or the family physician often can resolve encopresis by counseling with the parents and the child about any obvious stresses in the child's life. However, when the emotional problems of the encopretic child are severe, or when a trial of several months of counseling gives no improvement, the child and his parents should be referred to a child guidance clinic or an individually practicing child psychiatrist. The physician should refer encopretic adolescents promptly for psychiatric evaluation, for as a rule they are quite disturbed.

Learning Problems

We shall discuss here all the disorders of school learning except those caused by chronic organic brain damage, mental retardation, and sociocultural deprivation. (These three topics have been covered in Chapters 18 and 20.)

There is much controversy about various aspects of learning difficulties, but we shall try to present points of view which have the support of many authorities in this field.

Problems of school learning may be caused by:

1. Learning inhibitions produced by emotional turmoil generated in unhealthy interpersonal relationships between the child and his parents, or other close persons.

2. Mixed cerebral dominance, in which there is confusion of dominance between the right and left cerebral hemispheres, with absence of dominant right- or left-handedness and much difficulty in using symbols in writing and reading; this kind of problem is sometimes termed a strephosymbolic disorder, or a specific reading disability, or a specific learning disturbance.

3. Subtle, discrete brain damage that causes special learning difficulties, as of reading or arithmetic, in the presence of otherwise intact intelligence; this is a very controversial subject.

4. Miscellaneous problems such as inadequate teaching, debilitating physical diseases, poor vision and poor hearing.

Learning Inhibitions Caused by Emotional Problems. Interpersonal difficulties may cause learning blocks. For example, an inability to learn may be an avenue of unconscious rebellion by an emotionally neglected child against the stern demands of his parents that he do well in school. This particularly may occur in the passive child whose professional-class parents put a high value on education. By refusing to learn, the child unconsciously rejects the values and standards of parents who have given him little love but want him to be a social credit to themselves. In other families, the battle over school performance deteriorates into a chronic seige between a sullen, resistant child and strident, insistent parents. In other cases, an emotionally insecure child becomes frightened and inhibited in most areas of life, and carries his diffuse inhibitions into the learning process. As Harry Stack Sullivan pointed out, one of the characteristics of anxiety, whether it exists as a subtle interpersonal force or a symptom of a psychiatric disorder, is that it gravely impairs learning of all kinds, including school learning; the pain of anxiety prevents an individual from learning, both in interpersonal situations and in solitary study. Some psychiatrists feel that learning blocks may arise in children whose curiosity about sexuality has been rudely repulsed by harsh parents; the patient develops a fearfulness of all intellectual curiosity, which inhibits the learning process. Children with emotionally caused learning blocks need the expert evaluation and therapy offered by a child guidance facility.

Learning Difficulties Associated With Mixed Cerebral Dominance. In each person either the right or the left cerebral hemisphere is dominant in controlling and coordinating intellectual skills and physical agility. The left cerebral hemisphere is dominant in right-handed persons and the right cerebral hemisphere is dominant in left-handed persons. Thus, in a right-handed person the special agility of the right hand is coordinated in the left cerebral hemisphere, and the person's intellectual skills in speaking, reading, arithmetical calculation and many other activities also are lodged in the left cerebral cortex.

However, in some persons the dominance of one cerebral hemisphere over the other is not complete, and these persons have mixed cerebral dominance. An uneasy competition for dominance exists between the two hemispheres, and this lack of clear-cut dominance may cause difficulties in using the written symbols employed in reading and writing and the verbal symbols employed in speech. The causes of mixed cerebral dominance are not well understood. In former decades it often occurred when left-handed children were forced into right-handed writing in the early grades of school, but this is rarely done in modern schools. The cause of mixed cerebral dominance in most cases today is obscure. The technical name for mixed cerebral dominance is strephosymbolia, a term derived from the Greek words meaning the twisting of symbols; this difficulty sometimes is also called specific reading disability, or specific learning disturbance. For unknown reasons, it occurs mainly in boys, the percentages in various series running from 75 to 94 per cent; in six consecutive cases of strephosymbolic reading problems seen in our practice over a several year period, all were boys.

The child or adolescent with mixed cerebral dominance may be physically awkward and he often uses his left hand for some skilled acts and his right hand for others. He also is somewhat prone to develop stuttering. However, his most striking problems often arise in difficulties with the symbols used in reading and writing. He often has trouble with reversals of letters and words; he sees and writes them backwards. For example, he has trouble distinguishing the letter "b" from the letter "d," since the letters "b" and "d" are mirror-image reversals of each other. He reads the word "saw" as "was" and "on" as "no," reversing the order of the letters; normal children may have slight, transitory problems of this sort, but the strephosymbolic child's difficulties are severe and persistent. He often writes letters, numbers, words and whole sentences as they would appear if reflected back from a mirror. In occasional instances, the person with mixed cerebral dominance can write rapidly in a complete mirror-image reversal form, so that his writing can be read only if it is held up to a mirror and reflected back from it; his writing is an illegible scrawl if read without this device. As the stephosymbolic child struggles to write, he often writes from right to left or begins forwards or backwards in the center of the page.

The child with mixed cerebral dominance often has much difficulty learning to read and write, and occasionally he may be mistaken for being mentally retarded. We have seen strephosymbolic children with high intelligence who were in the third or fourth years of grade school and could read and write no better than a child with three or four months of school education. The child with mild or moderate mixed cerebral dominance usually learns to read and write after several years of schooling, but his penmanship is slovenly and his reading speed is slow. The child or adolescent with severe strephosymbolic difficulties may have much educational trouble throughout his school career if his problem is not diagnosed and given special attention.

A few simple tests are useful, but by no means infallible, in detecting strephosymbolia. To test a child *who cannot read*, the examiner shows the child simple line profile drawings of a person, a bird and a house. He then asks the child to draw similar things. In many, but not all, cases of mixed cerebral dominance the child draws the person, the bird and the house in a mirror-reversed fashion; that is, if the person and the bird are facing toward the right in the picture the child draws them facing toward the left, and all other details of the person, bird and house are similarly reversed. Sometimes the child draws them accurately upside down or crowds them, mirror-reversed, into the upper or lower right-hand corner of the page.

In testing strephosymbolic children and adolescents *who can read* but do so with painful slowness, the examiner writes a simple sentence, such as "All children like ice cream and chocolate," on a sheet of paper with a piece of carbon paper beneath it with the inked side facing upward. When the carbon sheet imprint, which is a mirror-image reversal, is shown to a person with mixed cerebral dominance, he often can read it without hesitation; a normal person must study it carefully to make it out, but can read it easily when he sees it reflected back from a small hand mirror. The examiner also examines carefully the spontaneous writing of these children and adolescents, and notes the kinds of errors they tend to make in reading aloud.

When the clinical evidence of mixed cerebral dominance is striking, the diagnosis is easy, but when the child has mild or moderate strephosymbolic problems he requires expert evaluation by psychiatrists, psychologists and educators who have experience with this type of problem. In our opinion, mild and moderate mixed cerebral dominance is a somewhat common cause of learning disability in children of normal intelligence; severe mixed cerebral dominance is less common but more striking when it is encountered. Special teaching technics are used to help the strephosymbolic child learn to read and write well, and the child should have such help. Large school districts often have specially trained teachers, reading therapists and speech therapists to work with these children.

The Question of Discrete Foci of Organic Brain Damage as a Cause of Learning Problems. The question sometimes arises whether a child of normal intelligence with a learning problem has subtle, discrete foci of cortical brain damage causing specific learning problems, such as special difficulties in reading, or writing or arithmetic. The evidence that prompts such speculations usually rests on controversial findings in psychological testing of the child. For example, these findings may suggest subtle difficulties in coordinating visual impressions with ideas and symbols, but the meaning of these findings is subject to much dispute. We are here speaking of children who have normal I. Q.'s and who do not have other evidence or history of organic brain damage; moreover, the popularization of the concept of minimal brain damage (MBD) as the cause of many kinds of difficulties in children has further confused this subject (as discussed in Chapter 18). This field is very controversial, and many clinicians doubt its validity. In our opinion, the causes of learning problems in children almost invariably should be sought in the other types of learning difficulties discussed in this section.

Other Causes of Learning Difficulties. Various other problems occasionally cause learning difficulties in children and adolescents. Inadequate teaching and a lack of motivation for education in culturally deprived groups sometimes are causes of learning problems. (This subject is considered in detail in Chapter 20.) Undetected poor vision and poor hearing may cause learning difficulties, and in most schools all children are checked for hearing and vision early in their school careers. Physical disorders such as undiagnosed frequent petit mal seizures during the day, or debilitating physical diseases and handicaps cause educational problems in some children, and very frequent changes of family residence, resulting in changes of school one or more times a year, may hinder a child's scholastic progress.

Speech Problems

Unclear speech, poorly formed sounds and special disorders such as stuttering are fairly common in children. Since they are much less common in adults, and most children with speech problems receive little or no specific therapy, it would appear that most speech problems in children resolve spontaneously as the result of emotional, social and physical maturation. Only a small percentage persist into late adolescence and adulthood.

Various factors may cause speech problems. Inadequate speech training in early life may play a role. In some instances the cause lies in neurologic disorders or hearing defects, and dysfunctions of the oral, the nasopharyngeal or the upper respiratory areas cause some speech problems. However, emotional factors are important in the etiology of many speech problems. In keeping with the scope of this book, we shall pay particular attention to the interpersonally caused disorders of speech.

Delayed Speech. Most children can use a few words by the age of 15 months and can express their needs reasonably well by the age of $2\frac{1}{2}$ years. However, the rate of speech development is variable, and normal children may lag as much as two years in their rate of speech development. Delayed speech occurs more often in single children, firstborn children and isolated children. Since a child learns much of his speech from other children, the child with few playmates often is slow in learning to talk. Delayed speech also may occur in insecure, emotionally inhibited children and shy, withdrawn children. In many instances, however, the reason the child is slow to talk is not clear.

The vast majority of children with delayed speech are of normal intelligence and eventually speak well; their speech often develops more rapidly if they are given more opportunities to play with other children, and attendance at a nursery school for half days several days a week often is helpful. However, in some instances delayed speech may be due to mental retardation, impaired hearing, early infantile autism, childhood schizophrenia, chronic organic brain damage and neurological defects that affect the complex neurological control of speech.

Stuttering. Stuttering is caused by tonic and clonic movements of the mouth, the tongue and the upper respiratory tract that produce interrupted speech with inhibited and repetitive sounds. Stuttering usually begins in early childhood, but it may commence in later childhood. It is more common in boys than in girls. Various features of stuttering have long aroused speculations that it is caused by emotional factors. For example, the stutterer may lose his stuttering for a few days when he is in a new locality or in an emotionally calm environment. Stutterers usually can whistle well, do not stutter when singing and have exacerbations of their stuttering when they are under emotional stress. Many mild or moderate stutterers recover spontaneously in later childhood, adolescence or early adulthood. Stuttering that persists into adulthood can be a major obstacle in the patient's vocational and interpersonal adjustment.

There are various opinions about the etiology of stuttering. Some speech therapists feel that stuttering is caused by incorrect articulation and breathing, and they treat stutterers with exercises to correct these defects. Stuttering also is prone to occur in persons with mixed cerebral dominance (discussed in the section on learning problems earlier in this chapter). However, most psychiatrists feel that in many patients stuttering is caused by emotional factors. The psychiatric studies of stuttering suggest that the stutterer releases much pent-up hostility in his short, staccato outbursts of explosive articulation, and his stammering pauses symbolize his need to inhibit expression of his turbulent anger. In addition, stuttering is a provocative symptom. The listener finds himself growing annoyed and impatient while waiting for the stutterer to get his words and sentences out. A child who begins to stutter quickly senses unconsciously that his stuttering annoys his parents and other close persons, and when the child has much pent-up resentment against other people the provocative nature of the stuttering may make it an entrenched symptom. In this way stuttering becomes the avenue through which a rejected child, an unloved child, or a passive child with pent-up anger torments his parents and others with an exasperating symptom. Thus, the nature of the parents' relationship with the child may determine whether stuttering is a mild, transitory symptom or a prolonged speech handicap. Many investigators of stuttering feel that this speech problem may be produced by the additive effects of emotional stresses, faulty training in articulation and mixed cerebral dominance.

Harry Stack Sullivan emphasized that the stutterer is using speech as a tool for "defiance and domination" rather than communication. The stutterer immobilizes and frustrates his hearer, who impatiently fidgets while awaiting the messages that emerge with tantalizing slowness and incoherence. The stutterer is thus "quite adhesive," both infuriating the hearer and grappling him in uncompleted communication in the context of a mutually hostile interpersonal relationship. The stutterer does not stutter while whistling and singing, since these are not primarily *interpersonal* activities.

Two major avenues of treatment are used to help stutterers. Speech therapists often aim at training the child in correct, relaxed articulation and breathing. On the other hand, some children are treated in child guidance clinics for emotional problems. Both methods are used in some cases. Each method helps many stutterers, and comparisons of results of these two avenues of treatment is difficult since children with severe stuttering tend to be seen in child guidance clinics, and mild or moderate stutterers often are treated in speech therapy clinics attached to schools. Moreover, many stutterers improve spontaneously as they grow older, and often it is difficult to know whether a child improved because of treatment or merely during it. In my opinion, a stuttering child or adolescent should be evaluated emotionally and should receive child guidance help when significant emotional problems are found. However, a large number of stutterers recover in speech therapy, and it may be recommended for patients who do not seem to have marked emotional problems.

Disorders of Speech Articulation. These disorders include slurred speech, lisping, excessively rapid speech, abnormalities of voice pitch and tone, and various other incorrectly formed sounds. These disorders may be caused by (1) faulty training during early speech development, (2) anatomic abnormalities or defective innervation of the upper respiratory tract, the pharynx, the tongue and the mouth, and (3) emotional factors.

Clinicians disagree about the role of emotional factors in disorders of articulation in children who do not have anatomical or neurological abnormalities. Whereas some clinicians feel that disorders of articulation usually are due to faulty speech training early in life, other clinicians feel that emotional factors often cause them. The specific disorder of articulation does not in itself indicate clearly one etiology or the other. For example, in two children with the same speech problem, such as slurring of speech, the difficulty might be caused by emotional factors in one case and by faulty speech training in the other. Most psychiatrists feel that disorders of articulation may be caused by either type of process, and proper treatment can be planned only after careful evaluation of the patient from the points of view of the otolaryngologist, the psychiatrist, and the speech therapist.

Other Disturbances of Language. Diffuse abnormalities of language may be caused by mental retardation, chronic organic brain damage, early infantile autism and childhood schizophrenia. These general subjects are discussed in other chapters. Aphasia, as a cause of speech difficulties in children, is a complex, controversial neurologic subject that lies beyond the scope of this book.

Acting-Out Behavior Disorders

The child with an acting-out behavior disorder expresses hostile feelings in rebellious, defiant acts; in severe cases the child or adolescent may engage in antisocial or illicit acts. In the history of the development of child psychiatry, the concept of acting-out behavior disorders was one of the earliest diagnostic categories to be carved out of the mass of interpersonal problems of children. The concept of acting-out behavior disorders is used by almost all schools of psychiatry, for it aptly describes both the emotional problems and the behavior of a large group of disturbed children. The acting-out behavior disorders include such disorders as stealing, fire-setting, marked lying, severe school truancy, repeated running away, destructiveness and vandalism, and physical brutality; in some cases blatant sexual promiscuity and flagrant drug abuse may be forms of acting-out behavior.

The main emotional force behind the various acting-out behavior disorders is hostility; the child or adolescent is releasing pent-up anger and resentment through his antisocial, defiant acts. The acting-out child's hostility may be obvious, as in cruelty and destructiveness, or it may be somewhat disguised, as in evasive stealing and lying. In addition to the simmering hostility within him, the child with an acting-out behavior disorder often has weak interpersonal bonds to his parents and the other adults in his life. He does not have the warm, close feelings toward his parents that bind most children to their parents' standards of socially acceptable behavior. Because of the harshness, the coldness or the negligence of his parents, the acting-out child or adolescent has not identified himself with his parents or other close persons, and has not adopted their moral standards. Since the child does not have within himself a sound model of socially acceptable behavior, he is prone to depart from the accepted ethical standards of society and to express his repressed hostile feelings in acting-out behavior such as lying, stealing, vandalism and sexual delinquency. In some instances, the behavior problems of the acting-out child arise, at least in part, from being reared in a culturally deprived socioeconomic environment, which gives the child corrupt or inadequate standards of behavior.

In the official nomenclature there are three diagnostic categories which, among them, encompass the acting-act behavior disorders; they are (1) unsocialized aggressive reaction of childhood, or adolescence, (2) group delinquent reaction of childhood, or adolescence and (3) runaway reaction of childhood, or adolescence. However, these terms from the standard nomenclature, other than in official statistical reporting, are much less used than the older term acting-out behavior disorder.

Various kinds of traumatic relationships during childhood and early adolescence may generate the hostility that lingers in the acting-out child or adolescent. In some instances the child is reared in a harsh, loveless environment, and in later childhood and adolescence he lashes back with antisocial behavior at his parents and other close persons, and at the social standards they represent. He emerges resentful and rebellious from an unaffectionate, stringent childhood, and he has no affectionate bonds with people to hold him to the requirements of sound social living. A pathetic yearning for love often lies beneath the surface, but reaching the dependent needs of the acting-out child or adolescent may be a difficult task. In other instances the acting-out child was entirely neglected by his parents and other close persons, and he comes out of his formative years with a bitter defiance and foot-dragging sullenness which he expresses at school, in the neighborhood and in most other social areas. Some acting-out children and adolescents come from homes where they never had realistic limitations and discipline set on their behavior; they have little feeling for the rights and needs of others, and they have a demanding insistence that each impulsive whim or fleeting urge be satisfied. Beneath the thorny crust of their hostile, reckless behavior most acting-out children have much anxiety and emotional insecurity.

Acting-out behavior disorders may be mild, moderate or severe, depending on the amount of emotional tumult within the child. A large part of the treatment case load of the average child guidance clinic or individual practicing child psychiatrist is occupied by acting-out behavior disorders. (These children and adolescents and their parents need the psychotherapeutic approaches outlined in Chapters 21 and 24.)

Juvenile delinquency is a sociologic and legal term embracing various acting-out behavior disorders that bring children and adolescents into conflict with the law. Most acting-out behavior disorders may cause legal trouble if they are severe enough. Social conditions in deprived sections of society also contribute to juvenile delinquency. Slum gangs with their deviant morality and antisocial codes lead children and adolescents toward delinquency. In recent decades the juvenile courts and other legal agencies that deal with delinquent children and adolescents increasingly have used psychiatric insights and therapeutic approaches. Many juvenile courts have psychiatric consultation services, and court officials work closely with family and children's service agencies. Many courts have psychiatrists, psychologists and psychiatric social workers on their staffs to work with delinquent children and their parents. Various private and governmental agencies work on the social, psychiatric and economic problems woven into the causes of juvenile delinquency.

Other Adjustment Problems of Childhood

The standard medical and psychiatric nomenclature contains six diagnoses listed under the general category "Behavior Disorders of Childhood and Adolescence." Three of these diagnoses have been mentioned in the preceding section on acting-out behavior disorders. We shall discuss the other three here. We shall not consider them in detail since, except in the statistical reporting of child guidance clinics and other child care facilities, psychiatrists and other mental health professionals customarily employ other terms in talking and writing about patients.

Overanxious Reaction of Childhood, or Adolescence. In the official nomenclature this diagnosis is designed to include children who have acute or chronic anxiousness, which often is accompanied by mild phobias, nightmares, sleeplessness and other minor expressions of emotional distress. In the standard nomenclature the overanxious child or adolescent is described as being passive, approval-seeking, fearful of expressing his feelings, apprehensive about the attitudes of others toward him, and ill at ease in unfamiliar situations. The symptomatology of the overanxious child or adolescent presumably is not sufficiently clear-cut to justify a diagnosis of anxiety neurosis, or phobic neurosis, or obsessive neurosis. Moreover, even when a child's symptomatology is severe, psychiatrists and other mental health professionals hesitate to use such terms as phobic neurosis and anxiety neurosis, since the child's personality is still in a state of fluid development in which his emotional structure cannot be neatly separated from his continual interactions with the close persons in his environment.

Most child psychiatrists and parapsychiatric professionals tend to use descriptive phrases in speaking of an emotional upset in a child; thus, a psychiatrist would tend to use the phrase, "phobic and anxious symptoms in a passive, dependent, rejected child, who has strong underlying feelings of inadequacy, hostility and guilt," than to say that he child had an "Overanxious reaction of childhood." The causes of anxiousness in children and adolescents are covered in our discussions of the interpersonal roots of anxiety and related problems (in Chapters 6, 7 and 8, as well as, in part, Chapter 1 and others).

Withdrawing Reaction of Childhood, or Adolescence. The official psychiatric nomenclature provides this diagnosis for children and adolescents who retire from close interpersonal relationships. They are described as being seclusive, shy, timid, and emotionally detached from others. However, these personality traits are not sufficiently ingrained to justify a diagnosis of schizoid personality. (The interpersonal roots of this kind of emotional reaction in children are the same as those described in the discussion of schizoid personality in Chapter 12.)

Hyperkinetic Reaction of Childhood, or Adolescence. A child with this type of disorder is overactive, restless and distractible and has a short attention span, as defined in the criteria of the standard nomenclature. A hyperkinetic reaction may be caused by interpersonal stresses in the child's life, or it may be a manifestation of minimal, diffuse organic brain damage. This type of disorder is said to diminish, or to clear entirely, during adolescence. (This diagnostic category is discussed in Chapter 18 in the section on organic brain syndromes in children.) As pointed out there, many psychiatrists and other mental health professionals shun this diagnosis because (1) it is based on a single feature of the child's total emotional functioning, and (2) it covers so broad a range of emotionally caused and organically determined conditions that it has no specific meaning. We agree with those psychiatrists who feel that it is desirable to diagnose the personality problems, or specific kind of organic brain damage, of the child, and to note in passing that physical restlessness is one of its main characteristics, than to make a diagnostic entity out of a single, superficial symptom.

Tics

We shall discuss tics here since, though they may occur in adults, they are particularly common in children. In the official nomenclature tics are accorded a separate diagnostic status under "special symptoms," and we agree that they merit this individual treatment. However, a few psychiatrists classify them under hysterical conversion disorders or compulsions.

A tic is a repetitive movement of a discrete group of small muscles. Examples of tics are eye-blinking, hunching of the shoulders, rapid twisting of the neck, twitching and bobbing of the head, licking of the lips, grimacing, throat-clearing and similar movements. A tic may occur from once every few seconds to several times a day. For unclear reasons they are much more common in boys than in girls; in a survey of all patients with tics seen in our practice over a 12-year period, over 90 per cent of the patients with tics were male.

Childhood tics have a different course, as a rule, than the statistically less frequent tics that appear after middle adolescence. Childhood tics usually disappear after several months or two or three years. Tics in children sometimes are multiple, diffuse and severe, but even these severe tics usually do not persist past puberty. The adolescent or adult patient with tics tends to have only one or two tics, which usually are milder than childhood tics, but adolescent and adult tics may persist for many years or several decades. Many persons who appear otherwise well adjusted have one or two tics that appear from time to time when they are under stress.

Tics are almost always of emotional origin. However, in rare cases they are residuals of encephalitis; a tic should not be diagnosed as postencephalitic unless the evidence for previous encephalitis is irrefutable. In the differential diagnosis, the weaving, jerking, athetoid movements of Sydenham's chorea must occasionally be distinguished from tics; Sydenham's chorea usually runs a self-limited course of several weeks' duration, occurs more often in girls than boys, and its movements are not truly tic-like if observed carefully. The muscular fibrillations and fasciculations that accompany various neurological illnesses can be distinguished from tics by similar careful clinical observation.

The repetitive movements of tics are partial expressions of muscular movements that would occur if the patient gave vent to some of his pent-up feelings and unconscious emotional problems. For example, aggressive feelings lie behind many tics; the hunching, jerking shoulder and body movements of many tics are similar to the initial parts of the muscular movements the patient would make if he were to fight physically with another person. His repressed hostile feelings find expression in tics symbolic of the aggressive urges lying behind them. Tics of the facial musculature are parital manifestations of the facial movements that would accompany the expression of repressed anger, joy, crying or grief.

Some psychiatrists feel that a particular type of tic often has a symbolic relationship to the nature of the pent-up emotional force expressed through it. Thus, an eye-blinking tic is said to express the patient's unconscious wish symbolically to blot out from his awareness, to refuse to see, emotionally painful things about himself and his relationship with others. A head-shaking tic may originate as a vigorous side-to-side shaking of the head in a negative response; it is as if the person symbolically were saying "no, no, no" to interpersonal pressures and demands. Hunching and twitching tics of the shoulders and arms often suggest the muscular movements involved in physical fighting.

Harry Stack Sullivan called tics "fragmented communicative gestures" which lie outside the individual's field of awareness and beyond his capacity for voluntary control. Thus, a tic betrays the beginning of a smile, a shrug of the shoulder, a wink of the eye, and other communicative physical movements. They have, Sullivan wrote, some relevance to the interpersonal situation which the patient is in, or his apprehensive interpretation of it. He felt that these "intrusions of unaware forces" into the muscular behavior of the individual are most obvious in tics of the vocal apparatus, such as throat-clearing tics, nasal snorting tics, and tics of the lips, mouth and tongue.

SPECIAL PROBLEMS OF SITUATIONAL ADJUSTMENT IN ADULTHOOD

In this section we shall cover five special types of adjustment difficulties which occur in adulthood. They are (1) grief reactions, (2) gross stress reactions, (3) emotional adjustments to physical illness, (4) adjustment problems of middle age and (5) adjustment problems of old age.

Grief Reactions

A grief reaction is the normal process of mourning for the loss of a beloved person by death, or by incapacitating illness, or by prolonged separation. For example, a grief reaction may occur when a person loses a parent or a marital partner in death or prolonged disease. A grief reaction also may be caused by the loss of things, such as the loss of possessions in a financial disaster or a devastating fire. Grief reactions may be mild or severe, and they are commonly seen in medical practice. The patient often presents himself, or is brought by relatives, for various physical complaints, behind which lurks his grief reaction.

Grief reactions differ in significant ways from neurotic depressions and severe depressions (which are discussed in Chapters 10 and 14). A grief reaction is, by definition and nature, self-limiting and self-healing. In pathological depressiveness the person's depression arises from deeply rooted personality problems, but the grieving individual is going through a normal period of catharsis of feelings. When a pathological depression is precipitated by the death of a close person, the patient usually had strong mixed feelings of both hostility and affection toward the lost person, but the individual with a grief reaction is working through the pain of loss of a person with whom he had a reasonably sound interpersonal relationship. The pathologically depressed person often feels worthless, guilty and sinful, whereas these feelings do not occur in grief reactions. Suicidal thoughts are common in severe depressions, but they are rare in grief reactions. The pathologically depressed person needs psychiatric help, whereas the person with a grief reaction recovers spontaneously, though he may benefit from a few services his family physician or internist can provide him.

A grief reaction has certain useful functions. It is the way in which the grieving person resolves his ties to the lost individual. Through his sobbing and distress he cuts one by one the bonds that joined him intimately to the person he has lost. Though some persons bear grief stoically, such suppression of feelings may not be healthy emotionally. Often it is healthier for the person to grieve openly and to give vent in words and tears to the desolation he feels.

Sullivan considered grieving the gradual termination of an interpersonal relationship. The griever at first idealizes the lost individual, and then proceeds to break the ties of the relationship and to work out any "unfinished business." The central problem in grieving, Sullivan felt, is that each person, no matter how intimate his relationship with another individual is, has only inaccurate and partial understanding of him. By transforming the lost individual into an illusory ideal, the griever can work out any residual misunderstandings, hostilities, inadequacies and unmet needs that existed in the relationship at the time it was broken by death. The griever does this by profound preoccupation with the lost person, by rehearsing old incidents, and by thinking through aspects of their relationship. Grief is the solvent that dissolves the bonds, one by one. Grieving thus releases the griever from one interpersonal relationship and enables him to form new ones to take its place.

In most instances the patient with a grief reaction does not seek medical aid, but when he does he usually consults his family physician or internist. Hence, our comments about managing grief reactions will refer mainly to measures that may be administered by these physicians. The first step in managing a grief reaction is to listen quietly while the patient expresses his feelings and tells of his loss; the physician should interview a close relative of the patient to fill in any details the patient does not mention. The doctor should indicate briefly that he understands what the patient is going through. Much talk tends to give the grieving patient the feeling that he is getting a cheery brush-off by an uninvolved person, or that the doctor is overly concerned. Grieving people usually are repelled by verbosity, and to offer banal advice about the ups and downs of life is rarely useful at such times. Those who can find consolation in religion will find this path themselves and are rarely led to it by doctors. Occasionally a physician may indicate to a religiously-inclined patient that the patient's faith or pastor may be of help at this time, but the doctor should not urge the point further.

A little medication sometimes helps the grieving person. He often sleeps poorly, and ruminating over his grief through long sleepless hours of the night aggravates his distress. An appropriate sleeping medication may be useful. Only a small total amount of the medication should be given in any one prescription, and when the grieving person is very distressed it may be best to put its administration in the hands of a relative with whom the patient lives. When the patient is anxious and restless during the day, a mild daytime calming medication, such as meprobamate, 400 mg., three times each day or amobarbital, 30 or 60 mg., three times each day, may be useful. Antidepressant medications such as imipramine and its derivatives rarely are useful in grief reactions.

The physician can help by explaining some features of the grieving process to the patient and his family. He can point out that grieving is normal and that expression of his feelings is emotionally helpful for the patient and should not be considered weak, annoying or unreasonable. The doctor also should point out that persons who are going through grief reactions should not make major decisions about financial matters, changes of residence, job retirement or changes, and similar matters. The grieving person should not be put through an elaborate medical workup to rule out improbable physical causes for his fatigue, apathy, poor appetite and other body distresses. After the patient emerges from his grief reaction he will be able to evaluate his situation more objectively and reach whatever decisions are in his best interests. Actions that seem necessary or compelling while going through a grief reaction may be seen later in quite a different light. As the patient emerges from his grief reaction he may find it useful to busy himself in his customary work, and his relatives and friends should try to fill in the interpersonal vacuum left in his life by the loss he has sustained.

Gross Stress Reactions

The term gross stress reaction embraces states of emotional turmoil in basically well-adjusted people who undergo overwhelming environmental stresses which may occur in civil disasters such as explosions, tornadoes, floods, major industrial disasters, automobile accidents and major fires; they also may occur in wartime military combat. Gross stress reactions are, by definition, transient; the patient recovers within a short time when he is removed from the environmental stress that caused his disturbance.

In a gross stress reaction the patient is flooded during a short period of time with more excitement and stress than he can master and resolve. The clinical features often present in a gross stress reaction are: (1) much acute and chronic anxiousness, (2) spells of uncontrollable emotions such as rage, sobbing tearfulness or panic, (3) inhibition and blocking of various emotional and intellectual activities, resulting in states of bewildered confusion, fainting, loss of appetite and sexual desire, and regression to states of helpless dependence on other people, (4) sleeplessness and severe disturbances of sleep with frightening dreams in which the patient repeatedly visualizes scenes of the traumatic experiences which precipitated his gross stress reaction, (5) marked preoccupation during his waking hours with memories of his traumatic experiences and with fearful daydreams related to them and (6) transient neurotic traits such as hysterical conversion symptoms, hysterical dissociative symptoms, phobias and obsessions.

These basic features of a gross stress reaction stem from the saturation of the person with excitement and terror he cannot handle; the symptoms also stem from the unhealthy ways in which the patient attempts to rid himself of the burden of these excessive stimuli. For example, as the individual feels himself flooded during a short period of time with stimuli with which he cannot cope and feels he is losing control of his emotional and intellectual processes, he has much acute and chronic anxiety. The outbursts of rage, grief or panic the gross stress reaction mobilizes are delayed expressions of feelings the patient cannot control. In addition, the patient's emotional energies are largely absorbed in attempts to resolve the turmoil within himself, and usual feelings such as hunger and sexual desires are neglected. Moreover, he may retreat into states of confusion, in which he clings to others in puzzled, helpless, childlike ways. The frightening dreams in which he revisualizes his stressful experiences and his daytime preoccupations with these experiences are unconscious attempts to rid himself of these memories by reliving them and thus releasing the associated terror. However, these various avenues of resolving the anxiety and terror are inadequate, and transient neurotic symptoms such as phobias or conversion symptoms result.

Obviously, the clinical distinction between a gross stress reaction and a neurotic disorder depends on the duration of the disturbance. When the patient's symptoms stretch out into a prolonged course he is diagnosed as having a neurotic disorder precipitated by major stress. When his symptoms clear up in from a few days to three or four weeks, he is said to have a gross stress reaction. The variables that determine whether gross stress precipitates a prolonged neurosis or a brief gross stress reaction are (1) the basic stability or instability of the patient's personality structure, (2) the severity and duration of the precipitating stresses and their particular emotional meaning for the patient and (3) the promptness with which the patient is removed from the stress and the kind of psychiatric management he receives.

In our discussion of the psychiatric management of gross stress reactions, we shall assume that in all instances the patient recovers within a short time, realizing that the decision as to whether he had a gross stress reaction or a neurotic illness often is made in retrospect after observing the course of the patient's disturbance. We shall divide our discussion of treatment of gross stress reactions into two parts—those occurring in civilian life and those occurring during military combat.

Management of Gross Stress Reactions Which Occur in Civilian Life. The two basic steps in the treatment of a gross stress reaction are (1) removal of the patient from the stressful situation, administration of sedation, and provision of a calm environment in which the patient can resolve his emotional turmoil, and (2) allowing the patient an opportunity to talk about his stressful experience and thus unburden himself of its effects.

The patient with a gross stress reaction in many cases is removed promptly from his stressful situation by relatives, friends or work associates, since the relationship of the patient's turmoil to the stressful situation frequently is obvious. When a gross stress reaction is mild or moderate the patient often is taken to his home where his family physician or internist can administer sedation. A nighttime sedative to assure sound sleep and a mild daytime sedative or antianxiety medication to assuage the patient's turmoil usually help much. The medication usually can be given by mouth, but when the patient is quite agitated the initial dose of the sedative may be given intramuscularly. Barbiturates are useful for such sedation. When the gross stress reaction is mild or moderate, a rest at home with appropriate sedation for from several days to two weeks usually suffices for recovery. The physician's attitude should be reassuring and optimistic, and he should explain the nature of the gross stress reaction to the patient and his family.

When a gross stress reaction is severe and resistant to the above measures, the patient should be admitted to the psychiatric division of a hospital where appropriate sedation can be given under medical supervision and the patient can reintegrate his personality in a protective setting. The psychiatrist should make available to the patient opportunities to talk about his stressful experiences and to unburden his terror, rage or grief; sometimes this can be done in group psychotherapy. The psychiatrist is reassuring and understanding, and he presents a gently optimistic attitude for recovery as the patient works through the turbulence aroused in him by the stressful experience. In our opinion, the patient should not be pressed to talk about his stressful experiences, but he should be given ample opportunity to do so if he wishes. As the patient recovers from his gross stress reaction he benefits from occupational therapy, ward recreational programs and other hospital group activities for patients. Barbiturate interviews (discussed in Chapter 5) formerly were much used to enable patients to relive and work out their traumatic experiences, but they now are rarely employed.

Management of Gross Stress Reactions Which Occur in Military Combat. Gross stress reactions are a significant cause of disability in soldiers, and the military services now pay much attention to the factors that decrease their incidence. Much attention is given to morale-building services such as periodic recreation and entertainment, occasional rest periods, good food supplies, prompt medical services for the injured, and prompt mail service from family and friends at home. Much effort is spent in orienting the soldier toward the stated purposes of the war and the goals for which his sacrifices and hardships are being requested.

The basic principles of management of gross stress reactions during wartime combat are the same as those for civilian gross stress reactions, but they are modified to fit the military situation. The soldier is removed from combat to an aid station near the fighting zone. He is given rest and mild nighttime and daytime sedation. The physician reassures him, explains the nature of his gross stress reaction and presents an optimistic attitude that the soldier will soon recover and return to his combat unit. Care must be taken not to allow the gross stress reaction to acquire the secondary gain of removing the soldier from battle for a prolonged period, for in such instances the gross stress reaction runs the risk of becoming the nucleus of a neurotic reaction, which may last for many months or even years. Obviously, the line between gross stress reactions and neuroses precipitated by combat stress is a fine one, and the differential diagnosis often is made in retrospect depending on whether the patient requires a number of days or a long period of time to recover. In addition to rest and mild sedation, the soldier with a gross stress reaction may be allowed an opportunity to talk out his stressful experiences. Often this can be done in group therapy sessions in an informal setting with other soldiers. The orientation of the therapist who moderates the group discussions should be that after talking out his feelings the soldier soon will be able to rejoin his combat unit.

Emotional Adjustments to Physical Illness

Physicians in all specialties encounter patients with physical diseases whose emotional reactions toward their illnesses cause major difficulties in treatment. In some instances, the patient's emotional reaction to his illness is a greater problem than the physical disease. Every patient has ideas and feelings about any physical illness he has, and physicians often must direct significant parts of their treatment efforts to dealing with these factors.

For example, a dependent, passive person with a chronic illness such as mild arthritis or heart disease may use his physical disease unconsciously as a means of retreating into a role of helpless dependency on others. The patient finds expression for his unhealthy dependent needs in the role of a chronic semi-invalid. He can retire back to a childlike situation in which people take care of him and make no demands on him, and he may become completely dependent on others. This reaction is not justified by the severity of the illness; it is largely the product of the patient's personality structure and emotional reaction to his illness. It may be very difficult to rehabilitate such a patient after this kind of dependent invalidism has become established. The opportune time for dealing with such a reaction is in its early stages. The physician should talk with the patient and his family about the emotionally unhealthy way the patient is reacting to his illness, and he should emphasize social and vocational rehabilitation of the patient as an important aspect of treatment. Psychiatric orientation may at times be useful for this kind of patient.

Occasionally a patient uses illness to dominate and manipulate his family. For example, an elderly patient may employ mild or moderate cardiac disease to control an adult child. The elderly person may refer ominously to his inability to tolerate emotional stress without a possibly fatal crisis each time his adult son or daughter wishes to do something the elderly person does not want. In other instances an elderly person may state that his daily care by a single child who lives with him is the crucial factor that prevents him from dying or entering a nursing home; the fear of possibly causing the parent's death by leaving him or of his consignment to a nursing home keeps the adult child chained. The child often has much repressed hostility and guilt toward the parent to whom he is bound. Persons of all ages, from childhood to old age, may use illness to control the people around them. They often become skillful at making their families feel guilty about any refusal to follow their wishes. Such situations are harmful both to the patient and to those he dominates; the patient becomes more firmly fixed in a semi-invalid role which is not justified by the severity of his illness, and the dominated relatives find their lives blighted by the demandingness of the patient and their bitterness toward him. A physician should carry out some prompt counseling with the patient and his family when an unhealthy situation of this kind begins to develop. Firm, clear counseling with the relatives may be more effective than talking with the patient in preventing this type of unhealthy symbiosis.

An occasional patient finds unconscious gratification in the role of a long-suffering martyr with chronic illness. Some of these patients have deeply rooted guilt feelings from which they find partial relief through the expiatory suffering of invalidism. In other instances, solicitous attention from relatives and friends gratifies the patient's unhealthy need to appear a brave, long-suffering martyr. These distorted gratifications from illness may exacerbate the symptoms of illness and prolong its duration. The resolution of this kind of reaction to illness requires psychiatric help which should come early in the process, for when a martyr reaction to illness becomes entrenched the patient often resists psychotherapy and does poorly in it.

In some instances the patient unconsciously uses illness as a tool to punish the people around him. We recall a 52-year-old passive, dependent woman who throughout her married life had been harshly treated by her domineering, callous husband. In her early 50's she developed emphysema and sank into invalidism which was caused more by her emotional reaction to the illness than by the severity of her pulmonary pathology. Through her invalidism she escaped from the demandingness and domination of her husband, and by her chronic nocturnal and diurnal distress she made home life miserable for him. She thus expressed through chronic illness the pent-up, unconscious hostility produced by 25 years of marital unhappiness from which she had never been able to rebel.

Surgeons and physicians in the various surgical specialties occasionally encounter patients who seek distorted emotional gratification by undergoing repeated surgical operations (sometimes called, loosely, polysurgical addiction). These patients press physicians to operate on them for relief of distresses that are emotional in origin. Various kinds of pelvic and abdominal pains are their most common complaints, but any area of the body may be involved. We recall a patient who had 18 major surgical operations in various parts of her body in a 22-year period, and we remember another patient who had seven abdominal operations in nine years. The emotional problems of patients who go from doctor to doctor seeking surgery are diverse. Some of them gain gratification from the attention and sympathy of relatives and friends which repeated surgery brings. Others find relief of guilt feelings through chronic surgical suffering, and some unconsciously seek escape from emotionally painful home situations in frequent major surgery and subsequent long convalescent periods. The surgeon should be alert to such problems, especially when the patient has had previous surgery for vague reasons. Psychiatric evaluation should be included in the comprehensive evaluation of these patients, but in our experience they rarely accept psychiatric help for their underlying personality difficulties.

In many instances, and especially in older people, the patient's attitude toward his illness has a significant effect on its outcome. For example, the optimistic, cheerful elderly person with a good relationship with his family is more likely to make a good recovery from a fractured hip than a depressed, apathetic, emotionally isolated old person whose alert cooperation in his rehabilitation cannot be aroused. Also, the emotional state of a patient has an effect on his postsurgical course; it affects his attitude toward eating, early ambulation, alert cooperation with the nursing staff and many other details affecting the postoperative course. Similarly, the final adjustment of an elderly patient after a stroke, or a patient after a serious injury in an automobile accident, or an adolescent after a disfiguring facial injury, is much affected by his motivation, his basic personality, his emotional attitude toward the illness or injury, and his interpersonal relationships with the significant people in his life. The diabetic who is optimistic and cooperates well in his medical regimen does much better than the discouraged, depressed diabetic who is careless with his diet and his medication. An oft-cited adage states that a physician should not treat a disease and ignore the patient who has it. The person, his disease and his interpersonal environment form a closely integrated whole.

Some patients have special emotional needs in carrying out various forms of treatment. For example, the patient who enters a program of *prolonged hemodialysis* needs careful explanations, reassurances and optimistic encouragement in facing the demanding regimen, periodic pain and anxieties of his treatment. In addition to dietary restrictions, alterations of life style, and other things, he must adjust to the fact that his existence is tied to periodic dependency on medical machinery. If the treatment team with whom he deals take time to form a good relationship with him, and if the treatment personnel remain fairly constant, and if they make the patient feel that both they and he are engaged in a common effort with a common challenge, the chance of success is much better than if these conditions do not prevail. Patients involved in prolonged hemodialysis programs have a sufficiently high rate of abandonment of treatment, carelessness in treatment details and direct suicidal attempts to make psychiatric participation in these programs useful.

Patients facing *transplant operations* also should be well prepared emotionally, and they should, with much reassurance and optimistic explanations, be aware of the experiences they will undergo; again, if the patient feels that he has the backing of a medical team whose members are fairly constant, he will more readily give the cooperation that is needed and undergo the suffering and uncertainties involved. Parapsychiatric personel, such as psychiatric nurses and clinical psychologists, can participate usefully in organ transplant units in meeting the emotional needs of these patients. [The psychiatric disturbances following *open heart surgery*, which are caused by a combination of organic factors (transient impairment of brain nutrition and oxygen supply) and the emotional stresses of facing hazardous surgery and undergoing a difficult postoperative period, have been discussed in Chapter 19.]

Adjustment Problems of Middle Age

We shall here discuss the normal problems of interpersonal adjustment which people face during middle age; we shall, somewhat arbitraily, define middle age as extending from 50 to 65. A person's success or failure in making these adjustments has marked effects on his emotional health, his physical well-being and his total socioeconomic welfare. In the standard psychiatric nomenclature, maladjustments in facing the stresses of middle age are included under *adjustment reactions of adult life*.

Interpersonal Stresses of Middle Age. Extensive changes take place in the interpersonal relationships of middle-aged persons. Many of these changes occur in the person's family environment. During middle age a person often loses his parents by death, and similarly he may lose siblings, other relatives, close friends and long-time work associates. Other family members and friends in the patient's age group begin to suffer from illnesses that are more common from middle age onward, and the individual witnesses an increased incidence of disease and incapacitation in his interpersonal circle. These deaths and illnesses also remind the middle-aged person that his own life span is drawing shorter and that his probability of illness is becoming greater.

During his middle-aged years the person's children arrive at adulthood, move out of the home and establish new homes of their own. The children develop their own interests and interpersonal circles and often they take up residence in distant cities. During the previous 25 years much of the middle-aged person's interpersonal life, emotional energy and time were occupied with rearing his children, and the absence of his children may create a large vacuum in his life.

Moreover, middle-aged persons face various other social changes. They often have difficulties establishing common grounds for friendship with the new generations entering their twenties and thirties. The person in late middle age often finds the ranks of his friends being thinned by death and chronic illness, and he may be unable to fill in these interpersonal gaps with new friends from younger age groups. Each generation has new preoccupations, new customs, new recreations and new ways of doing things, and the interpersonal gap between generations may be large. The middle-aged person may begin to feel he is being cast aside in the vigorous onrush of younger people at a time when his interpersonal circle with people his own age is growing smaller.

The middle-aged person often faces vocational and economic problems. Professional people and independent businessmen have less difficulty in this respect than white collar workers, semiskilled workers and unskilled laborers. For most people, however, earning capacity begins to drop as they proceed through middle age, and the margin of their economic security may become thinner. Employment opportunities diminish during middle age and the prospect of eventual economic dependence on others hovers on the distant horizon. Middle-aged people begin to lose some of their vocational flexibility; they find it hard to adjust to changing business methods, new industrial processes and new commercial practices. They may begin to fear the competitive push of younger, more vigorous people who sometimes displace them in their jobs.

In many instances the middle-aged individual must adjust to an increased incidence of physical illness, since the degenerative diseases become more common during this age span. Hypertension, cardiovascular diseases, diabetes, arthritis, carcinoma and many other illnesses may occur. In addition to causing physical suffering, these illnesses may cause emotional anguish. Moreover, by diminishing the patient's vitality they may constrict his customary interpersonal contacts with people and they may impair his vocational capacities.

In our consideration (in Chapter 15) of severe depressions that may occur during the involutional period we discussed the controversial subject of the influence of the female menopause on emotional functioning in middle-aged women. As pointed out there, the role of the endocrinologic menopause in the emotional problems of middle-aged women is probably of little significance. The emotional adjustments of middle-aged women are caused by the major interpersonal problems they face, not by the minimal endocrinologic changes they undergo. However, the experience of ceasing to menstruate and undergoing the various physical sensations common in the menopause may have a marked interpersonal meaning for a middle-aged woman. To her, they may signify loss of femininity, loss of beauty and attractiveness to men, loss of youth and childbearing capacity, and approaching old age. These fears are not caused by hormonal changes; they are emotionally unhealthy interpretations the middle-aged woman may place on the physical menopause. (In Chapter 15 we also mentioned the highly controversial subject of the so-called male menopause; most psychiatrists reject the concept and feel that the major stresses of middle age in men are interpersonal, not endocrinologic.)

Principles for Adjusting to the Interpersonal Stresses of Middle Age. Successful interpersonal adjustment to the changes of middle age often requires planned programs of work on these problems. An important principle is that the middle-aged person should keep active. He should not allow his usual interests and routines of activity to wither. This may require careful planning, for it is easy in middle age to drop activities one by one until life is barren and empty. The middle-aged person often receives trite advice to "take it easy" and "not to try to keep up with things the way you used to." Such advice more often is harmful than useful. Longevity and activity go hand in hand, and health and a good adjustment are tied to a reasonably busy life in middle age.

New interests and new ideas stir new vitality in a person and erase the barrenness of old routines. The middle-aged person should find new avocations and plunge into them with avid interest. Some of the activities he may take up are gardening, rose culture, home carpentry, cabinet work, painting, ceramics and bridge. Many middle-aged people develop an avid interest in watching sporting events and become fans of the hometown baseball team, football team and other teams.

The middle-aged person should use his new activities to create new interpersonal contacts with people. Every field has its group of enthusiasts, its clubs, its exhibitions, its journals and its associations. A dog raiser should be a member of the local kennel club and an amateur radio operator should spend time with others who are interested in that field. Some middle-aged people find stimulation in the evening educational programs many colleges offer for adults. Church study groups, language study groups, hobby groups and similar groups interest some middle-aged people and widen their interpersonal circle.

Usefulness to others keeps a person's interpersonal contacts vital and expands them. A golfer should teach a friend or two to play the game and should interest them in playing regularly. The middle-aged woman who develops tolerable skill in painting landscapes and still-life pictures should give them to friends who find them attractive home decorations, and she should exhibit her pictures at amateur shows. Hospital auxiliaries, church welfare groups, political parties, fund-soliciting groups for philanthropic purposes and other organizations need the assistance middle-aged people can give. Grandfathers who like to take their grandsons to baseball games delight their grandsons and earn the gratitude of the boys' parents who find themselves with free afternoons to go where they please without taking the children. An older man who learns how to repair television sets or plumbing fixtures will find himself in much demand by neighbors and friends. To feel that he is not needed by anyone and is of no use anymore is one of the grimmest feelings a middle-aged person can develop. If he finds new ways to be useful to people, the middle-aged person need not experience this devastating feeling.

The middle-aged couple should not abandon sexuality in their marriage, nor let it grow stale, for continued sexual activity is a useful stimulant to their morale. The importance of sexuality in middle age is more often emotional than physical; the middle-aged man is pleased that he is still sexually capable, and the middle-aged woman is flattered that her years have not diminished her husband's ardor for her. Continued sexuality reassures middle-aged people about their "youthful" vigor. We shall discuss this subject at more length later in this chapter.

In our opinion, a middle-aged person should be cautious about making major changes of residence, vocation and economic situation, or, at least, such changes should be very carefully planned. Extensive changes often tax the flexibility and resourcefulness of the middle-aged person, and such changes also require leaving an established set of friends or work colleagues and forming entirely new interpersonal circles at a time of life when the individual is beginning to find this difficult. Though in some instances middle-aged people make extensive changes successfully, in other instances they regret such changes and lack the flexibility and resources to return to their former situations.

A middle-aged person should take good care of his physical health. He should not put on excess weight and he should remain moderately active physically. For example, golf, moderate hunting and fishing, moderate swimming and bowling are physically healthy for the middle-aged person and lift his morale by giving him a sense of continued vigor and well being, especially if he occasionally outdoes younger people in some of these activities.

Systematic orientation of middle-aged people toward the problems they may face, and ways of adjusting to them, would improve both the physical and mental health of the vast section of the population that is in the 50- to 65-year age bracket.

Adjustment Problems of Old Age

Ten per cent of the American population now exceed the age of 65, the point we shall define as the beginning of old age. Moreover, because of the increased frequency of physical illness in old age, elderly people occupy a sizable segment of the treatment time of physicians, and understanding their special problems aids in their total management.

The interpersonal problems of old age in many ways form an accentuation and continuation of the difficulties of middle age. Thus, the elderly person often has marked changes in his interpersonal environment. He loses many of his relatives and long-time friends by death and incapacitating illnesses. Often the elderly person loses his marital partner, and his children frequently live in distant cities rearing families of their own. The elderly man retires from work and loses the companionship of the people with whom he worked. The elderly individual often finds himself drifting into interpersonal isolation at a time when his emotional health demands vibrant, supportive interpersonal contacts.

The elderly individual faces marked economic and vocational changes. Most older people retire from their jobs because of lack of physical vitality or because of company employment regulations which set mandatory retirement ages. In addition, many elderly people are not economically self-sufficient. Savings, pensions and social security payments do not meet their expenses and they must accept financial aid from their children and in some cases they must live with them. Their economic dependence frightens and discourages older people, and living with their children may cause interpersonal tensions.

Sociologic changes often have marked effects on the interpersonal adjustments of older people. They cling to their old ideas, customs and ways of doing things, while the new generations are developing different ideas and interests. Thus, the older person's interpersonal isolation is accentuated by loss of common grounds for interaction with people around him. Moreover, the older person often lacks the intellectual flexibility to close this interpersonal gap by adopting new ways of doing things and developing new interests.

The older person faces a rising incidence of chronic health problems. In addition to causing him physical distress, these problems often narrow his interpersonal circle by producing physical incapacitations. His ability to go places, to visit people and to drive his car may be restricted. Moreover, many older people, in addition to their interpersonal and socioeconomic difficulties, begin to suffer the subtle loss of brain tissue caused by senile brain degeneration and cerebral arteriosclerosis. (The chronic organic brain disorders produced by senile brain degeneration and cerebral arteriosclerosis are described in Chapter 18.) Long before the frank symptoms of brain damage occur, the older person has a narrowing of interests and a loss of intellectual flexibility, the earliest signs of minimal loss of brain cells. This loss of intellectual flexibility often robs the older person of the ability to make interpersonal changes gracefully at a time of life when difficult interpersonal pressures are impinging on him.

Principles for Adjusting to the Interpersonal Stresses of Old Age. The principles for making a good interpersonal adjustment in old age follow the same general pattern outlined for a successful interpersonal adjustment in middle age. However, the problems of the older person are more marked and his flexibility for resolving them is less. Hence, he more often needs the help of others in solving the adjustment problems he faces.

The older person should keep active, both intellectually and physically, to the comfortable limits of his capacities. The retired man should have a program of work about his home, and a light parttime job often is helpful. Many elderly women have less difficulty remaining active than elderly men, since elderly women can still remain occupied with the household activities in which they engaged much of the time during their entire adult lives. Psychiatrists and other mental health professionals have long observed that the elderly person who remains intellectually and physically active has less chance of psychiatric deterioration due to senile brain damage and cerebral arteriosclerosis than the intellectually and physically inactive old person. Presumably, the intellectually and physically alert elderly person continues to use undamaged parts of his cerebral cortex in more effective, more extensive ways than the older person who has drifted into intellectual and physical inactivity. With the same amount of brain damage, an interpersonally and intellectually active old person functions better than one who is interpersonally isolated and intellectually stagnant.

The elderly person should work hard to keep up his old interpersonal contacts and to form new ones, and he should make himself useful to other people in all possible ways, thus avoiding the desolate feeling of uselessness. Older people have a major asset which enables them to be useful; they have much time. They can make the many telephone calls necessary to remind people of a church dinner, and they can make the house-to-house visits required in soliciting funds for philanthropic purposes. They can baby-sit for younger friends, tend information desks in hospitals, call on people to urge them to register for voting, canvass neighborhoods for the political party of their choice and carry out many other tasks. There are endless jobs waiting to be done and the older person need never feel useless and unwanted.

The older person should develop new interests and new activities. Though developing new interests may be hard work, the rewards are great and the alternative is grim stagnation. Handicrafts such as cabinet work, ceramics, repairing electrical appliances, reupholstering furniture and many others are stimulating and useful. Games such as bridge, backgammon and chess form useful interpersonal links, and, if golf and tennis become prohibitively strenuous, shuffleboard and croquet are practical substitutes. Many community groups, church groups and colleges have afternoon and evening study groups and courses where avocations and cultural interests can be developed.

The elderly person should be cautious about making abrupt changes in his place of residence and his long-established habits and customs. He often lacks the resourcefulness and flexibility to make such changes successfully. In clinical practice one often sees elderly people who begin to deteriorate physically or mentally after making a radical change in residence or long-established customs. The older person often adjusts poorly to new circumstances. He has difficulty learning new names and faces, new streets, new closets and drawers and new arrangements of rooms. He tends to become confused and frightened in new surroundings, especially at night. Moderate modification of long-time customs may be stimulating, but radical changes often precipitate a gradual mental and physical decline.

SPECIAL PROBLEMS OF SEXUAL ADJUSTMENT

Problems of sexual adjustment are common complaints for which patients consult physicians in various medical specialties. We shall give particular attention to the most frequent sexual difficulties, which are (1) *premature ejaculation,* (2) *impotence* and (3) *orgasmic dysfunction,* the preferred name for the condition long called frigidity. We shall consider briefly the less common sexual problems, which are *ejaculatory incompetence, vaginismus* and *dyspareunia.* In a final section we shall discuss the special *sexual problems of the aging man and the aging woman.*

Premature Ejaculation

The man with premature ejaculation is able to achieve penile erection but he ejaculates spontaneously before insertion of his penis into the vagina or within 30 to 60 seconds after insertion. Premature ejaculation occurs occasionally in many men when they are anxious, when they have been sexually abstinent for some time, or when they are under various kinds of situational stresses. Premature ejaculation also is common in young men who are inexperienced sexually, and it often clears as the man gains more self-confidence and relaxation in sexual intercourse. The adoption of a relaxed position for the man during intercourse, as in side-by-side positions or with the woman lying on top of the man, resolves many cases of premature ejaculation. A simple measure that often helps premature ejaculation is the application of a mild topical anesthetic ointment to the glans penis and the prepuce shortly before intercourse. This decreases the intensity of erotic stimulation and often allows the man to delay ejaculation until satisfactory mutual intercourse with his partner occurs; allergic dermatitis reactions to such ointments, which sometimes are cited as a factor against them, are very rare and soon clear upon ceasing to use them.

However, in some men premature ejaculation is a more deeply rooted emotional problem caused by the patient's marked discomfort about sexual intimacy with women. Sexual intercourse holds certain anxieties for him which cause him to ejaculate and terminate the act when it has scarcely begun. These anxieties often arise in long-term traumatic interpersonal experiences with the close females in his life during childhood and early adolescence. These interpersonal causes of premature ejaculation are largely the same as those outlined in the following section on impotence; many psychiatrists consider premature ejaculation to be a variant form of impotence. Some investigators feel that premature ejaculation is a pattern that becomes ingrained during early premarital sexual activity in unrelaxed, clandestine, hurried and often physically awkward situations; later, the premature ejaculator's wife often has disappointment and irritable frustration which make him anxious each time he approaches sex and rob him of the capacity to maintain an erection for longer periods of time.

Although psychotherapy sometimes helps a man with premature ejaculation, the results are in general little better than the natural course of the problem; a fair number of men, especially recently married ones, improve gradually with the passage of time as they become more at ease with their marital partners. The most effective treatment technic is the sexual retraining process developed by Masters and Johnson, based on earlier observations of J. H. Semans. In this method the man's sexual partner diminishes his ejaculatory tendencies by repeated slightly painful squeezes to her partner's erect penis before vaginal entry. This is done by pinching the glans penis at its base between the thumb and first two fingers. After a few training sessions using this repeated squeezing technic, the man maintains the capacity to maintain an erection for a long period of time outside the vagina despite stimulating manual sex play by his partner. The wife then mounts her husband, who lies supine on his back; in a nondemanding, low stimulating way she inserts his penis into her vagina as she sits astride and above him. The wife remains motionless for periods up to half an hour, while the man develops physical and emotional comfort with the experience of prolonged vaginal containment of his penis. Intercourse can then begin with slow pelvic movements by the woman, perhaps with occasional interruptions to prevent ejaculation by vaginal withdrawal and a few repeated penile squeezes. In time, such reinforcing squeezes are not needed. The final step in such sexual retraining is a shift to a lateral (side-by-side) sexual position in which the man assumes a more vigorous pelvic thrusting role.

A number of therapists have reported cure rates running well over 90 per cent with this technic, and our experience has been similar. However, there are three limiting factors. Obviously, successful application of this technic requires a highly motivated, cooperative couple who can work well together in this procedure and will continue to engage in reinforcing sessions, with occasional penile squeezing, for a year or more after a satisfactory sexual pattern has been achieved. Also, this technic is couple-oriented; the man who solved his problem in this way with the partner with whom he carried out the retraining is usually still a premature ejaculator with other women. Thirdly, when the man is unmarried, the therapist finds himself supervising the sexual practices of unmarried persons; although in our permissive era this would not be a problem for most psychiatrists and other mental health professional workers, there are still therapists and patients for whom this is morally unacceptable, and objections also have been raised in some segments of the lay public about treatment procedures that encourage extramarital sexual activity.

Impotence

Sexual impotence is a common complaint about which men consult physicians. In an article on the subject of impotence written in 1912, Sigmund Freud stated that, after anxiety neuroses, psychogenic sexual impotence in men was the most common problem encountered in psychotherapeutic practice. Impotence still remains a common problem about which men consult psychiatrists, family physicians, urologists and other physicians. Impotence almost invariably is due to emotional factors; less than one per cent of all impotence is caused by physical defects or diseases. The infrequence of physical causes of impotence militates against elaborate physical workups while the patient becomes more despairing of resolution of his problem and neglects the emotional areas where solution to his problem lies. Impotence is defined as the inability to achieve penile erection and to maintain it for from 30 to 60 seconds after vaginal entry; as pointed out above, premature ejaculation is thus a special kind of impotence, by this definition. However, in most cases coming to medical attention the impotent patient cannot achieve erection at all, or he achieves erection only to lose it when he attempts vaginal penetration.

Impotence may be divided into three clinical categories: (1) *transient situational impotence*, in which a man who has long had satisfactory erectile capacities undergoes a brief period of impotence while under emotional stress, or fatigued, or in conflict with his sexual partner, (2) *primary impotence*, in which a man has never been able to achieve or maintain an erection adequate for complete vaginal penetration, and (3) *secondary impotence*, in which the man has had from several to a few dozen episodes of reasonably adequate sexual performance, but then develops persistent inability to achieve penile erection for weeks, months or years.

Transient Situational Impotence. Short periods of impotence are common in men who ordinarily function well in the sex act. These periods of impotence may last from a few days to two or three months. Transitory impotence may occur when a man is anxious, or depressed, or is worried about his job and his financial situation, or is having marital difficulties. Fatigue, or fear of discovery in illicit intercourse, or lack of self-confidence of a young man in his first few experiences with sexual intercourse may produce impotence of short duration. In the vast majority of cases, if the man is basically well adjusted, this period of impotence clears spontaneously in from a few days to a few months. Often the man attributes his recovery to some benign medication he took, or a restful vacation, or body building exercises, or some such measure, but his recovery actually occurred as he resolved the emotional stresses he was under. However, the suggestive effect of whatever therapeutic measure the man adopted often gave him a measure of self-confidence which helped his recovery.

In some instances a man who is relatively well adjusted fails a time or two in his ability to perform the sex act and becomes so upset about his failures that his period of impotence is prolonged. Sex is a prestige-laden activity for a man, and many complex factors of masculine pride are tied to reasonable sexual capacity. The man who after a few failures approaches each opportunity for intercourse with the question, "Can I, will I?" may find that his dread of failure prolongs his impotence for weeks or months. Frequently, such a man consults his family doctor or a urologist, and, with strong reassurances and a little counseling on sexual matters, he usually recovers in a short time. The doctor should explain to the patient that short periods of impotence are common and that the prognosis for return to his former level of sexual competence is good. The physician may suggest a trial of changes of position in sexual intercourse, or love-making at a different time of the day, but his reassuring attitude probably is more important than the specific advice he gives. The physician should explain that emotional tension, fear of failure and fear of humiliation in the eyes of his wife are common factors in brief periods of impotence, and that a return of self-confidence and repeated attempts at intercourse usually resolve the problem in a short while. Relatively few patients with this type of mild, transitory impotence are seen by psychiatrists and other mental health professional workers.

Primary Impotence. The man with primary impotence has never been able to achieve and maintain an erection adequate for full vaginal penetration. Such impotence usually is rooted in marked personality problems whose origins often stretch back to prolonged interpersonal trauma that occurred during the patient's childhood and adolescence.

Men with primary impotence usually have a deep-seated dread of sexual intimacy with women. They are not consciously aware of this dread; it is symptomatically expressed in their impotence. Some of these men unconsciously fear women as harsh, domineering, depreciating persons who use sexual intimacy as a tool to trap men and dominate them. Such a man basically fears that once he has been sexually united with a woman she will become hostile and will try to reduce him to a submissive role. In other instances, the primarily impotent man has immature personality characteristics that prevent him from achieving a mature sexual relationship with women; he in some cases is so emotionally dependent on his mother, or an older sister, or some other older woman, that any movement toward a mature sexual relationship fills him with a panic that prohibits sexual activity; his infantile personality characteristics preclude the development of comfortable sensuous feelings toward women.

Latent, unconscious homosexual strains are causes of primary impotence in a small number of men. Other men, for various reasons, are flooded by feelings of shamefulness, guilt or ridicule when they approach sexual intercourse and they are unable to perform sexually. As one of our patients expressed it, "I feel like my mother is standing at the foot of the bed shaming me and telling me it's all a dirty business."

Many kinds of interpersonal traumas during childhood and adolescence may contribute to primary impotence in adult life. Often the patient was made to feel inadequate by domineering, belittling parents and other close persons, and in many cases the patient's father was a distant, rejecting person or an ineffective, floundering individual who failed the patient in his paternal role. Careful study of a primarily impotent man often reveals that he was reared by a harshly controlling mother and a passive, anxious father, and that he had no other close relationships with adults during childhood and early adolescence to diminish the impact of these unhealthy relationships with his parents. Thus, the impotent man emerged into middle adolescence with marked feelings of inadequacy and a deep-seated dread of any kind of close relationship with women; he unconsciously fears sexual intimacy and marriage as the gateways to misery from which exit is impossible.

The causes of latent homosexual strains in a small number of primarily impotent men are the same as those outlined in our discussion of male homosexual (in Chapter 12), but in impotent men they are not strong enough to produce overt homosexual behavior. Some psychiatrists feel that in some cases the primarily impotent man was repeatedly shamed and made to feel guilty about sexual curiosity, masturbation, and other sexual cravings throughout childhood and early adolescence, and that as an adult he is unable to free himself of these feelings each time he approaches sexual activity.

In our experience, men with primary impotence who enter psychotherapy and persist in it have a somewhat better than 50 per cent chance of resolving their problem. Resolution of the problem, however, is much aided by a cooperative, encouraging, devoted sexual partner; conversely, a sexual partner who, because of personality difficulties of her own, wishes to keep the man in a humiliated, ineffective role much reduces the chance of psychotherapeutic success. A certain amount of joint counseling of the two partners together, even when the man is the major focus of psychotherapy, is, in our opinion, often useful.

The sexual retraining technics developed by Masters and Johnson for both primary and secondary impotence will be described at the end of our discussion of secondary impotence.

Secondary Impotence. A man who has had from several to a few dozen episodes of reasonably adequate sexual performance, but then develops persistent inability to achieve penile erection adequate for satisfactory intercourse, has secondary impotence. All the etiologic forces which produce primary impotence, as listed above, may contribute to secondary impotence; however, in secondary impotence they are of lesser degree and permitted a certain amount of satisfactory sexual activity before persistent impotence set in. Interpersonal stresses in his relationship with his sexual partner, and other current interpersonal problems, often play a large role in secondary impotence.

For example, in some instances the patient's wife plays a significant role in causing his impotence. If, after an episode of impotence due to fatigue, or alcoholic excess, or a quarrel between them, the wife taunts her husband with his inability "to be a man," or tearfully demands that he "do it now, after you've got me all excited," or apprehensively hammers him with questions if "it's always going to be like this," she may create so much anxiety in him that he fails to achieve an erection on subsequent occasions. After each failure she berates him and further erodes his confidence and erectile capacity. This may occur when the wife uses her husband's impotence as a tool for dominating him, or for getting revenge for his previous neglect or harshness toward her, or for avoiding sex, which she finds distasteful.

In their series of 213 cases of secondary impotence seen during a period of 11 years, Masters and Johnson found as contributing causes the following: a prior state of premature ejaculation which undermined the man's confidence in his sexual capcity, occasional bouts of acute alcoholic excess and sexual failure at such times, harsh maternal or paternal dominance which eroded the man's feelings of masculine adequacy, religiously based feelings that sexuality was a dirty or dangerous activity, and erroneous or inadequate counseling and orientation on sexual matters, often from ill-advised lay friends or from misleading or unsound reading material.

Psychotherapy, sometimes involving the man's wife in several sessions of joint counseling, resolves secondary impotence in about 60 per cent of cases, in our experience. Such psychotherapy often deals with current stresses in the patient's life, as well as predisposing experiences in his childhood and adolescent years. Also, this psychotherapy frequently includes a certain amount of direct couseling about stimulating kinds of love play, sexual technics and timing of intercourse.

The sexual retraining technics developed by Masters and Johnson resolve secondary impotence in about 70 per cent of cases. They employ a treatment format in which a male and female treatment team (as, for example, a male psychiatrist and a female clinical psychologist, or a male psychiatrist and a female psychiatric nurse) hold joint four-person counseling sessions with the patient and his wife. This approach assures both the man and his wife of an understanding therapist of his own sex in the treatment situation.

In these counseling sessions attention is not focused directly on the symptom, since, as Masters and Johnson emphasize, "no man can will an erection." Erectile capacity is developed gradually as the result of stimulating, desultory, relaxed sexual play in bedroom sessions over a period of time. Implicit in this approach are three principles: (1) The man's fears about his sexual performance are gradually dissolved in nondemanding (no demands are made by the wife for immediate sexual performance), relaxed sexual play. (2) The man slowly alters his role from that of an anxious spectator waiting for an erection to occur to that of a comfortable participant in mutually stimulating, affectionate love making. (3) The wife's apprehensiveness and sense of urgency are removed as she pays little attention to her husband's erectile capacity and enjoys their sex play, and her increased comfort is reflected in relaxed confidence in her husband; neither is watching and waiting for "him to perform."

The couple begin at home. using the orientation they have received from the therapists, to engage in sessions of nondemanding love play; their goal is merely to stimulate each other in the physical and verbal ways that each one finds most enjoyable, and each one indicates to the other, after trial and error exploration, what he finds most stimulating in terms of stroking and "teasing" attention to the skin, lips, mouth, breasts and genitals. Direct stimulation to the man's penis is often a late step in this process. Each one "gives to get"; satisfaction of the other is the main goal, and eventual development of strong, prolonged penile erections is the incidental, though important, side effect. When the time eventually comes for genital-to-genital sexual activity, the woman mounts astride the man, who lies supinely looking up at her and engaging in mutual fondling. Responsibility for insertion of the penis into the vagina lies with the woman, who gently directs the penis into her vagina as she sits downward, moving slightly forwards, on the man. After penile insertion no pelvic thrusting by either partner occurs, but the man is allowed a considerable period to enjoy the sensation of prolonged vaginal penetration. When the man, perhaps with repeated direct penile stimulation from the wife, can maintain his erection for a satisfactory period within the vagina, gentle pelvic thrusting by the woman can begin. In later sessions the man also engages in pelvic thrusting. In the final stages the couple may shift to a lateral (side-to-side) position, and after satisfactory sexual intercourse has occurred many times they may shift to the man-above position if they wish.

Obviously, this type of sexual retraining requires a well-motivated couple who are devoted to each other and are willing to work with patience and ingenuity to resolve the husband's impotence. When the marital relationship is contaminated with hostility, competitiveness and indifference to one another's needs, this type of sexual retraining is much less likely to work.

Orgasmic Dysfunction (Frigidity)

There is much misunderstanding about the nature of sexual responsiveness in women. Although some women have a fairly rapid decrease of tension after a gradual buildup of sexual excitement in the so-called classical orgasm, many other women have a more gradual resolution of sexual excitement with a lingering afterglow; both types of sexual pleasure must be considered within the range of normal limits. Moreover, very few women experience intense sexual pleasure and release of tension in all acts of intercourse. It is probable that the average women has orgasm (in either of the above senses) in only 50 to 70 per cent of episodes of intercourse. Understanding this has some importance, for many women mistakenly feel inadequacy and shame if they do not have intense feelings in all acts of intercourse. Unlike a man, a woman must have a gradual buildup during love play, must be in a reasonably relaxed and fresh state, and must have at least a certain degree of emotional commitment to achieve orgasm; all these things do not prevail during a sizable minority of occasions when the average woman has intercourse.

Although some psychiatrists and other

mental health professional workers still maintain that there are two types of orgasm, a clitoral orgasm which is somewhat immature in nature and a vaginal one which signifies greater emotional maturity, modern physiological studies of female sexual responsiveness indicate that such a distinction is not valid. Sexual responsiveness in women has a characteristic pattern, in terms of genital reactions, which may be divided into four phases: (1) An excitement phase in which there is vaginal lubrication, deep pelvic tissue vasocongestion, increased muscle tension and some distension of the vaginal barrel. (2) plateau phase in which there is venous congestion in the outer third of the vaginal barrel, increased muscle tension and flattening of the clitoris on the anterior surface of the symphysis. (3) The orgasmic phase, in which vascular engorgement and muscle tension in the outer third of the vagina increase, and, in some women, mild muscular contractions occur in the same region. (4) The resolution phase in which vasocongestion and muscle tension of the genital region decrease, at different rates in different women. These reactions in the genitals are, of course, only local physiological responses in the total emotional, interpersonal and physical commitment of the woman to the sex act. In considering sexuality in both men and women, one must always keep in focus the central, obvious fact that it is an *interpersonal* process.

A wide variety of factors can contribute to orgasmic dysfunction (frigidity), and they vary from superficial to profound, in terms of their emotional content and interpersonal determinants. Current circumstances and stresses may play a role. The skill of a woman's sexual partner in exciting her sexually and his capacity in performing the sex act in a gratifying way may be significant factors. The soundness of her affectionate relationship with her partner, and any recent gratifications or disappointments in it, affect her sexual responsiveness to him. Such factors as fear of pregnancy, fear of detection in illicit sexual activity, worry about a coughing child in the next room, lingering anger from a recent argument over a new washing machine and endless other situational distractions may inhibit a woman frequently or occasionally.

Despite the greater frankness about sexuality in our society in recent times, prudishness and depreciation of female sexual responsiveness still prevail in some homes, and a girl reared in such an environment may have much difficulty altering long-ingrained feelings on the night of her first sexual experience; such factors may also contribute to long-lasting discomfort in the sex act which prevents sexual arousal and pleasure.

Various kinds of personality problems and interpersonal traumas can lead to lack of orgasmic capacity. Some nonorgasmic women have an unconscious fear of men as exploiting persons who use sexual domination as a means of controlling and cruelly using women. Other women are so immature in personality structure and so fixed at childish levels of feeling and behavior that they are ill equipped emotionally for the relaxed, sensuous self-abandonment and commitment to a sexual partner that orgasmic capacity requires. Some women feel guilty and ashamed of sexuality and their nude bodies, and these feelings inhibit them in sexual intercourse. Women who are competitive with men and basically hostile and domineering toward them often cannot participate comfortably in sex, fearing it as a process in which an aggressive male assumes a dominant role with a submissive female; they cannot see sexuality as a mutually gratifying process in which two equal persons give each other pleasure. Latent, unconscious homosexual strains in a woman's personality structure are occasional contributants to orgasmic dysfunction.

Various kinds of prolonged unhealthy relationships during childhood and early adolescence may be conducive toward orgasmic dysfunction in adulthood. A girl whose father treated her throughout her formative years in harsh, depreciating, rejecting ways may fear that all close relationships with men are painful and hostility-ridden. For her, sexual intimacy signifies vulnerability to interpersonal suffering, and her dread leads to nonorgasmic dysfunction. A girl who was repeatedly seduced sexually by an adult man during her childhood or puberty may have a profound dread and revulsion toward sexual contact. Girls reared in loveless, strife-ridden, painful homes, who, in addition, had no other close interpersonal relationships to mitigate the impact of these traumas, may fear sexuality as the avenue that leads toward similar painfulness as a marital partner in adult life. Many other kinds of traumatic interpersonal relationships throughout a girl's formative years may predispose toward orgasmic dysfunction.

Orgasmic dysfunction (frigidity) is sometimes divided into *primary orgasmic dysfunction* and *situational orgasmic dysfunction*. The woman with primary orgasmic dysfunction has never experienced orgasm in any kind of sexual activity. The woman with situational orgasmic dysfunction has on one or more occasions achieved orgasms but cannot do so at the time she comes for treatment. In our opinion, this distinction is of much less importance than the division of impotence into primary and secondary types. The same kinds of emotional problems and interpersonal traumas can lead to either primary or situational orgasmic dysfunction; the distinction may reflect little more than the woman's marital status in many cases. The treatment results in primary and situational orgasmic dysfunction run nearly the same in large series of cases; the difference is only about 6 or 7 per cent.

Treatment of Orgasmic Dysfunction (Frigidity). In our experience, individual psychotherapy resolves orgasmic dysfunction in between a quarter and a half of cases; the large difference in results is caused by the ways in which patients are selected for treatment. For example, if the therapist undertakes treatment mainly with women who have cooperative, interested husbands his results will be much better than if he accepts all women regardless of the soundness of their marital relationships. Depending on the causes of the orgasmic dysfunction, psychotherapy may deal mainly with current and recent interpersonal stresses in the patient's life or it may deal with long-term interpersonal traumas in the patient's childhood and adolescence. Also, depending on causative factors and the therapist's technics, treatment may include some joint counseling sessions with both the patient and her sexual partner.

When the nonorgasmic woman and her sexual partner are well motivated and have sufficient personality flexibility to engage in the process, the sexual retraining approach of Masters and Johnson resolves orgasmic dysfunction in between about 75 and 80 per cent of cases. The details of such sexual retraining are given in the 1970 Masters and Johnson publication listed in the bibliography of this chapter, but we shall outline them briefly here.

The nonorgasmic woman and her partner must first of all view their goal as the development of a new point of view about sexual sensuousness and physical communication between themselves. In the first phase, the bedroom sessions are spent exploring, both verbally and nonverbally, the kinds of stimulation that most excite the woman; combinations of stroking, kissing, teasing and gently manipulating the breasts, mouth, tongue, neck, thighs and other body areas are carried out. This is sometimes called "sensate-focus" play. In the next phase, direct stimulation of the genitals is added to the previous love play. At this stage there is no emphasis on genital-to-genital penetration; the couple merely engage in nondemanding, pleasure-giving and pleasure-receiving physical and verbal communication. In the following phase (each phase consists of several or more bedroom sessions) the woman mounts astride the man and, in the manner most acceptable to her, inserts his penis into her vagina. Periods of time are spent in which no pelvic thrusting by either the man or woman occurs; the woman thus becomes progressively more comfortable with vaginal penile containment in a nondemanding way, and in time she becomes increasingly stimulated by it. In the final stages of sexual retraining the couple shift to a lateral (side-by-side) position and engage in pelvic thrusting in whatever way is best suited to the woman's needs to reach orgasm. After an extensive period of orgasmic success in many episodes of intercourse, other positions, such as the man-above position, may be employed. Success in this retraining therapy depends to a large extent on many details discussed by Masters and Johnson in the reference cited above, and they strongly recommend treatment of the couple by a male therapist and a female therapist in four-person counseling sessions.

Other Sexual Problems

We shall here discuss three types of sexual difficulty which are less commonly encountered in clinical practice. They are *ejaculatory incompetence, vaginismus* and *dyspareunia*.

Ejaculatory Incompetence. The man with ejaculatory incompetence is unable to ejaculate intravaginally, regardless of how long he continues the sex act; even an hour or two of active pelvic thrusting after vaginal penetration does not cause ejaculation. This is a rare disorder. In almost three decades of active psychiatric work, we have seen only one case. This patient was an extremely hostile late adolescent man who was verbally and physically brutal to women; ejaculatory incompetence was only one of his many emotionally caused problems. Persons who work exclusively in the treatment of sexual disorders see a small number of these cases.

The psychiatric literature on this subject is too small to permit a general discussion of the personality characteristics, interpersonal traumas and treatment of men with ejaculatory incompetence. Masters and Johnson in their 1970 publication give their observations on 17 men with this disorder whom they saw during an 11-year period. Masters and Johnson developed a sexual retraining technic, based largely on highly stimulative sex play by the man's sexual partner, which was successful in 14 of their 17 cases. However, as in all their other cases, these men were highly motivated and had very cooperative, flexible wives or other sexual partners with whom to work in the retraining process.

Vaginismus. Vaginismus is syndrome with either emotional or physical causes in which, when penile entry into the vagina is imminent or attempted, the outer third of the vaginal canal and the surrounding muscular structures enter into a prolonged spasm which prevents penile intromission. This condition is rarely the cause of psychiatric consultation; a patient with it usually consults a gynecologist or family physician. We have been consulted about vaginismus only twice in almost three decades of psychiatric experience, and both these patients were recently married women whose vaginismus was resolved by some superficial counseling. The psychiatric literature is too sparse on this subject to allow a general description of its causes and treatment, but presumably it occurs in women who, because of anxiety or old personality traumas, have apprehensiveness about sexual activity; in some instances it may be caused by hostile or competitive feelings toward the sexual partner, or toward men in general.

Persons who specialize in the treatment of sexual problems see occasional cases of vaginismus, but it still is a relatively rare cause of consultation with them. Care must be taken to be sure that the patient does not have a physical condition which is causing her vaginismus; however, in such cases the vaginismus usually is preceded by a period of short or long dyspareunia (discussed in the following section). Masters and Johnson report virtually 100 per cent recovery rates with a treatment regimen in which the vagina is dilated and relaxed by the insertion of graduated sizes of Hegar dilators, in combination with a careful educational and counseling program for the couple.

Dyspareunia. Painful sexual intercourse, whether caused by emotional factors or by vaginal or pelvic pathology, is called dyspareunia. It is much more commonly encountered in clinical practice than either of the two preceding conditions discussed in this section. Before accepting dyspareunia as an emotionally caused complaint, it is best to rule out gynecologic pathology. A wide variety of gynecologic problems may cause it; they include inflammatory and infectious processes of the vagina and surrounding genital structures, insufficient vaginal lubrication due to diverse factors, endometriosis, broad-ligament lacerations, postsurgical anatomical difficulties and various other problems. Nevertheless, the physician must be cautious in evaluating even obvious physical problems in any particular case of dyspareunia, for minor or even negligible discomforts may be used as the reasons for refusing intercourse by women who, for superficial or profound emotional reasons, find sexual intimacy repulsive.

In many cases persistent dyspareunia (as opposed to transient dyspareunia in newly married, tense and sometimes sexually inexperienced women) is caused by emotional problems. In general, they are the same as those discussed above in our consideration of orgasmic dysfunction (frigidity). Old interpersonal traumas or current stresses with the woman's sexual partner, and other factors, may lead to a profound dread or rejection of sexuality, of the female role, of the particular partner, resulting in dyspareunia. Psychotherapy is sometimes helpful in these cases. However, in our experience, many women who come to psychiatric consultation for dyspareunia have had it for from many months to several years or longer, and it often has become a fixed feature of a sick marriage; in these cases the patient usually does not persist in treatment, and when she does the results are frequently discouraging.

Sexual Problems of the Aging Man and the Aging Woman

In this section we shall consider briefly some sexual problems which are common in men and women after the age of 50; they become of greater importance after the age of 60 in most cases. Emotional and physiological factors are closely intertwined in these cases. These difficulties may have marked psychological impacts on how the aging person sees himself, his marriage, his social role and his total life experience in his later years.

The Aging Man. The first problem the older man faces is the culturally accepted myth that his sexual activity must decrease, or perhaps stop altogether, in his later years. Belief in this myth frequently leads the man and his sexual partner to decrease sexual activity, or to abandon it; in doing so they lose something that can give them feelings of vitality and self-esteem, and can also keep their marriage fresh and close.

The older man customarily requires a longer period of pre-intercourse love play to achieve an erection, but once he achieves an erection he tends to hold it longer. The aging couple should understand this, and not give up an attempt at intercourse because the man does not acquire an erection as quickly as he did in his earlier years. The older man usually takes longer to ejaculate after vaginal entry is accomplished and pelvic thrusting begins. This too should not discourage him or his partner. In fact, it prolongs the sex act and often allows the woman to achieve orgasm in a more leisurely manner. Whereas a younger man may ejaculate after a couple of minutes, or less, of pelvic thrusting, the older man may require five or 10 minutes to do so.

The older man's orgasm is briefer than a younger man's, and he ejaculates less seminal fluid. If he does not understand these things, the older man may falsely feel that he is losing his sexual capacity. In reality, his sexual pattern is merely changing. Finally, the older man requires more time to recover his erectile capacity after intercourse; whereas a man in his 20's or 30's may recover his ability to get an erection within 30 to 60 minutes after an act of intercourse, an older man may require from several hours to two or three days, depending on his age. If he recognizes this it ought not to stop his sexual activity, though it may decrease the frequency of intercourse. If the older man wishes, he may continue frequent intercourse by the simple expedient of not ejaculating during each act of intercourse; this can be easily done since, although he requires a longer period of pelvic thrusting to ejaculate than a younger man does, he has greater control over his ejaculations. In this way an older man can satisfy his partner and maintain his self-esteem by acts of fairly frequent intercourse, if this is needed for emotional reasons.

The Aging Woman. The aging woman may be affected by the same cultural myth that discourages the aging male in continuance of sexual intercourse; cultural prejudices hold that she must decrease her sexual life, or abandon it altogether, in her later age period, and acceptance of this false belief may lead her into sexual inactivity. In reality, if she understands the changes that occur in older women sexually and adjusts to them, she can continue her sexual life into her 60's and 70's.

The older woman, especially after the age of 60, requires a significantly longer period of nondemanding sexual play for the development of adequate vaginal lubrication; she may need five minutes or much more of sexual play before the has sufficient vaginal lubrication to allow comfortable, relaxed vaginal penetration. Also, the elasticity of the vaginal walls decreases, and some of the external genitals may become somewhat sensitive to pressure; these problems can be overcome by sound understanding of these changes by the older couple and simple expedients. A longer period of sexual play allows better lubrication and attainment of the maximal vaginal relaxation of which the older woman is capable. Also, the man takes care not to press brusquely on the clitoris and external genitals during penile entry, since these areas are sensitive to undue pressure. In selected cases the pre-intercourse use by the woman of a simple lubricant, such as the jelly used by gynecologists on their gloves before examinations, can further facilitate easy and pleasant intercourse.

The orgasm of the older woman is shorter than that of the younger woman, and its vascular and muscular features are less marked. This should be understood by the woman, and should not lead her to feel that her period of sexual activity is coming to a close. In a few cases the older woman has somewhat uncomfortable uterine contractions during orgasm. This is not a common complaint, however. Most of these physical changes can be much reduced, or eliminated, by prolonged steroid replacement therapy of postmenopausal women. However, gynecologists differ much in opinion about the wisdom and possible complications of this therapy. Psychiatrists and other mental health professional workers will find that in almost all cases they can do adequate counseling with older women on sexual problems by use of the adjustments in sexual technic and other simple expedients we have outlined above.

BIBLIOGRAPHY

Basch, S. H.: The intrapsychic integration of a new organ. A clinical study of kidney transplantation. Psychoanal. Quart., 42:364, 1973.

Burkowsky, M. R. (ed.): Orientation to Language and Learning Disorders. St. Louis, Warren H. Green, 1973.

Chapman, A. H.: The Physician's Guide to Managing Emotional Problems. Philadelphia, J. B. Lippincott, 1969.

———: Management of Emotional Problems of Children and Adolescents. Philadelphia, J. B. Lippincott, 1974.

Copel, S. L. (ed.): Behavior Pathology of Childhood and Adolescence. New York, Basic Books, 1973.

Ginsberg, G. L., Frosch, W. A., and Shapiro, T.: The new impotence. Arch. Gen. Psychiatry, 26:218, 1972.

Grayson, H.: Grief reactions to the relinquishing of unfulfilled wishes. Am. J. Psychother., 25:287, 1970.

Harrison, S. I., and McDermott, J. F.: Childhood Psychopathology. New York, International Universities Press, 1972.

Linksz, A.: On writing, reading and dyslexia. New York, Grune & Stratton, 1973.

Lowenthal, M. F.: Transition to the empty nest. Arch. Gen. Psychiatry, 26:8, 1972.

Masters, W. H., and Johnson, V. E.: Human Sexual Response. Boston, Little Brown, 1966.

———: Human Sexual Inadequacy. Boston, Little Brown, 1970.

Moldofsky, H.: A psychophysiological study of multiple tics. Arch. Gen. Psychiatry, 25:79. 1971.

Myklebust, H. R.: Identification and diagnosis of children with learning disabilities. Semin. in Psychiatry, 5:55, 1973.

Palmore, E. (ed.): Normal Aging. Durham, N. C., Duke University Press, 1974.

Parkes, C. M.: The first year of bereavement. Psychiatry, 33:444, 1970.

Stierlin, H.: A family perspective on adolescent runaways. Arch. Gen. Psychiatry, 29:56, 1973.

Viederman, M.: Adaptive and maladaptive regression in hemodialysis. Psychiatry, 37:68, 1974.

Volkan, V. D.: The linking objects of pathological mourners. Arch. Gen. Psychiatry, 27:215, 1972.

Wertheim, E. S.: Ego dysfunction in stuttering. Brit. J. Med. Psychol., 46:155, 1973.

Wishnie, H. A., and Hackett, T. P.: Psychological hazards of convalescence following myocardial infarction. J. A. M. A., 215:1292, 1971.

26

Legal Aspects of Psychiatry

Both psychiatry and the law are concerned with the interpersonal relationships of people. Psychiatry deals with understanding the individual's personality development and the emotional aspects of his interpersonal relationships. The law deals with his liberties and rights, his rights to acquire and use property, his social and economic obligations to others, his responsibility for crimes against other persons or against society as a whole, his capacities to make contracts and many other aspects of his interpersonal life.

However, psychiatry and the law differ fundamentally in their views of the person. Psychiatry seeks to understand the person and to help him solve his emotional problems; it does not judge him. Psychiatry does not attempt to decide whether any of his acts are moral or immoral, and it does not judge him bad or good; it attempts to understand how the lifelong development of his personality led him to do certain things in the context of his current interpersonal situation. Psychiatry does not censure the person, and it does not punish him; it studies the person and seeks to modify his personality problems and interpersonal functions in healthy ways.

The law, on the other hand, judges people. Though the law is interested in the person's intentions as well as his acts, it judges him to be right or wrong and may punish him according to the degree in which he is found wrong. The law views its capacity to judge and punish the person as necessary for keeping society orderly and morally sound. The law does not try to change the person's personality; it accepts his personality as it exists and holds him responsible for obeying the precepts which it sets up for all members of the society it regulates.

Psychiatry holds that a person is not consciously aware of the motivations of many of his acts. Psychiatry holds that unconscious motivations and personality forces that originate in the patient's childhood and adolescence affect his conduct in adult life in ways he often does not understand. Hence, psychiatry takes the view that the person who violates the civil or criminal laws of society often is more in need of treatment than punishment. Psychiatry often is skeptical that punishment is an effective force in deterring antisocial acts, and it wonders about the justice of punishing a person who is the product of a childhood environment he did not choose and interpersonal upbringing he could not control.

The law, however, assumes that the individual is responsible for his acts after a specific age in late childhood or early adolescence (depending on state law) and must answer for their consequences unless he is shown clearly to be mentally ill by definitely prescribed legal criteria. The law feels that each person has full freedom of choice and the ability to know right from wrong, and if he makes antisocial choices and does illegal things he must be prepared to suffer censure and punishment. The law feels that its power to punish offenders is a major social force in preventing society from lapsing into unbridled brutality, rampant deceit and civil disorder.

The psychiatric point of view has been pithily summarized by Sullivan, who wrote that psychiatry could find "nothing but dogma in the entity, free will." Sullivan pointed out that, especially in culturally deprived sections of society, a person rarely is fully aware of the nature and consequences of his acts, as the law assumes he is at all times. The concept that a person has full, or even adequate, insight into the nature of what he does and why he does it is "glaringly ridiculous." Moreover, it is artificial, Sullivan states, to view a criminal act, or any other act, divorced from the interpersonal setting in which it occurred; the act and the environment are one thing. Any type of legal offender or civil litigant should be seen in the context of the intimate interpersonal relations, the cultural circumstances and the socioeconomic environment which produced him and dovetailed with the action that is in question. The law, as Sullivan saw it, is "punitive-retaliatory," as opposed to psychiatry, which is exploratory, nonjudgemental and oriented toward therapy. The law consists of a set of convenient, more or less workable fictions which enable society to grind on, but it is not rooted in what is known scientifically of the nature of man and his society.

These differences of point of view may be made concrete by considering two specific examples. While dirving his automobile, an intoxicated alcoholic runs down and seriously injures a woman. The law investigates the facts of the case. It determines from witnesses and examination of the man shortly after the accident that he was drunk when the accident occurred. The law judges him to have done a wrong thing. It punishes him by depriving him of his license to drive a car, and it may fine him or imprison him for his misdeed against the woman and against society as a whole. In addition, upon her appeal to the law, it may force the man to pay her substantial sums of money for the injuries and suffering she had because of the accident. Psychiatry, on the other hand, asks other questions. It asks why this man needs to drink excessive amounts of alcohol. Psychiatry wonders what occurred in his childhood, adolescence and early adulthood to make him an alcoholic, and it examines the stresses in his current interpersonal life which contribute to his alcoholism. It seeks to treat this man so he will not drink excessively in the future and be a danger to himself and others. Psychiatry is skeptical that fining and imprisoning intoxicated drivers decreases the amount of alcoholism or much diminishes the number of automobile accidents caused by intoxicated motorists.

In another instance, a 65-year-old woman makes a will in which she leaves most of her property to her 42-year-old son and leaves only a token amount to her 32-year-old daughter. The law is interested only in knowing if at the time she made the will she knew (1) that she was making a will, (2) the amount and nature of the property she possessed, and (3) who were the possible heirs and other beneficiaries. If she knew these three things, her will is valid and the law takes no further interest in the matter.

Psychiatry, though it may have little to say about the legal rights and financial expectations of the son and daughter, looks deeper than the law if it is asked to study why this woman did what she did. Psychiatry may discover that the son, her firstborn child, was a wanted, cherished child. The woman may not have wanted more children after her son was born, and the conception, birth and upbringing of her daughter may have been repugnant to her. In addition, because of long-standing personality problems originating in her own childhood, this woman may have been affectionate toward her son and competitively hostile to her daughter. Hence, the daughter may have been treated with irritable coldness and criticism all her life while the woman lavished fond favoritism on her son. When the woman draws up a will disposing of her property to her son and daughter, both of whom are now married with children of their own, her long-standing emotional attitudes toward her children gravely affect the distribution of her property. Psychiatry views these family relationships as unhealthy and the distribution of the property as determined by the woman's unhealthy emotional attitudes whose origins she does not understand; moreover, from a strictly logical point of view, her attitudes toward her children are irrational. Psychiatry must agree that she was "mentally sound" in the legal sense of the phrase at the time she made the will, but psychiatry has an understanding of her actions that goes immensely beyond the interest of the law. Also, though the requirements of the law are met in this woman's will, it does a gross economic injustice to the daughter.

These two examples illustrate the basic differences between psychiatry and the law in dealing with the same interpersonal situations. These basic differences affect almost every area where psychiatry and the law meet. The full resolution of these differences still lies in the future. For the present, the psychiatrist must try to understand the law and work toward resolutions that are scientifically sound, interpersonally humane and legally just. Much thought, work and time will be needed before these goals are met.

We shall now review the most important legal aspects of psychiatry. We shall consider them in five broad categories: (1) the person and his responsiblities for criminal acts, (2) the person and psychiatric hospitalization procedures, (3) the person and his capacities for making wills, contracts and other important decisions, (4) the person and his privileged communications to psychiatrists and other mental health professional workers and (5) the legal responsibilities and liabilities of psychiatrists and other mental health professionals.

THE PERSON AND HIS RESPONSIBILITY FOR CRIMINAL ACTS

Until recently, the criteria for determining whether or not a person who had committed a crime was of sufficiently sound mind to be held responsible for his act were determined by the *M'Naghten rules* in most English-speaking courts; in the United States the *irresistible impulse test* was an added criterion in a minority of courts. In recent times, however, the criteria of the American law Institute's *Model Penal Code* have been rapidly supplanting these other criteria in American courts; though the M'Naghten rules are still more commonly employed, the balance is shifting steadily toward the rules of the Model Penal Code.

The M'Naghten Rules. In 1843 Daniel M'Naghten, a Scotsman, shot and killed Edward Drummond, the secretary to the British prime minister, Sir Robert Peel. M'Naghten for several years had suffered from paranoid delusions; he had spoken to various people about his delusions and had appealed to public authorities for protection against persons he felt were persecuting him and conspiring against him. M'Naghten waited outside Peel's house and when he saw Drummond coming out of the house shot him, thinking he was Peel. At his trial M'Naghten was acquitted on the grounds that he was mentally unsound and was committed to a psychiatric facility. This decision aroused much criticism in Britain, and the House of Lords drew up five questions which they submitted to the 15 common-law judges of England requesting a clear definition of the criteria for determining whether or not a person who committed a crime was mentally responsible for his act. The reply of the 15 judges can be condensed into two general principles which since then have been the basis for most legal criteria for determining mental responsibility for criminal acts in the English-speaking countries.

These two general principles are: (1) a person is not responsible for a criminal act if at the time he committed it he was "laboring under such a defect of reason, from disease of the mind, as not to know the nature and quality of the act he was doing," or (2) "if he did know it, he did not know he was doing what was wrong." Although the reply of the judges in the M'Naghten case contained other precepts, these two principles form the most important part of their ruling.

However, defects in the M'Naghten rules have been apparent from the time of their enunciation to the present. The M'Naghten rules do not attempt to base mental responsiblity for a criminal act on the presence or absence of psychiatric disease. They merely list two criteria, (1) knowing the nature and quality of the act and (2) knowing whether or not it was wrong, as the bases for criminal responsiblity. Many psychotic patients would have to be judged sane under the M'Naghten rules. For example, most psychotically depressed patients, many manic patients and many schizophrenic patients know the general nature and quality of the acts they are carrying out and know whether their acts would be considered right or wrong by a court. The M'Naghten rules apply most validly to patients with advanced organic brain disease who have marked defects of memory, orientation, judgement and other intellectual functions. A further difficulty in applying the

M'Naghten rules is the problem of determining what different people would consider "wrong." The problems of applying the M'Naghten rules have become increasingly difficulty as psychiatric knowledge has advanced during the 20th Century. The M'Naghten rules, of course, do not take into consideration unconscious motivations, disturbances of affect such as depressive or manic states, and many other concepts of modern psychiatry. Nevertheless, with a few exceptions, until relatively recently, when the American Law Institute's Model Penal Code has begun to be widely adopted, the M'Naghten rules have remained the cornerstone for determining mental responsibility for criminal acts in courts throughout the English-speaking world. In actual practice, the M'Naghten rules have worked better than their precise wording would lead one to expect, mainly because both judges and juries have used them as rough, rather than precise, guidelines.

The Irresistible Impulse Test. The one other principle which long has been used in American definitions of criminal responsibility is the irresistible impulse test, which is employed in some states as an addition to the M'Naghten rules. The irresistible impulse test states that a person is relieved of criminal responsibility for an act if he performed it because of an irresistible impulse caused by mental disease. However, the term irresistible impulse is difficult to define from a psychiatric point of view and is not harmonious with modern psychiatric concepts of emotional illness. Moreover, it does not take into account the fact that a paranoid psychotic patient may brood upon an act of violence for many weeks or months and then carry it out in a craftily conceived manner. For example, if Daniel M'Naghten were to be judged on the irresistible impusle test alone, he would probably be declared criminally responsible for the murder he committed. One of the early cases establishing the irresistible impulse test was in Ohio in 1834, and in the decades following the Civil War its use spread to a number of states. At its height, the irresistible impulse test was employed in about 15 states and in some other courts as an addition to the M'Naghten rules. Its use has declined in recent years as various federal and state courts and legislatures have adopted the Model Penal Code's criteria for use within their jurisdictions.

The Model Penal Code Criteria for Criminal Responsiblity. In 1955 the American Law Institute published its Model Penal Code after a nine-year study. The Model Code states, "A person is not responsible for criminal conduct if at the time of such conduct as the result of mental disease or defect he lacks substantial capacity either to appreciate the criminality of his conduct or to conform his conduct to the requirements of law. The terms 'mental disease or defect' do not include an abnormality manifested only by repeated criminal or otherwise antisocial conduct."

This definition of criminal responsiblity has been accepted by an ever-increasing number of American courts, and by some state legislatures. It is generally assumed that, with the passage of time, it will gradually replace the M'Naghten rules in American courts. The Model Code rule is sometimes referred to as the "Vermont rule" since the Vermont state legislature was one of the first bodies to vote it, with minor modifications, into statutory law. It also is occasionally referred to as the Currens formula, or rule.

Although some criticisms may be raised against features of the Model Penal Code's criteria, most psychiatrists and lawyers now feel that it is the best common ground on which psychiatry and the law can meet at the present time and is a decided advance over the M'Naghten rules and the irresistible impulse test. However, most courts in the English-speaking world outside the United States continue to employ the M'Naghten rules or variations of them.

Other Aspects of Criminal Responsibility

If a person accused of a crime is psychiatrically ill to the extent that he cannot participate well in his own defense, he cannot be tried until he recovers from his psychiatric illness. The definition of mental illness in this situation does not rest on the M'Naghten rules, or the Model Code, or any other rule used in determining criminal responsibility. The question is whether the patient is mentally ill to the extent that he cannot confer effectively with his attorneys and participate in preparing his own defense; the law specifies that he must be able to do these things before he can be brought to trial. After his mental illness is established by psychiatric examination, the person usually is committed by court order to a psychiatric hospital. When the psychiatrists caring for the accused person report to the court that he has recovered from his psychiatric illness, or has improved to the extent that he can participate well in his own defense, he can be brought to trial for the crime of which he is accused.

When a person is found not guilty of a criminal act because he was mentally ill at the time he carried it out, he usually is committed to a state psychiatric hospital by the court in which he was tried. In some states such commitment is mandatory by law, whereas in others it is left to the discretion of the judge. In some states the patient may be released from the hospital by the court which committed him when he recovers. In other states he may be discharged only by order of the governor. In addition, the patient, or persons representing him, can initiate litigation at any time claiming that he has recovered from his mental illness and should be discharged.

The criminal law of Massachusetts has a well known provision, the Briggs law, which requires that persons accused of various kinds of crimes must be examined psychiatrically by an impartial psychiatrist appointed by the state. The examiner makes his report to the court having jurisdiction over the person, and the report is also available to the prosecuting attorney and the defense attorney. The Briggs law has been much praised by psychiatrists as an approach to harmony between psychiatry and the law. It is stated that it tends to avoid the "battle of the experts" spectacle at criminal trials in which psychiatrists testifying for the prosecution and the defense say opposite things to a confused jury and public. However, the Briggs law has not spread to other states, since its opponents state that in it the law is abandoning too much of its authority to a medical specialty which they do not regard as an exact science.

THE PERSON AND PSYCHIATRIC HOSPITALIZATION PROCEDURES

Voluntary Admission. The vast majority of persons who are admitted to private psychiatric hospitals and to the psychiatric divisions of private general hospitals enter as voluntary patients. The patient signs the admission form and his closest relative usually signs it also. As a rule, the admission form contains a simply worded statement that the patient agrees to enter the psychiatric hospital and to abide by the regulations governing its care of patients. Only a small percentage of patients admitted to private psychiatric facilities enter by court commitment. The admission form a voluntary patient signs may contain a provision that if the patient wishes to leave the hospital against the advice of his psychiatrist he must give clear notice of his demand to leave 24 to 72 hours before he is discharged. However, the psychiatrist may not insist that the patient remain the full time specified in the prior notification stipulation.

The percentage of patients who enter public psychiatric facilities, especially state mental hospitals, voluntarily is much lower than in private hospitals. However, the legal trend in recent times has been to encourage voluntary admissions in all possible ways. Every state but one has legislation permitting conditional voluntary admission; "conditional" means that when he signs in voluntarily the patient agrees to give prior (often written) notice of his intention to terminate treatment and leave the hospital if he changes his mind, and to remain in the hospital for two to 10 days more before leaving. In effect, this opens the way for the hospital staff to initiate proceedings for a commitment if they feel the patient meets the criteria for commitment (discussed later) and should be committed. Eight states provide by law for unconditional voluntary admission; "unconditional" means that the patient can immediately terminate treatment and leave the hospital if he at any time demands it; this often means that the hospital does not have easy ways to institute commitment proceedings to stop him, even when they feel it is justified. In efforts to increase voluntary admissions, some state laws stipulate that all involved legal officers must strongly encourage patients and their families to use voluntary admissions, as opposed to admissions by court commitments, and that full information about the advantages of voluntary admission be laid before them.

If the psychiatrist in a private or public facility feels that a patient who entered voluntarily and later demands his release is so ill that he should not be discharged, he can (with the limitations mentioned above in some states) advise the patient's family to start court commitment proceedings immediately to allow the hospital to hold the patient for further treatment; as a rule, once the request for court proceedings is filed, the patient can be held legally in the hospital for the short period of time until the court hearing is held to decide the matter. However, such a court commitment is needed in only a very small percentage of voluntarily admitted patients; in the vast majority of instances, the voluntarily admitted patient remains voluntarily in the hospital until he is well enough to leave on his psychiatrist's recommendation.

In most states a child under the age of 14 to 18, depending on state statutes, may be admitted to a private or public psychiatric hospital if his parents or guardians sign the admission form; the willing consent of the child or adolescent is very desirable from the psychiatric point of view, but it is not legally necessary.

Admission by Commitment Procedure. From the psychiatric point of view, voluntary admission by the patient's own choice, or by application of his relatives and the acquiescence of the patient, is the most satisfactory arrangement. It places admission to a psychiatric facility on the same basis as any other type of hospital admission for medical or surgical purposes. However, in some instances a psychiatric patient who urgently needs psychiatric hospitalization rejects the advice of his doctors and the persuasion of his relatives. The health and welfare of the patient, the prevention of suicide and the protection of other people may make the patient's psychiatric hospitalization necessary. In such cases the patient may be committed to a psychiatric hospital only by legal procedure.

The viewpoints of psychiarty and the law differ much on the question of legal commitment procedures of psychiatric patients. Psychiatry feels that application of the patient's family to the court stating all the facts, accompanied by reports of two psychiatrists who recently have examined him, should suffice for issuance of a commitment order. Psychiatry disapproves of courtroom hearings before a judge, and perhaps a jury, with the patient present and interrogation of the patient and other people by opposing lawyers. Psychiatry feels that such commitment procedures are psychiatrically damaging to emotionally sick patients and often aggravate their psychoses; this is particularly true of paranoid schizophrenic patients with delusions of persecution. Such courtroom hearings put the patient in a position similar to that of an accused criminal who is brought into court to decide whether or not he should be deprived of his liberty.

However, almost all state laws specify that the patient must receive prior notice of the hearing and that he has the right to be present if he chooses. In some states the hearing is heard only by a judge, but the laws of some states specify that the patient may have a jury decide the matter if he wishes. The law views court hearings as necessary safeguards to prevent malicious people from unjustly incarcerating other persons in psychiatric hospitals and thus depriving them of their liberty. Psychiatry feels that unjust or unnecessary commitment of psychiatric patients is immensely rare. Moreover, after commitment to a psychiatric hospital, any patient may be discharged immediately by his attending psychiatrist or the head of the hospital if the patient is found not to require hospital care. However, the law protects the liberties and rights of each person against even the rarest kinds of infringements. The right of a court hearing at which he may be present if he chooses is considered to be an inalienable right of a person who is to be deprived of his liberty for any reason, including his own medical health.

This sometimes leads to ludicrous, and even tragic, results. Many years ago, while on a government assignment in Texas, I participated as an expert witness in the commitment hearing of a paranoid psychotic lawyer. He represented himself legally, and the prosecuting attorney's office, thinking the matter a routine chore, sent to the hearing an elderly clerk who was not a lawyer; the judge was an elected official who also was not a lawyer. After the hearing began it became apparent that the only lawyer in the courtroom was the patient, who proceeded to convince a six-

indefinite commitments. In recent years several states have enacted legislation that requires hospitals to make periodic reviews of indefinitely committed patients with particular attention to determining if they can be treated on an outpatient basis or discharged. These laws are designed to prevent possible neglect of long-term "back ward" patients in large psychiatric hospitals.

The indefinitely committed patient, like the temporarily committed patient, retains all civil liberties except the rights to leave the hospital at will and to refuse treatment.

4. **Emergency Commitment.** Many states have laws that permit emergency commitment of a disturbed patient for a few days while a temporary commitment or an indefinite commitment is being sought. A close relative or a public health officer files a petition with the hospital in which commitment is sought, and the petition is supported by the report of a physician who recently has examined the patient. In other states the petition and the supporting report are presented to a judge who issues the emergency commitment order. An emergency commitment usually allows the hospital to hold the patient three to five days. Within that period of time, proceedings for a temporary commitment or an indefinite commitment must be filed. Once the petition seeking temporary or indefinite commitment has been filed, the hospital can hold the patient until his court hearing has been held. However, most judges hold the hearing for a temporary commitment or an indefinite commitment promptly when the patient previously has been committed on an emergency basis.

Other Aspects of Commitment Procedures

In most instances the petition for a commitment is filed with the chief clerk of the court having jurisdiction in the matter. The clerk then sets the procedure in motion and schedules the hearing. In large cities the clerk's office usually has a staff of persons trained to outline the steps in a commitment procedure to the patient's family and to aid them in executing them. When a physician has doubts about his role in a commitment procedure or about the best way to proceed, he may call the attorney whose services are retained by the hospital to which he takes patients, and the attorney can orient him easily. In most states the patient's family, guided by the staff of the clerk's office or by their attorney, institute the commitment procedure and the psychiatrists merely provide the needed medical reports.

As noted above, even though he has been committed to a psychiatric hospital, the patient still retains all his civil rights except the right to leave the hospital without the permission of his psychiatrist and the right to refuse treatment. A patient loses his other rights only if he is judged *incompetent*, and this usually involves a separate *incompetency hearing*. However, in rare cases a commitment procedure and an incompetency hearing may be held at the same court session. An incompetency ruling is given by a court only after a careful hearing in which the patient's long-range, severe mental incapacitation is proved. After a patient is adjudicated incompetent, a guardian, who may be a relative, or a responsible interested person, or a bank, is appointed to handle his affairs.

Despite the fact that, by common law and prevalent practice, a patient who is committed loses only his rights to leave the hospital and to refuse treatment (most commitment orders give the hospital the right "to hold and to treat" the patient), the urgings of civil liberties advocates in recent years have caused state legislatures to pass a great deal of legislation specifically insuring that committed patients retain the right to enter contractual agreements, to execute wills, to have religious freedom during commitment, to keep reasonable amounts of personal clothing and other items, to communicate with persons outside the hospital by telephone, correspondence and visits from them, to manage and dispose of property, to be employed if feasible, to procure habeas corpus writs, to make purchases, to receive education, to retain civil service status, to have examinations by psychiatrists and other physicians besides the ones attending him, to retain licenses such as driver's licenses and professional licenses, to marry, to sue and be sued, and not to be subject to unnecessary mechanical restraints. Legislation also has been passed guaranteeing the patient's right to legal counsel, at state expense if necessary, in commitment hearings and any other legal matters in which he might become involved (writs of habeas corpus, and others). Many psychiatrists view such legislation as unnecessary, since a patient can lose a civil right only by a court action, and a commitment order deprives him of only the two rights listed above, but civil liberties advocates argue that such legislation protects patients in clearer ways.

However, in actual practice, with the exception of the rights to receive visitors, to correspond, to consult an attorney if he wishes, and to do other understandable, routine acts, patients rarely exercise most of these rights (to marry, to sign contracts, to start civil litigation, and others) during periods of commitment, unless they are approved by his psychiatrist and closest relatives. If a committed patient insists on entering into contractual agreements and conducting business when he is not psychiatrically capable of exercising reasonable judgement, his family may seek a court hearing to declare him incompetent and to have the court appoint a guardian to handle his affairs and to make any necessary decisions (sometimes with court approval) for him until he again has good judgement and reasonably sound mental health. Whereas a commitment order almost invariably is terminated automatically when the patient's psychiatrist discharges him from the hospital to which he was sent, a special court hearing usually is necessary to lift an incompetency ruling.

False Imprisonment. If a person is held against his will in a psychiatric hospital, or any other place, without a commitment or other legal procedure, he may sue the individuals who detained him on the grounds of *false imprisonment*. This is a civil action, and the plaintiff may claim financial damages for the false imprisonment and any economic losses he suffered as a result. In law, any period of illegal detainment, even for a few hours, is grounds for a false imprisonment suit, but such a suit is rarely instituted against a physician and a hospital unless the period of detainment was more than 24 hours.

Consent for Treatment. A patient who enters a hospital *voluntarily* must also sign papers for any special treatments. The papers he signs upon admission usually contain a statement in which he agrees to take the medications prescribed and to cooperate in other activities (group psychotherapy, activity programs and others) which are ordered for him. However, in almost all psychiatric facilities the patient, and often his closest relative must sign additional *consent for treatment* permits for special therapies such as electroshock therapy, new or particularly hazardous medications, and other such things. It is legally unwise for any hospital or psychiatrist to give such treatments without specific consent in writing. Most hospitals have printed forms for this purpose, and the legal department of the American Medical Association publishes a book of standard permit forms for all the various kinds of procedures. A parent signs for a minor child, and a guardian signs for a person who has been ruled incompetent in a court hearing.

The law further specifies that the patient, his relatives and any others who sign these papers must give "informed consent." Informed consent requires that the general nature of the procedure and all its possible risks are explained to the patient, or any other signing party, before he signs. This is a difficult medical point, for often it is not in the patient's best medical and psychiatric interests to be told all the possible complications and side effects of a procedure, such as electroshock therapy; he has little capacity to place such things in their proper perspectives, and, moreover, it has been experimentally shown that patients who know of the possible ill effects (nausea, backache, headache, and others) of a procedure have a decidedly greater chance of developing them. To tell a severely depressed patient with strong obsessive fears and worries all the possible complications of electroshock therapy, or even of antidepressant medication, submits him to much emotional suffering in many cases. Nevertheless, the physician who does not do so is vulnerable to lawsuits by an increasingly litigation-conscious public if an untoward effect occurs. Some hospitals have all the common complications of a treatment, such as electroshock therapy, printed as part of the permission form, and a nurse watches the patient read them and then countersigns the form. The legal and medical interests of patients often are at variance with each other. In the field of informed consent, statutory law and judicial precedent are conflicting and confusing, but most physicians are becoming increasingly cautious in this area.

Right to Treatment Decisions. Since the late 1960's a large number of suits and decisions have resulted in the "right to treatment" doctrine, which is still not a settled issue. Various courts have held that patients remanded to mental hospitals on commitments, or because they were found not guilty of crimes because of psychiatric illness, or were unable to stand trial because of psychiatric conditions, have a right to receive reasonable and appropriate psychiatric treatment. If they do not, these courts have reasoned, the patients' stays in hospitals amount to incarceration similar to that of imprisonment in a jail, rather than hospitalization in a treatment facility. Some courts have even stipulated specific ratios of hospital staff for patient totals, the minimum appropriations in money for state hospital systems, and the availability of various modes of treatment. Similarly, courts have held that mentally retarded persons in institutions for the mentally retarded have a "right to education," and have ruled that they must be given education adequate to their needs, either in the institution or in nearby public schools.

Although this movement has been hailed by many persons interested in the welfare of psychiatric patients, it has raised many problems. One high court, moreover, has held that all such court decisions are unconstitutitonal since they represent an undue invasion by the judicial branch of the government into the prerogatives of the legislative and executive branches of the government; the court held that the establishment and maintenance of standards in mental hospitals, and the services they render, should be determined by legislatures, and that reformers should, by direct appeal and election campaigns, secure such action from legislatures rather than courts. There are, moreover, the problems of how treatable many conditions are, especially those of persons who have been found not guilty of criminal actions because of psychiatric disease, and whether a daily phenothiazine antipsychotic medication and a good hospital activity program constitutes adequate treatment for a paranoid schizophrenic, or whether he has a right to group or individual psychotherapy. It undoubtedly will require many years of litigation before standard law, if any, is established in this field.

THE PERSON AND HIS CAPACITY FOR MAKING WILLS, CONTRACTS AND OTHER IMPORTANT DECISIONS

The Person's Capacity to Make a Will

In order to make a legally valid will a person must meet the three following criteria: (1) He must know that he is drawing up a will. (2) He must know the nature and amount of his property. (3) He must know who are his reasonable heirs or beneficiaries. If a person knows these three things and his judgement about them is reasonably sound, he can make a valid will. Thus, a patient can make a valid will even in the presence of a psychiatric illness, if the illness does not significantly affect these three mental capacities. The person need not know the exact amount of his property, but he must have a reasonable concept of its nature and extent. The person also must be able to name all the members of his family who are his reasonable heirs, and he must be able to state his relationship to them. In addition, he must be able to list any other institutions or persons to whom he wishes to bequeath property and he must know his reasons for doing so. The patient must not be influenced by delusions or by the manipulations of persons who exploit him when he is in an infirm or dependent state, for the courts have held that such influences distort his judgement about his reasonable heirs and the property he should give them.

A physician may be called upon to give an opinion about a patient's mental capacity to make a will under two circumstances: (1) in the case of a patient whom the physician attended at the time the will was made, and about whose mental state the physician therefore can give an opinion, and (2) in the case of a deceased patient whom the physician never saw, but whose mental state is described in a court hearing by witnesses who saw him at the time he made the will. Any physician may give an opinion about a patient's capacity to make a will, but the opinions of psychiatrists increasingly are sought today.

The opinion of the physician about the patient's fitness to make a will should be based upon whether the patient had the three mental capacities listed above. If a psychiatrist, or any other physician, is asked specifically to examine a patient who is making a will to determine if he has the sound mental capacity to do so, he should question the patient carefully about the three mental capacities discussed above and he should write down many of the patient's answers verbatim. He also should note the patient's emotional reactions to the questions and should carry out a systematic mental status examination of the patient (as outlined in Chapter 4).

The Person's Capacity to Make a Contract

When a person is severely ill psychiatrically and is unable to handle his affairs, his relatives or any other person interested in his welfare may file a petition in court to have the person declared mentally *incompetent* and to have a guardian appointed to look after his interestes. A person so ruled in an *incompetency hearing* loses all rights to enter into contracts, to buy or sell things, to render or receive services, and engage in other verbal or written contracts.

The central question in an incompetency hearing is not so much whether or not the person has a psychiatric illness, but whether a psychiatric illness has caused sufficient deterioration of his judgement to rob him of the capacity to make sound decisions in contractual matters. The presence of a psychiatric illness, even a fairly severe one, is not in itself sufficient to justify an ajudication of incompetency. In actual practice, incompetency rulings are most commonly sought for persons with permanent organic brain damage (especially due to cerebral arteriosclerosis and senile brain degeneration), moderate or severe mental retardation and prolonged schizophrenic illnesses. However, an incompetency hearing may be held on a patient with any type of psychiatric illness, even if the illness has a good prognosis within a reasonable time, if he has important financial or personal business requiring prompt action. The legal term *insane* is often used in these matters. The term insane has no precise medical meaning, but in general it implies a severe psychiatric illness in which the individual has marked defects of judgement and interpersonal incapacitation.

Incompetency hearings usually are held before a judge who makes the decision, but juries are impaneled in some states. The patient must be notified of the hearing in advance and he has the right to be present at the hearing and to be represented by counsel if he chooses. Written reports or personal testimony from one or two physicians are required, and psychiatric testimony often is necessary; in many instances the physician must appear in court, but in some cases a written report is accepted as evidence. When the patient has substantial property a disinterested agent, such as a bank, is often appointed the guardian. The court sometimes reserves certain decisions to itself; for example, in many instances a mentally retarded person cannot undergo a sterilizing operation without a further court order, and such orders are given sparingly.

The person who has been ruled incompetent loses his right to conduct business, make contracts, vote, drive a car and exercise many other rights which involve discretion and judgement. He usually is deprived of the right to marry, start divorce proceedings, practice a licensed profession and exercise other privileges. The guardian assumes responsibility for making all important decisions and managing the person's affairs. To lift an incompetency ruling requires a special hearing with medical testimony that the patient no longer has defective judgement and now can manage his affairs adequately.

If a person enters a contract, such as an agreement to buy or sell something or to perform certain services, at a time when he is psychiatrically ill and has defective judgement, his relatives may seek court action to void the contract and to ajudicate the patient incompetent. The contract usually can be set aside if it can be demonstrated that the patient had defective judgement because of psychiatric illness at the time he made the contract. However, all these general statements about contracts and mental competency are subject to variations that depend on the particular circumstances of each case and different state laws.

The Person's Capacity to Marry or Divorce

From the legal point of view, a person who marries enters a marriage contract in which he assumes certain obligations and duties toward his marital partner. A marriage sometimes can be annulled if it is demonstrated that at the time of the marriage the person did not understand the nature of the obligations and duties of the marriage contract because he was psychiatrically ill, severely intoxicated with alcohol, or in any other way mentally incapacitated. In general, a court is hesitant to annul a marriage unless the demonstration of mental incapacitation is clear-cut. In most states, psychiatric illness alone does not constitute grounds for granting a divorce to the marital partner of the psychiatrically ill person. However, many states allow divorce if the patient has been psychiatrically ill a specified number of years and recovery seems improbable in the foreseeable future. State laws vary much in this regard.

THE PERSON AND PRIVILEGED COMMUNICATIONS TO PSYCHIATRISTS AND OTHER MENTAL HEALTH PROFESSIONAL WORKERS

There is a fundamental conflict in attitude between psychiatry and the law about the degree of confidentiality of psychiatrists' information about patients. Psychiatry feels that what the patient tells the psychiatrist, or other mental health professional worker (clinical psychologist, psychiatric nurse, psychiatric social worker or others), and what the professional person observes about the patient, cannot be disclosed to any third party, including a court, without the patient's consent and, in some cases, only with the considered judgement of the professional person. Psychiatry feels that unless such protection exists the completely uninhibited nature of patient-therapist communication becomes much impaired and the patient's welfare is damaged. The patient will not feel comfortable in communicating freely with the therapist if he knows that at some future time his words and actions may be released to a third party, or even made public in a court hearing.

The law, on the other hand, while recognizing that reasonable privacy should exist in almost all patient-therapist dealings, often takes the position that crimes and civil misbehavior should not go uninvestigated and perhaps unpunished because therapists withold information from investigating bodies and courts. The law often feels that third parties, or society in general, will be damaged if illegal acts are allowed to flourish because psychiatrists and other mental health professional workers do not give the information they have. The pendulum of general opinion and action swings backs and forth, often from one decade to the next, as legislatures and courts reverse their attitudes. Current trends are hard to clarify, since each point of view has its vigorous proponents.

Professional *ethics* dictate that psychiatrists and other mental health workers shall not disclose any psychiatric information about a patient unless requested to do so by the patient or his guardian in writing. When this ethical principle is accepted in law, it becomes known as *privileged communication*; privileged communication is a legal, not an ethical, term. It indicates that information divulged by a person to certain types of professional workers cannot be disclosed in court hearings, and other procedures and business, without the patient's consent, except in rare circumstances. Persons who are covered by privileged communication include attorneys, clergymen, and, where laws provide for it, physicians and some other kinds of nonphysician therapists.

Under English and American common law privileged communication exists only when a legislature specifically votes a law to provide it. The first such law in the United States was passed by the New York state legislature in 1828, and at present about two-thirds of states have laws providing some degree of privileged communication. However, even these laws have, in some cases, limitations about what the physician can withold from the court. Two states, at the time of this writing, give privileged communication to "patient-psychotherapist" relationships, and this term could be construed to include any recognized mental health professional worker. Patient-nurse confidentiality has been legislated in only several states.

There is one notable extension of confidentiality. In some cases it has been held that nurses are covered by the privileged communication protection of physicians if the nurses are working as agents of physicians under their supervision. That is, if a psychiatric nurse is aiding a psychiatrist in the care of a patient, anything the patient tells the nurse, or anything she observes about him, is confidential if the laws of that state give privileged communication coverage to the physician. However, this exists in relatively few court jurisdictions and is based on the principle that nursing is a licensed profession. Although this principle could conceivably apply to psychiatric social workers, clinical psychologists and other mental health professional workers, it is hampered by the fact that only in a few states are any of these professional persons licensed to carry out their work.

The right of confidentiality, in law, resides with the patient, not the therapist. The patient may at any time request the psychiatrist to release information about him, and the psychiatrist is usually assumed to be required to do so if the patient's best interests, as the patient sees them, demand it. However, this has been contested by some psychiatrists lately, who feel that they also have certain rights to the information in their possession since that information involves not only what the patient did and said, but also what the psychiatrist thought about the patient's deeds and words. However, at present confidentiality rests, in law, only with the patient. Only he can deny information in the psychiatrist's hands to any third party or to a court.

The question of privileged communication (and its largely synonymous term, confidentiality) has been much complicated in recent times by the fact that the patient-therapist relationship has been breached by third parties who are paying for the patient's care; such third parties include insurance companies (often linked to the patient's employers), state or federal government agencies and, in rare cases, others. Since the patient has a signed or legislated contract with the third party to pay for his care only within certain limits, the third party feels that it has a right to certain basic data to be sure that the type of care the patient is receiving, for whatever problem he has, is actually covered by his contract. However, the information received by insurance companies and others is often fed into computers, which may be linked to other computers, and any break in confidentiality may set information on a course whose future is unpredictable. A person may be confronted by obstacles in gaining employment because of information released a decade or more before.

In all cases in which enacted legislation does not provide for it, privileged communication does not exist, and the therapist may be required to divulge information in court about a patient. This has happened in child custody suits, divorce hearings, criminal actions and other procedures. In actual practice a showdown between a judge and a psychiatrist, or other mental health professional worker, is rare; most judges treat psychiatric personnel with consideration and a compromise which meets the needs of the law and the integrity of the psychiatric professions is worked out. However, in the rare cases when such confrontation in court results in punitive action by an insistent judge toward a reluctant professional person, there is usually a good deal of publicity which disturbs the psychiatric professions and the many patients who are revealing intimate things to them.

When a psychiatrist or other mental health professional person faces a problem regarding confidentiality he should seek information about what the law, and common judicial practices, are in the district where he works. Often a good attorney to consult is the official attorney of the hospital to which the psychiatrist takes his patients. Social welfare agencies often have legal advisors who may be consulted by nonphysician mental health workers.

It also should be noted that insurance companies, business firms, potential employers and other third parties usually do not press psychiatrists and other mental health professionals about details; they tend to respect confidentiality. The psychiatrist usually can give them the data wanted without injuring his patient if he words his replies carefully and gives the inquiring party only the information it specifically is seeking.

A certain amount of caution should be exercised in the material that goes into hospital records, including any psychologists' reports, nursing notes, progress notes and workups. Hospital records can be subpoenaed into court and can be admitted as evidence. Laws of privileged communication rarely are construed to cover any material written on a patient's hospital chart. In this connection, the reader may consult the section on special precautions in handling psychiatric records (at the end of Chapter 5).

All the patient's rights of professional confidence are abandoned if he calls the psychiatrist, or other mental health professional worker, as a witness in a legal procedure, since the psychiatrist is automatically open to both examination and cross-examination in court; also, the patient abandons all rights of privileged communication if he takes any legal action against the psychiatrist, as in a malpractice suit.

THE LEGAL RESPONSIBILITIES AND LIABILITIES OF PSYCHIATRISTS AND OTHER MENTAL HEALTH PROFESSIONAL WORKERS

Negligence is a legal term applied to acts in which a professional person causes harm to a patient by not exercising the kind of care and caution generally exercised by similar professional persons in the particular community. For example, if a physician gives a patient an injection with a syringe and needle which the physician knows to be unsterilized, and if the patient develops an abscess because of this act, the physician was clearly negligent. *Malpractice* is a special kind of negligence carried out by a physician, or a lawyer, or, in some states, by a nurse; in practice, the terms malpractice and negligence often overlap and frequently are used interchangeably, but malpractice is the usual term employed in speaking of the negligent acts done by physicians.

Malpractice suits against psychiatrists usually fall in one of four categories: (1) Complications of electroshock therapy, (2) failure to take adequate suicidal precautions for a suicidal patient, (3) drug reactions and (4) accidents which occur to infirm or mentally irresponsible people under psychiatric care. In each case, however, the patient must suffer some kind of damage or loss because of the psychiatrist's negligent act, or lack of action.

Complications of electroshock therapy are much less common as causes of malpractice suits when adequate succinylcholine preshock muscle relaxation is attained; fractures have been the most frequent causes of malpractice suits in this procedure.

The self-injury or suicide of a clearly suicidal patient, when the psychiatrist did not recommend or take adequate suicidal precautions, is the second most common cause of malpractice litigation against psychiatrists. For example, if a patient is seen in an emergency room after slashing his wrists, and the psychiatrist who sees him does not recommend psychiatric hospitalization, or psychiatric hospitalization is carried out but the psychiatrist fails to order suicidal observation and precautions on the psychiatric ward, and the patient injuries himself in a further suicidal attempt, or commits suicide, a malpractice suit may result. Suicide in itself is not ground for a malpractice suit; it must be shown that the psychiatrist did not take reasonable steps to prevent it or to warn the patient and his relatives that the patient should be hospitalized to prevent it.

Drug reactions are occasionally the source of a malpractice suit in psychiatry. The patient as a rule must suffer long-term incapacitation, permanent damage or loss of income because of the drug reaction. Also, it must be shown that the physician did not observe the patient with sufficient care, or perform the necessary tests to detect the incipient reaction, or grossly erred in the dosage or means of administration of the drug.

A final category of malpractice suits focuses on accidents suffered by infirm or mentally irresponsible persons, usually while under hospital care. Thus, an elderly patient with senile brain deterioration who breaks his hip in a fall because of inadequate precautions, or who sets fire to his bed and suffers burns because he was allowed to have matches, or who suffers a hand injury in occupational therapy which was too complex for a person with his degree of mental incapacity, may become the center of a malpractice suit brought in his behalf by his family.

In many court jurisdictions, moreover, psychiatrists are held responsible for acts by their agents or employees. Thus, if an inexperienced hospital aide leaves a confused patient alone on a bed immediately after an electroshock treatment, and the patient rolls out of bed and suffers a fracture, the psychiatrist may be held responsible. The situation is more complex and variable when it involves a licensed professional person, such as a nurse, who is working under the direction of the psychiatrist. In some cases, responsibility and vulnerability for malpractice action devolves upon the nurse; if the psychiatrist orders suicidal precautions on a hospitalized patient, and the nurse takes no action and the patient commits suicide, the malpractice responsibility in some jurisdictions falls on the nurse (or on the hospital, as her employer) and sometimes on the psychiatrist who was assumed to be actively supervising the way in which she carried out his orders. In general, malpractice suits against nurses and physician assistants are much less common than against physicians and hospitals; hospitals often are assumed to assure the competence and diligence of their employees.

BIBLIOGRAPHY

Arens, R.: Insanity Defense. New York, Philosophical Library, 1974.
Bendt, R. H. Balcanoff, E. J., and Tragellis, G. S.: Incompetency to stand trial. Am. J. Psychiatry, *130*:1288, 1973.
Brakel, S. J., and Rock, R. S.: The Mentally Disabled and the Law. Chicago, University of Chicago Press, 1971.
Fingarette, H.: The Meaning of Criminal Insanity, Berkley, University of California Press, 1972.
Guze, S. B., Woodruff, R. A., and Clayton, P. J.: Psychiatric disorders and criminality. J. A. M. A., *227*:641, 1974.
Irvine, L. M., and Brelje, T. B. (eds.): Laws, Psychiatry and the Mentally Disordered Offender. Springfield, Ill., Charles C Thomas, 1973.
Levine, M.: Psychiatry and Ethics. New York, George Braziller, 1972.
McGarry, A. L., and Kaplan, H. A.: Overview: current trends in mental health law. Am. J. Psychiatry, *130*:621, 1973.
Matthews, A. R.: Mental Disability and the Criminal Law. Chicago, American Bar Association, 1970.
Sadoff, R. L.: Comprehensive training in forensic psychiatry. Am. J. Psychiatry, *131*:223, 1974.
Shaffer, T. L.: Death, Property and Lawyers: A Behavioral Approach. New York, Dunellen Company, 1971.
Zusman, J., and Shaffer, S.: Emergency psychiatric hospitalization via court order: a critique. Am. J. Psychiatry, *130*:1323, 1973.

Index

Abstinence syndrome. *See* Withdrawal syndrome
Accident neuroses, 164
Accidents, in malpractice suits, 505–506
Acetophenazine (Tindal), 420
 dosage of, 414t
 efficacy of, 412t
Acne, 192
Acrophobia, 125
Acting-out behavior disorders, 468–469
Addiction. *See also* Narcotic addiction; Alcoholism
 physical, to alcohol, 239–240
  to sedatives and antianxiety medications, 345
 polysurgical, 476
 substances producing, 252–253
Adler, Alfred, concepts from, 70
Adolescence, adjustment to, 87
 alcoholism in, 241
 changing interpersonal relationships during, 17
 encopresis in, 463
 homosexual experimentation in, 227–228, 230
 phobias in, 126
 psychotherapy in, 454, 455–456
 residential treatment in, 456–457
 sexual maturation during, 17–18
 special education for retardation in, 379–380
 suicide in, 290
 transvestitism in, 232–233
Adrenal corticosteroids, overuse of, 348
Adults, anxiety neuroses in, 118–119
 asthma in, 195
 intelligence tests for, 101
 mentally retarded, expected levels of adjustment of, 369–370

 personality changes in, 22–23
 phobias in, 129
 situational adjustment problems of, 471–481
Advice, in psychotherapy, 389
Affect. *See also* specific affects
 anxiety, tension, and panic, 46–47
 concept of, 45
 depersonalization, 47–48
 depressive and manic, 45–46
 emotion contrasted with, 45
 flatness of, 47
  in schizophrenia, 262, 269
 inappropriate, 47
  in schizophrenia, 262
 in mental status examination, 89
 with uncommunicative patient, 95
Affection, ability to express, 15
 need for, in etiology of anxiety neurosis, 116
  in etiology of asthma, 195
  in etiology of severe depressions, 285
  in etiology of peptic ulcer, 185–186
  in oral stage, 59
Affective disorders, lithium treatment of, 438
Affective personality disorder, 217
Age, Down's syndrome and, 371
 electroshock therapy and, 445
 severe depressions and, 283, 284, 287
 sexual activity and, 489–490
 at time of brain damage, 318
Aggressive instinct, 41
Aggressive personality, 216–217
Agitated depression, 281
Agoraphobia, 125
Agranulocytosis, phenothiazine-related, 423
Ailurophobia, 125

Akathisia, 420
Alcohol, physiological effects of, 239–240
Alcoholic deterioration, 342
Alcoholic hallucinosis, acute, 340–341
 chronic, 341
Alcoholic intoxication, definition of, 238
Alcoholics Anonymous, 243
Alcoholism, clinical course of, 241–243
 definition of, 238
 delirium tremens in, 57
 drinking patterns in, 238
 emotional causes of, 240–241
 incidence of, 237–238
 nutritional deficiencies accompanying, 338
 organic brain disorders associated with, 337–342
 severity of, 238–239
 treatment of, 243–246
Alcohol paranoid state, 341–342
Allergic effects, of tricyclic antidepressants, 429
Allergies, to antipsychotic agents, 422–423
 in etiology of asthma, 195
 in etiology of urticaria, 191
Alzheimer's disease, 357
Ambivalence, 72
American Journal of Psychiatry, 28
Amino acid metabolism, in mental retardation, 374–376
Amitriptyline, (Elavil), 173, 288
 central nervous system effects of, 429
 effectiveness of, 427, 426t
 for enuresis, 462
 sedative effects of, 427–428, 434
Ammonium chloride, for bromide intoxication, 344

Amnesia, 54, 55. *See also* Memory loss
  anterograde, 54
  evaluation under sedation, 102
  following head trauma, 324
  hysterical, 152, 155
    diagnosis of, 153–154
  organically caused, 55
  retrograde, 54–55
Amnesic-confabulatory syndrome, 326. *See also* Korsakoff's psychosis
Amobarbital (Amytal), 434, 435
  for grief reaction, 472
  for psychosomatic disorders, 205
Amphetamines, 254
  clinical use of, 439
  combination with chlorpromazine, 418
  contraindications for, 189, 430
  dependence on, 254
  in hyperactive brain-damaged children, 336–337
  organic brain disorders resulting from overuse of, 347–348
Amytal. *See* Amobarbital
Anaclitic relationships, 74–75
Anal stage, 59
Analytic psychology, 68–69
  concepts of, 69
Anankastic personality, 214
Anectine. *See* Succinylcholine
Anemia, hemolytic, 423
  pernicious, 351
Anesthesias, hysterical, 150
Anger, in etiology of migraine headaches, 195
  inability to express, 215–216
Angina pectoris, 194
"Animal magnetism." *See* Hypnosis
Animals, sexual activity with, 234
Anorexia, 189
Anorexia nervosa, 189–190
Anoxia, with seizures, 359
Antabuse. *See* Disulfiram
Anterograde amnesia, 54
Antianxiety drugs, 432–434
  addiction to, 252–254
  in brain-damaged children, 336
  effectiveness of, 433–434
  overdosage of, 345–347
Anticoagulants, interactions with other drugs, 436
Antidepressant drugs, 425
  combination of, 429
  combination with antipsychotic drugs, 418
  for depressive neuroses, 173–174
  development of, 35
  MAO inhibitors, 429–430
    side effects of, 430–431
  tricyclic, 173, 174, 425–429
    combination with phenothiazines, 418
    effectiveness of, 431
    for elderly brain-damaged patients, 323
    overdosage of, 429
    for severe depressions, 288–289
Antiparkinsonian agents, 420–421
Antipsychotic drugs, 345, 410–425
  combinations of, 417–418
    with other types of drugs, 418
  comparative effects of, 412–413
  dosage and administration of, 413–417, 414t
  efficacy of, 411, 412t
  electroshock therapy combined with, 417
  maintenance treatment with, 416–417
  side effects of, 419–425
  uses of, 424–425
Antisocial behavior, postencephalitic, 353–354
Antisocial personality, 221–224
  alcoholism associated with, 241
  etiology of, 222–223
Anxiety, avoidance of. *See* Defense mechanisms
  concept of, 46–47
  consequences of, 11
  definition of, 10
  encapsulation in obsessions, 139
  in etiology of conversion hysteria, 154, 155
  in etiology of neuroses, 122–123
  in etiology of phobias, 127–129
  free-floating, 47
  in hyperventilation syndrome, 196
  impairment of learning by, 464
  minor tranquilizers as treatment for, 433
  in obsessive compulsive patients, 144
  responses to, 10–11
  return of the repressed and, 61–62
  subclinical, 112
Anxiety neurosis(es), 112
  acute, 112–113
  chronic, 113–114
  clinical course of, 119–120
  consequences of, 114
  explanation to patients, 121
  interpersonal causes of, 114–115
    in adult experiences, 118–119
    in childhood experiences, 115–118
  treatment of, 120–122
Aphasia, 51
Aphonia, hysterical, 150

Apnea, respiratory, in electroshock therapy, 444
Appearance, in mental status examination, 88–89
  with uncommunicative patient, 94–95
Apperception, 53
Appetite loss, 189
  in anorexia nervosa, 189, 190
Aralen. *See* Chloroquine
Archetypes, Jungian concept of, 69
Artane. *See* Trihexyphenidyl
Arthritis, 198–199
Articulation disorders, 468
Aspirin, for elderly brain-damaged patients, 323
Assertion, expression of, 15
Association(s), free, 66–67
  in dream interpretation, 68
  in manic disorders, 295
  psychoses of, 308–309
  schizophrenic disturbances of, 261–262
Asthenia, 175
  neurocirculatory, 193
Asthenic personality, 224
Asthma, 195–196
Atabrine. *See* Quinacrine
Athletic body constitution, 57
Atopic dermatitis, 191–192
  treatment of, 192
Atropine, 348
  in electroshock therapy, 441
Attention, 53
Attention span, 53
Attitudes, of interviewer, 79, 80–82
Autism, early infantile, 269, 270–271
  return to phase of crude sensations in, 20
Autistic thought, 50
Autonomic effects, of antipsychotic drugs, 419–420
  of MAO inhibitors, 430
  of tricyclic antidepressants, 428
Autonomic nervous system, in psychosomatic disorders, 204
Aventyl. *See* Nortriptyline
Aversive treatments, for alcoholism, 244–245
Avoidance, conditioned, 395
  of phobic objects and situations, 124–125
Awareness. *See also* Consciousness
  interpersonal and Freudian approaches to, 16
  levels of, 15–17

Backache, psychosomatic, 196, 197

Index

Barbital (Veronal), 434, 435
Barbiturates, 252, 434
  addiction to, 253–254
  for amphetamine withdrawal, 254
  contraindications for, 250, 336, 351–352
  interactions with other drugs, 436
  minor tranquilizers compared with, 433
  overdosage of, 345, 435
Barbiturate sedation, examination under, 101–102
  in diagnosis of hysteria, 153–154
  psychotherapy under, 403–404
  for conversion symptoms, 162–163
Behavior, in mental status examination, 89
  with uncommunicative patient, 94–95
Behavioral modification, 389
Behavioral toxicity, of antipsychotic agents, 422
Behaviorism, 70
Behavior theory, 70–72
  origins of, 36
Behavior therapy, 58, 71–72, 395–396
  origins of, 36
  of phobias, 133–134
Belladonna, 348
Belligerence, in manic disorders, 295
Benadryl. *See* Diphenhydramine
Bender-Gestalt test, 99
Benzedrine. *See* Amphetamine
Benzene, 349
Benzodiazepine derivatives, 432–433
Benztropine (Cogentin), 420
Bestiality, 234
Bethanecol (Myocholine; Urecholine), for autonomic side effects, 428
Birth trauma, 70
Bladder training procedure, 463
Blame, transfer of, 306
"Bland indifference," in conversion hysteria, 151
Blindness, hysterical, 151
Blocking, 49–50
  in schizophrenia, 262
Blood, impaired supply to brain, 349
Blood pressure, 193–194
  with antipsychotic drugs, 419
  in disulfiram therapy, 245
  in drug overdosage, 346
  with MAO inhibitors, 430
Blushing, 191
Body constitution, personality structure related to, 57–58

Body delusions, in schizophrenia, 263–264
Body overconcern, psychiatric disorders indicated by, 178
Bowel functioning, ignorance concerning, 190–191
Brain abscesses, 353
Brain damage. *See also* Organic brain disorders
  in etiology of antisocial personality, 223
Brain surgery, 446–447
  psychoses following, 310
Brain tumors, organic brain disorders caused by, 350–351
Briggs law, 495
Bromide intoxication, 343–345
Bromidism, 344
Bromism, 344
Bronchial asthma, 195–196
Butaperazine (Repoise), 420
  dosage of, 414t
  efficacy of, 412t
Butyrophenones, 345. *See also* Haloperidol
  dosage of, 414, 414t

Caffeine, clinical use of, 439–440
  for dyskinesia, 420
  for hyperactivity, 337
Camphor, 349
Cannabis, 256
Carbohydrate metabolism disorders, mental retardation due to, 376
Carbon disulfide, 349
Carbon monoxide, organic brain syndromes caused by, 349
Carbon tetrachloride, 349
Cardiac complications, in electroshock therapy, 444, 445
Cardiac decompensation, 349
Cardiac neurosis, 193
Cardiovascular effects, of tricyclic antidepressants, 428–429
Carnosinemia, 376
Carphenazine (Proketazine), dosage of, 414t
  efficacy of, 412t
Castration complex, 61
Cataract removal, psychoses following, 310
Catatonia, 263
Catatonic schizophrenia, 268
Cat-cry syndrome, 372
Catharsis, in psychotherapy, 386
Catron. *See* Pheniprazine
Censor, 68
Central nervous system, degenerative diseases of, 356–358
  effects of alcohol on, 239, 240
  effects of antipsychotic drugs on, 422

effects of tricyclic antidepressants on, 429
  psychosomatic disorders of, 199–200
  syphilitic infection of, 355–356
Cerea flexibilitas, 262
Cerebral arteriosclerosis, 318–319
  brain pathology in, 319
  clinical characteristics of, 319–321
  course and prognosis of, 321–322
  management of, 322–323
Cerebral beriberi, 352
Cerebral cortex, damage to, 329
  effect of alcohol on, 240
  functions of, 204
  pathology in cerebral arteriosclerosis and senile brain degeneration, 319
  in psychosomatic disorders, 205
Cerebral dominance, learning difficulties and, 464–466
Cerebral palsy, 332
Changes, inadvisability during middle age, 479
  inadvisability in old age, 480
Character analysis, 67–68
Child guidance clinics, 449–450
  evaluation of child and parents in, 450–451
  treatment approach of, 451–452
Childhood schizophrenia, 269–271
Child psychiatry, development of, 32
Children, ability to sense attitudes, 5
  acute anxiety states in, 113
  atopic dermatitis in, 192
  compulsive neuroses in, 145
  depression in, 286
  effects of epilepsy in, 200
  evaluation in child guidance clinics, 450–451
  hysteria in, 157
  intelligence tests for, 100, 101
  minimal brain damage in, 334–335
  obsessive neuroses in, 144
  organic brain disorders in, 331–337
  phobias in, 125–126
  psychotherapy for, 452–456
  residential treatment for, 456–457
  special problems of adjustment in, 461–471
  subjected to incest, 235
  suicide in, 290
  TAT adaptations for, 98
  treatment in child guidance clinic, 451–452
  viral encephalitis in, 353–354

Chloral hydrate (Hydral; Noctec; Somnos), 252, 348, 435
Chlordiazepoxide (Libritabs; Librium), 253
  in amphetamine withdrawal, 254
  contraindication in narcotic withdrawal, 250
  for delirium tremens, 339
  dosage of, 433
  for organic brain disorders, 361
  overdosage of, 345
  for pathological intoxication, 337–338
  physical dependence on, 436
  side effects of, 435
Chloroquine (Aralen), 348
Chlorperazine, 420
Chlorpromazine (Chlor-pz; Thorazine), 35, 278, 422, 423
  for bromide intoxication, 344
  dosage of, 413, 414, 415, 416, 424, 414t
  efficacy of, 412t, 426t
  for elderly brain-damaged patients, 323
  for manic disorders, 299
  for MAO inhibitor overdosage, 431
  for MAO inhibitor side effects, 430
  metabolism of, 415
  for narcotic withdrawal, 250
  for porphyria, 351
  for schizophrenia, 277–278
  for severe depression, 289
  for suicidal patients, 293
Chlorprothixene (Taractan), 420
  dosage of, 414t
  efficacy of, 412t
Chlor-pz. See Chlorpromazine
Chromosomal abnormalities, mental retardation due to, 371–372
Circumstantiality, 51
Citrullinuria, 376
Civil rights, of hospitalized persons, 499–500
Clang associations, 295
Claustrophobia, 125
Clinical psychology, development of, 33
Clouding of consciousness, 56
Cocaine, 257
  effects of, 257
Cogentin. See Benztropine
Cognition, concept of, 45
Colic, 189
Colitis, adaptive, 187–188
  mucous, 187–188
  ulcerative, 186–187
Collective unconscious, 69
Coma, 56
  therapeutic use of, 35, 445–446
Commitment, by court hearing, 495, 496–497
  emergency, 499
  indefinite, 498–499
  nonjudicial, 497
  temporary, 497–498
  by voluntary admission, 495–496
Communication, in compulsive persons, 143
  nonverbal, 73, 74
  privileged, 503–505
Communication theory, 74
Community mental health, 407–408
Compazine. See Prochlorperazine
Compensation, 64
Compensation neuroses, 164
Compensation problems, in conversion hysteria, 164–166
  in organic brain disorders, 362
  in posttraumatic syndrome, 327, 328
Competition, in anxiety neurosis etiology, 116–117
Complex. See also specific complexes
  concept of, 61
Compulsion, definition of, 135
Compulsive neuroses, clinical characteristics of, 137–139
  clinical course of, 144–145
  interpersonal causes of, 141–143
  treatment of, 145–146
Compulsive personality, 214–215
Conation, concept of, 45
Concussion, 324
Condensation, in dreams, 68
Conditioned avoidance, 395
Conditioned reflex, 71
Conditioning therapy, for alcoholism, 244–245
Confabulation, 55
  following head trauma, 326
  in Korsakoff's psychosis, 339, 340
  in organic brain disorders, 316
Confidentiality, conflict between psychiatry and law over, 503–505
Conflict, extrapsychic, 66
  intrapsychic, 66
Confusion, 56
  following head trauma, 324
  postconvulsive, 358
Congestive heart disease, 194
Consciousness, clouding of, 56, 153, 155
  concept of, 44
  disturbances of, 56–57
  in mental status examination, 91
  in organic brain disorders, 315–316
Consensual validation, definition of, 8
  in maintenance of reality orientation, 272
  in mental retardation, 380
  in personality development, 8–9
  therapeutic use of, 9, 389
Constipation, 190–191
Continuous sleep therapy, 448
Contract, capacity to make, 502
Contusion, 324
Conversion, 62
Conversion hysteria, 148
  clinical characteristics of, 148–152
  clinical course of, 157–158
  compensation problems in, 164–166
  interpersonal causes of, 154–155
  treatment of, 158–163
  impact of, 157
Convulsion(s), 199–200
  in electroshock therapy, 442
  evaluation under sedation, 102
  grand mal, 358
  hysterical, 149
  lowering of threshold by antipsychotic drugs, 422
  during non-narcotic drug withdrawal, 253, 254
  organic brain disorders caused by, 358–359
  in tricyclic overdosage, 429
Convulsive therapy. See Electroshock therapy; Inhalation convulsive therapy
Coronary artery disease, 194
Counseling, supportive, 397–398
Countertransference, 67
Cretinism, 352
Cri du chat syndrome, 372
Criminality, association with narcotic addiction, 247
Crowd phobia, 188
Crude sensations phase, 19–20
Currens formula, 494
Cyclothymic personality, 217–218
Cystathioninuria, 376

Dalmane. See Flurazepam
Darkness, in organic brain disorders, 321, 360
Day hospital, 407
Deafness, hysterical, 150–151
Death, antipsychotic drugs and, 419–420
  depressive neuroses and, 172
  grief reactions and, 471–473
  manic disorders and, 296
  severe depressions and, 287
  suicidal risk and, 292
Death wishes, in anxiety neuroses, 116–117
  obsessions and, 140
Deconditioning. See Desensitization
Defense mechanisms, 62–64

as resistances, 67
security operations compared with, 11
Degenerative diseases, organic brain disorders caused by, 356–358
Déjà vu, 55
Delayed speech, 466–467
Deletion syndromes, 372
Delirium, 56–57
   febrile, 358–360
   hysterical, 153, 155
   traumatic, 325–326
Delirium tremens, 57, 338–339
   treatment of, 339
Delusions, of body distortions in schizophrenia, 263–264
   concept of, 48
   following electroshock therapy, 444–445
   grandiose, 49
      as cause of suicide, 291
      in manic disorders, 295
      in paranoia, 304
      in schizophrenia, 263, 267, 268, 269
   in mental status examination, 90, 95
   in organic brain disorders, 317, 325, 326, 338
   persecutory, 48–49
      in paranoia, 304
      in schizophrenia, 263, 267, 268
      in severe depressions, 281, 284
   in psychoses of association, 308
   in schizophrenia, 263–264
   self-accusative and self-depreciative, 49
      in schizophrenia, 263, 264, 269
      in severe depressions, 281, 284
   systematized, 48
Dementia, 55
Dementia, praecox, 265
Demerol. See Meperidine
Demonology, 25, 26
Denial, 62
Deodorant sprays, inhalation of, 255
Dependence, emotional, in narcotic addiction, 246
   physical, on alcohol, 239–240
      on barbiturates, 435, 436
      on minor tranquilizers, 432
      in narcotic addiction, 246
      on sedatives and hypnotics, 436
Dependency, in anaclitic relationships, 75
   of elderly persons, 479
   in inadequate personality, 221
   in passive-dependent personality, 216

as reaction to physical illness, 475
   in supportive counseling, 398
Depersonalization, concept of, 47–48
   in development of schizophrenia, 264–265
   hysterical, 152, 155
   as symptom, 175–176
Depersonalization neurosis, use of term, 47–48, 168, 175–176
Depression(s), agitated, 281
   concept of, 45–46
   effectiveness of tricyclic drugs for, 425
   in elderly persons, 321, 323
   lithium treatment of, 438
   in manic disorders, 295, 297–298
   neurotic versus psychotic, 168, 280
   in obsessive compulsive patients, 144, 145
   reactive, 46
   severe, clinical characteristics of, 281–284
      interpersonal causes of, 284–287
      suicidal risk in, 281, 287–288, 289, 291, 292
      treatment of, 284, 287–290, 431–432, 442–443
   situational, 46
   stuporous, 56, 281
Depressive neuroses, clinical course of, 172
   clinical features of, 169–170
   differentiated from depressive psychoses, 168, 280
   interpersonal causes of, 170–172
   treatment of, 172–175
   use of term, 168
Depressive reaction, 168
Dereistic thought, 50
Dermatitis, atopic, 191–192
   factitial, 193
Descriptive psychiatry, 43
Desensitization, 395
   in treatment of phobias, 133–134
Desipramine (Norpramin; Pertofrane), 173, 289
   efficacy of, 427, 426t
   for enuresis, 462
Desoxyn. See Methamphetamine
Dextroamphetamine (Dexedrine), 254
Diabetes, 199
   organic brain disorders and, 352
Diagnoses, descriptive, 105
   ethical considerations and, 107–108
   interpersonal, 105
   limitations of, 104–105

standard official classification of psychiatric disorders for, 105–106
"Diagnostic and Statistical Manual of Mental Disorders" (DSM-II), 105–106
Diazepam (Valium), 253, 433
   contraindication in narcotic withdrawal, 250
   as detoxification agent, 436
   dosage and effects of, 433
   for dyskinesia, 420
   overdosage of, 345
   side effects of, 435–436
Diet, in control of metabolic disorders, 375–376
Digitalis, 348
Dilantin. See Diphenylhydantoin; Phenylhydantoin
Diphenylhydantoin (Dilantin), in non-narcotic drug withdrawal, 254
Diphenhydramine (Benadryl), 420
Diplopia, hysterical, 151
Discipline, anxiety-producing, 7
Disorientation, 52–53
   in Korsakoff's psychosis, 340
   in organic brain disorders, 316
Displacement, 62
   in dreams, 68
Dissociation, 62
Dissociative hysteria, 148
   clinical characteristics of, 152–154
   clinical course of, 157–158
   interpersonal causes of, 155
   treatment of, 163–164
Distractibility, 53
Disulfiram (Antabuse), in treatment of alcoholism, 245–246
   dangers of, 245
Divorce, legal aspects of, 503
Diuretics, for bromide intoxication, 344
   with MAO inhibitors, 430
Dole-Nyswander treatment, 251
Dolophine. See Methadone
Dopamine, 430
Dopar. See Levodopa
Doriden. See Glutethimide
Down's syndrome, 371–372
Doxepin (Sinequan), efficacy of, 427, 431, 432, 426t
Draw-A-Person test, 99–100
Dream interpretation, 68
Dreams, symbolization in, 64
   in psychotherapy, 392
Dream states, hysterical, 153, 155
Dream work, 68
Drinalfa. See Methamphetamine
Drive, concept of, 42
Drug abuse, 252–257. See also Narcotic addiction
   associated with narcotic addiction, 250

Drug abuse (*continued*)
 organic brain disorders resulting from, 343–349
 visual hallucinations in, 52
Drug-drug interactions, 436
Drug holidays, 417
Drug reactions, in malpractice suits, 505
Drugs. *See also* Pharmacologic treatment; *specific drugs*
 addictable, 252–253
 combinations of, 417–418, 429
Dry mouth, with antipsychotic drugs, 419
 with tricyclic antidepressants, 428
DSM-II. *See* "Diagnostic and Statistical Manual of Mental Disorders"
Dyskinesias, 420
 tardive, 421–422
Dysmenorrhea, 201
Dyspareunia, 488–489
Dysplastic body constitution, 57
Dyssocial behavior, 224
Dysuria, 201

Early infantile autism, 269, 270–271
Echolalia, 89–90
 in schizophrenia, 262
Echopraxia, in schizophrenia, 262
Eclectic psychotherapy, 396
Economic determinism, in communist psychiatry, 38
Ectomorphs, 57
Eczema, 191
Effort syndrome, 193
Ego, 65
Ego analysis, 65, 393–394
Egocentricity, of homosexuals, 229
 of hysterical patients, 155–157
Ego-dystonic experiences, 65
Ego psychology, 65
Ego-syntonic experiences, 65
Ejaculation, delayed, 424
 premature, 481–482
Ejaculatory incompetence, 488
Elaboration, in dreams, 68
Elavil. *See* Amitriptyline
Elderly persons, adjustment problems of, 479–481
 antipsychotic side effects in, 424
 bromide intoxication in, 343, 344
 cataract surgery in, 310
 cerebral arteriosclerosis and senile brain degeneration in, 318–323
 depression in, 284
 treatment of, 323, 432
 electroshock therapy for, 445
 sexual problems in, 489–490
 use of illness to manipulate others, 475
Electroencephalogram, antipsychotic drugs and, 419
Electroshock therapy, antipsychotic drugs combined with, 417
 complications of, 444–445
 contraindications for, 445
 for depression in elderly persons, 323
 efficacy of, 431, 426t
 indications and results for, 442–443
 introduction of, 35
 malpractice suits concerning, 505
 for manic disorders, 300–301
 mode of action of, 445
 for schizophrenia, 278–279
 for severe depressions, 189–190
 side effects of, 443–444
 technic of, 441–442
Emotion, affect contrasted with, 45
 concept of, 45
Emotional difficulties, past, 84–85
Emotional lability, in organic brain disorders, 317, 320, 330, 333
Emotional maturity, definition of, 212–213
Emotional reaction(s), during mental status examination, 89
 with uncommunicative patient, 95
 of examiner, 81
 in schizophrenia, 262
Empathy, 73
Encephalitis, 352
 in etiology of antisocial personality, 223
 organic brain disorders caused by, 353–354
Encopresis, 463–464
 causes of, 463
Encounter groups, 403
Endocrine system, antipsychotic agent side effects on, 423–424
 psychosomatic disorders of, 199
Endomorphs, 57
Enuresis, 461
 causes of, 461–462
 treatment of, 462–463
Environment. *See also* Heredity
 for elderly brain-damaged persons, 322
 influence on personality development, 13–14
 psychotherapeutic, 405–408
Environmental change, inadvisable, during middle age, 479
 during old age, 480
 in treatment of schizophrenia, 276–277
Environmental deprivation, mental retardation associated with, 372–374
Ephedrine, 430
Epilepsy. *See also* Convulsions
 posttraumatic, 330
Epileptoid personality disorder, 225
Epinephrine, 430
 contraindication for, 419
Equanil. *See* Meprobamate
Erogenous zones, 59
 during oral stage, 59
 during phallic stage, 60
Eros, 65
Esidrix. *See* Hydrochlorothiazide
Eskalith. *See* Lithium
ESP. *See* Extrasensory perception
Ethchlorvynol (Placidyl), 253, 435
 overdosage of, 345
Ethinamate (Valmid), 252, 435
 overdosage of, 345
Ethology, influence on psychiatry, 57
Ethylene diamine tetraacetic acid (EDTA), for lead poisoning, 348
Etryptamine (Monase), effectiveness of, 426
Euphoria, 46, 296
Eutonyl. *See* Pargyline
Evipan. *See* Hexobarbital
Examination. *See* Psychiatric examination
Examiner, behavior and attitudes of, 79–82
Exhibitionism, 231
Existential psychiatry, 37
Expectations, of parents of mentally retarded child, 378–379
Exploratory group therapy, 401–402
Explosive personality, 225
Extinction, 71
 in behavior theory, 71
 in behavior therapy, 395
Extrapsychic conflicts, 66
Extrapyramidal side effects, with antipsychotic drugs, 420–422
Extrasensory perception, 53–54
Extrasystoles, 194
Extraversion, 69
Eye changes, with antipsychotic agents, 424

Factitial dermatitis, 193
Fainting, hysterical, 155

False imprisonment, 500
Falsification, retrospective, 55–56
Family. See Father; Mother; Parents; Relatives
Family physician, legal testimony of, 499, 501–502
  treatment of anxiety neuroses by, 120–121
  treatment of conversion disorders by, 163
  treatment of encopresis by, 464
  treatment of enuresis by, 462
  treatment of grief reaction by, 472
  treatment of narcotic addiction by, 251
  treatment of obsessive neuroses by, 145
  treatment of phobias by, 132–133
  treatment of suicidal patient by, 293
Family therapy, 455–456
Fantasy, 72–73
Father, in etiology of schizophrenia, 274
  secondary role during first year of life, 6
Fatigue, in chronic anxiety states, 113–114
  in neurasthenic neuroses, 175
  psychiatric disorders indicated by, 175
Fear(s), concept of, 47
  in etiology of anxiety neuroses, 117–118
  obsessive, 135–136
  compulsions and, 138
Febrile delirium, 359–360
Feelings, expression of in personality development, 15
  suppression of, 117, 119
Fetishism, 233
Fever, treatment of, 360
Fixation, 60–61
"Fixed ideas," 29
Flight of ideas, 50, 295
Fluphenazine (Prolixin), 416, 420, 422, 423
  dosage of, 413, 416, 414t
  efficacy of, 412t
  intramuscular depo forms of, 417
Flurazepam (Dalmane), 435
  advantages of, 434
Flurohydrocortisone, for postural hypotension, 428
Flurothyl gas, for inhalation convulsive therapy, 448
Folie à deux, 308
Formication, 257
Fractures, in electroshock therapy, 444
Fragmentation of thought processes, 50

Free association, 66–67
  in dream interpretation, 68
Freudian-psychoanalytic approach, 58–59, 392–395
  basis of, 157
  to compulsive neuroses, 143
  defense mechanisms in, 62–64
  development of, 31–32
  to hypochondriasis, 177
  outgrowths of, 68–70
  personality structure and, 64–66
  psychosexual development in, 58–62
  therapeutic concepts of, 66–68
  training for, 58
Frigidity, 485, 487
  causes of, 486–487
  in hysterical personality, 226
  treatment of, 487
Frontal cortex, surgery on, 447
Frontal lobe tumors, 351
Fructose intolerance, 376
Fugue, 152–153, 155

Gain, primary, 75
  in conversion hysteria, 154, 155
  secondary, 75
  in asthma, 195
  from hysterical symptoms, 151, 154–155, 158, 165
Galactosemia, 376
Ganser syndrome, 153
  prognosis for, 158
Gasoline, toxicity, 349
Gastric lavage, for overdosages, 346, 429
Gastrointestinal disorders, psychosomatic, 183–191
General paresis, 355–356
General systems theory, 73–74
Generation gap, 477
Genital period, 61
Genitourinary disorders, psychosomatic, 200–202
Gesell Developmental Schedules, 101
Glaucoma, 202
Glioblastoma multiforme, 351
Glucagon hydrochloride, 446
Glue sniffing, 255
Glutethimide (Doriden), 252
  contraindication in narcotic withdrawal, 250
  interaction with anticoagulants, 436
  overdosage of, 345
  physical dependence on, 436
  side effects of, 435
Glycerol derivatives, 432
Goodenough test, 100
Grandiose delusions, 49
  as cause of suicide, 291
  in manic disorders, 295

  in paranoia, 304
  in schizophrenia, 263, 267, 268, 269
Grief reactions, 471–473
Gross stress reactions, 473–474
  in civilian life, 474
  in military life, 474–475
Group psychotherapy, 400–403
  for adolescents, 455
  for alcoholism, 244
  for children, 454–455
  for parents, 336, 377–378
  for schizophrenia, 277
  types of, 401–403
Group residential programs, for narcotic addicts, 252
Guilt, as cause of suicide, 291
  in compulsive neuroses, 141–142
  development of delusions and, 48–49
  in obsessive neuroses, 139–141
  severe depressions and, 287
  superego and, 65
Gun-barrel vision, hysterical, 151
Gyrectomy, 447

Haldol. See Butyrophenones; Haloperidol
Halfway house, 407
Hallucinations, 51
  auditory, 51–52
    in alcoholic hallucinosis, 341
    evaluation of, 91
    in schizophrenia, 263, 267, 268, 269
  as cause of suicide, 291, 292
  cocaine-induced, 257
  following electroshock therapy, 444–445
  gustatory, 52, 267
  hypnagogic, 53
  hypnopompic, 53
  hysterical, 151
  LSD-induced, 255
  in mental status examination, 91, 95
  olfactory, 52, 263, 267–268
  in organic brain disorders, 317, 320–321, 325–326, 338, 351
  in severe depressions, 281, 284
  tactile, 52, 263
  visual, 52
    evaluation of, 91
    in schizophrenia, 263, 268
Hallucinogens, dependence on, 254–256
Hallucinosis, alcoholic, 340–341
Haloperidol (Haldol), 299, 420, 422
  dosage of, 413, 414, 424, 414t
  efficacy of, 412t
Harrison Narcotic Act, 252
Hartnup disease, 375
Hashish, 256

Headaches, in chronic anxiety states, 113
  following electroshock therapy, 444
  migraine, 194–195
  due to muscle tension, 113, 194–195, 196, 197–198
  in posttraumatic syndrome, 326–327
Head trauma, 323–324
  amnesic-confabulatory syndrome following, 326
  confusional state following, 324–325
  delirium following, 325–326
  permanent organic damage following, 328–331
  posttraumatic syndrome and, 326–328
Heart disease, fear of, 193, 194
  psychosomatic, 193–194
Heart surgery, psychoses following, 350
Hebephrenic schizophrenia, 271
Hemianesthesia, hysterical, 150
Hemodialysis, emotional adjustment to, 476
Hemolytic anemia, 423
Hemorrhoids, 190
Hepatic failure, 351
Herd instinct, 41
Heredity, of collective unconscious, 69
  of Down's syndrome, 372
  in phenylketonuria, 374
  role in emotional development, 42–43
Heroin. See also Narcotic addiction
  use by marijuana users, 256–257
Hexobarbital (Evipan), 434, 435
Hibernation therapy, 448
Histidinemia, 376
History taking. See Psychiatric examination
Histrionic personality disorder, 225
Homosexuality, 227–228
  alcoholism and, 241, 341
  etiology of, 13, 228–230
  heterosexual relationships and, 228
  impotence and, 483–484
  as life style rather than disorder, 230
  in paranoid disorders, 220, 307
  pruritis and, 192
  relationship to transvestitism, 232
  transsexualism and, 234–235
  treatment and prevention of, 230
  urinary dysfunctions and, 201
Hospital(s), choice of, for young narcotic addict, 251

Hospitals, development during 19th Century, 27–28
  early, 27
  interpersonal milieu therapy in, 276
  legal committment for narcotic addict, 251
  modern developments in, 34
  therapeutic environment in, 405–407
Hospitalization. See also Commitment
  for anorexia nervosa, 190
  for delirium tremens, 339
  for depressive neuroses, 174–175
  in disulfiram therapy, 245
  for drug overdose, 346, 347
  effect of drug therapy on, 410–411
  for gross stress reaction, 474
  for hysterical personality, 227
  for Korsakoff's psychosis, 340
  for manic disorders, 298
  for non-narcotic drug addiction, 254, 255–256, 257
  for organic brain disorders, 361
  partial, 407
  during rehabilitation in narcotic addiction, 250
  of schizophrenic patients, 276, 277
  for severe depressions, 287–288, 290
  for suicidal patients, 293, 505
  for traumatic confusional states, 325
  by voluntary admission, 495–496
  during withdrawal from narcotics, 249
Hospital records, precautions concerning, 505
Hostility, in acting out, 468–469
  as cause of suicide, 291
  in etiology of antisocial personality, 223
  in etiology of colitis, 187
  in etiology of compulsive neuroses, 142, 143
  in etiology of phobias, 128–129
  expression through peptic ulcer, 186
  inwardly directed, in depressive neuroses, 171
  maternal, in etiology of atopic dermatitis, 192
  in paranoid personality, 219, 220
  in severe depressions, 285, 286–287
  in stutterers, 467
House-Tree-Person (HTP) test, 100
Huntington's chorea, 358
Hydral. See Chloral hydrate
Hydrochlorothiazide (Esidrix;

HydroDiuril; Oretic), for bromide intoxication, 344
Hydrotherapy, 448
Hyperactivity, 470
  in brain-damaged children, 333
  in catatonic schizophrenia, 268
  treatment of, 336–337
Hyperhidrosis, 193
Hyperkinetic reaction, 333, 334, 470
Hypermnesia, 55
Hyperphenylalanemia, persistent, 374
Hyperpyrexic reactions, with MAO inhibitors, 430
Hypertension, 193–194
  with MAO inhibitors, 430
Hyperthyroidism, 199, 352
Hyperventilation syndrome, 196
Hypnagogic hallucinations, 53
Hypnoanalysis, 404–405
Hypnopompic hallucinations, 53
Hypnosis, interview under, 102–103
  Mesmer's use of, 28–29
  psychotherapy under, 404–405
  for conversion symptoms, 162
  for warts, 193
Hypnotic drugs, 434–435
  addiction to, 252–254
  side effects of, 435–436
Hypochondriacal neuroses, concept of, 176–177
  use of term, 168, 176, 178
Hypoglycemia, 352
Hypomania, 46, 296
Hypotensive crises, with MAO inhibitors, 430
Hypothyroidism, 352
Hysteria, Charcot's investigation of, 29
Hysterical neuroses, 62. See also Conversion hysteria; Dissociative hysteria
Hysterical personality, 225–227
  use of term, 224–225

Id, 64–65
Ideas, flight of, 50, 295
  obsessive, 135–137
  paranoid, 219
Ideas of reference, 49, 267
Identification, as defense mechanism, 64
  in etiology of homosexuality, 228
  healthy and unhealthy, 12–13
  process of, 12
  sexual orientation and, 13
  in transvestitism, 232–233
Illusions, 51
Imipramine (Presamine; Tofranil), 173, 288

action and efficacy of, 425, 427, 426t
central nervous system effects of, 429
combination with antipsychotics, 418
for enuresis, 462
Impotence, 482
primary, 483–484
secondary, 484–485
transient situational, 482–483
Imprinting, 42
Inadequate personality, 220–221
Incest, 235
Incompetency, commitment and, 499
determination of, 502
Incorporation, 64
Incubation period, of compensable symptoms, 165
of posttraumatic syndrome, 327
Independence, development of, during adolescence, 17
during late childhood, 14–15
Individual psychology, 70
Individuation, 70
Indoklon. See Flurothyl gas
Infancy, personality development during, 5–6
Infanticide, obsessive fears of, 136, 141
Infections, organic brain disorders caused by intracranial infections, 352–354
severe general infections, 359–360
syphilis, 354–356
Inferiority complex, 70
Information, evaluation of fund of, 91–92
Inhalation convulsive therapy, 448
Inhibition, reciprocal, 395
Insane, use of term, 502
Insanity, obsessive fears of, 136, 141
Insidon. See Opipramol
Insight, definition of, 92
in mental status examination, 92
in psychotherapy, 67, 386–387
Insomnia, treatment of, 323, 434
Inspirational group therapy, 402–403
Instinct(s), aggressive, 41
definition of, 40
of id, 65
to live in groups, 41
modification by interpersonal relationships, 40–42
self-preservative, 41
sexual, 41
Institutionalization. See also Hospitalization
for brain-damaged children, 337
for children and adolescents, 456–457
for elderly brain-damaged persons, 323
for mental retardation, 380–381
Insulin coma therapy, 35, 445–446
complications of, 446
for schizophrenia, 279
Insulin shock, 352
Intellectual impairment, in organic brain disorders, 316–317, 332–333
Intellectualization, 64
Intellectual materialism, in communist psychiatry, 38
Intelligence, concept of, 44–45
definition of, 368
judgment related to, 368–369
Intelligence tests, 100–101
for brain-damaged children, 335
early, 32
limitations of, 368
International Classification of Diseases (ICD-8), 106
Internist, treatment of anxiety neuroses by, 120–121
treatment of conversion disorders by, 163
treatment of grief reaction by, 472
treatment of narcotic addiction by, 251
treatment of obsessive neuroses by, 145
treatment of phobias by, 132–133
Interpersonal approach, 390–392
communist rejection of, 38
development of, 30–31
Interpersonal relationships, changing, during middle age, 477, 478
in old age, 479
corrective, 388–389, 400
effects of acne on, 192
effects of epilepsy on, 359
of elderly persons, 321, 479
in etiology of anxiety neuroses, 118, 120
in etiology of compulsive neuroses, 141–143
in etiology of depressive neuroses, 170–172
in etiology of hysteria, 154–157
in etiology of manic disorders, 297–298
in etiology of obsessive neuroses, 139–141
in etiology of phobias, 126–129
in etiology of psychosomatic disorders, cardiovascular, 193–194, 195
endocrine, 199
gastrointestinal, 186, 187, 189–190
musculoskeletal, 197, 198
seizures, 199–200
of skin, 191–192
in etiology of schizophrenia, 271–275
in etiology of severe depressions, 284–287
history taking and, 85–87
hypochondriasis as barrier to, 177
in psychotherapy, 4, 387–389
retardation and, 369
Interpretation(s), of dreams, 68
psychoanalytic, 67
Interview. See also Psychiatric examination; Psychotherapy
ending of, 92–93
length of, 82
opening of, 82
special technics for, 101–103
Interviewer, as participant-observer, 79–80
Intimacy, concept of, 213
definition of, 18
development of, 18–19
impairment of, 19
Intoxication. See also Alcoholism
definition of, 238
organic brain disorders caused by, 343–349
pathological, 337
treatment of, 337–338
Intrapsychic conflicts, 66
Introjection, 63–64
Introversion, 69
Involutional melancholia, 283–284
Involutional paranoid state, 307–308
Involutional paraphrenia, 308
Iproniazid (Marsilid), efficacy of, 430, 426t
I. Q., 100–101
levels of retardation and, 367–368
Irresistible impulse test, 494
Irritable colon syndrome, 187–188
Isocarboxazid (Marplan), 173, 289
efficacy of, 430, 426t
in treatment of angina pectoris, 204
Isolation, as defense mechanism, 64
Isoniazid, 431

Jamais vu, 55
Jaundice, phenothiazine-induced, 422–423
with tricyclic antidepressants, 429
Judgement, evaluation of, 92
impairment, in organic brain disorders, 316, 320, 329, 333

Judgement (*continued*)
  intelligence related to, 368–369
  legal, 491
Juvenile delinquency, 469
Juvenile era, personality development during, 13–15
Juvenile paresis, 356

Kemadrin. *See* Procyclidine
Kidney function, lithium and, 439
Kleptomania, 224
Korsakoff's psychosis, 326, 339–340

Laceration, 324
Language problems. *See* Speech disturbances
Larodopa. *See* Levodopa
Laryngospasm, in electroshock therapy, 444
Latency period, 61
Latent content, 68
Latent schizophrenia, 271
Law. *See also* Commitment; Malpractice suits
  criminal responsibility under, 493–495
  testimony of physicians and, 499–502
  view of person, 491–493
Lead, organic brain disorders caused by, 348–349
Learning problems, 464–466
Leptosomic body constitution, 57
Lesbians, 228
Leukotomy, 447
Levallorphane (Lorfan), use of, 250
Levodopa (Dopar; Larodopa), 348
Libido, 65
  concept of, 58
Libritabs. *See* Chlordiazepoxide
Librium. *See* Chlordiazepoxide
Lighter fluid, 349
Limitations, imposed during second and third years, 7–8
  inadequate, 8, 117
Lithium (Eskalith; Lithane; Lithonate), 348, 437
  clinical use and dosage of, 437–438
  contraindications for, 439
  for manic disorders, 299–300, 301
  side effects and toxicity of, 300, 438–439
Lobotomy, 446–447
Lorfan. *See* Levallorphane
Loss. *See also* Death
  as precipitating event in depressive neuroses, 170, 172
Love. *See also* Intimacy
  meanings attached to word, 6

Love object, mother as, 59
Lowe's syndrome, 375
LSD. *See* Lysergic acid diethylamide
Luminal. *See* Phenobarbital
Lupus erythematosus, 357
Lysergic acid diethylamide (LSD), dependence on, 254–256
  physiological effects of, 255

Machover test, 100
Male climacteric, 283–284
Malingering, 166
Malpractice suits, 505–506
Manganese, 349
Mania, 296
  concept of, 46
Manic affects, 46
Manic depressive illness, 282–283
Manic disorders, clinical characteristics of, 294–297
  interpersonal causes of, 297–298
  treatment of, 298–301, 443
Manifest content, 68
Mannitol (Osmitrol), 346
Maple syrup urine disease, 376
Marijuana, effects of, 256
  legalization of, 256
Marital problems, in paranoia, 305
Marplan. *See* Isocarboxazid
Marriage, expectations of, 18
  in history taking, 86
  of homosexuals, 228
  legal aspects of, 503
  of mentally retarded persons, 369, 370
Marsilid. *See* Iproniazid
Masochism, sexual, 234
Masturbation, compulsive guilt over, 142
Maturity, emotional, definition of, 212–213
Medical history, in psychiatric examination, 88
Medicine, integration of psychiatry into, 33–34
Mega doses, 416
Megalomanic delusions, 49
Mellaril. *See* Thioridazine
Memory, 54
  disturbances of, 54–56
  in early infantile autism, 270
  in mental status examination, 90
  unconscious, 54
Memory loss, following electroshock therapy, 443–444
  in Korsakoff's psychosis, 339, 340
  in organic brain disorders, 316, 319–320
Meningitis, 352–353
Meningoencephalitic syphilis, 355

Meningovascular syphilis, 356
Menopause, involutional disorders at time of, 283, 307–308
  male, 283–284
  meaning to woman, 478
Menstrual irregularities, 200–201
Mental illness. *See also specific disorders*
  criminal trial and, 494–495
  development of diagnostic system for, 28
  duration of, 83
  historical concepts of, 25–26
  incompetency and, 499, 502
  obsessive ideas of, 135–136
  onset of, 83
  role of heredity in, 42
  treatment during 17th and 18th Centuries, 26–27
  treatment prior to psychiatry, 26
Mental retardation, associated with psychosocial deprivation, 372–374
  causes of, 365
    chromosomal, 371–372
    metabolic, 374–375
  clinical features of, 365–369
  differential diagnosis of, 370–371
  emotional problems in, 380
  expected levels of adjustment in, 369–370
  false appearance in epilepsy, 200
  incest and, 235
  incidence of, 365
  I. Q. level and, 100
  levels of, 367–368
  management of, 376–381
  special education for, 379–380
Mental status examination, 88–92
Mepazine, 423
  efficacy of, 412t
Meperidine (Demerol), 430
Meprobamate (Equanil; Miltown), 253
  contraindication in narcotic withdrawal, 250
  dosage and effects of, 432
  efficacy of, 433
  for grief reaction, 472
  overdosage of, 345
  side effects of, 435
Mercury, 349
Mescaline, 255
"Mesmerism," 29
Mesomorphs, 57
Mesoridazine (Serentil), dosage of, 414t
  efficacy of, 412t
Metabolic disorders, mental retardation due to, 374–376
  organic brain syndromes caused by, 351–352

Methadone maintenance programs, 251–252
Methadone withdrawal, 249
Methamphetamine (Desoxyn; Drinalfa), 254
Methaqualone (Parest; Quaalude; Somnafac; Sopor), 253, 435
  physical dependence on, 436
Methylmalonic aciduria, 375–376
Methylphenidate (Ritalin), 439
  for dyskinesia, 420
  for hyperactivity, 336–337
Methyprylon (Noludar), 253
  overdosage of, 345
  side effects of, 435
Middle age, interpersonal stresses of, 477–478
  adjustment to, 478–479
  paranoia in, 307–308
  severe depressions in, 283–284, 287
Migraine headaches, 194–195
Milieu therapy, 405
Military service, in history taking, 87
Miltown. See Meprobamate
Mind, interpersonal approach to, 211–212
  unconscious, 61–62
Minimal brain damage (MBD), 334–335
Minnesota Multiphasic Personality Inventory (MMPI), 98–99
Misconnected experiences phase, 19, 20–21
MMPI. See Minnesota Multiphasic Personality Inventory
M'Naghten rules, 493–494
Model Penal Code, 494
Monase. See Etryptamine
Mongolism. See Down's syndrome
Monoamine oxidase (MAO) inhibitors, 173
  combination with antipsychotics, 418
  dosage of, 430
  efficacy of, 430, 426t
  overdosage of, 430–431
  for psychosomatic disorders, 204
  for severe depressions, 289
  side effects of, 430–431
Mood, in cyclothymic personality, 217–218
Morals, in antisocial personality, 221–222, 223
  dyssocial behavior and, 224
  identification in development of, 12
Moral treatment, 27
Morning glory seeds, 255
Mother. See also Parents
  in etiology of schizophrenia, 273–274

importance during first year of life, 6
infantile colic and, 189
obsessive fears in, 136, 141
during oral stage, 59
postpartum psychosis in, 309–310
Motion sickness, 188–189
Motor development, in retarded children, 366
Mouth, as erogenous zone, 59
Multiple sclerosis, 357
Multiple sensory learning, 335, 380
Muscle relaxation, 434
  for electroshock therapy, 444
Muscles, conversion symptoms in, 149–150
Muscle tension syndromes, 196–197
  headaches, 113, 194–195, 196, 197–198
Musculoskeletal disorders, psychosomatic, 196–199
Myocardial infarction, 194
  during electroshock therapy, 444
Myocholine. See Bethanecol
Myxedema, 352

Nalorphine (Nalline), use of, 250
Narcissism, 61
Narcoanalysis, 102, 404
Narcosynthesis, 102, 404
Narcotic addiction, 246–247
  clinical characteristics of, 247–248
  emotional causes of, 248–249
  incidence of, 246–247
  treatment of, 249–252
Narcotic antagonists, use of, 250
Narcotics Anonymous, 252
Nardil. See Phenelzine
Natal brain damage, 332
National Association for Mental Health, 34
Nausea, 188–189
  in aversive treatment of alcoholism, 244, 245
Navane. See Thioxanthene derivatives
Negligence, 505
Neisseria meningitis, 352
Nembutal. See Pentobarbital
Neologisms, 50
Neoplasms, organic brain disorders caused by, 350–351
Neurasthenic neuroses, 175
  usage of diagnostic term, 168, 175
Neurocirculatory asthenia, 193
Neurodermatitis, 191, 193
Neuroleptics, combination with

psychological therapies, 418
Neurophysiological approach, 37
Neurosis(es), 110–111. See also specific neuroses
  in brain-damaged children, 333–334
  cardiac, 193
  classification system for, 168
  discovery of, 28–29
  in elderly persons, 321
  hysterical, 62
  investigations of 19th Century, 29
  role of anxiety in, 122–123
  transference, 67
Neurotic depression, psychotic depression distinguished from, 168, 280
Neutrality, of examiner, 80
Niacin, deficiency of, 352
  for Hartnup disease, 375
Nialamide (Niamid), 173
  efficacy of, 430, 426t
Night hospital, 407
Nihilistic delusions, 49
  in schizophrenia, 264
Noctec. See Chloral hydrate
Noludar. See Methyprylon
Nonthrombocytopenic pupura, 423
Nonverbal communication, 73, 74
Normality, concept of, 212
Norpramin. See Desipramine
Nortriptyline (Aventyl), 173, 289
  effectiveness of, 427, 426t
Note taking, during interview, 81–82
Nurses, 33
  confidentiality and, 504
  malpractice suits against, 506
Nutmeg, 255
Nutrition, in alcoholism, 338, 339

Obesity, 202–203
Obsession, definition of, 135
Obsessive compulsive disorder, 138
Obsessive compulsive personality, 214
Obsessive neuroses, clinical characteristics of, 135–137
  clinical course of, 144
  interpersonal causes of, 139–141
  treatment of, 145
Oceanic stage. See Crude sensations phase
Oedipus complex, 59–60, 61
Oedipus conflict, identification in, 64
  superego development and, 66
Old age. See Elderly persons
One-genus postulate, 23

Operant conditioning, 395
Opipramol (Insidon), effectiveness of, 426t
Oral stage, 59
Oretic. See Hydrochlorothiazide
Organic brain disorders, in alcoholism, 243, 337–342
  basic symptoms in, 315–318
  caused by cerebral arteriosclerosis and senile brain degeneration, 318–323
  caused by circulatory disorders, 349–350
  caused by convulsive disorders, 358–359
  caused by degenerative diseases, 356–358
  caused by head trauma, 323–331
  caused by infections, general, 359–360
    intracranial, 352–354
  caused by intoxication by drugs and chemicals, 343–349
  caused by intracranial neoplasms, 350–351
  caused by metabolic disorders, 351–352
  caused during prenatal, natal, and postnatal periods, 331–337
  discrete foci of, 466
  in etiology of anxiety neuroses, 119
  incest and, 235
  incidence of, 318
  management of, 322–323, 325, 328, 330–331, 335–337, 360–362
  syphilitic, 354–356
  thought process disturbances of, 51
Organic drivenness, 329, 333
Organic illness, associated with alcoholism, 242
  emotional adjustments to, 475–477
  in etiology of anxiety neuroses, 119
  hysterical symptoms associated with, 151
  in middle age, 477–478
  obsessive ideas of, 135
  in old age, 480
Organic psychiatry, 43
Orgasm, female, 486
Orgasmic dysfunction. See Frigidity
Orientation, 52
  disorders of, 52–53, 316, 340
  in mental status examination, 90–91
Orthostatic hypotension, with antipsychotic drugs, 419
Osmitrol. See Mannitol

Overanxious reaction, of childhood or adolescence, 469–470
Overdetermination, in dreams, 68
Overdosage, of barbiturates, 435
  of MAO inhibitors, 430–431
  of sedatives and antianxiety medications, 345–347
  of tricyclic antidepressants, 429
Overeating, causes of, 202, 203
Oxazepam (Serax), 253
  dosage of, 433
  overdosage of, 345
Oxygen, in electroshock therapy, 442, 444
  impaired supply to brain, 349

Pain, hysterical, 150, 158
  of muscle tension, 197–198
  in porphyria, 351
Paint sprays, inhalation of, 255
Pancytopenia, 423
Panic, as cause of suicide, 292
  concept of, 47
  treatment of, 433
Panphobia, 125
Paradoxical excitement, 436
Paraldehyde, 253, 348
Paralysis, hysterical, 149
Paramnesia, 55–56
Paranoia, alcoholic, 341
  categories of, 303
  clinical characteristics of, 304–306
  interpersonal causes of, 306–307
  involutional, 307–308
Paranoid delusions. See Persecutory delusions
Paranoid personality, 218–220
Paranoid schizophrenia, 267–268
  alcoholic hallucinosis and, 340–341
Parapsychology, 53
Parasympathomimetic drugs, for autonomic side effects, 428
Parataxic stage. See Misconnected experiences phase
Parents, anxiety neuroses originating in childhood and, 116–118
  of brain-damaged children, 335–336
  in etiology of severe depressions, 285–286
  evaluation in child guidance clinic, 450, 451
  in family therapy, 455–456
  group psychotherapy for, 455
  in history taking, 85
  of hysterical patients, 156
  identification with, 12
  importance during first year of life, 5–6

of mentally retarded child, counseling with, 376–377
  feelings of, 377–378
  expectations of, 378–379
Oedipus complex and, 60
possessive, 14
role during second and third years, 7–8
self-image formation and, 12
sexual development and, 18
superego development and, 66
treatment in child guidance clinic, 451–452, 454
Parest. See Methaqualone
Paresthesia, hysterical, 150
Pargyline (Eutonyl), effectiveness of, 426t
Parkinsonian syndrome, 420
Parnate. See Tranylcypromine
Participant-observer(s), hospital personnel as, 406
  interviewer as, 79–80
  therapist as, 101
  in family therapy, 455
Passive personality, 215–216
  aggressive type, 216
  dependent type, 216
Pathological intoxication, 337
  treatment of, 337–338
Pediatrician, treatment of enuresis by, 462
  treatment of phobias by, 133
Pedophilia, 231–232
Pellagra, 352
Penicillin, for psychoses, 35
  for syphilis, 356
Pentobarbital (Nembutal), 434, 435
  as detoxification agent, 436
Pentothal. See Thiopental
Peptic ulcer, 185–186
Perception, concept of, 51
  disturbances of, 51–54
  extrasensory, 53–54
  in mental status examination, 91
  with uncommunicative patient, 95
Pernicious anemia, 351
Perphenazine (Trilafon), 278
  dosage of, 414t
  efficacy of, 412t
Persecutory delusions, 48–49
  in organic brain disorders, 317, 326, 338, 340, 341
  in paranoia, 304
  in schizophrenia, 263, 267, 268
  in severe depressions, 281, 284
Perseveration, 50, 89
Personality(ies), aggressive, 216–217
  anal, 59, 60–61
  antisocial, 221–224
    etiology of, 222–223
  asthenic, 224

Index 519

of brain-damaged children, 332, 333–334
changes in, associated with convulsive disorders, 358–359
in organic brain disorders, 317, 329–330, 350
compulsive, 214–215
concept in interpersonal terms, 211–212
cyclothymic, 217–218
definition of, 4, 211
explosive, 225
hysterical, 225–227
use of term, 224–225
inadequate, 220–221
malevolent transformation of, 306
multiple, 152
normality and maturity of, 212–213
oral, 59, 60
paranoid, 218–220
passive, 215–216
prepsychotic, in manic disorders, 283, 298
in schizophrenia, 274
schizoid, 213–214
treatment of, 214
Personality development. *See also* Psychosexual development
during adolescence, 17–18
during adulthood, 22–23
from age eight to puberty, 13–15
during ages three through seven, 9–10
anxiety and security in, 10–11
awareness and unawareness in, 15–17
consensual validation in, 8–9
expression of feelings in, 15
during first year of life, 5–6
history taking and, 85–87
identification in, 12–13
during phase of crude sensations, 19–20
during phase of misconnected experiences, 20–21
Rank's theory of, 70
in retarded children, 367
role of heredity in, 42
during second and third years, 6–8
self-image formation in, 11–12
associated with alcoholism, 237–246
associated with narcotic addiction, 246–252
associated with non-narcotic drug abuse, 252–257
sexual disorders associated with, 227–235
Personality problems, of others, in psychosomatic illnesses, 205–206

reduction of, from age eight to puberty, 13
consensual validation in, 8–9
Personality structure, body constitution related to, 57–58
in compulsive persons, 143
coronary artery disease and, 194
course of anxiety neuroses and, 120
course of conversion or dissociative hysteria and, 157
Freudian concept of, 64–66
of hysterical patients, 155–157
Jungian concepts of, 69
Personality tests, 97–100
early, 33
Personal unconscious, 69
Perspiration, excessive, 193
Persuasion, in treatment of conversion symptoms, 161–162
Pertofrane. *See* Desipramine
Phallic stage, 59–61
Pharmacologic treatment. *See also* Drugs; *specific drug names*
of alcoholism, 244, 245–246
contraindications for, 244, 245
of anxiety neuroses, 122
of brain-damaged children, 336–337
of compulsive neuroses, 146
of depressive neuroses, 173–174
development of, 35, 36
effect on psychiatry, 410–411
efficacy of, 411
of elderly brain-damaged persons, 322–323
of enuresis, 462
evaluation of, 411
of grief reaction, 472
of gross stress reaction, 474
of manic disorders, 299–300
of narcotic addiction, 250, 251–252
of obsessive neuroses, 145
of organic brain disorders, 361
of phobias, 133
postencephalitic, 354
of posttraumatic syndrome, 328
of psychosomatic disorders, 203–204
of schizophrenia, 277–278
of severe depressions, 288–289
Phenacemide (Phenurone), 348
Phenelzine (Nardil), 173, 289
effectiveness of, 430, 426t
Pheniprazine (Catron), effectiveness of, 426t
Phenobarbital (Luminal), 434, 435
efficacy of, 412t

in treatment of psychosomatic disorders, 205
Phenothiazines, 345
in amphetamine withdrawal, 254
for anxiety, 433–434
changes produced by, 411–412
to control hyperactivity, 336
development of, 35
early use of, 410
efficacy of, 411, 412t, 426t
for elderly brain-damage patients, 322–323
for head trauma, 325, 326
lithium combined with, 437
maintenance dosages of, 278
for manic disorders, 299
mode of action of, 278
during narcotic withdrawal, 250
for organic brain disorders, 361
for psychosomatic disorders, 204
for schizophrenia, 277–278
for seizures, 358
side effects of, 420
in treatment of effects of LSD use, 256
Phentolamine (Regitine), for MAO side effects, 430
Phenurone. *See* Phenacemide
Phenylalanemia. *See* Phenylketonuria
Phenylhydantoin (Dilantin), 422
Phenylketonuria (PKU), 374–375
atypical, 374
treatment of, 375
Phenylpropanolamine, 430
Phobia(s), clinical characteristics of, 124–125
in children, 125–126
clinical course of, 129–130
development of, 47
interpersonal causes of, 126–129
nausea and vomiting associated with, 188–189
role of anxiety in, 122
treatment of, 130–134
behavior therapy as, 71–72
imipramine as, 425
Phosphorous, 349
Photosensitive reaction, 423, 424
Physical behavior, in early infantile autism, 270
schizophrenic disturbances of, 262–263, 268
Physical contact, between examiner and patient, 80
Physical evaluation, 103–104
Physical illness. *See* Organic illness
Physical treatment. *See also specific treatments*
for schizophrenia, 278–279
Physiotherapy, 447–448

Physostigmine, for tricyclic overdosage, 429
Pick's disease, 357–358
Pilocarpine, for dry mouth, 419
Pipanol. See Trihexyphenidyl
Piperacetazine (Quide), dosage of, 414t
  efficacy of, 412t
PKU. See Phenylketonuria
Placebo, in drug trials, 411
Placidyl. See Ethchlorvynol
Plastic surgery, 311
Play therapy, 452–453
Pleasure principle, 65
Polioencephalitis, acute hemorrhagic, 352
Polysurgical addiction, 476
Porphyria, 351–352
Possessiveness, personality development and, 14
Postconcussion syndrome, 326–328
Postnatal brain damage, 332
Postoperative psychoses, 309, 310–311
Postpartum psychoses, 309–310
Posttraumatic syndrome, 326–328
  management of, 328
Postural hypotension, with tricyclic antidepressants, 428
Preconscious, 44
Prefrontal lobotomy, 447
Premature ejaculation, 481–482
Premenstrual tension, 201
Prenatal brain damage, 331–332
Prepsychotic personality, in manic disorders, 283, 298
  in schizophrenia, 274
Presamine. See Imipramine
Presenting problem, 83
Primary gain, 75
  in conversion hysteria, 154, 155
Primary process thinking, 50, 68
Prochlorperazine (Compazine), 423
  dosage of, 414t
  efficacy of, 412t
  for nausea and vomiting, 204
Procyclidine (Kemadrin), 420, 421
Projection, 63
  in paranoid thinking, 307
Projective tests, 97–100
Proketazine. See Carphenazine
Prolixin. See Fluphenazine
Promazine (Sparine), 423
  efficacy of, 412t
  for elderly brain-damaged patients, 323
Propranolol, for tricyclic overdosage, 429
Prototaxic stage. See Crude sensations phase
Protriptyline (Vivactil), effectiveness of, 427, 426t
Pruritis, 192–193
Pseudocyesis, 201

Pseudoretardation, 371
Psilocybin, 255
Psychasthenia, 175
Psychiatric disorders. See also Mental illness; specific disorders
  classification of, 37
  one-genus postulate and, 23
  sources of, 3
Psychiatric examination, of current functioning, 88
  ending interview in, 92–93
  interview length for, 82
  mental status examination in, 88–92
  note taking during, 81–82
  opening of, 82
  past history in, 84–88
  of patient's family, 93–94
  physical evaluation in, 103–104
  present problem in, 83–84
  psychological tests in, 97–101
  special technics for, 101–103
  of uncommunicative patient, 94–95
Psychiatric social worker, in child guidance clinic, 450
Psychiatric theories, bases of, 4–5
Psychiatrists, in child guidance clinic, 449
  legal responsibilities of, 500–501, 505–506
  legal testimony of, 499, 500–502
  training of, 392, 394
Psychiatry, in communist countries, 37–38
  definition of, 3
  descriptive, 43
  development during 19th Century, 27–29
  existentialist, 37
  modern developments in, 29–30, 35–37
    child psychiatry, 32
    clinical psychology, 32–33
    Continental European, 37–38
    Freudian approach, 31–32
    integration into general medicine, 33–34
    interpersonal approach, 30–31
    nursing, 33
    pharmacological and physical, 35, 36
    psychiatric social work, 33
  organic, 43
  origins of, 26–27
  position on commitment, 496, 497
  position on confidentiality, 503–505
  psychodynamic, 43
  view of person, 491–493
Psychoanalysis. See Freudian-psychoanalytic approach
Psychodrama, 380, 402

Psychodynamics, 43
Psychologist, in child guidance clinic, 449–450
Psychology, 43
  analytic, 68–69
  concepts of, 69
  individual, 70
Psychoneurosis. See Neurosis(es)
Psychoneurotic depression, 168
Psychopathic personality, 221
Psychopathology, of everyday life, 68
  use of term, 43
Psychosexual development, 58–59
  anal stage in, 59
  defense mechanisms and, 62–64
  genital period in, 61
  latency period in, 61
  phallic stage and Oedipus complex in, 59–61
  oral stage in, 59
  unconscious mind and, 61–62
Psychosis(es). See also specific psychoses
  amphetamine-induced, 348
  of association, 308–309
  following brain damage, 330
  development of, 11
  in obsessive compulsive patients, 145
  postoperative, 309, 310–311, 350
  postpartum, 309–310
Psychosocial factors, in mental retardation, 372–374
  treatment on level of, 206
Psychosomatic illnesses, cardiovascular, 193–195
  of central nervous system, 199–200
  concept of, 183
  conversion hysteria contrasted with, 149
  endocrine, 199
  gastrointestinal, 185–191
  genitourinary, 200–202
  levels of disorder in, 183–185
  musculoskeletal, 196–199
  obesity, 202–203
  respiratory, 195–196
  of sense organs, 202
  of skin, 191–193
  treatment of, 203–206
Psychosurgery, 446–447
Psychotherapeutic environments, 405–408
Psychotherapy. See also Freudian-psychoanalytic approach; Group psychotherapy
  for aggressive personality, 216–217
  for alcoholism, 243–244
  for antisocial personality, 223–224

for anxiety neuroses, 121–122
under barbiturate sedation, 403–404
for conversion symptoms, 162–163
basic processes in, 385–390
behavior therapy, 395–396
for children and adolescents, 452–456
for children subjected to incest, 235
for colitis, 187
combination with drug therapy, 417, 418, 418t
for compulsive disorders, 146, 215
for conversion hysteria, 158–161, 165
for cyclothymic personality, 218
definition of, 385
for depressive neuroses, 173
for drug addiction, narcotic, 250
non-narcotic, 254, 256, 257
eclectic flexible, 396
for elderly patients, 323
for exhibitionism, 231
for frigidity, 487
for homosexuality, 230
under hypnosis, 404–405
for conversion symptoms, 162
for warts, 193
for impotence, 484
for inadequate personality, 221
indications and complications of, 398–399
interpersonal approach in, 390–392
for manic disorders, 299, 301
for obsessive neuroses, 145
for paranoid disorders, 220, 306
for passive personality, 216
for pedophilia, 232
for phobic neuroses, 130–132
for postencephalitic brain damage, 354
for rheumatoid arthritis, 198–199
for schizoid personality, 214
for schizophrenia, 276–277
for severe depressions, 288, 290
supportive counseling as, 397–398
for transvestitism, 233
Psychotic depression, neurotic depression distinguished from, 168, 280
Punishment, as legal deterrent, 491
use of illness for, 475–476
Pyknic body constitution, 57

Quaalude. *See* Methaqualone
Quide. *See* Piperacetazine
Quinacrine (Atabrine), 348

Rationalizations, 63
for phobias, 124
Reaction formation, 62–63
Reactive depression, 168
Realistic appraisals phase, 19, 22
Reality orientation, in depression, 280
in schizophrenia, 261, 272–273
Reality principle, 65
Reassurance, for organic brain disorder patients, 360
Recall, 54
Reciprocal inhibition, 395
Reflex, conditioned, 71
Registration, 54
Regitine. *See* Phentolamine
Regression, 63
Rehabilitation programs, for alcoholics, 246
for brain-damaged persons, 330–331, 362
for narcotic addicts, 250–251
Reinforcement, 71
in behavior theory, 71
in behavior therapy, 395
negative, 395–396
Relatives, in commitment proceedings, 496, 497–498, 499
counseling in treatment of schizophrenic patients, 276–277
information obtained from, 93–94
interview of, for severely depressed patients, 288, 290
paranoia in, 304
psychoses of association in, 308–309
in psychotherapy, 391–392
Release of information, importance of, 84–85
Repoise. *See* Butaperazine
Repression, 61
in anxiety neuroses, 118
failure of, 61
Reserpine, efficacy of, 412t
Residential treatment, for children and adolescents, 456–457
Residual schizophrenia, 271
Resistances, 67
Respiration(s), complications in electroshock therapy, 444
in drug overdosage, 346
psychosomatic disorders in, 195–196
sighing, 196
Responsibility, Ganser syndrome as escape from, 153
legal, 491, 493–495
of psychiatrists, 500–501, 505–506
Restraints, for delirium tremens, 339
for organic brain disorder patients, 361

Retardation. *See also* Mental retardation
of thought processes, 50
Retention, 54
Retinitis pigmentosa, 424
Retrograde amnesia, 54–55
Retrospective falsification, 55–56
Return of the repressed, 61
Rheumatoid arthritis, 198–199
Rhinitis, 202
Ritalin. *See* Methylphenidate
Rituals. *See* Compulsive neuroses
Rorschach test, 33, 97–98

Sadism, sexual, 233–234
Sado-masochism, sexual, 234
Salicylates, 348
Schizoaffective disorders, 265
Schizoaffective schizophrenia, 268–269
manic disorders as, 297
Schizoid, schizophrenia distinguished from, 214
Schizoid personality, 213–214
treatment of, 214
Schizophrenia, amphetamine-induced, 348
antipsychotic dosages for, 413–414
Bleuler's study of, 35–36
in brain-damaged children, 334
catatonic, 263
return to phase of crude sensations in, 20
change produced by antipsychotic drugs in, 411–412
clinical characteristics of, 261–265
clinical course of, 265–267
early emotional deprivation and, 5
flatness of affect in, 47
hypochondriasis prior to development of, 176–177
incidence of, 261
in twins, 275
induced by LSD, 255
interpersonal causes of, 271–275
lithium treatment of, 438
organic causes of, 275
schizoid personality differentiated from, 214
treatment of, 270, 275–278
electroshock therapy in, 443
insulin coma therapy as, 445–446
pharmacologic, 411
types of, 266–267
acute episode, 271
catatonic, 268
childhood, 269–271
chronic undifferentiated, 271
hebephrenic, 271
latent, 271

Schizophrenia (*continued*)
   paranoid, 267–268, 340–341
   residual, 271
   schizoaffective, 268–269
   simple, 269
School, adjustment to, 87
   for mentally retarded children, 379–380
School phobias, 126, 188
   treatment of, 133
Scoptophilia, 233
Secobarbital (Seconal), 434, 435
Secondary gains, 75
   in asthma, 195
   from hysterical symptoms, 151, 154–155, 158, 165
Secondary process thinking, 68
Security, definition of, 10
Security operations, 11
Sedation, produced by antipsychotic agents, 422
Sedatives, 434–435
   addiction to, 252–254
   organic brain syndromes caused by overdosage of, 345–347
   side effects of, 435–436
Seizures. *See* Convulsions
Self-accusatory delusions, 49
   in schizophrenia, 263, 264, 269
Self-assertiveness, expression of, 15
Self-centeredness, of homosexuals, 229
Self-concept, early development of, 6
Self-depreciative delusions, 49
Self-esteem, anxiety neuroses and, 116, 118–119
   depressive neuroses and, 171–172
   severe depressions and, 285, 286
Self-image, definition of, 11
   distortions in, 11–12
   formation of, 12
Self-preservation instinct, 41
Self-punishment, in factitial dermatitis, 193
Senile brain degeneration, 318–319
   brain pathology in, 319
   clinical characteristics of, 319–321
   course and prognosis of, 321–322
   management of, 322–323
Sense organs, psychosomatic disorders of, 202
Sensitivity training groups, 403
Sensorium, clouding of, 56
Sensory symptoms, in conversion hysteria, 150–151
Sentence Completion Test, 99
Serax. *See* Oxazepam
Serentil. *See* Mesoridazine

Sexual behavior, in manic disorders, 295
   study of, 36
Sexual development, during adolescence, 17–18
   history taking and, 85–86
Sexual instinct, 41
Sexuality, anorexia nervosa and, 189
   Freudian concept of, 59
   menstrual irregularities and, 201
   in middle age, 478–479
   pruritis and, 192
   urinary dysfunctions related to, 201–202
Sexual masochism, 234
Sexual orientation, development of, 13
Sexual problems, 481–490
   of elderly persons, 489–490
   in etiology of anxiety neuroses, 119
   of orientation, 230. *See also* Homosexuality
   in personality disorders retraining for, 389–390
     for ejaculatory incompetence, 488
     for frigidity, 487
     for impotence, 484–485
     for premature ejaculation, 481–482
Sexual sadism, 233–234
Sexual trauma, in etiology of anxiety neuroses, 117
   in etiology of compulsive neuroses, 142
   in etiology of phobias, 128
Sharing, development of, 9
Side effects, of antipsychotic drugs, 413, 415, 419–425
   of lithium, 438
   of minor tranquilizers, 435–436
   of sedatives and hypnotics, 435–436
   of tricyclic antidepressants, 428–429
Sighing respirations, 196
Simple schizophrenia, 269
Sinequan. *See* Doxepin
Situational depression, 168
Skin, effect of antipsychotics on, 423, 424
   psychosomatic disorders of, 191–193
Sleep, continuous, as therapy, 448
Slovenliness, in senile and cerebral arteriosclerotic brain damage, 320
Slums, psychiatric services in, 34–35
Smoking, heart disease and, 194
Social workers, 33, 450
   confidentiality and, 504
Sociodrama, 380

Socioeconomic status, conversion hysteria and, 151–152
   I.Q. scores and, 368, 373
Sociopathic personality disorder, 221
Sodium chloride, for bromide intoxication, 344
Sodomy, 234
Solacen. *See* Tybamate
Solicitousness, in examiner, 80
Somnafac. *See* Methaqualone
Somnos. *See* Chloral hydrate
Sopor. *See* Methaqualone
Sparine. *See* Promazine
Spasmodic torticollis, 197
Special education, for mentally retarded children, 379–380
Speech, role in personality development, 6
Speech disturbances, 466–468
   delayed speech, 466–467
   early infantile autism, 270
   in psychosocial retardation, 373
   schizophrenic, 264
Spina bifida occulta, 461
Stanford-Binet test, 100–101
Status epilepticus, 358
Stelazine. *See* Trifluoperazine
Stereotyped movements, in schizophrenia, 262
Strephosymbolia, 464
Stress reactions, 473–474
   in civilian life, 474
   in military life, 474–475
Stupor, 56
   catatonic, 56
   hysterical, 153, 155
Stuporous depression, 56, 281
Stuttering, 467
   etiology of, 467
   treatment of, 467–468
Subcoma insulin therapy, 446
Sublimation, 63
Substitution, as defense mechanism, 64
Succinylcholine (Anectine), in electroshock therapy, 441
   prolonged paralysis following, 444
Suggestion, 390
   in treatment of conversion symptoms, 161–163
Suicidal risk, diazepam and, 435–436
   in elderly brain-damaged persons, 321
   electroshock therapy and, 443
   evaluation of, 90, 292–293
   in Huntington's chorea, 358
   in hysterical personality, 227
   in manic disorders, 298
   in narcotic addiction, 247–248
   in neurotic depressions, 170, 172

in schizoaffective schizophrenia, 269
in severe depressions, 281, 287–288, 289, 292
tricyclic antidepressants and, 429
Suicide, emotional causes of, 291–292
incidence of, 290–291
malpractice suits concerning, 505
rational, 292
self-accusatory and self-depreciative delusions and, 49
Superego, 65–66
Supportive counseling, 397–398
Supportive group therapy, 402
Surgery, emotional gratification from, 476
psychoses following, 309, 310–311, 350
transplant, emotional adjustment to, 476–477
transsexual, 234
Surmontil. See Trimipramine
Sydenham's chorea, 471
Symbiosis, 74
Symbolism(s), in hysterical symptoms, 154, 161
schizophrenic, 262
Symbolization, 64
in dreams, 68
Symptoms, primary and secondary gains of, 75
treatment in hysteria, 161–163
Synanon, 252
Syntaxic stage. See Realistic appraisals phase
Syphilis, organic brain disorders caused by, 354–356
Systems theory, 73–74

Tachycardia, 193
Taractan. See Chlorprothixene; Thioxanthenes
Tardive dyskinesia, 421–422
Taste, hallucinations of, 52
TAT. See Thematic Apperception Test
Telepathy. See Extrasensory perception
Temporal lobe tumors, effects of, 351
Tension, concept of, 47
premenstrual, 201
Tension headaches, 113, 194–195, 197–198
Terminal extrapyramidal insufficiency, 421
Tests, early, 33
intelligence, 100–101
of memory, 90
personality, 97–100

projective, 97–100
for strephosymbolia, 465
Tetrahydrocannabinal, 256
T-groups, 403
Thanatos, 65
Thematic Apperception Test (TAT), 33, 98
Therapeutic community, 405
Therapist, patient's relationship with, 387–389
Thiamine deficiency, 352
Thiopental (Pentothal), 434
in electroshock therapy, 441
Thiopropazate, efficacy of, 412t
Thioridazine (Mellaril), 278, 420, 422, 423
dosage of, 424, 414t
efficacy of, 412t, 426t
for manic disorders, 299
ocular pathology associated with, 424
Thioxanthenes (Navane; Taractan), 345
dosage of, 414, 414t
efficacy of, 412t
Thorazine. See Chlorpromazine
Thought disturbances, 49–51. See also Delusions
Thought processes, in mental status examination, 89–90
primary process, 68
schizophrenic disturbances of, 261–262
secondary process, 68
Thrombocytopenic pupura, 423
Thyroid disorders, 352
Thyrotoxicosis, 352
Tics, 470–471
Tindal. See Acetophenazine
Tofranil. See Imipramine
Toilet training, 59
in etiology of compulsive neuroses, 143
Tolerance, in narcotic addiction, 246
Topectomy, 447
Torticollis, 197
Touch, hallucinations of, 52
Toys, therapeutic use of, 453
Training groups, 403
Tranquilizers. See Antianxiety drugs; Antipsychotic drugs
Transference, 67, 393
negative, 67
positive, 67
Transference neurosis, 67
Transorbital lobotomy, 447
Transplant operations, emotional adjustment to, 476–477
Transsexualism, 234–235
Transvestitism, 232–233
relationship to homosexuality, 232
Tranxene. See Chlorzepate

Tranylcypromine (Parnate), effectiveness of, 430, 426t
side effects of, 430
Trauma, of birth, 70
sexual, 117, 128, 142
Traumatic confusional state, 324–325
treatment of, 325
Traumatic delirium, 325–326
Traumatic neuroses, 164
Treatment. See also specific forms of treatment
consent for, 500
right to, 501
Tremin. See Trihexyphenidyl
Tremors, hysterical, 150
Tricyclic drugs. See Antidepressant drugs, tricyclic
Trifluoperazine (Stelazine), 278, 420, 422, 423
dosage of, 413, 416, 414t
efficacy of, 412t
for manic disorders, 299
Triflupromazine (Vesprin), dosage of, 414t
efficacy of, 412t
Trihexyphenidyl (Artane; Pipanol; Tremin), 348
Trilafon. See Perphenazine
Trimipramine (Surmontil), effectiveness of, 426t
Trisomy D^1 (trisomy 13), 372
Trisomy E (trisomy 18) syndrome, 372
Tuberculosis, as contraindication for electroshock therapy, 445
Tuberculous meningitis, 353
Tunnel vision, hysterical, 151
Turpentine, 349
Twilight states, hysterical, 153, 155
Twin studies, of etiology of schizophrenia, 275
Tybamate (Solacen; Tybatran), 432
effectiveness of, 433
lack of physical dependence liability, 436

Ulcer, peptic, 185–186
Ulcerative colitis, 186–187
Ulcerlike disorders, 186
Ultrasonotomy, 447
Unconscious, collective, 69
concept of, 44
expression in dreams, 68
personal, 69
Unconscious memory, 54
Unconscious mind, 61–62
Unconscious, with head trauma, 324
Undoing, 64
Urea (Ureaphil; Urevert), 348

Urecholine. *See* Bethanecol
Uremia, 351
Urevert. *See* Urea
Urinary frequency, 201
Urinary retention, 201–202
  in catatonic schizophrenia, 268
Urine, maple syrup odor in, 376
Urine tests, for phenylketonuria, 375
Urogenital surgery, psychoses following, 310–311
Urticaria, 191

Vaginismus, 488
Valium. *See* Diazepam
Valmid. *See* Ethinamate
Verbigeration, 50, 264
Vermont rule, 494
Veronal. *See* Barbital
Verrucae, 193
Vesprin. *See* Triflupromazine
Vineland Social Maturity Scale, 101
Violence, obsessive ideas of, 136
Viral encephalitis, organic brain disorders caused by, 353-354
Visual disturbances, hysterical, 151
Visuomotor difficulties, in brain-damaged children, 333

Vitamin B_{12}, for methylmalonic aciduria, 375
Vitamin B deficiencies, 352
Vitamins, in Korsakoff's psychosis, 339, 340
Vivactil. *See* Protriptyline
Vocational adjustment. *See* Work adjustment
Vomiting, 188–189
  in anorexia nervosa, 189
  in aversive treatment of alcoholism, 244, 245
Voyeurism, 233

WAIS. *See* Wechsler Adult Intelligence Scale
Warts, 193
Waxy flexibility, 262
  in catatonic schizophrenia, 268
Wechsler Adult Intelligence Scale (WAIS), 101
Wechsler Intelligence Scale for Children (WISC), 101
Weight loss, in anorexia nervosa, 189
  in depressed patients, 174, 282
Wernicke's encephalopathy, 352
Will, capacity to make, 501–502
WISC, 101
Withdrawal, in childhood and adolescence, 470

  in early infantile autism, 270
  schizoid personality and, 213
  in schizophrenia, 261, 269
Withdrawal syndrome, alcoholic, 239–240, 338
  in barbiturate addiction, 253
  in narcotic addiction, 246, 249–250
  with tricyclic antidepressants, 429
Women, involutional melancholia in, 283, 307–308, 478
Words, magical quality in obsessions, 137, 140
  separation from feelings in compulsive neuroses, 143, 146
"Word salad," 50, 89, 264
Work adjustment, in anxiety neurosis etiology, 118
  conversion hysteria and, 164–166
  duration of posttraumatic syndrome and, 327
  in history taking, 87
  of mentally retarded adults, 369, 370
  in middle age, 477

York Retreat, 27